Jewish Medical Practitioners in the Medieval Muslim World

I0305532

Non-Muslim Contributions to Islamic Civilisation
Series Editor: Carole Hillenbrand and Myriam Wissa

Titles in the series include:

Jewish Medical Practitioners in the Medieval Muslim World: A Collective Biography
Efraim Lev

The Rise of the Western Armenian Diaspora in the Early Modern Ottoman Empire: From Refugee Crisis to Renaissance in the Seventeenth Century
Henry Shapiro

edinburghuniversitypress.com/series/nmcic

Jewish Medical Practioners in the Medieval Muslim World

A Collective Biography

Efraim Lev

EDINBURGH
University Press

Edinburgh University Press is one of the leading university presses in the UK. We publish academic books and journals in our selected subject areas across the humanities and social sciences, combining cutting-edge scholarship with high editorial and production values to produce academic works of lasting importance. For more information visit our website: edinburghuniversitypress.com

© Efraim Lev, 2021, 2022

Edinburgh University Press Ltd
The Tun – Holyrood Road
12 (2f) Jackson's Entry
Edinburgh EH8 8PJ

First published in hardback by Edinburgh University Press 2021

Typeset in 11/15 Adobe Garamond by
Servis Filmsetting Ltd, Stockport, Cheshire,
printed and bound by CPI Group (UK) Ltd,
Croydon, CR0 4YY

A CIP record for this book is available from the British Library

ISBN 978 1 4744 8397 1 (hardback)
ISBN 978 1 4744 8398 8 (paperback)
ISBN 978 1 4744 8400 8 (webready PDF)
ISBN 978 1 4744 8399 5 (epub)

The right of Efraim Lev to be identified as author of this work has been asserted in accordance with the Copyright, Designs and Patents Act 1988 and the Copyright and Related Rights Regulations 2003 (SI No. 2498).

Contents

Lists of Tables, Maps, Charts and Figures vii
Notes on Names, Transcription, Abbreviations, Citations, Bibliography, Main Historical Periods and Muslim Rulers ix

1 Preface and Acknowledgements 1
 1.1 Rationale and History of Research 1
 1.2 Chronology 4
 1.3 Acknowledgements 7
 Notes 8

2 Introduction 11
 2.1 Prosopography 11
 2.2 Methodology and Main Sources 13
 2.3 The Cairo Geniza 18
 2.4 Research Difficulties 21
 2.5 Medieval Arabic Medicine and Practitioners 24
 Notes 32

3 Prosopography of Jewish Medical Practitioners 38
 3.1 Biographies 38
 3.2 Jewish Pharmacists in the Muslim World 136
 3.3 Dynasties of Jewish Practitioners 145
 Notes 228

4 Professional, Social, Geographical, Religious and Economic Aspects of Jewish Medical Practitioners 277
4.1 Professional Aspects 282
4.2 Everyday Life 312
4.3 Moral Aspects, Fees and the 'Geniza Patient' 319
4.4 Religious and Inter-religious Aspects of Jewish Practitioners 326
4.5 Community Affairs 357
4.6 Geographical, Sectoral and Historical Aspects 368
Notes 406

5 Epilogue 447
Notes 456

Bibliography 459
List of Geniza Fragments 498
Index of People 500
Index of Places 511
General Index 514

Tables, Maps, Charts and Figures

Tables

1 Main periods and dynasties of Muslim rulers mentioned in the book xi
2 Main Muslim rulers mentioned in the book (chronological order) xii
3 Dynasties of Jewish practitioners in the Fatimid, Ayyubid and Mamluk periods 148
4 Jewish physicians working in Muslim hospitals 294
5 Jewish court physicians 296
6 Inter-religious transfer of medical knowledge 336
7 Practitioners who converted to Islam 344
8 Jewish physicians as chief leaders of the Jewish communities (Head of the Jews/*nagid*) 362
9 Karaite practitioners in the Muslim world 371
10 Samaritan practitioners in the Muslim world 375

Maps

1 Selected locations of Jewish medical activity in Andalusia, north Africa and Sicily 376
2 Selected locations of Jewish medical activity in Egypt 388
3 Selected locations of Jewish medical activity in Bilād al-Shām 395
4 Selected locations of Jewish medical activity in Iraq, Iran and Azerbaijan 403

Charts

1 Dispersion of Jewish pharmacists in the Muslim world by year and location 139
2 Religious affiliations of Jewish physicians in the Muslim world 368
3 Dispersion of Jewish physicians in the Muslim world by year and location 369
4 Number of Jewish physicians in the Muslim world over time 450

Figures

1 ENA 2591.8. List of donors (Hebrew and Arabic) from the 12th century 50
2 TS K 15.16. Part of a list of pledges to charity made at a wedding (11th–12th centuries) 122
3 TS 13J4.13. Legal document concerning a loan (1292) 123
4 TS NS J 151. List of contributors and their contributions (1230) 131
5 TS 24.6. Part of a letter (1030) from the Jewish community in Sicily to the Jewish communities in Qayrawān and al-Mahdiyya 133

Notes on Names, Transcription, Abbreviations, Citations, Bibliography, Main Historical Periods and Muslim Rulers

Patronymics are marked with 'b.' (for Arabic *ibn* or Hebrew *ben*); however, where *ibn* has become part of a family name through usage over a few generations, it is spelled *Ibn*.

The hierarchy of presenting Arabic names is: *kunya*, *ism*, *nasab*, *nisba*, *laqab*. A full explanation is to be found in Section 2.4 and there are examples at the beginning of Chapter 3.

In transliteration of Arabic names, I have followed the rules of the *International Journal of Middle Eastern Studies*; and in transliterating Hebrew I have followed the guidelines of the *Jewish Quarterly Review*.

Similar to previous works by Goitein, Gil and Rustow in dealing with Hebrew names from Geniza and Arabic sources, I present familiar Hebrew names in Anglicised forms (see the main ones below).

Family Name

ha- Kohen/Kohen
ha-Levi/Levi

First Name

Aaron
Abraham
Abūn
Azariah
Baruch
Benjamin

Berākhōt
Bezalel
Daniel
David
Elazar
Ephraim
Hananiah
Ḥalfon
Ḥasday
Ḥayyīm
Isaac
Israel
Jacob
Japheth
Jekuthiel
Jonah
Joseph
Joshua
Josiah (Isaiah)
Judah
Meʾir
Melekh
Menahem
Mishaʾel
Moses
Nadīv
Nehorai
Nethanel
Obadia
Petahya
Pinḥas
Rabīb
Saʿadya
Ṣadāqā
Samuel

Shabbetay
Shemarya
Solomon
Tiqva
Tobias
Yaḥyā
Yedūthūn
Yeshūʿā
Zadok
Zechariah

Class marks of Geniza fragments are mentioned only in cases where they have not been published or mentioned in earlier publications dealing with the person (practitioner) in question. For further reading and for the class mark the reader will have to consult the cited publication(s), usually the last one dealing with the information.

When published works in Arabic or Hebrew have a title page in a European language, it has been used, and the original language indicated; in the few cases that have no title page, the book is listed in the bibliography with the original name transliterated into English.

In order to make reading the book easier with minimum interruptions, especially for readers who are not familiar with the history of the medieval Middle East, Tables 1 and 2 below present basic information regarding the most important (and most-often cited) periods, dynasties and rulers.

Table 1 Main periods and dynasties of Muslim rulers mentioned in the book

Name	*Years*	*Capital/Main areas of activity*	*Remarks*
Umayyad	661–750	Damascus	Andalusia 756–1031
Abbasid	750–969	Baghdad	
Fatimid	969–1171	Cairo	
Almoravid	1062–1147	Morocco, Andalusia	
Almohad	1147–1212	Morocco, Andalusia	
Ayyubid	1171–1250	Cairo, Damascus	
Mamluk	1250–1517	Cairo	
Īl-Khānate	1256–1335	Tabriz	Muslim Mongol
Ottoman	1517–1917	Constantinople	

Table 2 Main Muslim rulers mentioned in the book (chronological order)

Name	*Years of reign*	*Dynasty*	*Capital*
Caliph ʿUmar b. ʿAbd al-ʿAzīz	717–20	Umayyad	Basra
Caliph al-Manṣūr	754–75	Abbasid	Baghdad
Caliph al-Mahdī	775–85	Abbasid	Baghdad
Caliph al-Mutawakkil	847–61	Abbasid	Samarra
Caliph Jaʿfar al-Muqtadir	908–32	Abbasid	Baghdad
Caliph ʿAbd al-Raḥmān III	929–61	Umayyad	Cordova
Caliph al-Manṣūr bi-Ilāh	946–53	Fatimid	Qayrawān
Caliph al-Muʿizz li-Dīn Allāh	953–75	Fatimid	Qayrawān
Caliph al-Ḥakam II	961–76	Umayyad	Cordova
Caliph al-ʿAzīz bi-Allah	975–96	Fatimid	Qayrawān
Caliph al-Ḥākim bi-Amr Allāh	996–1021	Fatimid	Cairo
Caliph al-Mustanṣir biʾllāh	1036–94	Fatimid	Cairo
Caliph al-Mustaʿlī	1094–1101	Fatimid	Cairo
Caliph al-Āmir	1101–30	Fatimid	Cairo
Caliph al-Ḥāfiz li-Dīn Allāh	1130–49	Fatimid	Cairo
Caliph ʿAbd al-Muʾmin	1130–63	Fatimid	Cairo
Sultan Nūr al-Dīn Zengī	1154–74	Seljuk	
Caliph al-ʿĀḍid li-Dīn Allāh	1160–71	Fatimid	Cairo
Caliph al-Mustanjid biʾllāh	1160–70	Abbasid	Baghdad
Sultan Salaḥ al-Din (Saladin)	1171–93	Ayyubid	Damascus and Cairo
Sultan al-Malik al-ʿAzīz	1193–8	Ayyubid	Cairo
Sultan al-Malik al-Afḍal	1193–6	Ayyubid	Damascus
Sultan al-Malik al-Kāmil	1218–38	Ayyubid	Cairo
Sultan al-Ẓāhir Baybars	1260–77	Mamluk	Cairo
Sultan al-Manṣūr Qalāwūn	1279–90	Mamluk	Cairo
Sultan al-Nāṣir Muḥammad ibn Qalāwūn	1293–4, 1298–1308, 1310–41	Mamluk	Cairo
Sultan al-Nāṣir Ḥasan	1347–51, 1354–61	Mamluk	Cairo
Sultan al-Ẓāhir Barqūq	1382–9, 1390–9	Mamluk	Cairo
Sultan al-Nāṣir Faraj	1399–1411	Mamluk	Cairo
Sultan al-Mu'ayyad Sheikh	1412–21	Mamluk	Cairo

1

Preface and Acknowledgements

1.1 Rationale and History of Research

The idea of researching the social history of medieval Jewish practitioners in the eastern Mediterranean through their life stories dawned on me in 2003, while working on the medical documents in the Cairo Geniza collections. During the time in which I was studying the practical *materia medica* of the Geniza people, their prescriptions, lists of drugs and medical notebooks, as well as their medical literature, I was also collecting every bit of available information on the medical practitioners (both physicians and pharmacists). I was curious about the people behind the practice of medicine: the ones who wrote the prescriptions I examined; the ones that bought and sold the various medicinal substances I studied, which were found in the list of *materia medica*; the people who had actually prepared the compound drugs that were mentioned in the prescriptions, letters and notebooks.

Other scholars, working on cataloguing the various Geniza collections at the Taylor-Schechter Genizah Research Unit at Cambridge University Library, shared with me materials they found while studying new fragments, and the data accumulated slowly. By 2012, with information on more than 200 physicians and 30 pharmacists, it transpired that I could no longer regard this project as one of secondary importance, and consequently, I began a systematic study of this subject.

Medical historical literature contains many publications dealing with individual or groups of practitioners from all geographical areas and periods. This literature is important, since through the life stories of the practitioners and their medical activity, we learn much about the medical status and history of a period, culture, ethnic group or geographical zone. However, as stated by Peter Pormann and Emilie Savage-Smith, 'history often only remembers the conquerors, not the conquered. One is therefore scarcely astonished that our sources record the names of distinguished doctors and recount stories of success while usually avoiding mentioning their failure.'[1] They added that

> the status of the physicians differed greatly. The best and the brightest could certainly rise to considerable esteem and wealth. Others may have belonged to the 'upper middle class'. Yet, not all doctors belonged to this middle class, and there must have been many who struggled to make a living. They are the ones who history often forgets, who disappeared as if they have never existed, and about whom we know very little. Unlike their illustrious colleagues, they may well have practised in the market rather (than in) the palace or (in) the hospital.[2]

Various scholars have written about Jews and medicine in general[3] and Jewish physicians in particular.[4] However, this book aims to shed light on medieval Jewish practitioners across all the socio-economic strata, living in urban as well as in rural locations in the Muslim world. It deals mainly with physicians and pharmacists (druggists) and is an attempt to learn about their daily and personal life and their families, as well as their successes and failures, while, moreover, clarifying their communal and even financial affairs as well as their inter-religious relationships. This is mainly based on the wealth of primary sources found in the Cairo Geniza, and in Muslim Arabic sources too.

In the current chapter, I deal with necessary introductory issues, namely chronology and geography. In the Introduction, I elaborate on some methodological aspects such as prosopography, the main sources of this work and research difficulties, and I offer a brief introduction to medieval Arabic medicine and its practitioners.

In the beginning of the third chapter, I will discuss and fully present 496 biographies of Jewish physicians, followed by the biographies of 111 Jewish pharmacists (apothecaries, perfumers and druggists).[5] Related issues, such as potion makers and commercial aspects of drugs, will also be dealt with. Making up a third group are the dynasties of Jewish practitioners, a phenomenon that will be explained and discussed. Forty-nine dynasties consisting of 139 practitioners will be presented, including the biographies of the members[6] and in most cases a chart of the family tree, along with detailed discussion of the dynasties, their role in the Jewish communities and their relationship with the Muslim administrations and rulers throughout the relevant periods.

The fourth chapter is a discussion based on the total number of biographies, and the medieval as well as the contemporary literature available. There, I will discuss professional, social, geographical, religious and economic aspects of the Jewish medical practitioners (mainly physicians). In this chapter, I deal with places of medical practice, the practitioners' professional education, intellectual workshops (i.e. libraries), and their professional roles, mainly that of 'Head of the Physicians'. Another subject that will be dealt is the everyday life and activity of Jewish practitioners (their possessions, means of transportation and commercial activity). Moral aspects, fees and the 'Geniza' patients will be discussed, as well as religious and inter-religious aspects of Jewish practitioners, inter-religious intellectual and professional relations, the high-ranking positions Jewish practitioners held, the issue of conversion to Islam, and famous Jewish scholars, authors, poets and diplomats who were simultaneously practitioners. A few more insights will be related to community affairs, such as the socio-economic position of Jewish practitioners, their role in the leadership (*nagids* and Heads of the Jews), their place and share in charity activities, and the inter-community posts they held (judges and *ḥazzānim* or cantors). The last section of this chapter will endorse sectoral aspects (Karaite and Samaritan practitioners) of related geographical aspects (Jewish practitioners in Andalusia, north Africa, Sicily, provincial Egyptian towns, Syria, Iraq, Iran and Azerbaijan); these are set in geographical order, as near as possible, from west to east.

The attention given by medical historians to the importance of medical biographies as an approach to the history of the medical profession is mainly due to the publication of the *Dictionnaire biographique des médecins en France au moyen age* by Ernest Wickersheimer as early as 1936 and, almost thirty years later in 1965, *The Medical Practitioners in Medieval England: A Biographical Register* by Charles Talbot and Eugene Hammond. These books cover hundreds of practitioners in large European countries that have a long-standing tradition of keeping records of medical care and treatment.

As an historian of medicine, dealing with the eastern Mediterranean, I was exposed to these important works only when I began my study of Jewish practitioners in the Muslim world. However, both books encouraged me to continue with my research and with the plans for publishing the current book. I learnt the research methods used by these authors and others that dealt with prosopography in general; the methods were much improved in my book, especially concerning the focus on analysis and detailed discussions, as well as the final layout.

Later, three works of strong prosopographical character; mainly dealing with physicians in France between the twelfth and fifteenth centuries, were published by Danielle Jacquart. All are of great scientific value and influenced my research. The first deals with the medical milieu of France at this time.[7] The second is an annexe to Wickersheimer's work from 1936,[8] and the third focuses on the medical cadre of medieval Paris.[9] These books were based on contemporary sources and include detailed analyses and discussions.

The primary aim of my research is therefore to bring together all available biographical data on Jewish medical practitioners in the medieval Muslim world: the Middle East (including Iraq and Iran), Egypt, north Africa, Sicily and Andalusia.[10] By doing so, I intend to provide the basis for a clearer understanding, and for a more complete picture, of the social, economic and intellectual aspects of medicine during that period in the Jewish communities and their relations with their host societies. Hopefully, this project will lead to a better understanding of both the profession and the public health issues of the Jewish community in the medieval Muslim world. Moreover, since according to S. D. Goitein, those communities were 'to a certain extent representative of their class in the Mediterranean world in general, and its Arabic section in particular',[11] the discussion and the conclusions could contribute to the study of Jewish communities in locations such as north Africa, Andalusia and Sicily, as well as of Muslim and Christian communities at Egypt, Syria and Iraq in this period.

1.2 Chronology

The current book covers a time span of hundreds of years, between the eighth and the sixteenth centuries, although the vast majority of the practitioners whose biographies are presented here are from the eleventh to the thirteenth centuries (the classical Geniza period, under the rule of the Fatimid and Ayyubid dynasties).

The Jews, who were always the smallest of the minority communities in the Middle East before Islam, were mostly liable to persecution; according to Stephen Humphreys, they became 'most durable and culturally vital' under Islamic rule.[12] In the earliest years of the Islamic regimes, Jewish professionals immigrated to the caliphal centres of power, and offered their various skills.[13] According to Steven Wasserstrom, the caliphs took advantage of these readily available skilled persons; and indeed, Jewish astrologers, poets, physicians and *wazīrs* (ministers) attended to their affairs in court, and sometimes even directly to the caliph. By the tenth century, Jewish middle classes of Egypt and Iraq enjoyed the advantage of being powerful community members in the courts.[14]

The Fatimid caliphate in Egypt and Syria (969–1171) is considered a golden age for *dhimmīs* (the protected non-Muslim communities living under Islamic rule).[15] Interestingly enough, the *dhimmīs* in this period were not subjugated to discriminatory laws and managed to occupy even the highest bureaucratic positions in the state.[16] Thanks to dozens of Cairo Geniza documents, we may deduce that the discriminatory laws against *dhimmīs*, known as the 'Pact of ʿUmar',[17] were not fully enforced during most of this period, and that Jews did not fulfil most of these humiliating requirements.[18] The heretical Shīʿī-Ismāʿīlī sect, to which the Fatimid belonged, was more tolerant towards their non-Muslim subjects.[19] At the same time, the Fatimid rulers were suspicious of their Sunni counterparts, who formed the majority among their Muslim subjects during their entire period of rule.[20]

The tenth century, in Goitein's words, was 'the golden age of the high bourgeoisie' for the Muslim and the Jews. The period was even called at the time the 'bourgeois revolution', that is, an economic boom in the wake of the Arab conquests. This led the Jewish community towards a 'religious democracy', where the rich cared for the poor through efficient social services.[21] Jews were heavily involved in almost all economic, commercial, administrative and other professional spheres; Goitein counted about 250 manual occupations and 170 types of commercial, professional, educational and administrative activities.[22] This period was indeed a golden age for Jewish practitioners in general, and Jewish court physicians in particular.[23]

The Ayyubid period marked a general deterioration in the status of Jews and Christians in Egypt and Syria, due to the removal of Shīʿī rule in favour of Sunni Islamic rule, established by Saladin (r. 1171–93). The *jihad* (holy war) propaganda which this sultan conducted against the Crusaders definitely contributed to a general animosity towards Christians and Jews, both by the government and by the people. However, Jews continued to serve in the government bureaucracy, perhaps in lesser numbers and in lower positions than they had under Fatimid rule.[24]

It is important to note that throughout this period, there were ups and downs in a sense due to the behaviour of local rulers, geographical events and even personal relationships between the Muslim local regime and the leaders of the Jewish community. Openings and closings of synagogues in this period are one type of evidence among others that can be found in the Geniza.

It is generally accepted among scholars that the Mamluk period (1250–1517) marked the deterioration in the position of *dhimmīs* in Egypt and Syria, and that of Jewish physicians in particular. External threats, in addition to internal crises and political developments, brought about the rise of zealous Islamic orthodoxy and the adoption of more aggressive policies and attitudes towards *dhimmīs*, both by the rulers and by the people. The offensive policy against the remains of the Crusaders Kingdom, conducted by the first Mamluk sultans, increased the hate Muslims felt not only towards Christians, but also against the infidel Jews. The Jewish communities of the Middle East and north Africa lost some of their members to Islam due to conversion.[25] The Mongol invasions from the north, in addition to the Black Death and other natural disasters such as droughts,[26] brought about economic crises, which, as usual in history, only increased religious persecution. The Mamluk rulers, who were originally non-Muslim military slaves, were anxious to prove their loyalty to their new religion, and to gain the support of the Muslim religious scholars (*ʿulamāʾ*), in order to legitimise and strengthen their rule. Hence, they tended to accept the demands of the *ʿulamāʾ* and the people, and to increase the burden on the *dhimmīs*. As a result, during the Mamluk period, the sultans and emirs[27] enforced more strictly the humiliating restrictions on non-Muslims.[28]

It seems that during the first half of the fourteenth century, the persecution of Jews and Christians by the Muslim people and the regime reached its peak. In 1301, for example, the Mamluk sultan Baybars al-Jāshnakīr intensively enforced the restrictions of the Pact of ʿUmar all over the sultanate. Synagogues and churches were closed for long periods, and many *dhimmīs* had to convert (*masālima*) to Islam.[29]

1.3 Acknowledgements

This book would not have been possible without the existence of the Taylor-Schechter Research Unit, under the management of Prof. Stefan Reif. I worked there first as an overseas visiting scholar at St John's College from 2003 to 2004, and then for several weeks each year, until my next overseas visiting scholarship in 2011–12.

In my research for this book, I made use of the studies of many Geniza researchers and scholars that predated me, I would like to thank them all deeply. Hopefully, younger scholars in the future will make similar use of the data in this book for their scholarly research projects.

Many thanks go, first and foremost, to my volunteers and friends Sara Kemp (England), for her help with editing the text, and Abraham Latty (Israel), for all his help in conducting the research, mainly for the great work he has done on the Muslim Arabic sources. My gratitude also goes to my personal and academic friends who shared with me their vast knowledge and expertise, for their good ideas, comments, critique and friendship over the years, primarily Dr Amir Ashur, Dr Amir Mazor and Dr Leigh Chipman. My research assistants during long years of research deserve individual acknowledgment: Dr Eyal Meyer, Aya Evron, Atalya Shienfeld, Adam Hefetz, Boaz Gorfinkel and Uri Giron. My special thanks go to Prof. Stefan Reif, founder, and then director, of the Unit, who was a constant source of encouragement to me; and for supporting my idea and helping me to fulfil my academic dreams, also to Dr Ben Outhwaite, the current director. Warm thanks equally go to members of the Unit during that time and today: Dr Rebecca Jefferson, Dr Avi Shivtiel, the late Dr Friedrich Niessen, Dr Esther-Miriam Wagner, Dr Gabriele Ferrario, the late Mrs Shulie Reif and Mrs Sarah Sykes. I would also like to thank Mr Peter Jones of King's College, Cambridge for his good advice that always turned out to be highly beneficial; and Prof. Simcha Levyadun, Oranim College and University of Haifa, for his constant help and support, excellent remarks and his sharp eyes.

The research on this book was mainly funded by the Landy Foundation at Cambridge. I thank Barry and Ros Landy for their great support, and the Faculty of Humanities and the Research Authority of the University of Haifa for financial backing for the production of this book.

I thank Dr Tirza and the late Prof. Norman Bleehen from the bottom of my heart for all their patronage during the years, and particularly for the first Bleehen Visiting Scholar Award, which enabled me to spend the term in Cambridge in 2011–12, working on the research and writing of this book.

I would like to thank the Syndicate of Cambridge University Library for permission to publish the Cairo Geniza fragments presented in this book and on the cover (TS K 15.16, TS 13J4.13, TS NS J 151, TS 24.6, TS Ar. 45.40 and TS NS 97.20).

Last but not least, I wish to thank my dear wife Dr Michal Lev and our children Hagar and Itamar, Amitay and Erel, Avigail and Ilay, who for the last decade and a half have accepted the Geniza research as an important part of my life, and I dedicate this book to them with much love and appreciation.

Efraim Lev
Zichron Yaakov, Haifa, and Cambridge 2020

Notes

1. Pormann and Savage-Smith, *Medieval Islamic Medicine*, pp. 81–3.
2. Ibid., p. 95; for hospitals in the Christian and pre-Christian periods see for example Risse, *Mending Bodies, Saving Souls*.
3. See for example Friedenwald, *The Jews and Medicine*; Berger, *Jews and Medicine*; Heynick, *Jews and Medicine*; Nevins, *The Jewish Doctor*; Shatzmiller, *Jews, Medicine, and Medieval Society*.
4. To name a few: Assis, 'Jewish Physicians and Medicine'; Weisz, 'The Jewish Physicians'; Shefer, 'Physicians in Mamluk and Ottoman Courts'.
5. The names and basic details of the pharmacists that were members of dynasties are mentioned in this section; however, their detailed biographies are presented in Section 3.3.2.
6. The names and basic details of the physicians that were part of dynasties are mentioned in this section; however, their detailed biographies are presented in Section 3.3.2.

7. Jacquart, *Le Milieu médical en France.*
8. Jacquart, *Le Milieu médical en France: en annexe.*
9. Jacquart, *La Médecine médiévale dans le cadre parisien.*
10. The Jewish physicians and pharmacists that practised in Ottoman Turkey deserve separate attention due to their special conditions and characteristics; I hope that another scholar, equipped with the right research tools, will deal with this project soon.
11. Goitein, *A Mediterranean Society*, vol. I, p. viii.
12. Humphreys, *Islamic History*, p. 262.
13. On the role of the Jews in the economy of Muslim countries see in depth Gil, *Jews in Islamic Countries*, pp. 615–721.
14. Wasserstrom, *Between Muslim and Jew,* pp. 19–20.
15. On the Jews in the Muslim world see Lewis, *The Jews of Islam.*
16. On the role and status of the *dhimmī* in Muslim society, see Humphreys, *Islamic History*, pp. 255–61.
17. Restrictions that were imposed on non-Muslims referred to dress, social behaviour, transport, religious practices, and secular as well as sacred architecture.
18. Stillman, 'The Non-Muslim Communities', pp. 207–8.
19. Ibid., pp. 206–7; Ashtor, *The History of the Jews in Egypt and Syria*, vol. I, pp. 28–30.
20. Ashtor, *The History of the Jews in Egypt and Syria*, vol. I, p. 28; Lane-Poole, *A History of Egypt in the Middle Ages*, pp. 122–40; Goitein, *A Mediterranean Society*, vol. II, pp. 345–407; Gil, *The Tustaris*, p. 10.
21. Goitein, 'The Rise of the Near-Eastern Bourgeoisie'; Goitein, *A Mediterranean Society*, vol. II.
22. Goitein, 'Jewish Society and Institutions under Islam', p. 175.
23. Lewicka, 'The Non-Muslim Physician', p. 505.
24. Stillman, 'The Non-Muslim Communities', p. 207; cf. Ashtor, *The History of the Jews in Egypt and Syria*, I, p. 31.
25. Humphreys, *Islamic History*, p. 262; see also Lewicka, 'The Non-Muslim Physician', p. 505.
26. See for example Ellenblum, *The Collapse of the Eastern Mediterranean.*
27. Emirs or amirs are military office holders; see Shefer, 'Physicians in the Mamluk and Ottoman Courts', p. 114.
28. Stillman, *The Jews of Arab Lands*, pp. 68–72; Meyerhof, 'Medieval Jewish Physicians in the Near East', p. 457.
29. For more on this wave of persecutions see Ashtor, *Toledot ha-Yehudim*, vol.

I, pp. 84–103; Little, 'Coptic Conversion to Islam', pp. 554–8. For the most detailed list of restrictions that was imposed on the *dhimmīs* see al-Nuwayrī, *Nihāyat al-Arab*, vol. XXIII, pp. 417–18. On the closure of synagogues in Egypt in 1301 for ten years, see Ashtor, *Toledot ha-Yehudim*, vol. I, pp. 93, 96–8; on their closing again in 1316, see al-Maqrīzī, *Kitāb al-Sulūk*, vol. II, p. 157.

2

Introduction

2.1 Prosopography

There are several definitions of prosopography in the literature; and in the last decade, there have been many publications dealing with this field and its various methods. There are a number of interpretations of the concept of prosopography, thus presenting copious examples of the possible uses of this genre.

So, what is prosopography? According to the Merriam-Webster online dictionary, it is 'a study that identifies and relates a group of persons or characters within a particular historical context'; from a philological point of view, it comes from new Latin *prosopographia*, based on Greek *prósōpon* (person) + New Latin *graphia* (-graphy).[1]

Forty years ago, Lawrence Stone wrote that prosopography, which is a collective biography or multiple career-line, 'has developed into one of the most valuable and most familiar techniques of the research historian'.[2] Another interpretation of prosopography which has become important in recent years was initially introduced by the French sociologist Pierre Bourdieu. This was explained by Donald Broady as a kind of collective biography, with the following main characteristics: it is 'a study of individuals belonging to the same field', and it is based on comprehensive collections of data about these individuals (social origin, educational background, position in their field or society, their resources from different aspects and so on). The same set of data should as far as possible be collected for each individual, and – last but not least – the main object of the study is not the individuals *per se*, but rather, the history and structure of their field.[3] Robin Fleming described prosopography as a 'multiple biography' and claimed that this method has since proven fruitful: 'analyzing gross and generalized patterns across dozens of contemporary lives is almost always more feasible than reconstituting a single life in detail'.[4] Lately, Avraham Elmakias in another definition portrayed prosopography as a 'detailed research of a defined historical group whose members share a common denominator'.[5]

The set of prosopographical study is chosen according to the research one wishes to carry out. Therefore, the individuals are selected either because they have one or more characteristics in common, or because they belong to a particular profession, or geographical or ethnic origin.[6]

Although modern scholars and researchers such as Lois Banner and Fleming do not discuss prosopography *per se*, they nonetheless analyse the theoretical pros and cons of biographies for the historian.[7] Their extensive experience of delving into and writing about diverse biographies from different eras can help us to present and deal with the theoretical complexity of prosopography. Certain aspects which these authors considered while recording the biography of an individual are also reflected in the task of writing collective ones.

Many scholars have written about the advantages of prosopography as a tool for historical research, but it is not free from difficulties. Elmakias stated that in some cases there is abundant data regarding certain individuals, while for others it will be missing. He also claimed that 'the danger, therefore, lies in drawing conclusions and generalisations based on fragmented information'. Therefore, he rightly suggested that researchers who use prosopographic methodology should be aware of its challenges when it comes to writing the conclusions and insights from all the gathered details.[8]

The prosopographic method, which was developed as a scientific tool for historical studies in the first half of the twentieth century, was shortly after used in historical research on the Roman and Byzantine empires[9] and on medieval and early modern countries.[10] Reviews on the genre of biographies, and their contribution to the research of Arab-Islamic medieval culture, were written by Manuela Marín and Claude Gilliot.[11] Patricia Crone also demonstrated the use of prosopographical approach and method in her early research on Islamic history.[12] On prosopographic methodology within the field of Islamic studies we can learn from the early thoughts of Jacqueline Sublet on the prosopography of the Arabs and Asad Ahmed's research on the religious elite of the early Islamic Hijaz.[13]

Recent studies have used biographical dictionaries as a unique source for the reconstruction of the world of Islamic knowledge, tracing scholarly networks, the place of scholars in urban life, their connection with political power, and their professional careers.[14] Michael Lecker showed what the benefits of a computerised database of biographies can be. His project on 'The Prosopography of Early Islamic Administration', which contains biographical data about more than 1,600 persons, has proved to be a strong and efficient research tool.[15] Elmakias used a prosopographical approach in writing about the naval commanders in early Islam.[16]

Two more works that used and were inspired by this database and method should be mentioned here. The first, written by Michael Ebstein and dealing with the Shuṭra chiefs in Baṣra during the Umayyad period, gives a description of prosopography as 'biographical analysis of a given group of individuals from various aspects: genealogy, marital relationship, and progeny, political, military or administrative offices, estates and economic activity, political and religious loyalties etc.'[17] The second, written by Yaara Perlman, dealt with the bodyguard of the Umayyad and Abbasid caliphs.[18]

A recent piece of prosopographical research done by Luigi Andrea Berto dealing with 'the first Venetians' is another example of how beneficial and instrumental such an historical study can be.[19] Paolo Brezzi and Egmont Lee demonstrated in their study the importance of the contribution of private records to social history. A case in point is that of Italy in the late Middle Ages where private performances were used to write about social and economic history.[20] In this respect, one definition of social history is 'history that concentrates upon the social, economic, and cultural institutions of a people'.[21]

2.2 Methodology and Main Sources

Constructing the biography of a person that lived and was active 1,000 years ago is never an easy task. The well-known and famous are usually better recorded in books dealing with their period, and in the national or ethnic ethos as legends, mainly due to the works they wrote, if and when they become known and applied. Equally important is their fame, which has survived to modern times. But in medieval times, and especially concerning those living in the East, where public records were almost non-existent, there was little chance for 'simple' ordinary people to leave traces of their existence or achievements behind them.

As mentioned above, the main sources for the current research are the documents found in various collections of the Cairo Geniza around the world.[22] It is important to note that the information is of neither archival nor medical records. It is a repository of daily and private documents as well as inter-communal formal and bureaucratic ones, of both religious and secular characteristics. The vast number of Geniza documents include private letters, commercial documents, court orders, marriage agreements, memorial lists and lists of charity donors. They enable us to collect authentic bits and pieces of information regarding the lives and activities of various ordinary people, including medical practitioners.[23] Indeed, precious pieces of information were accumulated for this research during a decade and half of my study of the Cairo Geniza, mainly on medical issues.[24] Catalogues of the various Geniza collections, as well as online databases,[25] were screened and studied for names of, or data about, Jewish practitioners. Accordingly, specific fragments were studied to extract the information. During that time, friends and scholars studying Geniza documents and knowing about my project (mainly Dr Amir Ashur) provided me with more information, names and data. Moreover, for the purpose of the current research, dozens of books and hundreds of articles that were written by other Geniza scholars were studied and surveyed for hints and information regarding Jewish practitioners in the medieval Muslim world.

Whereas the Geniza documents supply intimate, unmediated social information regarding Jewish practitioners, usually in the context of the Jewish community, Muslim historians often provide 'objective' social information concerning the medical and political career of Jewish doctors within the elite of Muslim society. This integration of Jewish and Muslim Arabic sources brings our prosopographical study to its maximal fruition: to quote Marín, 'through the careful study of many individual biographies, a collective portrait of these groups can be drawn'.[26] Banner suggested regarding the individual (as portrayed in historical biography) as 'text' and the surrounding culture as 'context'; therefore, she claimed that the 'text' reflects the 'context' and influences it in a 'dialogic' interaction.[27] In her opinion, 'collective' biographies involving a comparison or analysis of several lives are linked to a central theme.[28] In our book the theme is 'Learned medical practice in the medieval Muslim world'.

With the help of my colleagues, Avraham Latty and Dr Amir Mazor, I therefore studied Muslim Arabic sources of all sorts: descriptions of medieval Egypt and Syria, historiography of the Middle East, geographers, travellers, Muslim scholars, biographies of physicians and more. Thousands of biographies, mainly of Muslim scholars, poets, scientists, and high officials and administrators, were inscribed in dictionaries of biographies. These were the basis of works on medieval Muslim cities such as Damascus and Baghdad, countries such as Andalusia, and the study of prominent men in the urban Muslim community.[29]

One important piece of work that should be mentioned here was published by Richard Bulliet as early as 1970.[30] This article, based on his PhD thesis, was the beginning of a line of highly informative research works, from which prosopographical methods could and should be learnt, including the use of the quantitative approach. Interestingly, some of Bulliet's ideas were not easily accepted by the research community, for example his theory that 'a bell-shaped curve of overtly religious Islamic naming' is related to the conversion to Islam of the studied population.[31]

And indeed, biographies and autobiographies of Muslim physicians had been studied in the past. Biographical dictionaries in the Muslim Arabic tradition and culture were very popular around the thirteenth century, and some of them are being used in this book, for example those by Ibn Abī Uṣaybiʿa (d. 1270) and Ibn al-Qifṭī (d. 1248).[32] For the Jews, unfortunately, we have no biographical dictionaries at all. Interestingly enough, some of the Muslim scholars wrote stories about their private and professional life, out of which biographical data was extracted.[33]

All the small details found in the Cairo Geniza documents and Muslim Arabic sources were carefully double checked, collected, analysed, separated and distributed to the various entries (i.e. biographies) of Jewish practitioners presented in this book.[34] This realisation of several years is similar to an artist's work of many scenes constructing one big picture or dozens of small puzzles collectively composing a single, harmonious whole.

In order to identify Jewish practitioners in the Muslim Arabic sources and literature, we searched mainly for the epithets ***al-Yahūdī*** and ***al-ʾIsrāʾīlī***.[35] These are almost synonyms. However, according to David Wasserstein *al-Yahūdī* regularly means a Jew, but *al-ʾIsrāʾīlī* can also be used to refer to a non-Jew when they happen to be a former Jew as well.[36]

While searching both Geniza and Muslim Arabic sources, we were looking for the following Arabic titles and descriptions for physicians: ***al-Ṭabīb*** and ***al-Mutaṭabbib*** (physician);[37] ***al-Ḥakīm*** (physician as well as philosopher);[38] ***Kaḥḥāl*** (ophthalmologist, oculist), ***Jarāʾiḥí*** (surgeon) or ***Mujabbir*** (orthopaedist).[39] These were the common titles for medical practitioners in the Arabic culture; however, there is also a name in Hebrew that was sometimes attached to a Jewish physician: ***ha-Rōfē***. The names considered for the professions of pharmacy were ***ʿAṭṭār*** (which originally designated a perfumer)[40] and ***Ṣaydalānī*** or ***Ṣaydanī*** (usually translated as pharmacist, apothecary, or seller of medicine, drugs and perfumes).[41] Names denoting other paramedical professions, such as ***Sufūfī*** (specialist preparer of medical powders), ***Kallām*** (wound specialist) and ***Sharābī*** (potion maker), were collected and studied, but were not included in the current book.[42]

As with other occupations, being a physician was a source of pride, and sons of physicians continued to carry not just their fathers' names but also their professions; therefore, a man would be called 'the son of the doctor', like 'the son of the clan of sieve makers', 'the son of the clan of indigo dyers', 'the son of the clan of scarf makers' or 'the son of the judge'.[43]

Gathering the information, and constructing the biographies of the medieval Jewish practitioners, was both the 'concept' and the 'target' of this research; besides presenting the biographies, this allowed me to discuss professional as well as social issues in the history of medicine of communities – in the cities and rural regions (mainly but not only Jewish) in Egypt, the Mediterranean and other Muslim territories.

Banner stated that biographies are often categorised as inferior or even second-rate history by some historians.[44] In her opinion, both modern genres (history and biography) are based on 'archival research, [interweave] historical categories and methodologies, [reflect] current political and theoretical concerns, and [raise] complex issues of truth and proof'.[45] Moreover, she added that 'studying the life story of an individual might be seen as akin to studying the history of a city, a region, or a state as a way of understanding broad social and cultural phenomena'.[46]

The biographical information that has been gathered and presented in this book rarely consists of medical affairs, but it supplies much information regarding the life, achievements, actions, relations, social status and many other aspects of each practitioner. Collectively, it provides us with a better and detailed picture of their status, their socio-economic position within the Jewish communities and among their Muslim/Christian neighbours and colleagues.

In his book *Jews, Medicine, and Medieval Society*, Joseph Shatzmiller raised several questions, some of which are relevant to my research: How many Jewish physicians were practising during the period under investigation, and what proportion of the profession did they represent? From where did the Jewish doctors obtain their education? What were the social and economic conditions that gave birth to this professional opportunity (a lucrative profession that awarded its practitioners power and prestige)? How was it then that Christians and Muslims accepted the Jewish doctor and allowed him to inspect their bodies, to prescribe medication for them, to prepare drugs, and consequently, to determine their survival? And last but not least, did the law come to their defence when misunderstandings occurred?[47] Our sources and the analysis of the hard-won facts we have collected can answer only a few of these important questions regarding the Jewish practitioners of the medieval Islamic world.

The research questions, listed below, that I faced when I started my work were many and varied; and they were not always answered by the biographies alone. In some cases, the query was never solved.

- Who were the Jewish practitioners in the medieval Muslim world?
- Where did they actually practise? Did they operate privately or were they somehow organised?
- What fees did they charge for their medical work?
- How many Jewish practitioners were active in each generation? What was their geographic distribution?
- Did Jewish practitioners treat Muslim and Christian patients in their private practices? What was the essence of such a relationship?

- Were there any professional interactions with Muslim and Christian practitioners? If so, of what nature were these relations?
- What was their socio-economic status in the communities within which they operated?
- Were there any dynasties among the medical practitioners?
- What other kinds of duties did Jewish practitioners carry out in their communities?
- How often did Jewish physicians serve in the courts of the rulers and what was their relationship with the authorities?
- Did each practitioner have his own library? What works did it contain?
- How many Jewish practitioners actually worked in the city hospitals, and in what capacity?
- How did medieval Jewish practitioners acquire their medical skills and expertise? What was their professional standard?
- What was the theoretical background associated with the training of the Jewish practitioners?
- Where did they specialise in various fields of medicine?
- What were the common medical problems with which our practitioners had to deal?
- What was the intellectual contribution of the Jewish practitioners – medical, religious, literary etc. – to the Jewish and other communities?
- How widespread was conversion to Islam among the practitioners? Did it change throughout the periods the book deals with?

2.3 The Cairo Geniza

For hundreds of years, especially during Fatimid, Ayyubid and Mamluk rule, Egypt in general, and Cairo in particular, was the centre of the Muslim world. The strategic location that joined the Indian Ocean and the Mediterranean trade made it a commercial hub. Moreover, Cairo looked eastward to Iraq and Iran, and westward to southern Spain and north Africa. Therefore, the Jewish community of Old Cairo (Fusṭāṭ) became one of the most important centres of Jewry, particularly in the East, but also throughout the world. This community had close relations with other Jewish communities (in the east: Babylon, Palestine, India and Yemen; and in the west: Spain, Sicily, Morocco, Algeria, and Tunisia), with whom it maintained extensive internal and international ties and engaged in widespread social, economic and religious activities.

The Jews of Fusṭāṭ worshipped in several synagogues, one of which was named Ben-Ezra. It served as a hub for the 'Syro-Palestinian' Jewish community, which used the same building as their religious centre for almost a millennium. During that time, one of the upper store-rooms in the synagogue was utilised as a *geniza*, or repository for discarded handwritten material, from about the tenth to the nineteenth century.

In accordance with Jewish religious practice, sacred books no longer in use were not idly discarded, but were either committed to such a *geniza* or buried. The community in Fusṭāṭ made use mainly of the first option and deposited not only sacred works such as the Bible, Rabbinical literature and liturgies, but also sectarian and secular literature, palimpsests, *responsa*, poetry and a range of other documents. Consequently, almost every piece of writing, whether secular or religious, printed or in manuscript form, from early or later periods, containing scholarly research or reading exercises for children, which passed through the hands of its members was consigned to the Geniza.

The extraordinary circumstance of its preservation for this long period against the ravages of time and decay was due to the exceptionally dry climate of Egypt, and the unique dust blowing in from the hills around the city; indeed, vast quantities of these manuscripts were preserved.[48]

While dated documents found in the Geniza range from about 870 to 1887, most of the material comes from two periods. The major part of this material is from the 'classical' Geniza period, which extends from the refounding of the Ben-Ezra synagogue in 1040 until the fire that broke out there in 1260. These documents, from the Fatimid and Ayyubid periods in Egypt, were written in various languages, but primarily in Arabic and Judaeo-Arabic, as well as in Hebrew. The other group of documents, which was far less studied, dates to the 15th–17th centuries, immediately after the expulsion of the Jews from Spain. Many Jews immigrated to the Ottoman Empire, including to Egypt, and transformed Jewish society there. The documents are largely in Hebrew and Ladino and are readily distinguishable from documents of the 'classical' period, due to the difference in handwriting.

The existence of the Cairo Geniza was known to European scholars long before it was formally 'collected'. Some even visited it, but superstitious tales prevented them from touching or removing any fragments. During the nineteenth century, the 'spell was broken', and manuscripts were bought from the synagogue officials and guards.

The largest collection of documentary Geniza material is held by Cambridge University Library. This collection owes its existence to Dr Solomon Schechter (1847–1915) and Dr Charles Taylor (1840–1908), who were responsible for recovering the majority of Geniza manuscripts from Cairo in 1896, and it is known as the Taylor-Schechter Geniza Collection. It was offered to the Cambridge University Library Syndicate with certain conditions in 1898. Other significant collections can be found at the John Rylands University Library, Manchester; the Saltykov-Shchedrin Public Library, St Petersburg; the Bodleian Library, Oxford; the British Library, London; the Alliance israélite universelle, Paris; Westminster College, Cambridge; the Bibliothèque nationale et universitaire, Strasbourg; the Academy of Science, Budapest; the Annenberg Research Institute, Philadelphia; the Jewish National and University Library, Jerusalem; and the Hebrew Union College, Cincinnati; in the Mosseri family collection, Cambridge; in Vienna, Washington, DC, Birmingham, Frankfurt and Berlin; and in a few private collections.[49]

In 1973, the Geniza Research Unit at Cambridge University Library was established, and since then it has conducted numerous research projects. Individual fragments have been published, catalogues compiled,[50] and much research focusing on a wide variety of matters has yielded a wealth of articles and books.

Among the main fields that have been studied are various religious and Biblical subjects, such as Jewish law, education, poetry, economic aspects, social life, trade and communal organisation, including medicine, in medieval Mediterranean communities. Islamic historians praised the potential of the Geniza and its research; for example, Stephen Humphreys described the Geniza as 'a body of sources unequalled in medieval Islamic studies for its range, coherence, and intimacy'.[51] Moreover, Marina Rustow claimed that 'the Geniza has changed and is still changing the way the history of the Near-East is written'.[52] This book is another link in the chain of publications that validates these observations.

The importance of the Geniza for research on medieval Mediterranean communities, supplying information on almost every aspect of life, has been amply demonstrated by the research of many Geniza scholars such as S. D. Goitein, Moshe Gil, Menahem Ben-Sasson and many others.[53] It is important to note here that the significance of the Geniza is also due to the fact that hardly any archives have survived from the Near East before Ottoman rule (sixteenth century). The importance of the discoveries is further highlighted by the fact that Jews constituted one of Egypt's significant minorities. The community not only mirrored Mediterranean society as a whole, but was also famed for its medical heritage and its learned physicians.[54]

Today, we have a high-quality digitised database and a collective catalogue of most of the hundred thousand Geniza documents from seventy-two collections,[55] enabling researchers to study better and share their finds with other scholars. This database was built and is operated by the Friedberg Genizah Project.[56]

2.4 Research Difficulties

Various scholars claim that Arab anthroponomy is one of the more developed systems of identifying individuals. According to Manuela Marín and Annemarie Schimmel, the Arab-Islamic name system offers information about ethnic and geographical origins, family ties and religion; its complexity and richness have few parallels, if any, in other cultures.[57]

In general, Arabic names are formed according to a strict pattern: each name consists of (a) the *kunya* (agnomen, designation of a person as father), (b) the *ism* (personal proper name, which could be an adjective, noun or verb), (c) the *nasab* (one's relations to one's forefathers), (d) the *nisba* (cognomen, one's native place, or national or religious allegiance) and (e) the *laqab* (nickname, given to a person to distinguish them from another; it can be an honorific title), which sometimes develops into a proper name, or a family or clan name which could also, according to Schimmel, be an honorific designation; this sequence was usually applied.[58]

The names of the Jewish practitioners presented in this book were extracted from historical sources and original documents (Cairo Geniza documents and Muslim Arabic literature) written in three different languages: Hebrew, Judaeo-Arabic and Arabic.[59] As was customary in the Arab tradition, each person, including Jewish physicians and pharmacists, had, as mentioned above, a long name: his own name, the names of his father and his son, a professional name/names, occasionally a nickname, and sometimes the name of his geographical origin,[60] for example Abū al-Barakāt Hibat Allāh b. ʿAli b. Malkā (or Malkān) al-Baladi al-Tabib al-Faḍl[61] and Abū al-Makārim Abū al-Hibat-Allāh b. Zayn b. Ḥasan b. Ephraim b. Yaʿqūb b. Ismāʿīl Ibn Jumayʿ al-ʾIsrāʾīlī (Nethanel b. Samuel).[62]

In most cases, the names are given in a brief and unstandardised form, that is, only a few of the components of the name of the person appear in each source or document, and to make things even more complicated, since these practitioners were active in both societies and cultures (Jewish and Muslim), in many cases they had two sets of names – a Hebrew name and an Arabic name, such as Abū al-Ḥajjāj Yūsuf b. Yaḥyā b. Isḥāq al-Sabatī al-Maghribī = Joseph b. Judah b. Simon ha-Maghribī[63] or Yaḥyā b. Sulaymān al-ʾIsrāʾīlī al-Ṭabīb al-Ḥakīm = Zechariah b. Solomon.[64] Not only were the names of the practitioners written in different languages; the sources from which we collected the information about them were written in different periods (from the eighth to the sixteenth century), by people of various socio-economic strata, in many locations around the Muslim empire. I had to face a similar problem regarding the secondary sources. The publications I used were written by dozens of scholars, coming from various disciplines and schools that have been studying the Geniza and the Muslim Arabic sources of the last 150 years. They used different systems of transliteration in their academic works, published in several languages in numerous journals and books (by many publishers).

Therefore, great care was taken to identify the number of variants of each practitioner's name, and in some cases, when too little of the name was given to confirm an identification, I left practitioners with the same name in separate biographies (entries) since I could not find clear-cut evidence that they were actually the same person.

A few more observations regarding decision making while writing the book:

a. In most cases I have used translations of the medieval sources; these were made by the scholars that published the information, hence, I critically checked each one of them with the help of members of my research group and specialists (linguists, Geniza scholars and scholars of medical Muslim Arabic sources). The same specialists worked with me on the sources that had not been published before. Due to the vast amount of materials processed, studied and presented in this book, inaccuracy or mistakes might be found. In that case, I am responsible for each one of them!

b. I have included in the book some practitioners that practised out of the Muslim world (in Crete or Byzantium); however, in those cases, their origin and medical training took place in the Muslim world. The time span this book covers is considerable, and the histories of the regions it encompasses are diverse, and people, especially Jews, moved from place to place (in some cases from Muslim to Christian lands) in order to find refuge or make a living. This phenomenon was especially evident in Andalusia, and I might have missed some practitioners that worked on both sides.[65]

c. In this book, I present biographies and information about practitioners that were identified as such and where the information about their professional medical activity was proven; dozens of biographies have not been included since the evidence was not clear enough.

d. In some cases, due to the wealth of information, not all the sources and publications regarding the practitioners are cited. In such cases, mainly concerning well-known physicians such as Maimonides, Ḥasday b. Shaprūṭ, Isḥāq b. Sulaymān al-ʾIsrāʾīlī and Ibn Jumayʿ, I decided to present only the relevant pieces of information from selected sources. Therefore, the size of a biography has nothing to do with the importance of the practitioner! Information about the important figures is usually available in the academic literature (published in known languages); however, in case of the less-known ones, for the benefit of readers, I have tried to include as much information as possible (in most cases from Muslim Arabic sources and Geniza documents).

e. When information that was extracted from publications of previous scholars, using Geniza fragments, is cited, I have omitted the class-mark of the documents, in an attempt to make the book more readable.

Readers are invited to send more information about Jewish practitioners in the Muslim world between the eighth and the sixteenth century, in case we have missed any names or pieces of information. Any comments, references or pieces of additional information will be greatly appreciated!

2.5 Medieval Arabic Medicine and Practitioners

Most scholars studying the history of medicine agree that Arabic medicine is in fact the Hippocratic–Galenic system or legacies in its 'Arabised' form, meaning the inclusion of medical knowledge from mainly Indian and also Iranian medicine. Moreover, the new drugs from the East that were introduced and inserted into the system fitted into the overall pattern.[66]

In general, Arabic medicine was to a large extent rational; as Leigh Chipman wrote: 'All things ultimately may have come from the Master of the Universe, but proximate causes and cures for illness were sought in this world.'[67] The basic theory was that the body consisted of four humours (blood, black bile, yellow bile, phlegm), composed like all other things of the four basic elements (water, air, fire, earth), and the state of which depended on two qualities out of the four characters (hot, cold, humid, dry) and their varying degrees (1–4). Diseases resulted from the disturbance of the equilibrium between the humours and were treated accordingly by restoring it. Each person had their own equilibrium, which was dependent on their individual nature, such as their diet, and the specific qualities of the environment in which they lived. The humoral theory was also the basis for the classification and application of remedies. Other themes and fields of Arabic medicine were anatomy, ophthalmology, fertilisation, embryos, treating of wounds, physiology, pathology, diagnosis, prognosis, dietetics, surgery, therapy, psychology and pharmacology.[68]

For many decades, historians of medicine and historians of the Arab world studied Arab medicine of the classical Muslim period (from the early eighth century to the late twelfth century).[69] Several scholars studied the biographies of medieval physicians while they were learning, editing or translating their medical books, for example Colin Baker (Saʿīd ibn Hibat Allāh),[70] Charles Burnett (Ibn Biklarish),[71] Leigh Chipman (al-Kohen al-ʿAṭṭār al-ʾIsrāʾīlī),[72] Michael Dols (Ibn Riḍwān),[73] Sami Hamarneh (Ibn al-Quff),[74] Oliver Kahl (Ibn al-Tilmīdh, Sābūr b. Sahl),[75] Efraim Lev (Ibn Jazla),[76] and Martin Levey (al-Kindī, Ibn Māsawayh and al-Samarkandī).[77]

The main sources of our knowledge of Arab practitioners are biographies and autobiographies of Muslim scholars, including physicians, and especially biographical dictionaries or encyclopedias, which were very popular in the thirteenth century in the Muslim Arabic tradition and culture. Doris Behrens-Abouseif, who studied the image of physicians in Arab biographies of the post-classical age (13th–18th century), claimed that there are two categories of encyclopedias in which biographical information about physicians can be found. The first and early genre consists of biographical encyclopedias that were dedicated exclusively to medical practitioners and scientists, some of which, as in the case of the example by Ibn Abī Uṣaybiʿa,[78] were written by a physician belonging to a family (dynasty) of doctors. Another one is by Ibn al-Qifṭī.[79] Mohamed Meouak asserted that 'because of the difficulties surrounding the study of classical Islamic society, due to the nature of the extant sources and the almost complete absence of documentary archives, biographical texts are documents of the greatest importance for the study of the *'ulmā'*.[80] These two works supply us with details mainly of the physicians of Egypt and Syria, from the early and classical periods, until the end of the Ayyubid period (thirteenth century). They give a positive picture of the status of the medical profession at these locations, mainly under the Ayyubid rulers.[81] Based on his deep knowledge and long-term study of the Mediterranean society Goitein described the medieval doctors of the Mediterranean area as 'the torchbearers of secular erudition, the professional expounders of philosophy and the sciences', and added that they wore a 'halo of social prestige'.[82]

The second category, general biographies, consists of encyclopedias that deal with physicians along with other professions. In both categories, there are biographical details of only prominent physicians; in Behrens-Abouseif's words, 'those attached to the service of the ruling class, and those who became famous either through their outstanding scholarly achievements, their medical skills, or both'.[83]

Both Ibn Abī Uṣaybiʿa and Ibn al-Qifṭī mention Arab physicians who were philosophers, astronomers, mathematicians and astrologers, a combination that was inherited from the Greek tradition. These physician-scholars received their education sometimes within the family, or in some cases in hospitals, with private teachers, in specialising schools, and even in religious institutions.[84] Moreover, in most cases their education also included literature, poetry and music, and often these were part of their activities. Interestingly enough, despite the wide range of interest of these physicians, they were familiar with theoretical and also practical medicine. Most of them worked in hospitals and taught medicine as well. Early physicians as recorded by the medical biographies were sometimes also druggists.[85]

Some of the Muslim physicians were Sufis,[86] and some of them even held office in religious institutions. Others were involved in trade, which contributed to their income. Neither Ibn Abī Uṣaybiʿa nor Ibn al-Qifṭī saw religious affiliations 'as [a] handicap to the medical practice and research under Islam'. Therefore, they also reported on non-Muslim physicians who took an important part in the field of medicine, praised some of them in the same way they praised Muslim physicians, and considered others as friends.[87]

According to the description in the medical biographies, physicians were highly respected and appreciated by the rulers, and sometimes even managed to get influential positions at the sultan's court; some received huge salaries, others were married to women of the court. The Ayyubid rulers promoted medicine and sponsored hospitals, did not hesitate to take physicians who had previously worked for the Fatimid court, and surrounded themselves by physicians whom they esteemed as scholars, including non-Muslim ones, since they did not consider themselves religious fanatics. Behrens-Abouseif suggested that since the twelfth and thirteenth centuries were characterised by the warfare with the Crusaders, 'physicians were badly needed to treat wounded soldiers which may also have enhanced their prestige at that time'.[88] However, in the fourteenth and fifteenth centuries, when the Arab world faced a violent plague, religious awareness of its cause spread at the expense of medical understanding, as in the case of other catastrophes, unfortunately lessening the competence of the physicians.[89]

A different picture of the medical profession is portrayed by the second category, that is, the general biographies. This is mainly due to the fact that the physicians were only one of many other scholarly professions. The main focus of this genre is men from the religious and ruling establishment. Therefore, its references to practitioners are brief and scarce, unless they belonged to the religious elite. Interestingly, the physicians are rarely referred to as *Ḥakīm*, but instead as *Ṭabīb*, *Kaḥḥāl* and *Jarāʾiḥī* (surgeon). Many of these physicians were attached to religious institutions (a physician who would be involved with philosophy was suspect); and sometimes the name of the teacher of a physician was mentioned and/or a few words described their reputation as practitioners. From the general biographies, we learn that some scholars, mainly during the Mamluk period, studied medicine without practising it; and, on the other hand, we learn about non-physician scholars who wrote medical books. Behrens-Abouseif claimed that this might be the reason why Mamluk authors made a distinction between a good medical scholar and a proficient practitioner.[90]

And indeed, in the Mamluk period, there were two distinct orientations of medicine: a theoretical one (with a higher status due to its aspect of erudition) and a practical one. According to Behrens-Abouseif, this distinction might indicate that 'general medicine was a subject which a *sufi* could be familiar with, mainly through reading, whereas surgery and ophthalmology needed more specialised and practically oriented craftsmen who could not acquire their skills within a religious institution'. Non-Muslims were not mentioned in this genre, unless they were converts to Islam.[91] This reflects the Mamluk attitude towards *dhimmīs*, which was less tolerant in comparison with the Ayyubid dynasty. However, other sources, including the Cairo Geniza, inform us that non-Muslims continued to be part of the medical profession throughout the Mamluk and Ottoman periods; their education was probably in the 'non-religious private sector'. Likewise, engineering and architecture were also studied besides medicine by both Muslims and non-Muslims. The Mamluk court physicians, especially those of the fifteenth century, did not belong to the immediate circle of the sultan's entourage; they enjoyed neither the privileges, nor the prestige, of the Ayyubid court physicians.[92] Miri Shefer raised and discussed various questions and aspects of the phenomena of court physicians, for example: how did physicians gain a foothold in their patron's house? How could an anonymous physician make himself noticed by an influential ruler? One of the ways, for example, was to write a book and present it to the patron.[93]

An important issue regarding promotion of Arab physicians of all periods, and especially from the Mamluk period, was patronage: physicians could be promoted and receive a regular income through positions either at religious institutions or at courts. Otherwise, they could not become wealthy, and had to take on other jobs (as we see in the case of many Jewish practitioners of that period).[94] According to Behrens-Abouseif, positions in the judiciary or administration in the Mamluk establishments were more prestigious and lucrative than that of an average medical doctor; a physician who had other qualifications might have abandoned medicine for such a post. These phenomena deprived medicine of its scholarly grounding; moreover, they depreciated the image of the physician on the one hand, and on the other, left the field of medicine open to non-Muslims.[95] According to Prosper Alpin, a Venetian physician who lived in Cairo during the late sixteenth century, even then the ruling class already employed European physicians; he added that the medical craft was poorly supervised, the status of the local physicians was low, and since the society was totally controlled by religion, the sciences were neglected.[96]

Based on medieval Muslim Arabic literature, it appears that the ideal Arab physician was therefore 'competent, well-spoken, properly dressed, kind, righteous, and discreet – at least in the view of the doctors who laid down the guidelines in writings on medical ethics'. Moreover, he ought to inspire confidence.[97] Shefer added that court physicians had been described at the biographical dictionaries as 'good-looking people and skilled debaters who provided intellectual entertainment and stimulation for their patron'.[98] Many Muslim doctors were only following in the footsteps of their fathers. This phenomenon of the ancestry of physicians (dynasties) created generations of practitioners belonging to the same family. One example, and maybe the best one, is the renowned Bukhtīshūʿ family of Christian doctors from Baghdad, which can be traced over two and a half centuries.[99] A similar situation was recorded in medieval Europe, with for example the Plateanus family of Salerno on the northern shore of the Mediterranean.[100] The phenomenon of medical dynasties among Jewish families in the Muslim world was recorded and studied, and will be discussed in the next chapter.

Physicians in the Islamic world acquired their medical knowledge in a number of ways, namely by self-teaching, familial tuition, private tutoring, apprenticeships, attendance at *majlises* and hospital training.[101] They were tested later and received official graduation diplomas from management and governing bodies.[102] The graduation was recorded, thus affording the physician recognition as qualified to work in his field; this was intended to establish the profession, and mainly to prevent imposters from causing irreparable damage to both hospitals and patients. Moreover, this process led to a more advanced level of achievement. Renowned physicians would have often served in such a hospital, not only for the financial benefits, but for the sake of the approbation which the position generated and in order to train new young doctors.[103]

There were different views regarding physicians' training and practice. Ibn Sīnā claimed that you 'can be a good physician without having had a patient sitting in front of you whom you tried to help through bloodletting or feeling his pulse'. However, Ibn Jumayʿ al-ʾIsrāʾīlī (d. 1198) criticises him, saying that medicine is not theory alone, or just pure scholarship or knowledge, it is also practice. Actually, Ibn Jumayʿ adopted the classical trend that medicine is a practical art, and therefore the physicians need to practise it 'as carpenters or goldsmiths practice their craft'.[104]

In general, hospital physicians treated patients that were hospitalised, or they came to work in the outpatient clinic in the morning. Teaching took place later in the afternoon, by the senior physicians, including the head physician in the hospital, in a remote corner of the central space. The junior physicians and students of medicine gathered around the seniors and read medical texts together. The good teachers explained the content, especially the unclear issues, and could correct mistakes. The medical texts were taken from the hospital's library, or from the senior physicians' private libraries. An apprenticeship at the hospital was another important foundation for the professional education of the young medical students and practitioners.[105]

Peter Pormann and Emilie Savage-Smith dealt with several issues regarding Arabic physicians in their *Medieval Islamic Medicine*: medical education, medical regulations, medical ethics, the status of physicians, places of medical practice, Islamic hospitals, inter-religious relations (Muslim, Christians and Jews), female practitioners, women patients, medicine in rural settings, public health care and more.[106] And indeed, the information from the Muslim Arabic sources clearly portrayed the historical figures of the medieval Arabic medical milieu, mainly famous physicians and pharmacists that were serving the elite and their court members, treating the rulers and generals, working in the best hospitals in the most important capitals, writing famous and lengthy medical treatises and teaching students, some of whom became renowned.

Another interesting issue is how effective was the medical treatment given by the medieval physicians. W. V. Harris claimed that the average patient in the classical world was at least partially aware that physicians' treatments did more harm than good.[107] It is reasonable to extend this hypothesis to medieval Arabic medicine as was described by Franz Rosenthal.[108] Luke Yarbrough described a few cases of Arabic poets publicly (by using ridicule) criticising doctors for killing patients and making off with their money.[109] A medieval specialist insight on this issue was written by Maimonides: 'And [since] most physicians are incompetent, the result is as Aristotle has said – namely, that most people die as a result of medical treatment.'[110]

Most modern scholars agree that physicians played an important role in Muslim societies and could enjoy very high status; Shefer wrote about what made Mamluk and Ottoman physicians part of the elite, to which elite they belonged, and in what way they could became success stories.[111]

Another issue can be learnt from Maimonides' criticising of the people in Egypt for their habit of skipping from one physician to another; however, he recommended treatment on the basis of consensus by multiple physicians.[112] Sometimes, circles of physicians were formed around an institution, as in the case of al-Bīmāristān al-Nūrī, in Damascus, under the guidance of Muhadhdhab al-Dīn al-Naqqāsh (d. 1178). This circle was described by Ahmed Ragab in his book on Islamic hospitals; he claimed that the true success and prominence of this group, namely shaping the medical elite in the Levant and in Egypt for more than a century, happened under the guidance of al-Dakhwār (d. 1231) thanks to his distinguished court position, *bīmāristān* (hospital) service and medical madrasa. Members of this group were committed to Ibn Sīnā's philosophical and theoretical writings and 'rediscovered' *al-Ḥāwī* of al-Rāzī in the Levantine and Egyptian contexts. Moreover, they placed more emphasis on practical writings derived from their own experience.[113] The *bīmāristān* relied on the collective practice of practitioners of the art of medicine and 'neighbouring' medical arts and crafts. In general, collective practice was not a new idea; it was applied in Islamic courts, having many physicians consulting together and giving more than one opinion. In the case of healthy patients or in the court, the patient was the final judge regarding the right treatment. In hospital, where the patient lost their right and ability to judge between the physicians' suggestions of treatment, the *bīmāristān* bureaucracy and hierarchy gave one physician precedence over the others for the sake of faster and better process of diagnosis and treatment.[114] Based on Muslim Arabic medieval medical sources such as al-Rāzī,[115] Ragab portrayed the medical encounter between physician and patient, and the examination process. He claimed that the majority of patients sought medical help mainly when symptoms persisted for a long time, if new symptoms appeared, or in cases of severe pain. During his examination, the physician detected the signs of illness by questioning the patient, and observing their colour, movement, facial features and the three cardinal signs (urine, pulse and stool). These would yield information about the patient's regular and normal complexion, and about the changes occurring during the illness. Thereafter, the physician determined the nature of the illness and prescribed a diet, treatment or evacuation.[116]

Similar to other scholars, Paulina Lewicka suggested that the bulk of physicians in the medieval Near East were non-Muslim. Based on Muslim Arabic sources and medieval Christian chroniclers (mainly from the Crusaders period), she claimed that between the tenth and the thirteenth centuries, Christian physicians prevailed among the medical practitioners in Syria and Egypt. Cautiously she suggested that

> the relatively high demand for their services might have been the reason, why Christian and Jewish practitioners were not only allowed to stay in business, but also to maintain numerical advantage over Muslims almost throughout the Middle Ages, in the otherwise less-than-friendly circumstances notwithstanding.[117]

The main importance of the current book is that it presents the biographies of various kinds of Jewish practitioners, based on both the Jewish sources (mainly the Cairo Geniza) and the Muslim Arabic sources. These include not only the well-known Jewish practitioners that were treating their community members, but also the ordinary Muslim people in the hospitals and the Muslim elite in the courts. But it is mainly dedicated to the non-illustrious and unknown Jewish practitioners, and highlights their names, deeds and life stories. These practitioners carried on their shoulders the responsibility of supplying medical care, firstly to the members of their Jewish communities all over the Muslim world, and equally to their fellow citizens, Muslim and Christians alike.

The next section presents the findings; that is, biographies of Jewish physicians and pharmacists and Jewish practitioners who were part of medical dynasties.

Notes

1. 'Prosopography', Merriam-Webster, http://www.merriam-webster.com/dictionary/prosopography (accessed 4 August 2020).
2. Stone, 'Prosopography'; for another view see Beech, 'Prosopography'; for an example of a dozen studies in medieval prosopography and various methodologies see Bulst and Genet, *Medieval Lives and the Historian.*
3. Broady, 'French Prosopography'; for detailed introductions to the field see Keats-Rohan, *Prosopography Approaches and Applications*, pp. 1–32; Murray, 'Prosopography'.
4. Fleming, 'Writing Biography at the Edge of History', p. 607.
5. Elmakias, *The Naval Commanders of Early Islam*, pp. 135–8.
6. For a few examples see Berto, *In Search of the First Venetians*, p. 1, nn. 2, 3. For more examples see the annotated bibliography in Keats-Rohan, *Prosopography Approaches and Applications*; for works regarding the later Roman Empire, Byzantium and beyond see Cameron, *Fifty Years of Prosopography.*
7. Banner, 'Biography as History'; Fleming, 'Writing Biography'.
8. Elmakias, *The Naval Commanders of Early Islam*, p. 21; for further views on the advantages, challenges and disadvantages of this method see for example Stone, 'Prosopography'.
9. See for example Martindale, 'The Prosopography of the Byzantine Empire'; Rebenich, 'Mommsen, Harnack, and the Prosopography of Late Antiquity'.
10. See in depth Elmakias, *The Naval Commanders of Early Islam*, p. 22; for some thoughts about the use of prosopography in research on the Middle Ages see Bachrach, 'Introduction'.
11. Marín, 'Biography and Prosopography'; Gilliot, 'Prosopography in Islam'.
12. Crone, *Slaves on Horses.*
13. Sublet, 'La Prosopographie arabe'; Ahmed, *The Religious Elite of the Early Islamic Hijaz.*
14. Marín, 'Biography and Prosopography', p. 8; see also Qāḍī, 'Biographical Dictionaries'.
15. Lecker, 'The Prosopography of Early Islamic Administration'.
16. Elmakias, *The Naval Commanders of Early Islam.*

17. Ebstein, 'Shurṭa Chiefs in Baṣra'.
18. Perlman, 'The Bodyguard of the Caliphs during the Umayyad and Abbasid Periods'.
19. Berto, *In Search of the First Venetians.*
20. Brezzi and Lee, *Sources of Social History*, mainly pp. 99–104.
21. 'Social history', Merriam-Webster, http://www.merriam-webster.com/dictionary/social%20history (accessed 4 August 2020). For a more detailed quick review see 'Social history', Wikipedia, https://en.wikipedia.org/wiki/Social_history (accessed 4 August 2020).
22. Regarding the Geniza and its story see Reif, *A Jewish Archive from Old Cairo.*
23. According to Marina Rustow's estimation, there are about 15,000 documents in total preserved in the Cairo Geniza; see Rustow, Heresy and the Politics *of Community*, p. xx.
24. The main works dealing with history of medicine in the Geniza are: Goitein, *A Mediterranean Society*, vol. II, pp. 240–72; Goitein, 'The Medical Profession'; Isaacs, *Medical and Para-medical Manuscripts*; Baker, 'Islamic and Jewish Medicine in the Medieval Mediterranean World'; Cohen, 'The Burdensome Life'; Lev and Amar, 'Practice versus Theory'; Lev and Amar, *Practical Materia Medica*; Lev, 'A Catalogue of the Medical and Para-medical Manuscripts'; Lev, 'Medieval Egyptian Judaeo-Arabic Prescriptions'; Lev, 'Work in Progress'; Lev, 'An Early Fragment of Ibn Jaziah's Tabulated Manual'; Lev and Niessen, 'Addenda to Isaacs's "Catalogue"'; Lev and Smithuis, 'A Preliminary Catalogue'; Lev, Chipman and Niessen, 'A Hospital Handbook for the Community'; Lev, Chipman and Niessen, 'Chicken and Chicory Are Good for You'; Lev and Chipman, 'Texts/Documents/Translations'; Lev and Chipman, *Medical Prescriptions*; Chipman and Lev, '"Take a Lame and Decrepit Female Hyena"'; Chipman and Lev, 'Arabic Prescriptions'; Serry and Lev, 'A Judaeo-Arabic Fragment'; Chipman and Lev, 'Syrups from the Apothecary's Shop'; Ashur and Lev, 'Medical Recipes'.
25. For example Freidberg Jewish Manuscript Society, https://fgp.genizah.org; Princeton Geniza Lab, https://www.princeton.edu/~geniza (both accessed 4 August 2020).
26. Marín, 'Biography and Prosopography', p. 3.
27. Banner, 'Biography as History', p. 582.
28. Ibid., p. 583.
29. See in depth Marín, 'Biography and Prosopography'.

30. Bulliet, 'A Quantitative Approach to Medieval Muslim Biographical Dictionaries'.
31. Bulliet, 'The Conversion Curve Revisited'.
32. Ibn Abī Uṣaybiʿa, *ʿUyūn al-Anbāʾ*; Ibn al-Qifṭī, *Taʾrīkh al-Hukamaʾ*.
33. Reynolds, *Interpreting the Self.*
34. See Section 3.1.1 for physicians, Section 3.1.2 for pharmacists and Section 3.3.2 for members of dynasties.
35. Wasserstein, 'Ibn Biklarish'.
36. Wasserstein, 'What's in a Name?'
37. Cohen, 'The Economic Background and the Secular Occupations of Muslim Jurisprudents and Traditionists', pp. 55, 59.
38. Behrens-Abouseif, 'The Image of the Physician', p. 333.
39. Cohen, 'The Economic Background and the Secular Occupations of Muslim Jurisprudents and Traditionists', p. 34.
40. Ibid., p. 48.
41. Ibid., p. 58.
42. Similarly, barbers were excluded from the book on physicians in Britain; see Talbot and Hammond, *The Medical Practitioners in Medieval England.*
43. Goitein, *A Mediterranean Society*, vol. I, p. 79.
44. In her words 'historians in general'.
45. Banner, 'Biography as History', p. 580.
46. Ibid., p. 582.
47. Shatzmiller, *Jews, Medicine, and Medieval Society*, pp. x–xi.
48. Reif, *A Jewish Archive from Old Cairo*, pp. 1–22.
49. Richler, *Guide to Hebrew Manuscript Collections*, pp. 63–4.
50. Gottheil and Worrell, *Fragments from the Cairo Genizah*; Reif, *Published Material from the Cambridge Genizah Collections*; Khan, *Arabic Legal and Administrative Documents*; Baker and Polliack, *Arabic and Judaeo-Arabic Manuscripts*; Jefferson and Hunter, *Published Material from the Cambridge*; Shivtiel and Niessen, *Arabic and Judaeo-Arabic Manuscripts in the Cambridge Genizah Collections.*
51. Humphreys, *Islamic History*, p. 262.
52. Rustow, *Heresy and the Politics of Community*, p. xxi.
53. Goitein, *A Mediterranean Society*; Goitein, *Palestinian Jewry*; Gil, *In the Kingdom of Ishmael*; Gil, *Jews in Islamic Countries*; Ben-Sasson, *The Jews of Sicily.*
54. Goitein, *A Mediterranean Society*, vol. I, pp. 153–4, 209–24, vol. II, pp. 240–72.

55. For more about the various Geniza collections and how to find, learn and understand Geniza fragments, see Zinger, 'Finding a Fragment in a Pile of Geniza'.
56. https://fjms.genizah.org
57. Marín, 'Anthroponymy and Society'; Schimmel, *Islamic Names.*
58. Schimmel, *Islamic Names*, pp. 1–13.
59. For more about Arabic naming see Beeston, *Arabic Nomenclature*; Bareket, 'Jewish First Names'.
60. Bareket, 'Jewish First Names'; Bareket, 'Note on Jewish Naming Patterns in the Cairo Geniza'; Goitein, *A Mediterranean Society*, vol. I, pp 357–8; Goldberg, *Trade and Institutions*, pp. xv–xvi.
61. Poznański, 'Die jüdischen Artikel in Ibn al-Qifti's Gelehrtenlexikon', p. 52.
62. Miller, 'Doctors without Borders', p. 112; Ashtor-Strauss, *Saladin and the Jews*, p. 310; see biographies in Chapter 3 of this volume.
63. Ibn al-Qifṭī, *Taʾrīkh al-Ḥukamāʾ*, p. 392.
64. Tobi, 'Ben Solomon'.
65. See for example, Shatzmiller, *Jews, Medicine, and Medieval Society.*
66. See in depth Amar and Lev, *Arabian Drugs*, pp. 1–12.
67. Chipman, 'The Jewish Presence in Arabic Writings', p. 394.
68. See in detail Brentjes, *Teaching and Learning*, p. 71; Pormann and Savage-Smith, *Medieval Islamic Medicine*, pp. 41–79; Lev and Chipman, *Medical Prescriptions*, pp. 7–9; Chipman, 'The Jewish Presence in Arabic Writings', pp. 394–5.
69. See for example Campbell, *Arabian Medicine and Its Influence on the Middle Ages*; Ullmann, *Islamic Medicine*; Dols (trans.) and Gamal (ed.), *Medieval Islamic Medicine*; Conrad, 'Arab-Islamic Medicine'; Pormann and Savage-Smith, *Medieval Islamic Medicine.*
70. Baker, ''Abū al-Ḥasan Saʿīd's *Maqāla fī Khalq al-ʾInsān*'.
71. Burnett, *Ibn Baklarish's Book of Simples.*
72. Chipman, *The World of Pharmacy and Pharmacists.*
73. Dols (trans.) and Gamal (ed.), *Medieval Islamic Medicine.*
74. Hamarneh, *The Physician. Therapist and Surgeon Ibn al-Quff.*
75. Ibn Sahl, *The Small Dispensatory*; Kahl, 'Sābūr b. Sahl'; Kahl, *The Dispensatory of Ibn al-Tilmīḏ*; Kahl, *Sābūr ibn Sahl's Dispensatory.*
76. Lev, 'An Early Fragment'.
77. Levey, *The Medical Formulary*; Levey, 'Ibn Māsawaih and His Treatise on

Simple Aromatic Substances'; Levey and al-Khaledy, *The Medical Formulary of al-Samarqandī.*

78. Ibn Abī Uṣaybiʿa, *ʿUyūn al-Anbāʾ*.
79. Ibn al-Qifṭī, *Taʾrīkh al-Ḥukamāʾ*.
80. Meouak, 'Prosopography of the Political Elites'.
81. Behrens-Abouseif, 'The Image of the Physician', p. 333.
82. Goitein, *A Mediterranean Society*, vol. II, pp. 240–1.
83. For details see Behrens-Abouseif, 'The Image of the Physician'.
84. For a detailed presentation of the classification of Muslim biographical dictionaries, and the part of the biographies of physicians, see Gilliot, 'Prosopography in Islam', especially p. 31.
85. Behrens-Abouseif, 'The Image of the Physician', pp. 333–4.
86. Sufism is Islamic mysticism.
87. Behrens-Abouseif, 'The Image of the Physician', pp. 332–3.
88. Ibid., p. 333–4.
89. Dols, *The Black Death in the Middle East*, pp. 109–42.
90. Behrens-Abouseif, 'The Image of the Physician', p. 334.
91. From the point of view of the current research this means that much important data regarding Jewish practitioners has not come down to us.
92. Behrens-Abouseif, 'The Image of the Physician', p. 336.
93. Shefer, 'Physicians in the Mamluk and Ottoman Courts', p. 116.
94. Behrens-Abouseif, 'The Image of the Physician', pp. 336–8. For an interesting description of the life stories of two very rich Muslim physicians from the fifteenth and sixteenth centuries, see Shefer, 'Physicians in the Mamluk and Ottoman Courts', p. 114.
95. Behrens-Abouseif, 'The Image of the Physician', pp. 336–8.
96. Alpin, *La Médecine des Égyptiens*, vol. I, p. 9.
97. Ragab, *The Medieval Islamic Hospital*, pp. 89–90.
98. Shefer, 'Physicians in the Mamluk and Ottoman Courts', p. 119.
99. Sourdel, 'Bukhtishūʿ'.
100. See in detail Goitein, *A Mediterranean Society*, vol. II, pp. 245–66.
101. Hazan, 'Medical, Administrative and Financial Aspects', pp. iv–v, 90–9; Pormann and Savage-Smith, *Medieval Islamic Medicine*, pp. 81–3; Leiser, 'Medical Education in Islamic Lands'.
102. Karmi, 'State Control of the Physicians in the Middle Ages'.
103. Hazan, 'Medical, Administrative and Financial Aspects', pp. v–vi, 101–9.
104. Nicolae, 'Jewish Physicians at the Court of Saladin', p. 28.

105. Brentjes, *Teaching and Learning*, p. 122.
106. Pormann and Savage-Smith, *Medieval Islamic Medicine*, especially ch. 3.
107. Harris, 'Popular Medicine in the Classical World', p. 11.
108. Rosenthal, 'The Defense of Medicine in the Medieval Muslim World'.
109. Yarbrough, *The Sword of Ambition*, pp. 56–7.
110. Bos, *Maimonides on Asthma*, pp. 93–4.
111. Shefer, 'Physicians in the Mamluk and Ottoman Courts'.
112. Bos, *Maimonides on Asthma*, pp. 108–9. Interestingly, Ahmed Ragab, citing al-Rāzī, offers a similar idea but with no geographic specification: Ragab, *The Medieval Islamic Hospital*, pp. 220–1.
113. Ragab, *The Medieval Islamic Hospital*, pp. 173–5.
114. Ibid., pp. 220–2.
115. al-Rāzī, *Kītāb al-Tajārib.*
116. Ragab, *The Medieval Islamic Hospital*, pp. 201–9.
117. Lewicka, 'The Non-Muslim Physician', pp. 501–2.

3

Prosopography of Jewish Medical Practitioners

3.1 Biographies

Readers will realise that the information in our entries is not all strictly medical. This issue has already been raised by Charles Talbot and Eugene Hammond: 'The biographer of medieval medical practitioners is soon aware of the non-medical nature of the bulk of his finding.' They concluded this issue by stating: 'And thus one comes to understand the importance of every type of evidence in constructing the total account of the medical profession.'[1]

Thanks to the integration of the information we studied from both genres of sources – that is, the Cairo Geniza fragments and the various Muslim Arabic sources – the biographies I present in this book reflect various aspects of the lives and deeds of the Jewish practitioners. The Muslim Arabic sources mainly supply us with information regarding places in which Jewish practitioners practised, rulers they were serving, or their teachers or students. In some cases, we learn about their medical education, salaries, size of their libraries and other details. The documents of the Cairo Geniza provide us with information regarding their families, everyday life, the religious aspect of their lives, their involvement in community affairs, their patients and so on. These hundreds of integrated biographies presented bellow allow us to analyse the hard-won facts and learn about various socio-economic aspects of the Jewish practitioners.

In the following biographies the names are loaded with various meanings. For the benefit of the readers, I hereby present the most common and therefore important ones with the translations of their original names:

a. Ethnic origin (part of the *nisba*): **al-ʾIsrāʾīlī** (Jewish), **al-Yahūdī** (Jewish), **al-ʿAnānī** (Karaite), **al-Sāmirī** (Samaritan).
b. Professional honorific titles (*laqab*): **al-Sadīd** (sound), **al-Muwaffaq** (successful), **al-Muhadhdhab** (accomplished, courteous, decent), **al-Mudawwar** (admired), **al-Sheikh** (leader, elder, old), **Asʿad al-Dīn** (happy, successful – indicates high status in the Jewish and Muslim populations), **al-Wajīh** (honourable), **Shams al-Ḥukamāʾ** (sun of the doctors), **al-Ḥakīm al-Ṣafī** (the loyal physician), **al-Thiqa** (reliable), **Awḥad al-Zamān** (one of a generation). An honorific title ending with **al-Dawla** (state or dynasty) was awarded mainly to Jews and other non-Muslims.[2] In the Mongol Īl-Khānate in Iran, Iraq and Azerbaijan (1256–1335), this title was already applied to Jews in official high positions.[3]
c. Social honorific titles and Hebrew professional occupations (*laqab*): **Atteret ha-Rōfēim** (crown of the physicians), **Hadrat ha-Rōfēim** (glory of the physicians), **Tifēret ha-Rōfēim** (splendour of the physicians), **ha-Dayyān** (the judge), **ha-Shōfēt** (the judge), **ha-Ḥasid** (the devout person, the pious God-fearing person), **ha-Zaqēn** (old, wise), **ha-Talmīd** (the student), **ha-Ḥākhām** (the intelligent one, scholar, or rabbi), **ha-Melammēd** (the teacher, of young boys), **ha-Sar** (notable, distinguished), **ha-Nikhbad** (respected, important, honoured), **ha-Yaqar** (dear, beloved), **ha-Mahir** (quick, fast), **ha-Nāsī** (the president, the leader), **ha-Mefoar** (magnificent, splendid), **ha-Nehedar** (magnificent, wonderful), **ha-Bāḥūr ha-Ṭōv** (the good person), **ha-Sōfer** (the writer, the author).

The names are arranged in alphabetical order. If the biography has a twofold name, the Arabic name appears first followed by the Hebrew name (as well as any honorific titles and synonyms). If one or more parts of the Arabic name are missing, the entry will be set according to the next one in the hierarchy (see below). If there is no Arabic name, the biography will start with and be set according to the Hebrew name.

As mentioned in Section 2.4 above, the hierarchy of presenting the Arabic names is as follows: (1) *kunya* (agnomen, for example Abū al-Barakāt), (2) *ism* (personal name, for example Hibat Allāh), (3) *nasab* (one's relations to one's forefathers, for example Ibn Malkā ʿAlī), (4) *nisba* (one's native place, national or religious allegiance, for example: al-Ṭabīb, al-Maghribī, al-Yahūdī), (5) *laqab* (nickname or honorific title, for example al-Faḍl, al-Muhadhdhab. The *laqab* sometimes develops into a proper name, a family or a clan name which could also, according to Annemarie Schimmel, be an honorific designation.[4]

The hierarchy of presenting the Hebrew names is as follows: (1) first name, for example Moses b. Yaḥyā, (2) family name and relations to one's forefathers, for example: ha-Levi, (3) nickname/ancient origin, for example Ibn al-ʿAmmānī, (4) occupation, for example ha-Rōfē], (5) geographical origin, for example Iskandarī, (6) honorific title, for example ha-Zaqēn.

In general, most of the practitioners whose geographical origin is unknown are from Egypt, since they were probably mentioned in the Cairo Geniza documents. Moreover, it is important to note here that the vast majority of the Geniza documents are from the eleventh to the thirteenth centuries, so, when there are no dates, it is most probable that the information, and the practitioner, are from those centuries.

The biographies of members of dynasties have been extracted from their places in the biographies of physicians (Section 3.1.1) and pharmacists (Section 3.1.2), and are presented in Section 3.3.2 together with other members of their dynasty. However, for the sake of readers, the names of the subjects have been retained in their places and set in *italics*.

Some notes regarding abbreviations, titles, origins and more

Chronological abbreviations: a. (active), b. (born), c. (circa), d. (died), r. (ruled).

Geographical origin: An. (Andalusia), Eg. (Egypt), EY (Eretz-Israel), Iq. (Iraq), Ir. (Iran), In. (India), Ma. (Maghrib), Mo. (Morocco), It. (Italy), Si. (Sicily), Sy. (Syria), Ye. (Yemen).

Sectarian origin: K. (Karaite), S. (Samaritan).

The word 'Ibn' is capitalised in order to indicate an individual's affiliation to a family or dynasty; whereas uncapitalised 'b.' (for Arabic *ibn* or Hebrew *ben*) denotes the son of an individual.

3.1.1 Biographies of Jewish physicians

Aaron b. Zedaqa b. Aaron ha-Rōfē al-ʿAmmānī [Eg., Alexandria, 11th century]

Aaron ha-Levi ha-Rōfē ha-Sōfer ha-Mahir [K., Eg., 12th century]
A Karaite physician, from the al-Sakanī family, mentioned in a memorial list.[5]

Aaron ha-Rōfē al-ʿAmmānī [Sy., Amman, Eg., Alexandria, 11th century]

Aaron ha-Rōfē al-Kāzrūnī [K., Eg., Sy., 12th century]
A Karaite physician. It is reported that he was buried in the Holy Land. He is mentioned in a genealogy list.[6] According to his name, his or his family's origin is the city of Kāzrūn, Iran.

Aaron ha-Rōfē b. Samuel Ibn al-ʿAmmānī [Eg., Alexandria, Cairo, 13th century]

Aaron ha-Rōfē b. Yeshūʿā Ibn al-ʿAmmānī [Eg., Alexandria, Cairo, 13th century]

Aaron ha-Rōfē b. Yeshūʿā ha-Rōfē Ibn al-ʿAmmānī [Eg., Alexandria, 12th century]

ʿAbd Allāh (Taqī al-Dīn) b. Dāʾūd b. Abī al-Faḍl b. Abī al-Munajjab (or al-Mūnā) b. Abī al-Fityān (or al-Bayān) al-Dāʾūdi [K., Eg., 14th–15th centuries, convert]

ʿAbd al-ʿAzīz b. Maḥāsin al-Muwaffaq al-ʾIsrāʾīlī al-Mutaṭabbib (Uziel b. Obadia) [Iq., al-Bīra, 14th century]

ʿAbd al-Dāʾim (al-Muwaffaq) b. ʿAbd al-ʿAzīz b. Maḥāsin ʾIsrāʾīlī al-Mutaṭabbib (Jekuthiel b. Uziel b. Obadia ha-Dayyān) [Eg., Iq., al-Bīra (Birecik), 14th century]

ʿAbd al-ʿAzīz ha-Ḥazzān al-Ḥakīm [Eg., Cairo, 16th century]
A physician, one of the representatives of the Mustaʿarabi Jews who stood in front of the Radbaz (Rabbi David b. Zimra, 1479–1573/1589), for a discussion following a dispute that broke out in 1527 between them and the Maghribis in Cairo. Beside him are mentioned as 'Ḥakīm' also Zakī and ʿAbd al-Wāḥid ha-Kohen. He is also mentioned in Arabic documents of the Cairo Geniza: a *waqf* bill (1519–20) written by ʿAbd al-Wāḥid al-Mutaṭabbib who is called 'Ibn al-Sīqānīyya'.[7]

ʿAbd al-Karīm b. ʿAbd al-Laṭīf [K., EY, Jerusalem, 16th century]
A Karaite physician, practised medicine in Jerusalem (1550–61).[8]

ʿAbd al-Karīm b. Mūsā [K, EY, Jerusalem, 16th century]
A Karaite physician, practised medicine in Jerusalem (1532–52) and reached the level of 'Head of the Physicians'. Additionally, he was one of the leaders of the Karaite community and in charge of the Jewish *waqf* in Jerusalem. In 1547, when the 'Head of the Physicians' in the hospital in Jerusalem went to Constantinople for several months, ʿAbd al-Karīm took his place.[9]

ʿAbd al-Laṭīf b. Ibrāhīm b. Shams al-Baghdādī [Eg., Cairo, 15th century]
A physician, apparently the leader of the Jewish community in Cairo in the mid-fifteenth century. In a legal document that was preserved by the Karaite community in Cairo, he is mentioned as one of the non-Muslim community leaders, who, in 1442, were summoned to appear in front of the Mamluk sultan Jaqmaq, regarding a violation of an order forbidding the construction of new ritual buildings and the renovation of old ones. It is possible that ʿAbd al-Laṭīf was the Head of the Jews (*Raʾīs al-Yahūd*)[10] and that while he served in this position, he was, similarly to the Christian patriarch, to testify before the sultan. It is also told that in the struggle for leadership of the Jewish community, Rabbinical Jews turned to the government and accused him of denying Islam.[11] Being a physician makes it more reasonable that he was the Head of the Jews. This position was usually assigned to Jewish physicians who, thanks to their valued service in the court of the Muslim rulers and other senior officials, became the most suitable representatives for the Jewish minority.[12] Eliyahu Ashtor asserted that in a governmental document, the description '*Raʾīs Ṭāʾifa al-Yahūd*' ('Head of the Jewish Sect') was added to his name, and therefore he was a *nagid*.[13] In another source, al-Laṭīf, the physician from Mesopotamia, is described as a great scholar who lived for long periods in Syria and Egypt and came into contact with the Ben Maimon family. He described his impressions of the architecture of the city of Cairo and expressed great knowledge of the wonders of nature, and wrote about how in Cairo he had the opportunity to review and explore skeletons and mummies and how he was happy to share his discoveries in his reports.[14]

ʿAbd al-Sayyid b. Isḥāq b. Yaḥyā al-Ḥakīm al-Faḍl Bahāʾ al-Dīn b. al-Muhadhdhab, al-Ṭabīb al-Kaḥḥāl [Sy., Damascus, 13th–14th centuries, convert]

ʿAbd al-Wāḥid (Ibn al-Sīqānīyya) b. ʿAfīf b. ʿAbd Allāh al-Yahūdī al-Rabānī al-Mutaṭabbib ha-Kohen al-Ḥakīm [Eg., Cairo, 16th century]
A physician, one of the representatives of the Mustaʿarabi Jews who stood in front of the Radbaz (Rabbi David b. Zimra, 1479–1573/1589), for a discussion following a dispute that broke out in 1527 between them and the Maghribis in Cairo. Beside him are mentioned as 'Ḥakīm' also Zakī and ʿAbd al-ʿAzīz ha-Ḥazzān. He is also mentioned in Arabic documents of the Cairo Geniza, such as a *waqf* bill (1519–20) written by ʿAbd al-Wāḥid al-Mutaṭabbib who is called 'Ibn al-Sīqānīyya'.[15]

Abraham b. al-F[...] [Eg., 12th–13th centuries]
A physician, possibly died in 1239. It is possible that he is the *wazīr* Abū Isḥāq.[16]

Abraham b. Hananiah ha-Rōfē [Eg., 11th–12th centuries]

Abraham b. Hillel ha-Ḥasid [Eg., Cairo, 12th–13th centuries]
A scholar, physician and a poet from Fusṭāṭ (d. 1223). He came from a high-class family; his grandfather was the presiding judge of the Jewish court in Egypt. He owned a large library of medical writings and religious Jewish writings. He was close to the ben Maimon family and Abraham ben Moses ben Maimon cited him in his writings.[17]

Abraham b. Isaac ha-Kohen b. Furāt [Eg., Cairo, EY, Ramle, 11th century]

Abraham b. Maimon (Maimonides) [Eg., Cairo, 12th–13th centuries]

Abraham b. Meʾir Ibn Qamniʾel [An., Ma., 12th century]

Abraham b. Moses ha-Rōfē [Eg., 11th century]
A physician, mentioned in a bill (1056) alongside Yeshūʿā ha-Rōfē b. Aaron al-ʿAmmānī.[18]

Abraham b. Saʿadya [K., Eg., 15th century]

Abraham b. Saʿadya ha-Rōfē Darʿī [K., Eg., Alexandria, 11th century]

Abraham b. Yijū [Ma., In., Eg., 12th century]
A man of many talents with medical knowledge;[19] born in al-Mahdiyya in Tunisia, travelled to India where he was active (1132–49)[20] and finally settled in Egypt in 1153. He was a Jewish scholar, wrote Halakhic responsa[21] and was also a merchant and a poet. Abraham had some medical education since two prescriptions were found in his handwriting. He served as the 'head of the community' in Dhū Jibla. His daughter Sitt al-Dār married Peraḥya b. Joseph.[22] Abraham's descendants were associates and supporters of the family of Maimonides.[23]

Abraham ha-Kohen b. Isaac [Eg., Cairo, 11th century]
Possibly Abraham ha-Kohen ha-Rōfē b. Isaac ha-Kohen. An important physician from Fusṭāṭ. The addressee of a letter written by Zakkay Nāsī b. Yedīdyāhū Nāsī.[24]

Abraham ha-Levi [K., EY, Jerusalem, 14th century]
A Karaite physician, lived in the fourteenth century, possibly in Jerusalem.[25]

Abraham ha-Levi ha-Rōfē [K., Eg., 13th century]
A Karaite physician and possibly Karaite *nāsī* (leader). His son Samuel dedicated a book to him in 1245.[26]

Abraham ha-Rōfē [Eg., 11th century]

Abraham ha-Rōfē b. ʿAlī [Eg., 11th century]
A physician, mentioned in a Geniza document.[27]

Abraham ha-Rōfē b. Isaac al-Ghazūlī [Eg., 13th century]
A physician, mentioned in a Geniza document.[28]

R. Abraham ha-Rōfē b. Jacob [Eg., 14th century]

Abraham ha-Rōfē b. Simḥā ha-Kohen [Eg., 13th century]
A physician; operated as the Kohanim deputy who was in charge of the Torah scrolls and Halakhic literature. His father is Simḥā ha-Kohen.[29]

Abraham Sakandarī [Eg., Cairo, 16th century]

Abraham ha-Sar ha-Rōfē [Eg., 12th century]
A physician, mentioned in the Blessing of the Dead. The document was written by Samuel b. Saʿadya ha-Levi (1163–1205).[30]

Abraham the Karaite [K., Eg., 12th century]
A Karaite physician. His son Yaḥyā married the widow Raʾīsa in Fusṭāṭ in 1117.[31]

Abū ʿAlī Ḥasan al-Mutaṭabbib al-Barqī [Eg., Cairo, 11th century]
A physician; mentioned in a letter sent from Alexandria by Yeshūʿā b. Ismaʿīl to Naharay b. Nissīm Abū al-Faraj at Fusṭāṭ (1062). The author sent him greetings.[32]

Abū ʿAlī al-Ṭabīb [Eg., 12th century]
A physician, mentioned in a letter, possibly from the twelfth century.[33]

Abū ʿAmr al-Ṭabīb [Eg., 12th century]
A physician, mentioned in a document from the beginning of the twelfth century.[34]

Abū Asʿad al-Mutaṭabbib ha-Zāqēn [Eg., 13th century]
A physician, mentioned in a document dated 1217.[35]

Abū al-ʿAshāʾir Hibat-Allāh b. Zayn b. Ḥasan b. Ifrāʾīm b. Yaʿqūb b. Ismāʿīl Ibn Jumayʿ al-ʾIsrāʾīlī (Nethanel b. Samuel) [Eg., Cairo, 12th century]

Abū Ayyūb al-Yahūdī (al-ʾIsrāʾīlī) (Solomon b. al-Muʿallim) [An., Seville, Ma., Marrakesh, 12th century]
A physician, native of Seville, that lived and practised medicine at the time of the Moors in Spain between 1105 and 1171.[36] He was mentioned by Maimonides, in his *Treatise on Asthma*, as one of the four physicians that served in the court of the Almoravid emir ʿAlī b. Yūsuf b. Tāshufīn (1106–1142) in Marrakesh, and mistakenly killed him due to the wrong dosage of theriac. One of the four physicians was another Sevillian Jewish practitioner, Abū al-Ḥasan Meʾir Ibn Qamniʾel. The two other physicians were the Saragossan Abū ʿAlī ʿAlāʾ b. Zuhr and one Sufyān.[37] Solomon served in the court of ʿAlī b. Yūsuf b. Tāshufīn with another Jewish physician, Abraham

b. Meʾir Ibn Qamniʾel, and they were jointly in charge of collecting the *jizya* tax from the Jewish community.[38] Solomon was also a Jewish scholar and a poet;[39] he carried the titles of *wazīr* and prince and was praised by Jewish dignitaries such as Moses b. Ezra, Judah ha-Levi and Judah al-Ḥarīzī (d. 1225) (in the third chapter of the *Taḥkemoni*).[40]

Abū al-Barakāt Hibat Allāh [Ir., 12th century, convert]

A physician and philosopher, who converted to Islam at the end of his life. David Wasserstein claimed that Isaac the son of Abraham b. Ezra and Abū Naṣr Samawʾal b. Judah b. ʿAbbās al-Maghribī were part of a circle of intellectuals with shared interests and paths to Islam. As all three were acquainted, there have been suggestions that Abū al-Barakāt may have acted to influence the other two to convert.[41]

Abū al-Barakāt Hibat Allāh b. ʿAlī b. Malkā (or Malkān) al-Baladī al-Ṭabīb al-Faḍl (Nethanel Baruch b. Melekh) [Iq., Baghdad, 12th century, convert]

A physician (1087–1165) known as ʻAwḥad al-Zamānʼ (one of a generation), appeared in Ibn Abī Uṣaybiʿa as native of al-Balad, a city on the Tigris near Mosul. He was a resident of Baghdad and served as a military physician and later as a court physician of the caliph al-Mustanjid biʾllāh. He was loved and respected by him. Afterwards, he was blamed by the sultan Muḥammad b. Malik-Shāh[42] for medical neglect and was arrested by him for a while.[43]

Abū al-Barakāt was knowledgeable in the sciences and was blessed with excellent thinking ability. He learnt medicine under Abū al-Ḥasan Saʿīd b. Hibat Allāh, who usually abstained from teaching Christians and Jews. He persuaded Abū ʼl-Ḥasan, via messengers, to permit him to listen to his lessons from the hall, and by that means he learnt medicine. After a year, a scholarly discussion took place between students concerning a question raised by Abū ʼl-Ḥasan. The students were unable to solve the problem, whereupon Abū al-Barakāt entered the room from the hall and asked Abū ʼl-Ḥasan for his permission to answer the question. Abū al-Barakāt's answer, which was based on Galen, was liked by Abū ʼl-Ḥasan, following which he included him among his permanent students. Abū al-Barakāt was more knowledgeable than all of his predecessors and delved into their writings.[44]

Abū al-Barakāt's own writings include *Kitāb al-Muʿtabar* (which covers logic, natural sciences and religion; it was considered one of the best of its time on these topics); a summary of *Kitāb al-Tashrīḥ*;[45] a summary of Galen; *Kitāb al-Aqrābādhin*; an article concerning a medicine he concocted named *Ṣifat Barsha'thā'* (an Indian medicine); and *Risāla fī al-'Aql wa-Māhiyatihi* ('The Brain and Its Essence').

Al-Ẓahīr al-Bayhaqī, a physician, mathematician and astronomer in Iraq (d. 1170), called Abū al-Barakāt 'the philosopher of the Iraqis' and compared him to Aristotle.[46] In al-Ṣafadī's and al-Ghuzūlī's books, there is a description of a treatment that Abū al-Barakāt gave to a melancholic person who imagined having a ceramic pot permanently seated on his head. He 'cured' him from his delusions using a quasi-psychological method.[47] Ibn al-Qifṭī wrote that when one of the Seljuk sultans was ill, he summoned Abū al-Barakāt from Baghdad and he treated him until he became healthy. In return, the sultan gave him many gifts, money, expensive clothing, chariots and other valuables.[48]

Despite his status and medicinal prestige, a poem was written about Abū al-Barakāt which said, among other things, that a dog had a higher status than he did. Following this, it became clear to him that if he wanted a good life, he would have to convert to Islam. He had daughters that did not convert with him, although they knew they wouldn't inherit from him when he died. Only after he ensured through the caliph that they would be financially secure did he agree to convert to Islam. The story of Abū al-Barakāt's conversion was told by al-Ṣafadī, and al-'Umarī described an event in which Abū al-Barakāt arrived at the caliph's. All of those present stood in his honour, except for the *qadi*, who refused to get up in honour of a *dhimmī*. Abū al-Barakāt turned to the caliph and said to him that if the reason for the *qadi*'s refusal to stand up was because of him being of another faith, then he was willing to convert to Islam, and that is what happened. After his conversion, Abū al-Barakāt avoided and disapproved of Jews, and even cursed them and his Jewish origin. For example, in a sitting with Amīn al-Dawla b. al-Tilmīdh (a physician, author and poet, the head physician of numerous Abbasid caliphs and a hospital manager who died in 1168),[49] Abū al-Barakāt cursed the Jews and Amīn al-Dawla also cursed their sons. Ibn Abī Uṣaybi'a noted that the two were rivals.[50] After his conversion his status rose, he began teaching medicine and treatment and 'many learnt from him'. Many of the physicians at this time would consult him on medicinal issues; he would answer them in writing and the physicians would circulate his answers.

Abū al-Barakāt lived well into old age. Towards the end of his life he suffered from illnesses and bodily defects which he was unable to overcome. He became blind, his hearing was damaged, and eczema spread in his body. According to Ibn Khallikān,[51] Abū al-Barakāt had leprosy and cured himself by laying snakes on his body but he became blind from the leprosy,[52] while Moritz Steinschneider had it that he became blind and deaf from an elephantiasis (lymphatic filariasis) treatment.[53] When he felt himself getting close to his death he dictated the sentence to be written on his gravestone: 'This is the burial place of Awḥad al-Zamān, the author of *Kitāb al-Muʿtabar*'. Those who have seen his grave confirm that that was indeed written there.[54] He died at the city of Hamadān, from where his coffin was carried to Baghdad.[55]

Abū al-Barakāt al-Quḍāʿī al-Muwaffaq [Eg., Cairo, 12th century]
A physician, served ʿUthmān, the son of Saladin. Ibn Abī Uṣaybiʿa mentioned that he also practised ophthalmology and was considered one of the best in this field. He died in Cairo in 1193.[56]

Abū al-Barakāt al-Ṭabīb b. al-Sharābī [Eg., Cairo, 12th century]

Abū al-Barakāt Ibn Shaʿyā al-Muwaffaq [K., Eg., 12th–13th centuries]

Abū al-Bayān Mūsā b. Abī al-Faḍl (Moses b. Mevōrākh b. Saʿadya) [Eg., Cairo, 11th–12th centuries]

Abū al-Bayān b. al-Mudawwar al-Sadīd [K., Eg., 12th century]

Abū al-Bishr b. Aaron ha-Levi al-Kirmānī al-Ḥakīm [K., Eg., Cairo, 14th century]

Abū al-Faḍāʾil (Jekuthiel b. Moses) [Eg., Cairo, 12th century]

Abū al-Faḍāʾil (Jekuthiel II b. Moses II ha- Rōfē) [Eg., 12th century]

Abū al-Faḍl (Ḥasday b. Joseph b. Ḥasday) [An., Saragossa, 11th century, convert]

Abū al-Faḍl Dāʾūd b. Sulaymān b. Abū al-Bayān al-ʾIsrāʾīlī al-Sadīd (David b. Solomon) [K., Eg., Cairo, 12th–13th centuries]

Abū al-Faḍl al-Sharīṭī al-Ḥalabī ha-Rōfē (Benjamin al-Sharīṭī ha-Rōfē) [Sy., Aleppo, 12th century]

A physician, mentioned in a comment in ʿAzrā Ḥaddād's book, in which he noted several famous physicians who lived in Aleppo while Benjamin of Tudela passed there. Also mentioned in the same comment is the poet Judah b. Ayyūb b. ʿAbbās al-Fāsī al-Maghribī (Judah b. Abūn) (d. 1183).[57] Ibn al-Qifṭī tells of a Jewish physician from Aleppo called Abū al-Faḍl ben Yāmīn who was known as 'al-Sharīṭī'. Ibn al-Qifṭī, who did not know Hebrew, probably divided up the name Benjamin into to 'ben' and 'Yāmīn'. Ibn al-Qifṭī wrote that Benjamin learnt from Sharaf al-Ṭūsī[58] the foundations of medicine as well as other domains that he mastered such as geometry, determining the calendar according to the stars, and the prediction of the future. Ibn al-Qifṭī also noted that Benjamin mainly treated 'ordinary' people (meaning the middle class – the translator). Benjamin died in 1207 from melancholy. He did not leave descendants.[59]

Abū al-Faḍl al-Ṭabīb [Eg., 11th–12th centuries]

A physician, appeared in a list of donors alongside Abū al-Munā al-Sharābī and Abū Saʿīd al-ʿAṭṭār.[60]

Abū al-Faḍl al-Ṭabīb 2 [Eg., 11th–12th centuries]

A physician, appeared in a list of donors headed by the *nagid* Mevōrākh b. Saʿadya (d. 1111) alongside Abū al-Munā al-ʿAṭṭār, Ibrāhīm ha-Rōfē, Abū Naṣr al-ʿAṭṭār 2, Salāma al-ʿAṭṭār, (anonymous) ʿAṭṭār and Abū al-Surūr al-Sharābī.[61]

Abū al-Faḍl (Abū al-Faḍāʾil) b. al-Nāqid b. Obadia, al-Ṭabīb al-Muhad-hdhab (Mevōrākh ha-Kohen) [Eg., Cairo, 12th century]

Abū al-Faḍl b. al-Ṣarīḥ [Eg., 12th–13th centuries][62]

A physician, lived in Damascus; al-Ḥarīzī praised his qualities as a physician and as a person.[63]

Abū al-Faḍl Mubārak (Mevōrākh b. Saʿadya) [Eg., Cairo, Alexandria, 11th-12th centuries]

Abū al-Faḍāʾil al-Ṭabīb [Eg., 12th century]

A physician, appeared in a list of donors (1180) alongside Abū al-Ḥasan

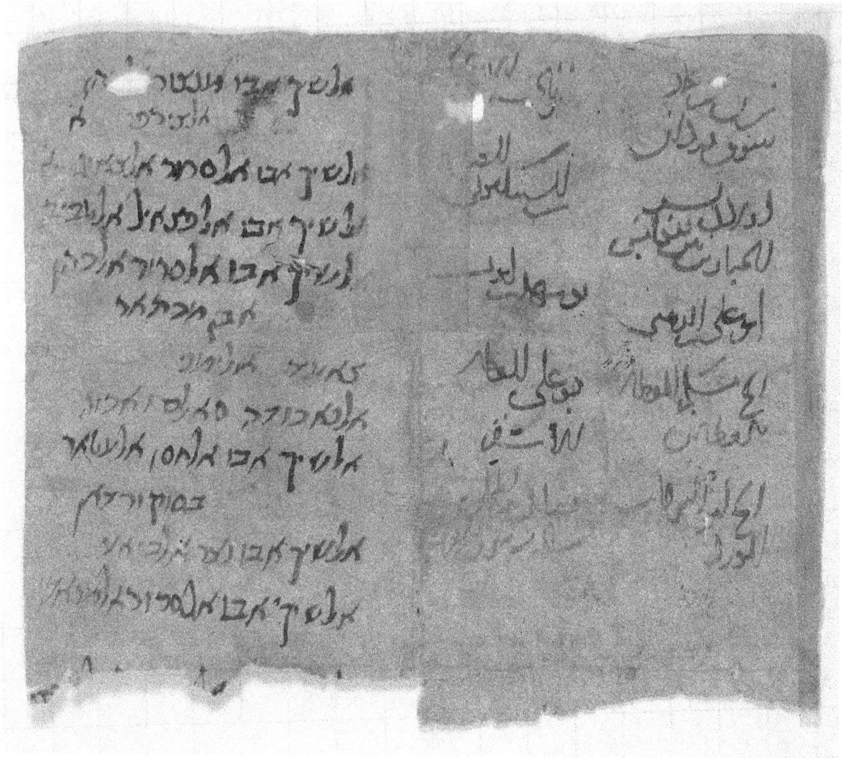

Figure 1 List of donors, Hebrew and Arabic (1180), including the names of a few pharmacists and physicians, among them Abū al-Ḥasan al-ʿAṭṭār, Abū al-Faḍāʾil al-Ṭabīb and al-Sheikh Abū al-Faḍāʾil al-Ṭabīb (ENA 2591.8). Image provided by the Library of the Jewish Theological Seminary, USA.

al-ʿAṭṭār 2 and al-Sheikh (A)bū al-Faḍāʾil al-Ṭabīb. It is possible that the document was written by the judge Samuel b. Saʿadya ha-Levi (see Figure 1).[64]

Abū al-Fakhr (Yeshūʿā ha-Rōfē) [Eg., 12th century]

A physician, mentioned in a memorial list.[65]

Abū al-Fakhr al-ʿAṭṭār b. al-Amshāṭī (Saʿadya b. Abraham) [Eg., 12th century][66]

A physician (and probably a pharmacist as well), active at the time of the Fatimid caliph al-ʿĀḍid li-Dīn Allāh (r. 1160–71). In the writings of Muslim Arabic historians, he was known as a specialist in healing snake bites. It was not mentioned that he was a Jew, but he did become famous for treating anyone, regardless of their religion.[67] Abū al-Fakhr is mentioned in a letter from July 1156, which was sent by Samuel ha-Melammēd b. Joseph ha-Melammēd b. Yijū from Sicily to his brother in Egypt.[68] He was the head of the al-Amshāṭī family in Egypt, a distinguished family that was in marriage contacts with Moses Maimonides.[69]

Abū al-Fakhr al-Ṭabīb [Eg., 12th century][70]

His name appears in *Warrāq's Notebook*, the diary of a book merchant.[71] The notebook includes medical prescriptions, commercial bills and records of book loans. Abū al-Fakhr's name is mentioned in the context of book purchases and it is written that he lent ten books, among them four copies of a book called *The Craft of Healing*, two parts of *The Power of Medicines* and *The Spiritual Medicine*. He also had in his possession two booklets, one an abridgment of *The Physician Is a Philosopher* and the other an abridgment of *The Craft of Healing*, as well as another booklet entitled 'Being and Loss'. Some of the books' prices are noted.[72] The list of books he purchased is dated c.1157.[73]

Abū al-Fakhr b. Abī al-Faḍl b. Abī Naṣr b. Abī al-Fakhr al-Yahūdī (Aaron ha-Levi Ibn al-Kirmānī, al-Kaḥḥāl) [K., Eg., Cairo, 13th–14th centuries]

Abū al-Faraj al-Ṭabīb [Eg., 12th century]

A physician (a. 1140–59), his wife turned to the *nagid* Samuel b. Hananiah asking him to assist her to redeem half of her mortgaged house, so she could remarry a man of her own status.[74]

Abū al-Faraj al-Uṣṭūl [Eg., 12th century]

A physician, mentioned in a legal document written and signed by Nathan ha-Kohen. In the document he permitted Abū al-Ḥasan b. Muʿammar b. al-Baṭṭ to repay him a debt in the sum of 22 dinars 70 dirhams, a quarter of a dinar a month, beginning in December 1129. The document also noted his arrival at Damietta.[75]

Abū al-Faraj b. Abū al-Barakāt [Eg., Cairo, 12th–13th centuries]

Abū al-Faraj b. Abū al-Faḍāʾil b. al-Nāqid [Eg., Cairo, 12th century, convert]

Abū al-Faraj b. al-Raʾīs (Elijah b. Zechariah) [Eg., Alexandria, Cairo, EY, Jerusalem, 12th–13th centuries]

Abū al-Futūḥ al-Ṭabīb [Eg., 13th century]

A physician, whose son's name appeared in a list of donors (c.1220), alongside Abū Manṣūr b. Abū al-Futūḥ al-Ṭabīb.[76]

Abū al-Ḥajjāj Yūsuf b. Yaḥyā b. Isḥāq al-Sabatī al-Maghribī (Ibn Samʿūn) (Joseph b. Judah b. Simon) [Ma., Eg., Sy., Ir., Iq., 12th–13th centuries]

A physician and a merchant, born in Ceuta, Morocco, studied medicine and mathematics in which he excelled. In 1182–4, Yūsuf moved to Egypt after the caliph ʿAbd al-Muʾmin (1094–1163) forced the Jews and Christians to choose between exile and conversion to Islam. At first, he resided in Alexandria, where he wrote letters and *maqāmāt* to Maimonides, and later moved to Fusṭāṭ, where he met Maimonides and heard him give lectures in astronomy, mathematics and philosophy. Together with Maimonides, he worked on exegesis of the Holy Scriptures and astronomy. A few years later (c.1185, and earlier than 1190), he left Egypt for Aleppo, where he started practising medicine and served Saladin. Either in Aleppo, or afterwards when he travelled to Iraq, he started to work as a merchant, an occupation that brought him to India. During his journeys as a merchant, he arrived at Baghdad where he had a dispute with Samuel b. ʿEli, the head of the yeshiva there, and Maimonides' opponents. Yūsuf defended Maimonides on additional occasions as well and the latter dedicated *The Guide for the Perplexed* to him. During his travels, he acquired a lot of medical knowledge. In his later years, he returned to Aleppo and while working as a merchant he also practised medicine, teaching the profession and serving as a private physician to the Ẓāhirī rulers, among them al-Malik al-Ẓāhir al-Ghāzī,[77] the second son of Saladin. Some believe that before he fled to Egypt, or maybe even later, in Aleppo, Yūsuf had converted to Islam, but it is uncertain. Yūsuf died in Aleppo in 1226.[78] Yūsuf was on friendly terms with Ibn al-Qifṭī, who dedicated to him a chapter in his book *Taʾrīkh al-Ḥukamāʾ* ('History of Physicians'). Ibn al-Qifṭī noted that Yūsuf was clever and highly perceptive, and described his arrival in Egypt and his meeting with Maimonides. He wrote that after the death of Yūsuf's first wife, with whom he had two girls, he got married again and had two boys (another boy died) and a girl.

Additionally, Ibn al-Qifṭī described how he and Yūsuf confided in personal matters as well; the personal problems concerned Yūsuf's inheritance, which he was worried would be taken by the government and wouldn't get to his daughters, and also his hopes for a son. Yūsuf and Ibn al-Qifṭī had a pact in which it was stated that the first one to die would return to tell the other one what occurs after death. Ibn al-Qifṭī reported that Yūsuf visited him in a dream, two years after his death, and they discussed the evolution of the body and soul.[79] Al-Ḥarīzī, who met Yūsuf in Aleppo, wrote about him in several of his poems, and he is a prominent figure in the Aleppo chapter in his book about his journeys. In one of his poems, al-Ḥarīzī described Yūsuf's criticism towards Elazar the king's physician, for desecrating Shabbat in order to take care of the king.[80] It is possible that Joseph b. Simon is 'Joseph ha-Nāsī' from Aleppo, who translated several medical writings and composed at least one medical treatise (in Arabic) which was not published, a commentary on Hippocrates' *Aphorisms*, and a philosophical essay of which only a translated Hebrew version remains, filled with mistakes.[81] There is a great confusion among scholars[82] between Joseph b. Simon and Ibn ʿAknīn (Joseph b. Judah b. Jacob). Many refer to the former's works as belonging to the latter, and vice versa.[83]

Abū al-Ḥasan [Eg., 12th–13th centuries]

Abū al-Ḥasan (Judah b. Samuel ha-Levi) [An., Toledo, Granada, Eg., Cairo, 12th century]

A poet, religious thinker and physician (d. 1141). Born in Toledo between 1070 and 1080, he travelled as a youth to Granada, where he joined the circle of Jewish public figures and intellectuals around Moses b. Ezra. He practised as a physician in Castile and Andalusia, and for most of his life he was a sought-after physician and a prominent, well-connected and well-adjusted member of the Andalusian Jewish aristocracy.[84] According to Oded Zinger, writing about Goitein's legacy, he was a merchant-physician-scholar-poet.[85] Judah's leadership, diligence and religious devotion were praised by a young friend of his in a document sent from Granada in 1130 and found in the Cairo Geniza.[86] Judah's writings showed his wide knowledge of Hebrew grammar, literary tradition, the Bible, Rabbinic traditions, Muslim Arabic literature, Sufism, philosophy and medicine. He was also active in Jewish communal affairs, donating to, and raising funds for, communal causes; moreover, he was employing his literary skills on behalf of the head of the Rabbinic academy in Lucena (Joseph b. Migash). In the summer of 1140, he left Spain and sailed for Egypt with the intention of dying in Eretz-Israel. Shortly before leaving, he completed his treatise *Kitāb al-Radd wa 'l-Dalīl fī 'l-Dīn al-Dhalīl* ('The Book of Rejoinder and Proof in Support of the Neglected Religion'), commonly known as the *Kuzari*. This book was translated into Hebrew in Provence by Judah b. Tibbon in 1167 and in this form has had great influence ever since. Judah arrived in Alexandria on 9 September 1140, and he spent over three months there as the guest of, or in company with, a prominent leader of the local Jewish community, Aaron Ibn al-ʿAmmānī. Later, in Fusṭāṭ, he was hosted by a wealthy businessman, Ḥalfon Abū Saʿīd b. Nethanel ha-Levi. There, Judah met such dignitaries as Samuel b. Hananiah, the *nagid*, Samuel's secretary and Nathan b. Samuel. Returning to Alexandria in the spring, Judah was denounced and sued by an apostate for attempting to compel his return to Judaism by withholding funds belonging to him. Judah was acquitted thanks to his connections and to a legal subterfuge.[87]

Abū al-Ḥasan ʿAmmār ha-Rōfē [EY, Jerusalem, 11th century]
A physician, mentioned in a letter in which Salāma b. Joseph al-Hārūnī turned to Abū al-Faraj Shmaya for help. In the letter he mentioned that he had also turned to Abū al-Ḥasan ʿAmmār ha-Rōfē (and to Abū al-Faraj Hārūn, who might also have been a physician).[88]

Abū al-Ḥasan b. Abū al-Sahl b. Abraham [Eg., Cairo, 13th century]
A physician,[89] mentioned in a document in which Abū Sahl b. Ibrāhīm gives his son a house as a gift.[90] Abū al-Ḥasan was asked (according to Marina Rustow, probably by a prospective high-ranking patient) for a certificate attesting to his professional qualifications and good conduct. Three separate drafts of the testimony have survived. Rustow claimed that Abū al-Ḥasan's attempt to procure the certificate suggests that he was adept at negotiating the channels of the Islamic judiciary, and the fact that the drafts survived in the Geniza suggests even more.[91]

Abū al-Ḥasan b. al-Muwaffaq b. al-Najm b. al-Muhadhdhab Abī al-Ḥasan b. Samuel (al-Sheikh al-Muhadhdhab) [Eg., Cairo, 13th century]
A physician and *nagid* of the Jews, apparently closely associated with the sultan and his physicians. Al-Maqrīzī mentioned that on 13 June 1285 he was appointed as a *nagid*. He received a letter of appointment as a *nagid* of all the Jews – Rabbanites, Karaites and Samaritans – who dwelt in Cairo, Fusṭāṭ and all the districts of Egypt. Versions of the appointment are mentioned by several of the Muslim authors of that time, wherein this Jewish *nagid* is called al-Sheikh al-Jalīl al-Ra'īs al-Kāfī al-Muqarrab al-Ḥākim al-Muhadhdhab Tāj al-Ḥukamā' Thiqāt al-Mulūk wa al-Salāṭīn (the old, accomplished, capable, closed to ministers, scholarly physician, crown of doctors, man in the confidence of kings and sultans). Hence the new *nagid*, who took over the position of Maimonides' grandson, David, was a physician and apparently was one of the sultan's advisers and maybe even one of the his physicians. If so, this *nagid* interrupted, for some time, the continuity of Maimonidean leadership. Ashtor found an echo to this dismissal in a Hebrew source and concluded that some informers in Egypt had told the authorities about the *nagid* David b. Abraham b. Moses b. Maimon and so he was removed from his position. David was made to leave Egypt and moved together with his family to the Crusaders' port of Acre. While he was there, he visited the cave of Hillel and Shammai at Meron in Galilee and there he banned the informers.[92]

Abū al-Ḥasan ha-Rōfē [Eg., Cairo, 11th century]
A physician, mentioned in a letter sent by Moses b. Jekuthiel to his acquaintances in Fusṭāṭ c.1040.[93]

Abū al-Ḥasan b. Sa'īd al-Ṣārīfī Ibn al-Maṣmūdī [Eg., Cairo, 12th–13th centuries]
A physician, addressee of a letter naming him as *ṭabīb al-Murabba'a ila al-Maṣṣaṣa*; according to Goitein, sent to the 'neighbourhood adjoining what the literary sources call district, *khuṭṭ*, of the perfumers'.[94]

Abū al-Ḥasan al-Ṭabīb [Eg., 11th century]
Mentioned in a document written in David b. Yefet's hand, dated c.1040.[95]

Abū al-Ḥasan al-Ṭabīb 2 [Eg., 12th century]
A physician, mentioned in a document from the twelfth century.[96]

Abū al-Ḥasan Yūsuf b. Josiah al-Tunisī (Joseph b. Isaiah) [Eg., ?11th–12th centuries]

A physician, mentioned in a document in which he undertook to pay a debt to a silk merchant.[97]

Abū Ibrāhīm b. Muwaril [An., 12th century][98]

A physician, mentioned as the one who told Joseph b. ʿAqnīn of the effort of Meʾir (Abū al-Ḥasan) Ibn Qamniʾel to convince the Almoravid ruler that the Biblical Song of Songs was holy, against another Jewish physician that claimed that it was a secular book of love songs.[99]

Abū Ibrāhīm b. Qasṭār (Isaac b. Yashush) [An., Toledo, 10th–11th centuries]

A physician, born in Spain (probably Toledo) in 982, and died there c.1056. He was identified by Steinschneider with the physician Isḥāq b. Qasṭār.[100] According to Ibn Abī Uṣaybiʿa, Ibn Qasṭār was praised as a person of acute intelligence and genteel manners, well versed in grammar, philosophy, the Hebrew Bible and Jewish law, and in addition a confirmed bachelor. He was the physician in ordinary of Muwaffaq Mujāhid al-ʿĀmirī and of his son Iqbāl al-Dawla, kings of the *taifa* of Dénia, a maritime power on the eastern coast of al-Andalus.[101] He was well trained in logic, and was conversant with the opinions of the philosophers. Moses b. Ezra called him and Abū al-Walīd (Ibn Janāḥ) the two sheikhs of Hebrew grammar.[102] His reputation went far beyond his medical role and reflects the literary and scholarly activities that bolstered Dénia's place in the *taifa* court. He was recognised as one of the premier Hebrew grammarians of the Middle Ages. His work circulated throughout al-Andalus in dialogue with many of the notable Jewish scholars of his age.[103] The *Kitāb al-Taṣārif* ('Book of Conjugations'), a grammatical opus known in Hebrew as *Sefer ha-Ṣerufim*, is Ibn Qasṭār's most famous work.[104] Abraham b. Ezra, who praised Ibn Qasṭār's philological work, wrote that the exegetical book he wrote should be burnt.[105]

Abū ʿImrān al-Ṭabīb (Ben Sumsuma) [Eg., 12th century]

A physician, mentioned in the Blessing of the Dead from 1201. His son's name is Abū al-Mufaḍḍal.[106]

Abū ʿImrān b. al-Lawī al-Ishbīlī (Moses b. Joseph ha-Levi) [An., Seville, 13th century]

A physician and a Jewish philosopher (probably of the Abulafia family), served the last Moorish king of Seville (d. 1255).[107] His work has survived mainly thanks to extensive quotations by the famous fourteenth-century philosopher Joseph b. Abraham b. Waqār, who admired him, in his book *Treatise on the Harmony between Philosophy and the Revealed Law* (c.1340). His most important work was a metaphysical treatise entitled *Maʾamar Elohi* ('Divine Treatise' or 'Metaphysical Treatise') and two minor works, one of them, entitled *ʿA lā Ṭarīq al Fuṣūl*, containing a metaphysical dissertation composed as a series of aphorisms.[108] Moses also wrote (assuming that Steinschneider's identification is correct) a work on musical harmonies, a short section of which is quoted by Shemtov Shaprūt b. Isaac of Tudela in his Hebrew commentary on Ibn Sīnā's Qānūn. Moses described the mathematical relations of musical intervals as well as some arithmetical operations carried out with them.[109]

Abū Isḥāq (Abraham b. Meʾir b. Muhājir) [An., Seville, 11th–12th centuries]

An expert physician, son of a well-established Jewish family of Seville.[110] He was also an astronomer, and an important clerk at the court of King al-Muʿtamid (the last ʿAbbāsid ruler of the *taifa* of Seville). He was mentioned in the *dīwān* (collection of poems) of Moses b. Ezra, with the title *wazīr*. According to some scholars Ohev b. Muhājir, mentioned by Abraham b. Daʿud as a poet, and Joseph Ben Meʾir b. Muhājir were probably his brothers. Like Meʾir, their father, Ohev and Joseph both had the title of *Nāsī*. Another relative of the same family was Abū Sulaymān David, a well-known poet. The whole family was apparently known by the unexplained name of Ibn Shortmeqash.[111] Abraham was praised in his time as highly cultivated and as a defender of the Jewish people. Moses b. Ezra and Judah ha-Levi were both very close to him. Ibn Ezra wrote of his aid to the Jews in times of crisis, especially, his redemption of captives; he also dedicated his *Sefer ha-ʿAnaq*, also known as the *Tarshish*, to Abraham, and sent it to him with a panegyric.[112]

Abū Isḥāq al-Ḥasid al-Ṭabīb [Eg., 13th century]

A physician, appeared in a list of donors (c.1210) which includes several physicians and practitioners.[113]

Abū Isḥāq Ibrāhīm b.ʿAṭā (Abraham b. Nathan) [Ma., Qayrawān, al-Mahdiyya, 9th–10th centuries]

A physician and *nagid* of Qayrawān. In 1015 he received the title of 'Nagid ha-Gola' from Hai Gaon,[114] of the Pumbedita Academy, probably in recognition of diverting to him half of the sum of a fund raised for the Babylonian academies. Abraham donated to the fundraise about thirty dinars, a heavy sum at that time.[115] He was physician to two emirs in al-Mahdiyya, Bādīs (r. 996–1016) and his son al-Muʿizz (r. 1016–62), and joined their war campaigns.[116] In a letter to a big merchant, Joseph b. ʿAwkal, who may have been a physician as well,[117] Abraham thanks him for transferring his father's body for burial in Eretz-Israel. In a letter from 1050 that Berechiah's sons sent to the merchant Joseph b. Jacob b. ʿAwkal, the writers refer to the Babylonian academies during the Geonic reign of Dosa, the son of Saadia Gaon and discussed the rising power of Abū Isḥāq Ibrāhīm b.ʿAṭā.[118]

Abū al-ʿIzz al-Kaḥḥāl [Eg., 12th–13th centuries]

An ophthalmologist, appeared in a list of taxpayers or donors for fundraising, redemption of captives etc. Also in the list are al-Nafīs al-Sharābī, (anonymous) al-Wajīh ('honourable') al-Ṭabīb, (anonymous) al-Sheikh al-Muhadhdhab al-Ṭabīb, Abū al-Faraj b. al-Nashādirī, Makārim al-Kaḥḥāl, Abū al-Thanāʾ and Abū Naṣr al-Sadīd.[119] He also appeared in a list of donors to aid payment of a *jizya* (head tax), alongside Abū ʿImrān Levi ʿAṭṭār, Abū ʿImrān Kohen ʿAṭṭār, Abū al-ʿAlā Levi, Abū al-Fakhr Levi ʿAṭṭār and Makārim al-Kaḥḥāl.[120]

Abū al-ʿIzz al-Ṭabīb[121] [Eg., 13th century]

A physician, the brother of Abū al-Mufaḍḍal al-Muhadhdhab (a physician); both appeared in a list of donors dated c.1210.[122] An inheritance document of Abū al-ʿIzz was also found.[123]

Abū al-ʿIzz Ṭabīb[124] [Eg., 13th century]

A physician, mentioned in a document alongside four other practitioners: Abū ʿImrān ʿAṭṭār, Mufaḍḍ(al) Ṭabīb, Makārim Ṭabīb and Abū al-Ḥasan ʿAṭṭār.[125]

Abū Jaʿfar Joseph b. Aḥmad b. Ḥasday [An., Saragossa, 12th century]

Abū al-Jūd Tobias [Ma., 12th century]

A physician, mentioned as working 'in the service of Kings' that paid him well to preserve their lives. We learn from a document (c.1140), that the ruler Gabès in Tunisia became very ill and sent his *qadi* to Tripoli to bring the Jewish physician called Abū al-Jūd Tobias. He was paid 100 golden pieces before he even left his house, and he was promised to be paid a thousand coins after providing a successful treatment.[126]

Abū al-Khayr al-Muhadhdhab b. al-Jalābnī [Eg., 13th century]

A physician, mentioned in a list of donors and their donations, c.1210, including several physicians and practitioners.[127]

Abū al-Khayr Salāma b. Mubārak b. Raḥmūn b. Mūsā al-Ṭabīb (Salāma b. Raḥmūn) [Eg., Cairo, 11th–12th centuries]

Abū al-Khayr al-Ṭabīb [Eg., Cairo, 12th–13th centuries]

A physician, mentioned in a list of rent payments written by Joseph ha-Levi b. Samuel, who was active c.1180–1220.[128]

Abū al-Maʿālī (Abū al-ʿAlā) Tammām b. Hibat Allāh b. Tammām [Eg., Cairo, Alexandria, 12th century]

A physician, student of Maimonides. He served under two Ayyubid rulers: Saladin (r. 1171–93), alongside Ibn Shūʿa, Abū al-Makārim Hibat-Allāh (Nathanael) Ibn Jumayʿ al-Isrāʾīlī, Ibn al-Mudawwar and Maimonides,[129] and his brother al-Malik al-ʿĀdil (r. 1199–1218). He wrote a number of books on medicine, among them *Taʿlīq Mujarrabāt fī al-Ṭibb* ('Remarks and Experiences in Medicine'). Some of his children converted to Islam.[130] He appeared as an addressee of a request to be accepted as an intern in a hospital at Alexandria.[131] He is also mentioned in a family letter sent by Amram b. Isaac from Alexandria to Ḥalfon ha-Levi b. Nethanel in Fusṭāṭ. The letter, which includes much detail about Bar Isaac's wife's illness and the methods of treating it, is dated to February 1141.[132] In another document we find Abū al-Aʿlā b. Tammām Ṭabīb, which is probably the same person.[133]

Abū al-Maʿānī [Eg., 13th century]

A physician, appeared in a list of future donors dated to the time of Abraham

Maimonides. Other physicians that appeared in the list are (anonymous) al-Mawlī al-Muhadhdhab, (anonymous) Awlād al-Raʾīs, (anonymous) al-Gaon al-Munā, Mufaḍḍal al-Mashmiʿa, al-Sheikh Joseph, another al-Sheikh Joseph and his son, Ibn al-Julājilī, R. Yeshūʿā, Abū al-Maʿānī 2, Najīb Kohen Kamukhī, al-Rabīb Kohen, al-Taqī Ibn al-Gadal and Makārim Ibn al-Gadalī.[134]

Abū al-Maʿānī 2 [Eg., 13th century]
A physician, appeared in a list of future donors dated to the time of Abraham Maimonides. Other physicians that appeared in the list are (anonymous) al-Mawlī al-Muhadhdhab, (anonymous) Awlād al-Raʾīs, (anonymous) al-Gaon al-Munā, Mufaḍḍal al-Mashmiʿa, al-Sheikh Joseph, another al-Sheikh Joseph and his son, Ibn al-Julājilī, R. Yeshūʿā, Najīb Kohen Kamukhī, al-Rabīb Kohen, al-Taqī Ibn al-Gadal, Makārim Ibn al-Gadalī and Abū al-Maʿānī.[135]

Abū al-Maḥāsin al-Sheikh al-Thiqa (Mishaʾel b. Josiah (Isaiah) ha-Levi ha-Rōfē ha-Sar) (b. Daniel, ha-Bāḥūr ha-Ṭōv) [Eg., Cairo, 11th century]

Abū al-Maḥāsin b. al-Kāmukhī b. Abū al-Faḍāʾil [Eg., Cairo, 13th century]
A physician, mentioned in a legal document (c.1241), probably his will, in which he granted a modest sum (10 dinars) to his widow. The document indicates that not all medical practitioners enjoyed high incomes.[136]

Abū Manṣūr b. Abī al-Futūḥ [Eg., 13th century]
A physician,[137] appeared in a list of donors c.1210, which include several physicians and practitioners.[138]

Abū Manṣūr (Isaac) [Eg., Cairo, 12th century]

Abū Manṣūr Muhadhdhab al-Dawla [Ir., Tabriz, ?13th century]
A physician and the governor of Tabriz. He was a relative of the physician Saʿd al-Dawla b. Ṣafī b. Hibat Allāh b. Muhadhdhab al-Dawla al-Abharī.[139]

Abū Manṣūr al-Mutaṭabbib (Elazar b. Yeshūʿā ha-Levi) [Eg., Qūṣ, 13th century]
A physician, mentioned in a document[140] from Qūṣ in Egypt, in the year 1216, concerning a donation he gave to his daughters.[141]

Abū Manṣūr al-Mutaṭabbib (Shemarya b. ʿAlī ha-Rōfē) [Eg., Cairo, 12th century]

Abū Manṣūr al-Ṭabīb [Eg., Cairo, 12th century]

A physician (possibly the same person above), appeared in the list of books and equipment of the Babylonian synagogue in Fusṭāṭ (1181–2) that were transferred from the *shamash* (synagogue clerk) Maḥfūẓ to the *shamash* Abū al-Faraj b. Abū Saʿd.[142]

Abū Manṣūr al-Ṭabīb 2 [Eg., 12th century]

A physician, appeared in a list of books in his possession (c.1157).[143]

Abū Manṣūr, the Karaite [K., Eg., Cairo, 12th century]

A physician, mentioned in a list concerning a debt of 120 dirhams.[144]

Abū Manṣūr Sulaymān b. Ḥaffāẓ (Solomon ha-Kohen) [K., Eg., 13th century]

A Karaite physician.[145] The seventeenth-century historian Ḥājī Khalīfa mentioned briefly that Abū Manṣūr wrote a book in Arabic named *al-Muntakhab fī al-Ṭibb* ('Selected Material on Medicine'), a medical encyclopedia which was written in the style of Ibn Sīnā's *al-Qānūn*. According to Ashtor, Abū Manṣūr died in 1295 or 1296, before he succeeded in finishing his book. The date of his death is quite problematic, since a book by Abū al-Munā b. Abī Naṣr b. Ḥaffāẓ (al-Kohen al-ʿAṭṭār al-ʾIsrāʾīlī), *Minhāj al-Dukkān*, which was written in 1260, quotes Sulaymān's *Muntakhab*.[146]

Abū al-Mufaḍḍal al-Muhadhdhab [Eg., 13th century]

A physician, appeared in a list of donors (c.1210) which includes several physicians and practitioners, including the brother of Abū al-ʿIzz al-Ṭabīb.[147]

Abū al-Muḥāsan (Samuel b. Khalīfa) [Eg., 13th century]

A physician, mentioned in a document (1220) giving a loan to a broker who was active in Fusṭāṭ and Cairo. The loan was to be paid back five years later (1225).[148]

Abū al-Munā al-Ṭabīb [Eg., Cairo, 12th century]

A physician, mentioned in a legal document (1127–38) written by Ḥalfon ha-Levi b. Manasseh. In an agreement between a couple on the verge of divorce it was agreed that the couple would move to the Jewish neighbourhood of Mamṣūṣa in Fusṭāṭ on the same floors on which Abū al-Munā al-Ṭabīb lived.[149] His name also appeared in two additional documents: a long list of names with varying amounts of money[150] and a list of donors and their donations.[151]

Abū al-Munā al-Ṭabīb 2 [Eg., 12th century]
A physician, mentioned in a document (c.1140).[152]

Abū al-Munajjā (Solomon b. Shaʿyā) [Eg., 11th–12th centuries, ?convert]

Abū al-Murajjā [Eg., 13th century]
A physician, appeared in a list of donors alongside Abū Naṣr al-Ṭabīb.[153]

Abū al-Murajjā b. Daniel [Eg., 11th–12th centuries]
A physician, mentioned in a statement of claim from 1129, in which he gave a 24-dinar loan to Sitt al-Ḥusn, daughter of Saʿadya, in return for the deposition of a gold object (a turban, headpiece or tiara). A witness testified that Abū al-Murajjā b. Daniel, who had just died, gave up the loan.[154]

Abū Naṣr Hārūn b. Saʿadya [Eg., Cairo, 11th century]
A physician, appeared in a lawsuit (1021).[155]

Abū Naṣr al-Sadīd [Eg., 12th–13th centuries]
A physician, appeared in a list of taxpayers or donors to a fund raised for the redemption of captives etc. Alongside him are mentioned al-Nafīs al-Sharābī, Abū al-ʿIzz al-Kaḥḥāl, (anonymous) al-Sheikh al-Muhadhdhab al-Ṭabīb, Abū al-Faraj b. al-Nashādirī, Makārim al-Kaḥḥāl, Abū al-Thanāʾ and (anonymous) al-Wajīh ('honourable') al-Ṭabīb.[156]

Abū Naṣr Samawʾal b. Yaḥyā al-Maghribī (Samuel b. Judah b. ʿAbbās al-Maghribī) [Ir., Iq., Baghdad, 12th century, convert]

Abū Naṣr al-Ṭabīb [Eg., 13th century]
A physician, appeared in a list of donors alongside Abū al-Murajjā.[157]

Abū Naṣr al-Ṭabīb 2 [Eg., 13th century]
A physician, mentioned in a letter sent by Judah ha-Melammēd Ibn al-ʿAmmānī to Abraham Maimonides in 1217.[158]

Abū Naṣr al-Ṭabīb 3 [Eg., 12th century]
A physician, mentioned in a document written by Ḥalfon ha-Levi b. Manasseh.[159]

Abū Naṣr al-Ṭabīb b. al-Tinnīsī [Eg., Cairo, 12th century]
A physician, mentioned in two documents: one of them is a matchmaking contract signed in Fusṭāṭ in 1146;[160] the other, dated 1143, mentioned his daughter, Sitt al-Sāda, who was married to Abū al-Barakāt b. Joseph Lebdī.[161]

Abū Riḍā al-Ṭabīb [Eg., 12th century]
A physician, mentioned in a document alongside Abū Zikrī al-Ṭabīb 2, another physician and the son of a wound specialist (*kallām*).[162]

Abū al-Riḍā al-Ṭabīb (Joseph ha-Levi) [Eg., Minyat Ziftā, 12th century]
A physician, mentioned in several documents. He is Maimonides' nephew and is mentioned by Ibn al-Qifṭī.[163] In a letter addressed to him, a patient described the symptoms from which he was suffering, and asked for a prescription. Abū al-Riḍā and his brother Abū al-Ḥasan appeared in a document originating in the peripheral city of Minyat Ziftā, from which it can be learnt that the two brothers took care of an orphan.[164] An additional document contained a list of Abū al-Riḍā's possessions, which was written at the request of Moses b. Maimon and under the supervision of the court in Fusṭāṭ, on 13 April 1172, probably shortly after Abū al-Riḍā's death. Following Moses b. Maimon's orders and under the same supervision, the possessions were moved to Abū al-Ḥasan's house, who declared in writing that he had received them. Later on, the possessions were given to the orphan son ʿImrān.[165] Goitein assumed, based on Abū al-Riḍā's list of possessions, that he served as a physician in one of Egypt's provincial towns and wasn't wealthy. However, Ora Molad-Vaza, in her research on clothing in Jewish society, came to the conclusion that Abū al-Riḍā was actually a well-off physician of high social status.[166]

Abū Saʿd al-Ṭabīb (al-Sadīd) [Eg., Cairo, 12th century]
A physician, died c.1190. Mentioned in a document concerning the sale of books from his estate, the revenue from which was allocated to his widow.[167]

Abū Saʿd al-Ṭabīb 2 [Eg., 12th–13th centuries]
A physician, mentioned in a letter sent to Abū Sahl Yedūthūn ha-Levi (Yedūthūn ha-Levi ha-Rōfē b. Levi ha-Levi).[168]

Abū Sahl Dūnash b. Tamīm [Ma., Qayrawān, 10th century]
A physician and linguist, born and grew up in Qayrawān and was educated in a family originating in Iraq. He was known among the Jews as 'Adūnīm' and was nicknamed 'al-Shaflajī'. He served as a court physician for two Fatimid rulers, al-Manṣūr b. al-Qāʾim and his son al-Muʿizz li-Dīn Allāh. He wrote numerous works about medicine, arithmetic and astronomy, some of them for the Fatimid rulers, as well as about the Jewish religion and Hebrew grammar. The scholar Ḥasan Ḥusnī ʿAbd al-Wahhāb noted twelve writings and letters that Dūnash had written, including *Kitāb al-Talkhīṣ* (a summary of basic drugs). According to ʿAbd al-Wahhāb, Ibn al-Bayṭār relied on this book four times in his own famous book (referring to him as Duways b. Tamīm). Dūnash was the student of Isḥāq b. Sulaymān al-ʾIsrāʾīlī, who incorporated him into the translation of the 'Book of Creation', which is one of the foundations of the Jewish religion. Dūnash was knowledgeable in the Jewish religion and its rule to the extent that he was one of its greatest scholars and even ruled on some religious issues for Eastern and Western Jews. One of Dūnash's important books, in the field of linguistics, compares Arabic and Hebrew, among other things as an attempt to use Arabic in order to understand unclear topics in the Torah. Dūnash's death date is not precisely known, but according to most scholars, he died in 971. According to a story by the Jewish linguist from Granada, Saʿadya b. Danān, Dūnash was Muslim when he died.[169]

Abū al-Surūr al-Ṭabīb (Sasson ha-Levi) [Eg., 12th century]
A physician, gave his daughter one-eighth of a house he owned with his brother for her wedding. The gift was provided he did not have to sell the apartment to make a living for himself. Later, the father did claim that he had to sell the house. The daughter and her possessions were with her father's brother, who had been appointed her trustee.[170]

Abū Yaʿqūb al-Ḥakīm (Jekuthiel b. Moses ha-Rōfē) [Eg., Cairo, 11th–12th centuries]

Abū Zechariah b. Sa'ada [Eg., 10th–11th centuries]
A physician, lived during the era of the physician Moses b. Elazar, his sons Isḥāq b. Mūsā b. El'āzār and Ismā'īl b. Mūsā b. El'āzār, and his grandson Ya'qūb b. Isḥāq.[171]

Abū Zechariah Yaḥyā b. Sulaymān al-Dhamārī [Eg., 15th century]
A physician (c.1430), wrote religious essays influenced by Samuel b. Solomon al-Maghribī.[172]

Abū Zikrī al-Sadīd b. Elijah b. Zechariah [Eg., Alexandria, EY, Jerusalem, 12th–13th centuries]

Abū Zikrī al-Ṭabīb (Judah b. Sa'adya) [Eg., 11th century]

Abū Zikrī al-Ṭabīb 2 [Eg., 12th century]
A physician, mentioned in a document in which his brother-in-law received or donated two *qīrāṭs*. The document mentioned several other medical practitioners, including Abū Riḍā al-Ṭabīb, a physician and the son of a wound specialist (*kallām*).[173]

Abū Zikrī Yaḥyā (Sar Shālōm) (Zūṭā) [Eg., Cairo, 12th century]

'Afīf (R. Joseph b. Ezra al-Miṣrī) [EY, Safed, 16th century]
A physician who immigrated to Eretz-Israel and lived in Safed. He is referred to as 'al-Miṣrī'. He is mentioned in a letter sent to the last Jewish *nagid* of the Mamluk period, R. Isaac Sholel (held the position 1502–17).[174]

'Afīf b. 'Abd al-Qāhir Sukra al-Yahūdī al-Ḥalabī al-Ṭabīb [Sy., Aleppo, 12th century, ?convert]

al-'Afīf b. Abī Sa'īd al-Sāwī [Eg., 15th century]
A physician, mentioned in a journal from the al-Azahar mosque as the head physician of Egypt and the author of the book *Kitāb al-Lamḥa fī al-Ṭibb*.[175]

'Alī b. Nathan [Eg., 13th century]
A physician, sent a letter to the *nāsī* in Cairo, probably Solomon b. Jesse, in which he complained that the *ḥazzān* had returned only two of the three dinars he had deposited with him.[176]

'Alī ha-Rōfē [Eg., Cairo, 12th century]

Amīn al-Dawla Abū al-Ḥasan b. Ghazāl b. Abī Saʿīd al-Sāmirī (Wazīr al-Ṣāliḥ, and Sharaf al-Milla 'Glory of the Nation') [S., Sy., Baalbek, 13th century, convert]

R. Amram b. Saʿīd b. Mūsā [Eg., Cairo, 11th century]
A physician, mentioned in a court document as working in the shop (*dukkān*) of a potion maker named Nethanel ha-Levi b. Amram Abū al-Faraj b. Maʿmar al-Sharābī.[177] Together with Amram there worked a Christian physician named Abū al-Ghālib (called *ṭabīb* and also *mutaṭabbib*), who wrote prescriptions in the shop owner's office. Amram was witness to an affair which developed between a Jewish lady and Abū al-Ghālib. Amram paid attention to the fact that the lady would come to the shop and meet with the Christian physician; after a while Amram discovered that she was Jewish, and even that she came from a respectable Jewish family. Not only did Amram follow the affair, Muslims did as well. The issue was discussed, as mentioned, in the Jewish court and three more Jewish witnesses' signatures were added to Amram's. The signatures are in Arabic, maybe a sign that this testimony in court was supposed to be passed on to the Muslim authorities.[178]

Amram ha-Kohen ha-Rōfē b. Aaron [EY, 11th century]
A physician, mentioned in a letter from Abraham b. Samuel III in Ramle to Solomon b. Judah in Jerusalem. The letter is dated around 1040 and signed with the name Amram.[179]

Araḥ ha-Rōfē [Eg., Cairo, 12th–13th centuries]
A physician; his son, Japheth b. Araḥ ha-Rōfē, is mentioned in a Geniza document.[180]

al-Asʿad Abī al-Barakāt al-Ṭabīb [Eg., 13th century]
A physician, in a list of donors c.1210 including several physicians and other practitioners.[181]

Asʿad al-Dīn (Ibn Ṣabra) al-Maḥallī al-Mutaṭabbib (Jacob b. Isaac) [Sy., Damascus, Eg., Maḥalla, Cairo, 13th century]
A physician from the Ṣabra family from al-Maḥalla in northern Egypt. He is also mentioned by Ibn Abī Uṣaybiʿa for being a friend of one of his uncles and successfully healing one of the women in his household at a time

when all other attempts had failed. In addition to being a physician, Asʿad wrote a number of medical books on optical issues, primary health care and comparisons between medical issues in Cairo and Damascus (where he stayed c.1200 and met the famous physicians of the time). He also carried on a scientific correspondence with the Samaritan physician from Damascus Ṣadaqa b. Munajjā b. Ṣadaqa al-Sāmirī.[182] In a testimony from 1217 it is mentioned that Asʿad raised in his house a girl named Akramiyya from 'disreputable' ancestry. This means she was bought as a slave when she was a baby, probably named after her previous owner, al-Sheikh al-Akram, grew up in Asʿad's house and was released when she was mature – an act of kindness known from other places and cases as well. With her release, Asʿad wished to find her a husband.[183] Asʿad's daughter married a physician[184] who came to al-Maḥalla in order to study under Asʿad and be cured of a chronic illness he was suffering from. Asʿad died in Cairo.[185]

al-Asʿad al-Ṭabīb [Eg., 13th century]

A physician, mentioned in lists of donors and their donations (c.1210), which included several practitioners.[186] He might be identical with al-Asʿad al-Mutaṭabbib.

Asad al-Yahūdī (Usayda) [Eg., Cairo, Sy., Hama, Saged, Damascus, Aleppo, 13th–14th centuries]

A prominent physician in Egypt and Syria under the Mamluks. He worked as a general physician and as an ophthalmologist but was known especially as a surgeon who healed fractures. He treated the military and political elite of the Mamluks. In addition to his medical education, he was knowledgeable in science, especially in metaphysics and physics. He was in contact with scholars of his time, including the famous Muslim theologian Ibn Taymiyya. His patron was the historian and Ayyubid prince of Hama al-Malik al-Muʾayyad Abū al-Fidāʾ (d. 1331). According to al-Ṣafadī, Asad died after the year 1330.[187]

ʿAwḍ [Sy., Damascus, 14th century]

A physician and a *dayyān*, had a great name in his time, treating the elite. He devoted himself to learning Arabic grammar and tried to express himself according to the literary Arabic rules, but he was not successful and spoke with rough mistakes.[188]

Azariah b. Ephraim [Eg., Cairo, 12th century]
A physician, active in Cairo during the Ayyubid period (c.1172). After he recovered from an illness, Mevōrākh b. Nathan, the court clerk, sent him a letter of congratulation written in rhymed Hebrew prose. In the letter he is described as a known practitioner among the Muslim physicians, and his recovery was a day of jubilation.[189]

Badīʿ (Ṣadr al-Dīn) b. Nafīs b. Dāʾūd b. ʿAnān al-Dāʾūdi al-Tabrīzī [?K., Ir., Tabriz, Eg., Cairo, 14th century, convert]

Barbosa the physician [EY. Jerusalem, 16th century]
A famous Portuguese-born physician, a Christian who converted to Judaism. He sailed to Ancona, from there moved to Turkey and in the end settled in the Jewish community in Jerusalem. In about 1560, the Portuguese traveller Pantaleo de Aveiro met him in Jerusalem and noted that 'Barbosa is a great physician'. Amato Lusitano, in his writings about medicines, wrote of him that he is 'a learned and excellent physician with much experience'.[190]

Baruch (the physician from Damascus) [Sy., Damascus, 12th–13th centuries]
A physician, severely criticised by al-Ḥarīzī in his book of travels, for his seclusion from the public during holidays and Sabbaths. Baruch worked as an astronomer-astrologer.[191]

Ben bū ʿ[…]ā al-Ṭabīb [Eg., 13th century]
A physician, mentioned in a list of donors along with: Abū al-Khayr al-ʿAṭṭār, Abū al-Riḍā al-ʿAṭṭār and al-Muwaffaq al-Kohen al-Ṭabīb.[192]

Benjamin ha-Rōfē [Eg., 13th century]
A physician, mentioned in a document. In earlier page of the document 'Sar ha-Rōfē' is mentioned, who is probably the same person, with his address.[193]

Berākhōt b. Samuel [Eg., 13th century]
A physician, mentioned in several documents.[194]

Berākhōt ha-Rōfē [Eg., 12th century]
A physician; his son, Yeshūʿā b. Berākhōt ha-Rōfē, is mentioned in a document.[195]

Berākhōt ha-Rōfē b. Sar Shālōm [Eg., 13th century]
A physician, mentioned in a document along with his brother (Tiqva ha-Rōfē b. Sar Shālōm).[196]

Burhān al-Dīn Ibrāhīm [K., Eg., 14th century, probably convert]

Dāniyāl (Daniel) Ibn Sha'yā [K., Eg., 11th century]

David [Sy., Homs, 12th–13th centuries]
A physician; al-Ḥarīzī described him as being 'of spotless character and gentle disposition'.[197]

David al-Mukhammas [K., Sy., ?10th century]
A Karaite physician who is mentioned in Ibn al-Hītī's chronicle.[198]

David b. Abraham b. Moses b. Maimon [Eg., Cairo, 13th century]

David b. Jacob [Eg., 14th–15th centuries]

David b. Joshua Maimon (al-Maimūnī) [Eg., Cairo, Sy., Aleppo, Damascus, 14th–15th centuries]

David b. Samuel Ibn Ṣaghīr [K., Eg., 13th–14th centuries]

R. David b. Shushan [EY, Jerusalem, 16th century]
The physician of the Jewish community and the head of the Spanish yeshiva in Jerusalem. In a letter written by R. Israel Ashkenzī from Jerusalem in 1517, David is mentioned as one who dealt in medicines.[199]

David ha-Rōfē [K., Eg., ?12th century]
A Karaite physician who is mentioned in a memorial list.[200]

Elazar (the king's physician) [Sy., Aleppo, 12th–13th centuries][201]
A physician, apparently served al-Malik al-Ẓāhir al-Ghāzī, Saladin's son and the ruler of Aleppo between 1186 and 1216. Elazar attracted criticism from the Jewish community after travelling on the Sabbath to treat the ill king. He also transgressed by condescending the great physician Joseph b. Simon al-Maghribī, who shamed him in public. In later editions of al-Ḥarīzī's 'Book of Travels', Elazar is praised for assisting the maintenance of good relations with the authorities. His sons Moses, Daniel and Joseph are praised as well.[202]

R. Elazar [Eg., Cairo, 14th century]
In a letter sent from Jerusalem by Joseph b. Eliezer to the *nagid* Amram in Cairo in 1380, the author sent his regards to the physicians R. Elazar and R. Joseph and the other physicians. Ashtor assumed that the author was R. Joseph b. Eliezer, who was sitting in Jerusalem at the time.[203]

Elazar b. Tiqva ha-Levi ha-Sar ha-Nikhbād ha-Rōfē [Eg., 12th–13th centuries]

Elazar ha-Levi ha-Zāqēn ha-Nikhbād ha-Rōfē [Eg., 12th century]
A physician, mentioned in a document from the time of the *nagid* Samuel b. Hananiah, between 1140 and 1153.[204]

Elazar ha-Rōfē [Eg., 12th century]
A physician, his son Abraham signed a letter sent from Alexandria at the end of the twelfth century, in which he reported on the arrival of a ship from Marseille containing questions to Maimonides, and complained of new decrees by the sultan as well as about the poverty of the local community. Elazar was no longer alive when the letter was written.[205]

Elazar Sakandarī [Eg., Cairo, 16th century]

Elias b. al-Mudawwar b. Ṣaddūd al-Yahūdī al-Ṭabīb al-Rundī (of Ronda) [An., Ronda, 12th century]
A physician and a poet in the time of the Moorish rulers of Spain. He was especially known by the Arab historians as a poet; and al-Maqqarī related the following anecdote of him: there was at Ronda another physician with whom Elias used to quarrel, as is generally the case between members of the same profession. One day, Elias became the master of a secret concerning his rival, which if made public might ruin him, and sent him in Arabic the following distich: 'Do not blame me; for no friendship can exist between two members of the same profession. Look at the two moons [that is to say, the sun and moon]: is there any light when a collision occurs between them?'[206]

Eliezer ha-Rōfē b. Obadia ha-Rōfē [Sy.. Tripoli, 14th century]

Elijah ha-Kohen ha-Rōfē [K., Sy., Damascus, 12th century]
A Karaite physician, mentioned in a memorial list.[207]

Elijah ha-R[ō]fē b. Samuel ha-Melammēd [Eg., 14th century]
A physician, mentioned in a colophon, apparently from the fourteenth century.[208]

Elisha ha-Rōfē [K., Eg., 12th century]
A Karaite physician, mentioned in a memorial list.[209]

Ephraim b. al-Ḥasan b. Isḥāq b. Ibrāhīm b. Yaʿqūb Abū Kathīr al-Zaffān (Ephraim b. al-Zaffān) [Eg., 11th century]

Ephraim b. Japheth [Eg., Cairo, 11th century]
A physician, mentioned in a document from 1066 in Fusṭāṭ.[210]

Ephraim ha-Rōfē b. Isaac [Eg., Cairo, 11th century]
A physician, mentioned in a document (c.1090).[211]

Ephraim ha-Rōfē b. Japheth b. Isaac [Eg., Cairo, 12th century]

Faḍl b. Khalaf al-Raʾīs al-Sadīd [K., Eg., ?Alexandria, 12th century]
A Karaite physician, apparently lived in Alexandria, or in another city some distance from Cairo. Judah ha-Maghribī, who was married to the physician's sister, sent him a letter[212] in which he asked his wife, who had fled to her brother, to return to Cairo.[213]

Faraj Allāh (Yeshūʿa) Ibn Ṣaghīr [K., Eg., Cairo, 13th–14th centuries]

Fatḥ Allāh b. Muʿtaṣim b. Nafis (Fatḥ al-Dīn) [K, Ir., Tabriz, Eg., 14th–15th centuries, convert]

Furāt b. Shaḥnāthā (Shaḥāthā) al-Yahūdī [Sy., Iq., 8th century]
A virtuous physician in his time who served al-Ḥajjāj b. Yūsuf[214] in that capacity, among others. At the end of his life, Furāt befriended ʿIsā b. Mūsā al-ʿAbbāsī, the heir to the throne in the days of al-Manṣūr, the Abbasid caliph, who used to consult him about everything, since he liked the nature of his opinions and thought. The two had a good and tight relationship.[215] Furāt died during al-Manṣūr's time. ʿIsā b. Mūsā used to mention him often after he died.[216]

Ḥalfon ha-Levi b. Nethanel [Eg., Cairo, Alexandria, Ye., 12th century]
One of the most important Jewish Indian trade merchants. There are some

indications that Ḥalfon had some medical education. Three sections of the book *al-Ṭibb* ('Medicine') are mentioned to have been sent to him during his time in Yemen by one of the local leaders. In addition, it seems that Jacob ha-Rōfē sent him a letter, addressing him a question about medicine. Amram b. Isaac wrote to Ḥalfon with a detailed description of his wife's illness and noted its similarity to an illness mentioned in the medical book *al-Ṭibb al-Manṣūrī* by Abū Bakr Muḥammad b. Zakariyya al-Rāzī.[217] According to Zinger, writing about Goitein's legacy, he was a merchant-physician-scholar-poet.[218]
It is possible that Ḥalfon met with the *nagid* Samuel b. Hananiah regarding the diagnosis of a disease and its treatment.[219]

Ḥalfon ha-Rōfē [Eg., Alexandria, 11th–12th centuries]
A physician; his son Samuel is a signatory of a document from 1100, in Alexandria.[220]

Hananiah b. Bezalel [Sy., Aleppo, 12th–13th centuries][221]
A physician, described by al-Ḥarīzī thus: 'A physician heavy on Goodness' scale – R. Hananiah, son of Bezalel, his people's praise: with lowered eyes he walks down wisdom's ways. Scholars, his door is open wide: enter and see virtue shining on every side.'[222] He was praised for his charitable activity.[223] It is possible that this is Abū al-Barakāt b. Abū al-Kathīr.[224]

Hananiah ha-Rōfē [Eg., 12th century]

al-Ḥaqīr al-Nāfiʿ al-Ṭabīb (al-Jirāḥī al-Miṣrī) [Eg., 10th–11th centuries]
A physician and surgeon who dealt mainly with healing wounds (al-Jirāḥī al-Miṣrī = the Egyptian Surgeon). According to Ibn Abī Uṣaybiʿa, al-Ḥaqīr al-Nāfiʿ (the Wretched and Helpful)[225] is not his real name, but was given to him by the caliph al-Ḥākim bi-Amr Allāh, when he successfully treated a wound in the caliph's leg in only three days, after his private physicians failed to do so. In return for his successful treatment, the caliph gave him a thousand dinars and honorary clothes, and appointed him among his personal physicians.[226]

Hārūn (Aaron) b. Isaac of Cordova [An., Cordova, 10th century]
A physician, practised in Cordova under the Moorish rulers of Spain. According to the sources he was a teacher and the author of medical work

(commentaries on Ibn Sīnā). He is known for his contribution to a song that was written by Ibn Sīnā on fever.[227]

Ḥasan Abū Kanū? [An., 12th century]
A physician, practised at the court of the Almoravid emir ʿAlī b. Yūsuf (r. 1106–42).[228]

al-Ḥasan Hibat Allāh Mufaḍḍal al-Yahūdī [Eg., Cairo, 12th century]
A physician, active in Cairo.[229]

al-Ḥasan Ṭabīb [Eg., 13th century]
A physician, mentioned in a list of donors written by Solomon b. Elijah. Al-Asʿad al-Ṭabīb is also mentioned in the list.[230]

Ḥasday b. Shaprūṭ [An., Cordova, 10th century]

Ḥayyīm b. Joseph Vital [EY, Safed, 16th–17th centuries]
A physician and Kabbalist (1543–1620), his family was originally from Italy, but he was probably born in Safed and was part of the Jewish scholars and revered Kabbalists of Safed and Jerusalem. Ḥayyīm Vital is considered the most prominent and important student of Isaac Luria. He studied Kabbala and the Torah, as well as alchemy, astronomy and medicine. During the years 1577–84 and 1591–4 he lived on and off in Jerusalem and taught the Torah. After his stay in Jerusalem he sojourned in Damascus, c.1610–20, where he wrote a book on medicines, talismans and supernatural care.[231]

Ḥazqīl [?An., ?9th–10th centuries]
A physician, apparently a prominent one, mentioned in a list of Jewish physicians in Jonah Ibn Janāḥ's book *Kitāb al-Talkhīṣ*.[232]

Hibat Allāh (Nethanel b. Moses ha-Levi) [Eg., Cairo, 12th century]

Ibn Aḥmad b. al-Maghribī [Eg., 13th–14th centuries, convert]

Ibn ʿAknīn (Joseph b. Judah b. Jacob) [An., Barcelona, Mo., Fez, 12th century]
A Jewish physician and scholar from the time of Maimonides. He was born in Barcelona, and immigrated to Fez during the Almohad period. Ibn ʿAknīn wrote several essays including *Ṭibb al-Nufūs al-Salīma wa-Muʿalaāt al-Nufūs*

al-Alīma (1190), not published at the time except for one chapter about education. This unique work is, as far as we know, the only one that focused on psychology and was written by a Jewish physician in the Middle Ages. He also wrote *Sefer ha-Musar*, a commentary on Perke Avot.[233] Ibn ʿAknīn was a pupil of Maimonides in Fez during the period of forced conversion of Almohads. He described how he lived as a Muslim with feelings of guilt, and secretly observed the commandments and studied the Torah with Maimonides. He remained in Fez when his master Maimonides left. Afterwards, he described the persecutions of the ruler Abū Yūsuf b. Yaʿqūb (r. 1184–99).[234]

There is much confusion among scholars[235] between Ibn ʿAknīn and Abū al-Ḥajjāj Yūsuf b. Yaḥyā b. Isḥāq al-Sabatī al-Maghribī (Joseph b. Judah b. Simon) (Ibn Samʿūn), Maimonides' pupil to whom he dedicated *The Guide for the Perplexed*. Arturo Prats suggested that Ibn ʿAknīn wasn't born in Barcelona and never claimed he was. He never left Spain, he never visited Fez, never met Maimonides, and never received letters from him.[236]

Ibn al-Julājilī [Eg., 13th century]

A physician, appeared in a list of future donors from the time of Abraham Maimonides alongside (anonymous) al-Mawlī al-Muhadhdhab, (anonymous) Awlād al-Raʾīs, (anonymous) al-Gaon al-Munā, Mufaḍal al-Mashmiʿa, al-Sheikh Joseph, another al-Sheikh Joseph and his son, Ibn al-Julājilī, R. Yeshūʿā, Abū al-Maʿānī 2, Najīb Kohen Kamukhī(?), al-Rabīb Kohen, al-Taqī Ibn al-Gadal, Makārim Ibn al-Gadalī and Abū al-Maʿānī.[237]

Ibn Kūjik [K, Eg., 13th century]

Ibn Qarqa (or Ibn Qirqah) [Eg., 12th century]

A physician, served as the head of the Jewish community after Samuel ha-Nagid b. Hananiah (Abū Manṣūr).[238] The Muslim writers al-Maqrīzī, Ibn Taghribirdī and Ibn al-Athīr disagree about his religion.[239] According to al-Maqrīzī, Ibn Qarqa was the owner of the bathing house known as Hammām al-Ṭabīb Abū Saʿīd ben Qarqa, in the Jewish neighbourhood of Zuwayla, adjacent to the al-Masʿūdī market in Cairo, and his own house was nearby.[240] But he had to sell both properties in order to avoid their confiscation by the ruler. Ibn Qarqa was also an engineer who worked for the caliph al-Ḥāfiẓ. He is noted to have prepared a poison, at the request of al-Ḥāfiẓ, in order to kill the caliph's son Ḥasan. By contrast, Samuel ben Hananiah (Abū Manṣūr) refused to make the poison for the caliph. Due to his consent to prepare the poison and Ḥasan's death, his possessions were confiscated and transferred over to Abū Mansur. In 1134 al-Ḥāfiẓ ordered Ibn Qarqa's execution.[241]

Ibn Ṣaghīr Abī Faraj Allāh [K, Eg., 14th century]

Ibn Shūʿa (al-Muwaffaq) [Eg., 12th century]
One of Saladin's physicians, alongside Abū al-Maʿālī Tammām b. Hibat-Allāh b. Tammām, Ibn al-Mudawwar, Ibn Jumayʿ al-ʾIsrāʾīlī and Maimonides. Ibn Abī Uṣaybiʿa further added that Ibn Shūʿa was knowledgeable in general medicine, ophthalmology and surgery. He was easygoing and funny, and played the guitar. An incident is mentioned in which a Muslim zealot threw a stone that uprooted one of Ibn Shūʿa's eyes, because he was riding a horse in violation of the laws restricting the *dhimmīs*. Ibn Shūʿa in response wrote a humorous poem against him. In addition, Ibn Abī Uṣaybiʿa mentioned a scornful poem written by Ibn Shūʿa against his Jewish colleague Ibn Jumayʿ. Ibn Shūʿa died in Cairo in 1183.[242]

Ibrāhīm [?K., Eg., Cairo, Sy., Damascus, 14th century]
The Karaite poet from Safed Moses b. Samuel wrote in one of his poems (after 1354) about his difficult situation in Damascus and his desire to find a livelihood in Egypt. He pinned his hopes on Ibrāhīm the physician, who was in Cairo, to help him. On his way to Egypt, however, he met Ibrāhīm in Jerusalem, and spent four days with him. Afterwards, Ibrāhīm went to Damascus, while Moses continued to Cairo, where he was supported by the Karaites.[243]

Ibrāhīm al-Mutaṭabbib b. Mukhtār (Ibn al-Yām) [Eg., 13th century]
Testimony of his death was signed in the court of Solomon (Sulaymān) ha-Sar ha-Rōfē b. […] ha-Rōfē.[244] Ibrāhīm the physician bequeathed all his property, including money and medicine books, to the famous synagogue in Dammūh.[245]

Ibrāhīm al-Rōfē [Eg., 11th–12th centuries]
A physician, appeared in a list headed by the *nagid* Mevōrākh b. Saʿadya

(d. 1111) alongside: Abū al-Munā al-ʿAṭṭār, Abū Naṣr al-ʿAṭṭār 2, Abū al-Faḍl al-Ṭabīb 2, Salāma al-ʿAṭṭār, (anonymous) ʿAṭṭār and Abū al-Surūr al-Sharābī.[246]

Ibrāhīm b. Faraj Allāh b. ʿAbd al-Kāfī al-ʾIsrāʾīlī al-Yahūdī al-Dāʾūdi al-ʿAffānī (al-ʿAnānī) [K., Eg., Cairo, 14th–15th centuries]
A physician (d. 1441, when he was over seventy years old). According to Muslim sources, after he died there were no other Jewish physicians who were familiar with the Torah. Ibrāhīm acknowledged Muhammad as a prophet, yet only as an Arabic apostle. Moreover, he believed that Jesus was a pious man, unlike the Jewish position regarding him.[247] Al-Maqrīzī mentioned that Ibrāhīm had an extraordinary memory. He was a judge of the Jews and he told al-Maqrīzī that the Ibn al-Banā mosque in Fusṭāṭ had previously been a Karaite synagogue called Shem b. Noah, since according to the Karaite people Shem, the son of Noah, was buried there. The Fatimid caliph al-Ḥākim bi-Amr Allāh turned the synagogue into a mosque.[248]

Ibrāhīm b. Faraj b. Mārūth al-Sāmirī al-Ṭabīb (al-Ḥakīm) (Abū Isḥāq Ibrāhīm al-Muṣannif) (Shams al-Ḥukamāʾ) [S., Eg., 12th century]
A physician of Saladin, and a known medical teacher. The writer ʿAṭiyya al-Qūṣī mixed him up with the physician Yūsuf b. Abī Saʿīd b. Khalaf al-Sāmirī al-Muhadhdhab al-Ṭabīb, claiming that the latter was nicknamed Shams al-Ḥukamāʾ and operated in the service of Saladin. According to Ramaḍān, Ibrāhīm al-Sāmirī is the one who was Saladin's physician and was nicknamed Shams al-Ḥukamāʾ. Ramaḍān based his claim on Ibn Abī Uṣaybiʿa, who wrote that Yūsuf b. Abī Saʿīd al-Sāmirī was indeed a specialised physician (and also that he was a successful writer) but that he studied medicine under the physician (al-Ḥakīm) Ibrāhīm al-Sāmirī, known as Shams al-Ḥukamāʾ, who worked in the service of Saladin. Ibrāhīm is the author of *Kitāb al-Mīrāth* and the grammar book *Kitāb al-Tawṭiʾa*. He was one of the teachers of the Samaritan physician Yūsuf b. Abī Saʿīd b. Khalaf. His father, Abū al-Ḥasan Isḥāq b. Faraj b. Mārūth al-Ṣūrī, was a known writer.[249]

Ibrāhīm b. Khalaf al-Sāmirī (the Samaritan) [S., Eg., Damascus, 12th–13th centuries]

Ibrāhīm b. Nūḥ al-Ṭabīb ha-Ḥākhām [K., Eg., EY, 10th century]
A physician; mentioned in al-Tamīmī's book about theriac, in the reign of the caliph Jaʿfar al-Muqtadir (r. 908–32), he was one of the notable physicians (he established a *beit midrash* in Jerusalem in which Karaite scholars convened). It is highly possible that he was the father of Abū Yaʿqūb al-Baṣīr (Joseph b. Abraham) b. Nūḥ.[250]

Ibrāhīm b. Shūmalī [EY., Jerusalem, 16th century]
A Jewish physician, mentioned in a document concerning a treatment he gave to a Muslim patient.[251]

Ibrāhīm b. al-Tharthār [An., Granada, Castile, Mo., 14th century]
A physician, practised in the court of Muḥammad V al-Naṣrī in Granada (r. 1354–9, 1362–91). He was the object of hatred for a Muslim physician named Muḥammad al-Lakhmī al-Shaqūrī, who wrote a book against the Jews. In 1359, when Muḥammad V moved to Morocco, Ibrāhīm took off to Castile and from there to Morocco. He later returned to Granada with his patron.[252] He is apparently identical to Ibrāhīm b. Zarzar, who was mentioned by Ibn Khaldūn for refusing, as the court physician of the ruler of Granada, to travel to Fez in 1356 to take care of Abū ʿAnān, the sultan of Fez. The king of Granada, Muhammad V al-Naṣrī, asked for Abū ʿAnān's forgiveness.[253]

Ibrāhīm b. Yaʿqūb al-ʾIsrāʾīlī al-Ṭurṭūshī [?An., ?Ma., 10th century]
A Jewish traveller (merchant), born in Tortosa to a judge and lived in the time of Menahem b. Sarūq, a Jewish linguist and philologist (920–70). Al-Ṭurṭūshī is mainly known for making a long journey in Europe in 965.[254] He crossed the Adriatic Sea, went to the countries of the West Slavs, visited Prague and eastern Germany, and later on at Magdeburg, he met Bulgarian ambassadors at the court of Otto I. He then travelled along the right bank of the Elbe, through more Slavic countries and farther northward to Schwerin. Due to the number of times al-Ṭurṭūshī is cited by later writers, it seems that there once existed an account of his journey, known mainly through al-Bakrī and al-Qazwīnī.[255] Some scholars expressed the view that Ibrāhīm was a physician or translator attached to a diplomatic mission to the court of the Holy Roman Emperor. However, the possibility exists that he was sent by

the caliph al-Ḥakam II, known to have been a supporter of research activities, on an exploratory expedition.[256] His story, known mainly from *al-Masālik wa-l-Mamālik* by the Arab geographer al-Bakrī (d. 1074),[257] is distinguished by its comprehensive character. Al-Ṭurṭūshī showed interest in many spheres: in the distances between towns, plants, economic life, the people's diet, the system of medicine and religious customs. Occasionally he mentioned the Jews who lived in the countries that he visited, and he also wrote about a salt mine near Magdeburg that was operated by Jews.[258]

ʿImād al-Dawla Abū al-Khayr b. Muwaffaq al-Dawla Abū al-Faraj ʿAlī b. Abī al-Shujāʿ al-Hamadānī [Ir., Tabriz, 13th century]

ʿImrān b. Ṣadaqa al-ʾIsrāʾīlī al-Ḥakīm Awḥad al-Dīn al-ʾIsrāʾīlī (Moses b. Ṣedāqā) [Sy., Damascus, Homs, 12th–13th centuries]

Isaac [K., Eg., Cairo, 15th century]
A Karaite physician, mentioned by the physician Moses b. Abraham b. Saʿadya, in a *maqāma* (work of rhyming prose) of his. Among the Cairo community's notables.[259]

Isaac b. Baruch ha-Rōfē [Sy., Damascus, 12th–13th centuries]
A physician, mentioned by al-Ḥarīzī, who criticised his poetry for having grammatical mistakes, among other things.[260]

Isaac ha-Kohen ha-Rōfē [Eg., 11th century]

Isaac ha-Kohen ha-Rōfē b. Furāt [Eg., Cairo, EY. Ramle, 11th century]

Isaac ha-Rōfē [Eg., 11th–12th centuries]
A physician, probably from Alexandria, mentioned in the *dīwān* of Moses b. Abraham b. Saʿadya ha-Rōfē Darʿī. Also included in Moses Darʿī's circle of friends (i.e., mentioned in his *dīwān*) are Moses ha-Rōfē b. Isaac ha-Rōfē, Samuel ha-Kohen ha-Rōfē, Moses ha-Levi, Elijah b. Samuel and Samuel b. Elijah al-Sinnī.[261]

Isaac ha-Rōfē 2 [EY, Jerusalem, Sy., Karak, 16th century]
A physician, born in Jerusalem, in 1507 he was practising in Karak.[262]

Isaac ha-Sar ha-Adīr ha-Talmīd ha-Nikhbād ha-Rōfē ha-Ḥākhām [Eg., 13th–14th centuries]
A physician, mentioned in a Geniza document.[263]

Isḥāq b. Mūsā b. Elʿāzār (Abū Yaʿqūb al-Ṭabīb) (al-Mutaṭabbib) [Ma., Mahdiyya, Eg., Cairo, 10th century]

Isḥāq b. Sulaymān al-ʾIsrāʾīlī (Isaac b. Solomon) [Eg., Ma., Qayrawān, 9th–10th centuries]
Apparently the best-known Jewish physician that preceded Maimonides. Born in Egypt (apparently in 832). Isaac was advanced in his profession and was the student of Isaac b. ʿImrān. Additionally, he was a philosopher, skilled in logic and in several branches of science. In Qayrawān he served as the court physician of the Aghlabī emir and of the Fatimid caliph. He served al-Mahdī ʿUbayd Allāh, the ruler of Ifrīqiyya, at whose request he wrote several medical essays in Arabic.[264] Isaac wrote books in Arabic on medicine and philosophy, yet only the Hebrew and Latin translations of them have survived. His medical writings were studied for hundreds of years in Europe during the Middle Ages and the Renaissance. His philosophical writings were influenced by Neoplatonism and he was considered one of the earliest Jewish philosophers of the Middle Ages. His main contribution was introducing Neoplatonism to the world of Jewish thought. Despite the critical attitude Maimonides held towards him and towards the greater publicity of his compatriot Saʿadya Gaon, Isaac influenced Solomon Ibn Gabirol and Joseph Ibn Ṣaddiq, as well as mystic Jews.[265] Among his main medical writings are a 'book of components', a 'book on dietetics', a 'book on fevers' (which was praised by the Muslim physician ʿAlī Ibn Riḍwān,[266] translated in the Middle Ages into Spanish and Latin, and introduced into the medical schools' curriculum during that time), a 'treatise on urine' (which became an important source of information for this form of diagnosis), treatises on 'elements and on definitions and outlines', 'ethical guidelines for physicians' (which have survived in Hebrew translations but have not received much attention), and a book titled *The Garden of Knowledge*, which deals with metaphysical matters. Ibn Janāḥ quoted three of Isaac's books in his *Kitāb al-Talkhīṣ*.[267] Isaac lived to the age of 100 and died in Qayrawān. He never got married or accumulated any wealth.[268] Ibn Khaldūn mentioned a story about how Isaac

saved Caliph al-Manṣūr Ismāʿīl's life after a Muslim physician gave him too strong a soporific.[269]

Ismāʿīl [Iq., Baghdad, 9th century]
A physician, contemporary of the poet Ibn al-Rūmī (836–96).[270]

Ismāʿīl b. Faddād [An., 11th century]
A physician, mentioned by Ibn Ḥazm (994–1064).[271]

Ismāʿīl b. Mūsā b. Elʿāzār [Ma., Mahdiyya, Eg., Cairo, 10th century]

Ismaʿīl b. Yūnis [An., Almeria, 11th century]
A physician; according to Ibn Ḥazm he was trained in physiognomy, and was able to detect a person in love by looking at their face.[272]

Israel b. Zechariah al-Ṭayfūrī [Iq., 9th century]
A physician, served at the court of the Abbasid caliph al-Mutawakkil. He received enormous sums of money and also lands from his employer, and he was even allowed to walk around with his retinue, which included a bodyguard.[273]

Jacob [Eg., 14th century]

Jacob b. Joseph [Eg., 14th–15th centuries]
A physician, mentioned in a notarial act (1407), where he is said to have purchased a white 'toga'.[274]

Jacob b. Meiʾr [An., Toledo, 12th–13th centuries]
A physician, lived in Toledo. Al-Ḥarīzī described him as 'the doctor and seer, Master Jacob ben Meʾir, light divine bright ore lifted from discernment's mine' and mentioned he was the cousin of R. Joseph ha-Dayyān.[275]

Jacob ha-Rōfē [An., 12th century]
A physician, lived and practised in Andalusia (c.1138). He was closely associated with Ḥalfon ha-Levi b. Nethanel, of the milieu of Judah ha-Levi. Two letters he wrote were preserved in the Geniza and have been found and studied lately.[276]

Jacob ha-Rōfē 2 [EY, Jerusalem, 16th century]
A physician; he and his legal representatives, Moses ha-Rōfē 3 and Samuel ha-Rōfē, are mentioned in a document from the Muslim court of Jerusalem,

dated 8 January 1550. Jacob rented a shop in Jerusalem from the Muslim *waqf*, which was used as a clinic.[277]

Jacob ha-Rōfē b. Ayyūb [Sy., 14th century]
A physician, wrote/copied a commentary and interpretation of the book of Ecclesiastes, authored by Abū al-Barakāt Hibat Allāh b. ʿAli b. Malkā al-Baladi al-Tabib. Jacob completed this work in 1335, in Madīnat Miṣyāf (probably the village of Miṣyāf, which is located on the way from the Banias to Hama, in the Nuṣayrīs mountains).[278]

Jacob ha-Rōfē b. Ḥalfon [Eg., 12th century]
A physician, signed a bill, apparently from the twelfth century.[279]

R. Jacob ha-Rōfē ha-Sar ha-Nikhbād ha-Zāqēn ha-[...] ha-Rōfē ha-[...] [Eg., 14th century]

Jalāl al-Dīn b. al-Ḥazzān [Ir., Tabriz, 14th century]
A physician, served in the court of Öljeitü Khān, from the Īl-Khānate dynasty in Azerbaijan. Jalāl al-Dīn testified in court against Rashīd al-Dīn Ṭabīb Faḍl Allāh b. al-Dawla Abū al-Khayr b. ʿAlī Abū al-Hamadānī, following which he and his son were executed.[280]

Jamāl al-Dīn Dāʾūd b. Abī al-Faraj b. Abī al-Ḥusayn b.ʿImrān al-Ṭabīb [Sy., Damascus, 13th–14th centuries, convert]
A physician (1275/6–1337), lived under the reign of al-Malik Naṣīr Naṣr Allāh, probably in Damascus. Converted to Islam alongside some other Jews: ʿAbd al-Sayyid the Dayyān and his son, and Nissim the Tanner and his sons.[281] Al-Jazarī provided us with details regarding his life and death:

> The great sheikh [al-Ṣāliḥ al-Faḍl Jamāl al-Dīn Dāʾūd b. Abī al-Faraj b. Abī al-Ḥusayn b.ʿImrān al-Ṭabīb] died and was buried in the cemetery of Bāb al-Ṣaghīr in Damascus. He was a blessed man, entered wholeheartedly into Islam and left his family and relatives for the sake of Allah. He engaged in learning [Islam], copying essays and worshipping God. He persisted until his death. He heard the famous Ḥadith written by ʻṢaḥīḥ al-Bukhārī.[282]

Jamāl al-Dīn ʿAbd Allāh b. ʿAbd al-Sayyid b. Isḥāq b. Yaḥyā [Sy., Damascus, 13th–14th centuries, convert]

Jamāl al-Dīn Ibrāhīm b. Shihāb al-Dīn Aḥmad (Sulaymān) al-Maghribī [Eg., 14th century, convert]

Japheth b. David b. Samuel Ibn Ṣaghīr (al-Ḥakīm al-Ṣafī) [K., Eg., Cairo, 13th–14th centuries]

Japheth ([Abū] al-Maḥāsin) ha-Kohen b. Josiah [Eg., 13th century]
A physician, mentioned in a legal document (1220–1) in which he is said to be the partner of a sugar merchant named Abū al-ʿIzz b. Abū al-Maʿānī in operating a sugar factory. The document mentioned that they can no longer pay the high governmental taxes.[283] Possibly the same person as Japheth ha-Rōfē or Japheth ha-Rōfē b. Joseph ha-Parnās.

Japheth Levi ha-Rōfē b. Judah ha-Sōfer [Eg., 12–13th centuries]
A physician, mentioned in a document, dating from earlier than the thirteenth century.[284]

Japheth ha-Rōfē [Eg., 13th century]
A physician, mentioned in a bill issued by the court of Alexandria (1220), in the time of Abraham Maimonides.[285] Possibly the same person as Japheth ha-Rōfē b. Joseph ha-Parnās or Japheth ([Abū] al-Maḥāsin) ha-Kohen b. Josiah.

Japheth ha-Rōfē b. Joseph ha-Parnās [Eg., 13th century]
A physician, mentioned in a document with his father, Joseph ha-Parnās.[286] Possibly the same person as Japheth ha-Rōfē or Japheth ([Abū] al-Maḥāsin) ha-Kohen b. Josiah.

Jekuthiel ha-Levi b. Petahya [K, Sy., Damascus, 13th century]

R. Joseph [EY. Jerusalem, 14th century]
In a letter sent from Jerusalem by Joseph b. R. Eliezer to the *nagid* Amram in Cairo in 1380, the writer asked about the physician R. Elazar, the physician R. Joseph and the rest of the physicians. Ashtor assumed the writer was R. Joseph b. Eliezer, who lived in Jerusalem during these years.[287]

Joseph 2 [Sy., Damascus, 15th century]
A physician, mentioned as the head of the community of Damascus during the visit of the traveller Meshullam of Volterra (1481).[288]

Joseph 3 [Eg., Cairo, 13th century]

A father and his son, both physicians, are mentioned in a list of future donors dated to the time of Abraham Maimonides. Also mentioned in the list are (anonymous) al-Mawlī al-Muhadhdhab, (anonymous) Awlād al-Raʾīs, (anonymous) al-Gaon al-Munā, Mufaḍḍal al-Mashmiʿa, al-Sheikh Joseph, Ibn al-Julājilī, R. Yeshūʿā, Abū al-Maʿānī 2, Najīb Kohen Kamukhī, al-Rabīb Kohen, al-Taqī Ibn al-Gadal, Makārim Ibn al-Gadalī, Abū al-Maʿānī. Abraham Maimonides wrote a note calling for help from the Jewish community in Fusṭāṭ and the surrounding area in finding a certain physician and warning that whoever knows his whereabouts and will not inform the Jewish court will be excommunicated, and it is possible that Joseph is that physician.[289] Maybe identical with Joseph al-Ṭabīb.

Joseph al-Gazī [Candia, 15th century]

A physician and Kabbalist, who settled in Candia, Crete, at the end of the fifteenth century.[290]

Joseph al-Ṭabīb [Eg., Cairo, 13th century]

A physician, mentioned in a document written between 1210 and 1220.[291] Maybe identical with Joseph 3.

R. Joseph b. Abraham Sakandarī (Iskandarī or Iskandarānī) [An., Eg., Alexandria, Cairo, EY, Jerusalem, Safed, 15th–16th centuries]

Joseph b. Isaac [EY, Jerusalem, 16th century]

A Jewish physician with a high professional rank. He was active in Jerusalem and mentioned in a document from 1575.[292]

Joseph b. Nissīn ha-Rōfē [Eg., 10th century]

A physician, mentioned in a mortgage bill from 969, in which it is mentioned that Malka b. Amram ha-Levi and her husband Maimon b. Japheth, who have provided as guarantee a court in Fusṭāṭ to Joseph (taking fifty dinars as a loan from him), are releasing the court and providing as a guarantee another court instead.[293]

Joseph from Damascus [Sy., Damascus, Crete, Candia, 15th century]

Joseph ha-Nagid b. Khalīfa [Eg., Cairo, 14th–15th centuries]
A *nagid* and possibly court physician of the sultan.[294] According to Ashtor, Joseph served as the *nagid* during the 1450s and 1460s. His origin was from the eastern Arab countries, according to Meshullam of Volterra, who travelled from Italy to Egypt in the second half of the fifteenth century. From a document we learn that Joseph was a *nagid* in 1458.[295] Apparently, he served as a *nagid* for many years. In 1465, the *nagid* R. Joseph b. Khalīfa was mentioned and it should be assumed he is the same Joseph. Joseph was a respectable man in the eyes of both the Jews and the Muslims. He was buried in the capital of Egypt.[296] Joseph's son, Solomon ha-Nagid b. Joseph ha-Nagid, took over his father's position as the *nagid*. It is not completely clear from Meshullam of Volterra's writings about Solomon ha-Nagid from 1481 whether it was Solomon or his father who served as the sultan's physician. Ashtor, based on Meshullam, mentioned that it was Joseph who was the sultan's physician. On the other hand, Mark Cohen sees both the father and the son as physicians, while Solomon is explicitly mentioned as the sultan's physician.[297]

Joseph ha-Parnās ha-Rōfē [Eg., Cairo, 11th century]
A physician, active in Cairo around the eleventh century.[298]

Joseph ha-Rōfē [K., 12th century]
A Karaite physician, mentioned in a memorial list.[299]

Joseph ha-Rōfē b. Isaac [Eg., 13th century]
A physician, mentioned in a Geniza document from the thirteenth century.[300]

Joseph ha-Sar ha-Nikhbād ha-Rōfē [Eg., 13th century]
A physician, mentioned in a document from the thirteenth century.[301]

Joseph (Abū ʿAmr) Ibn Qamniʾel [An., 11th–12th centuries]

Judah [Eg., Cairo, 11th century]
A physician and a *nagid*, maybe identical with Judah ha-Nāsī, son of Josiah ha-Nāsī, who came to Egypt from Damascus and became a *nagid*.[302]

Judah b. Joseph b. Abī al-Thanā [Sy., Raqqah, 9th–10th centuries]
A philosopher and a physician from al-Raqqah, Syria, mentioned by the

Muslim Arabic historian al-Masʿūdī (d. 957) as a student of the Muslim scholar Thābit b. Qurra (826–901).[303]

Judah b. Mūsā b. Jacob [Eg., EY, Jerusalem, 16th century]
A physician, mentioned in a document (1548), regarding the sale of an orchard in al-Māliḥa to a Muslim.[304]

Judah from Alexandria [Eg., Alexandria, 15th century]
A physician and surgeon, employed by the Venetian colony of Alexandria (15th century).[305]

Judah from Damascus [Sy., Damascus, Crete, Candia, 15th century]

Judah ha-Rōfē [Sy., Aleppo, 12th–13th centuries]
A physician, described by al-Ḥarīzī in the following words: 'Let stranger seek his coin and lo, he hasn't any – not a penny. There, too, lives R. Judah, the physician, blessed with piety and tact, and master of the righteous act.'[306]

Judah ha-Rōfē 2 [Eg., 15th century]
A physician; his son, Joshua from Alexandria, finished copying an essay written by the Kabbalist Abraham b. Samuel Abulafia about the Priestly Blessing (1473); he is mentioned in some other colophons from this period. Judah was no longer alive in 1473.[307]

Judah ha-Rōfē b. Abraham Taurīzī [K., Eg., Cairo, 16th century]
A Karaite physician who served also as a cantor (*ḥazzān*) in the Karaite synagogue in Cairo. He is mentioned in a document dated 1575.[308] His *nisba* implies his family's origin – Tabriz.

Kamāl al-Dawla Abū ʿAlī b. Abī al-Faraj, Ibn al-Dāʿī al-ʾIsrāʾīlī al-Irbilī al-Ḥakīm [Mongolia, 13th–14th centuries]
The historian Ibn al-Fuwaṭī, who lived during the Mongol Īl-Khānate reign (1244–1323), mentioned a biography of a Jewish *ḥakīm* (meaning physician/philosopher; the intention here is probably a physician, even one in the Mongol court). It is unclear whether or not he had converted to Islam. He was knowledgeable in mathematics, astronomy and Muslim Arabic literature (*adab*). The sultan, Khan Hülegü, sent him to his brother Möngke Khan in 1259, to serve as a physician in his court in Mongolia.[309]

Kamāl b. Mūsā [EY, Jerusalem, 16th century]
A physician (expert ophthalmologist) and *dayyān* from Jerusalem. His clinic was located in a rented store in the Sūq al-ʿAṭṭārīn. Since he was 'Head of the Physicians' of Jerusalem, he received his salary from the public treasury. On 16 July 1571, he got his supervisor's approval to be absent from Jerusalem for a short time, after he had found himself a suitable substitute.[310]

Khalaf al-Kaḥḥāl [Eg., 15th century]
An ophthalmologist, mentioned in a document (1436).[311]

Khiḍr [Eg., 15th–16th centuries]
A physician; the Muslim Arabic source noted that he 'claimed to be knowledgeable in medicine'. It is mentioned that in 1514 he treated one of the Mamluk emir's sons, Awlād al-Nās, who was ill. He ordered him to be treated with an enema, but the patient died after two days. Khiḍr was arrested, but he managed to escape death by bribe. It is unclear if he converted to Islam.[312]

Maḥāsin (Obadia ha-Dayyān) [Iq., al-Bīra, 14th century]

Maḥāsin al-Ṭabīb [Eg., 13th century]
A physician, mentioned in a note written by Abraham Maimonides (a. 1212–37).[313]

Maḥfūẓ al-Ṭabīb [Eg., 12th century]
A physician, mentioned in a document (1185) reporting that his granddaughter, Muʿzziza/Muʿzzaza b. Abū al-Faḍl, was getting married.[314]

Maḥfūẓ ha-Rōfē [Sy., Aleppo, 11th century]
A physician, mentioned in a letter as one of Aleppo's notables.[315]

Makārim ibn al-Gadalī [Eg., 13th century]
A physician, appeared in a list of future donors from the time of Abraham Maimonides alongside (anonymous) al-Mawlī al-Muhadhdhab, (anonymous) Awlād al-Raʾīs, (anonymous) al-Gaon al-Munā, Mufaḍḍal al-Mashmiʿa, al-Sheikh Joseph, another al-Sheikh Joseph and his son, Ibn al-Julājilī, R. Yeshūʿā, Abū al-Maʿānī 2, Najīb Kohen Kamukhī, al-Rabīb Kohen, al-Taqī Ibn al-Gadal and Abū al-Maʿānī.[316]

Makārim b. Isḥāq b. Makārim [Eg., Cairo, 13th century]

A physician and ophthalmologist, active in Cairo c.1245. According to Goitein, this might be the physician Makārim b. Isḥāq who sent a petition to the Ayyubid sultan, accompanied by recommendations from two of his personal physicians, to receive a lifetime appointment in the hospital of Cairo with the salary of three dinars per month.[317] Maybe the same person as Makārim al-Kaḥḥāl.

Makārim al-Kaḥḥāl [Eg., 12th–13th centuries]

An ophthalmologist, appeared in the list of taxpayers or donors for a fund-raising, redemption of captives, etc. Also in the list are al-Nafīs al-Sharābī, (anonymous) al-Wajīh ('honourable') al-Ṭabīb, (anonymous) al-Sheikh al-Muhadhdhab al-Ṭabīb, Abū al-Faraj b. al-Nashādirī, Abū al-ʿIzz al-Kaḥḥāl, Abū al-Thanāʾ and Abū Naṣr al-Sadīd.[318] Maybe the same person as Makārim b. Isḥāq b. Makārim.

Makārim Ṭabīb [Eg. 13th century]

A physician, mentioned in a document written by Solomon b. Elijah,[319] and in a document alongside Abū al-Ḥasan ʿAṭṭār, Abū ʿImrān ʿAṭṭār, Mufaḍḍ[al] Ṭabīb and Abū al-ʿIzz Ṭabīb.[320]

Makīn (al-Sheikh) al-Ṭabīb [Eg., 13th century]

A physician, relative of al-Sheikh al-Bakr, mentioned in a document from the thirteenth century.[321]

Manṣūr b. Abī al-Futūḥ b. Abī al-Ḥasan (Elazar b. Judah b. Japheth he-Levi) [Eg., Cairo, 12th–13th centuries]

A physician, said to have given his son 'charity' – a house on Chain Street in the Mamṣūṣa quarter in Fusṭāṭ.[322]

Marwān (Abū al-Walīd) Ibn Janāḥ al-Qurṭubī (R. Jonah Marinus) [An., Cordova, Lucena, Saragossa, 10th–11th centuries]

A Jewish intellectual, grammarian (Spanish Hebrew), Hebrew lexicographer and physician (985/990–1040). He was an expert in logic, and was talented in Arabic and Hebrew linguistics. Born at Cordova or Lucena, a song that was dedicated to him teaches us that he had at least one son.[323] Ibn Janāḥ was educated in Lucena, where he studied interpretations of the Bible and the Quran in Arabic, Hebrew and Aramaic, as well as traditional Rabbinical sources. He returned to Cordova, where he apparently studied medicine, which provided him with a livelihood throughout his life. Ibn Janāḥ left Cordova when it was besieged by the Berbers (1012–13), and settled, after much wandering, in Saragossa, where he practised medicine for the rest of his life.[324] In a letter to a friend, sent from Cordova, he explained Biblical phrases and referred to the deportation of Jews from Cordova to Saragossa following the Berbers' rebellion. In Saragossa, he worked with Menahem b. al-Fawwāl, who was also a physician and scholar of logic.[325] Ibn Abī Uṣaybiʿa mentioned that Ibn Janāḥ was interested in logic and had an extensive knowledge of Arabic and Hebrew philology, and ascribed to him a book, *Kitāb al-Talkhīṣ* ('The Book of Commentary'), which was a medical dictionary that dealt with simple drugs and weights and measurements that were used in medicine. The dictionary, which contained about 830 columns and hundreds of synonyms in different languages,[326] was frequently cited by later authors. Ibn Janāḥ was one of the most prominent Jewish authors of the time and contributed to the field of herbal medicine research. But the popularity of his dictionary dropped towards the end of the thirteenth century, when more detailed dictionaries appeared.[327] Several historians have declared the book as lost, but in fact there is a copy of it in Istanbul.[328] In the front page it is noted that Ibn Janāḥ wrote the book at the request of one of his 'brothers' in Saragossa, apparently referring to the request of another physician or another Jew, possibly Menahem b. al-Fawwāl or Abū al-Faḍl (Ḥasday b. Joseph b. Ḥasday), who were both active at the time in Saragossa. It is also documented in his book that in his search for information on drugs he consulted with tanners, pharmacists, physicians and even sorcerers and wandered in and around Saragossa to collect minerals and herbs.[329]

In Saragossa, Ibn Janāḥ formed a circle of young scholars interested in linguistic questions. Ibn Janāḥ was a scholar who made the quest for truth the sacred duty of his life.[330] His main works were *Kitāb al-Mustalḥaq* ('The Book of Criticism'), *Risālat al-Tanbīh* ('The Book of Admonition'), *Kitāb/Risālat al-Taqrīb wa al-Tashīl* ('The Epistle of Bringing Near and Making Easy'), *Kitāb al-Taswiya* ('The Book of Rebuke'), *Kitāb al-Tashwīr* ('The Book of Shaming') and *Kitāb al-Tanqīḥ* ('The Book of Minute Research'). In the shaping of Hebrew philology, Ibn Janāḥ's influence has no parallel in extent, depth and persistence. He was already mentioned by a few scholars of the eleventh century. Thus, from the twelfth century some or all of his works were known not only to philologists, and to writers who had recourse to philology, but also to exegetes, both Rabbanites and Karaites, whether they wrote in Arabic or Hebrew.[331]

Māsarjawayh [Iq., Basra, 7th–8th centuries]

An Aramaic Jewish physician (683–750), practised at Basra as the physician of the Umayyad caliph ʿUmar b. ʿAbd al-ʿAzīz (r. 717–20).[332] He was among the first to translate writings into Arabic and was one of the main figures in the translation enterprise.[333] Māsarjawayh was knowledgeable in medicine and according to Ibn Abī Uṣaybiʿa, it was he who translated *Kunnāsh Aaron*, one of the ancient medical books, from Syriac to Muslim Arabic. According to Ibn Juljul al-Andalusī, Māsarjawayh lived in the time of the Umayyads and was appointed to translate the book for them during Marwān b. al-Ḥākam's rule. The book was kept in a bookcase until ʿUmar b. ʿAbd al-ʿAzīz, when ruler, found it in the library and ordered it to be presented publicly so that all Muslims could benefit from it.[334] According to the Arabic sources, when Māsarjawayh translated *Kunnāsh Aaron*, he added two articles of which only a few copies have survived. Based on these articles, Māsarjawayh was considered, apart from being the first translator of medical books into Arabic, also the first writer in the field of Arabic medicine. A number of writers and physicians relied on these copies, including al-Rāzī in his book *al-Ḥāwī fī al-Ṭibb* and ʿAlī b. Sahl Rabban al-Ṭabarī in his book *Firdaus al-Ḥikma*. Among the physicians who quoted *Kunnāsh Aaron* using Māsarjawayh's translation were Ibn Sīnā, al-Bīyrūnī, al-Qalānisī and Ibn al-Bayṭār. Among Māsarjawayh's writings, we should mention *Kitāb Quwwā al-Aṭʿima wa-Manāfiʿihā wa-Maḍārihā* ('The Power of Food, Its Benefits and Demerits') and *Kitāb Quwwā al-Aqāqīr wa-Manāfiʿihā wa-Maḍārihā* ('The Power of Drugs, Their Benefits and Demerits').[335]

Masīḥ b. Ḥakam al-Dimashqī (ʿIsa) [Iq., 8th–9th centuries]

A physician in the court of Hārūn al-Rashīd (r. 786–809). Ibn Abī Uṣaybiʿa mentioned that he, his father, and his grandfather were Christian, but Tzvi Langermann claimed that Masīḥ apparently belonged to a Judaeo-Christian sect, the ʿIsawiyya. Masīḥ was the author of a medical text named *al-Risāla al-Hārūniyya*. In the introduction to this text, Masīḥ mentioned that it is based on three authorities – Hippocrates, Galen and Falaṭīs the Indian. Masīḥ's medical writings deal with a variety of subjects in the philosophy of nature with metaphysical and religious implications.[336] There are three references to Masīḥ in Jewish writings, among them a collection of chemical and alchemical prescriptions written in Judaeo-Arabic,[337] some of which are attributed to Masīḥ b. Ḥakīm, and a quote from Masīḥ's 'Kunnāsh' which appeared in the medical dictionary of Jonah b. Janāḥ.[338]

Maṣlīaḥ [Sy., Harran, 12th–13th centuries]

A physician from Harran. Al-Ḥarīzī described him thus (*sic*): 'There the physician R. Matsliaḥ (Succeeds) arose by wisdom's stream this blessed lily blows; he cries, yea, roars, prevails against his foes.'[339]

Me᾽ir (Abū al-Ḥasan) Ibn Qamni᾽el [An., Saragossa, Seville, Mo., Marrakesh, 11th–12th centuries]

Me᾽ir b. Isaac Aldabi [An., Toledo, EY, Jerusalem, 14th century]

A physician and religious philosopher, born in Toledo (probably 1310). He was a son of Isaac Aldabi ha-Ḥasid, and grandson of Asher Ben Jehiel. He received a comprehensive education in Biblical and Rabbinic literature, and afterwards he turned to philosophical and scientific studies. He left Toledo in 1348 and settled in Jerusalem, where, in 1360, he finished his work *Shevilei Emunah* ('Paths of Faith').[340] Aldabi wrote his book in the belief, prevalent in the Middle Ages, that the Greek philosophers (especially Plato and Aristotle) derived the essentials of their knowledge from Jewish sources. He determined to assemble the documents of ancient Jewish wisdom scattered throughout the various works of the philosophers and natural scientists and to trace them back to their original sources. The book is merely a compilation of subjects and theories, some of them translated by him from foreign languages, and culled from different works. He borrowed mainly from Hebrew literature and to some extent, particularly in the fields of medicine and astronomy, from Muslim Arabic literature. Aldabi's book is divided into ten 'paths' (*netivot*), of which the second deals with the creation of the world, geography and astronomy and the elements; the third with the creation of man and family life; the fourth with embryology, anatomy and human physiology (a digest of the accepted theories on anatomy and physiology in medieval medicine, presented on the basis of the comparison between the microcosm and the macrocosm); the fifth with the rules for physical and 'spiritual' hygiene (on the nature of anger, joy and the like); and the sixth with the nature and faculties of the soul.[341]

Menahem [Eg., Cairo, 13th century]

A physician, wrote to Abraham Maimonides about his experiences travelling to Tanān village (close to Cairo) to visit a patient.[342]

Menahem ha-Kohen ha-Rōfē b. Zadok [Eg., 11th–12th centuries]

A physician, the uncle of Yaḥyā ha-Kohen ha-Rōfē b. Mevōrākh, active at the end of the eleventh and beginning of the twelfth centuries.[343]

Menahem Ṭabīb [Eg., 13th century]

A physician, mentioned in a document probably written by Emanuel b. Yechiel (13th century). Also mentioned are Abū al-Rabī' 'Aṭṭār, al-Rashīd b. al-'Ajamī 'Aṭṭār, Rashīd Ṭabīb and al-Thiqa Ṭabīb.[344]

Mevōrākh ha-Rōfē [K., 12th century]

A Karaite physician, mentioned in a memorial list.[345]

R. Mishael ha-Rōfē [Eg., Cairo, 11th century]

Moses b. Abraham b. Sa'adya [K., Eg., Alexandria, Cairo, 15th century]

Moses b. Abraham b. Sa'adya ha-Rōfē Dar'ī [K., Eg., Alexandria, 11th–12th centuries]

Moses (Abū Sa'd) b. Nethanel ha-Levi [Eg., Cairo, 12th century]

Moses b. Peraḥya b. Yijū [Si., Mazara, Eg., Minyat Ziftā, Minyat Ghamr, 13th century]

A physician, had at least two brothers and a sister. He was a *dayyān* in Minyat Ziftā and Minyat Ghamr and there are many documents and letters written by him between 1220 and 1234, including a correspondence with Abraham Maimonides. Moses' family left Tunisia in 1148 and settled in Mazara, a port city located on the southern shore of Sicily. Peraḥya, Moses' older brother, mentioned him in a letter which tells the story of a trip they both took to

Egypt. After many hardships the two arrived at their destination and later on they were joined by their family members.[346] Moses b. Peraḥya is mentioned in a letter from R. Hananel, a relative of Abraham Maimonides. In another letter, Me᾽ir Ibn al-Hamadhānī asked Moses 'ha-Shōfēṭ, al-Sheikh al-Sadīd' to accept his son as a student. It is possible that his handwriting appeared on the verso of a collection of funds (1225–6).[347]

Moses b. Yerushalayim ha-Kohen [Eg., Cairo, 14th–15th centuries]
A physician, mentioned in a bill from about 1409, written in Judaeo-Arabic, which was preserved in the community archive in Cairo. Also mentioned are the physicians David b. Jacob and Ṣadaqa b. Abraham ha-Kohen.[348] In the bill it is mentioned that because of a debt that the community of Cairo held, the *parnāsim* (community leaders) sold to David a third of the ownership rights of the land the community had. On the margins of the bill an addition has been written where it is mentioned that Ṣadaqa, Moses and others have arrived at David's house and received a hypothecation that they gave him as a deposit.[349]

Moses ha-Rōfē [Eg., 12th–13th centuries]
A physician, had already passed away by 1232. He had a son named Abū al-Bahā᾽.[350]

Moses ha-Rōfē 2 [Eg., 11th century]
A physician, his son, Abraham, is signed on a 'remains of a guardianship' bill (1056). In that year Moses was no longer among the living. In the bill Yeshū῾ā ha-Rōfē b. Aaron al-῾Ammānī is also mentioned.[351]

Moses ha-Rōfē 3 [EY, Jerusalem, 16th century]
A physician, the official representative of Jacob ha-Rōfē 2 together with Samuel ha-Rōfē. The three of them are mentioned in a document of the Muslim court from 8 January 1550.[352]

Moses ha-Rōfē b. Isaac ha-Rōfē [Eg., Alexandria, 11th–12th centuries]
A physician of the Tarifi family. He was a member of the circle of the Karaite physician and poet Moses b. Abraham b. Sa῾adya ha-Rōfē Dar῾ī, who dedicated a wedding song to him.[353]

Moses Rōfē [Eg., 16th century]
A physician who lived in Egypt and was apparently also a merchant.[354]

R. Moses Vidalish ha-Rōfē [EY, Jerusalem, 15th–16th centuries]
A physician, mentioned in a will he edited (1502). At the beginning of the sixteenth century, apparently, he moved to Jerusalem where he acquired many assets.[355]

Mubārak b. Salāma b. Mubārak b. Raḥmūn b. Abū al-Khayr [Eg., 12th century]

Mubārak ha-Rōfē [Eg., 11th century]
A physician, mentioned in the margins of a document, where it is said that he was buried on 18 November 1050.[356]

Mufaḍḍ(al) Ṭabīb [Eg., 13th century]
A physician, mentioned in a document alongside Abū al-Ḥasan ʿAṭṭār, Abū ʿImrān ʿAṭṭār, Makārim Ṭabīb and Abū al-ʿIzz Ṭabīb.[357]

Mufaḍḍal al-Mashmīʿa [Eg., Cairo, 13th century]
A physician, appeared in a list of future donors from the time of Abraham Maimonides alongside Mawli al-Muhadhdhab, (anonymous) Awlād al-Raʾīs, (anonymous) al-Gaon al-Munā, al-Sheikh Joseph, another al-Sheikh Joseph and his son, Ibn al-Julājilī, R. Yeshūʿā, Abū al-Maʿānī 2, Najīb Kohen Kamukhī, al-Rabīb Kohen, al-Taqī Ibn al-Gadal, Makārim Ibn al-Gadalī and Abū al-Maʿānī.[358]

Mufaḍḍal b. Mājīd b. Abī al-Bishr al-ʾIsrāʾīlī (al-Kātib) [13th century]
A physician, known through Ḥājī Khalīfa and some manuscripts, among them a medical poem written in 1268 named *Arjūza fī al-Ṭibb* and a work named *Naqʿ al-Ghalal wa-Nafʿ al-ʿIlal* ('Breaking/Quenching the Thirst for Medical Knowledge and the Benefit of Drinking for the Second Time'). According to Ashtor he also wrote an educational poem on the wisdom of medicine (*manẓūma*) in the *rajaz* style, which is customary for this purpose, and this is the reason his essay is called *Arjūza fī al-Ṭibb*. The essay is divided into short chapters which are dedicated to anatomy, diseases and healing methods. The essay was preserved in several manuscripts. In one manuscript that was preserved in the al-Khālidī family's library in Jerusalem, the author

is called al-Miṣrī and from this we learn he came from Egypt or lived there. In the Paris manuscript, which maybe the autograph, the date in which it was written is found, 1268–9.[359]

al-Muhadhdhab [Eg., Minyat Ziftā, 13th century]

A physician, known only by his honorific title (the accomplished). He was mentioned in a letter to Abraham b. David, the grandson of Abraham Maimonides, in which a struggle was described between him and the physician al-Sadīd over a key position in the community. The two were supported by different groups in the town. Al-Muhadhdhab and his supporters stopped going to the synagogue.[360]

Munā al-Ṭabīb [Eg., 12th century]

A physician, mentioned in a document from the 1140s.[361]

Munajjā al-Ṭabīb b. Hiba [Eg., 12th century]

A physician, mentioned in a document from 1185.[362]

Munajjam (Menahem) b. al-Fawwāl [An., Saragossa, 11th century]

One of the most important Jewish physicians in Andalusia. He lived and practised at Saragossa during the Moorish period in Spain. Menahem wrote a book, *al-Adawiya al-Mufrada* ('On the Simple Drugs'), and another on innovations regarding the measurements and weights used in medicine, and drugs dosages. He also dealt with astronomy and philosophy, but mainly logic. He wrote a work named *Kanz al-Muqal*, edited in a style of questions and answers on the rules of logic and the principles of nature. Marwān Ibn Janāḥ, a physician and scholar of logic, was practising medicine and living in Saragossa parallel to Menahem.[363]

Mūsā b. ʿAbd Allāh al-ʾIsrāʾīlī al-Qurṭubī (Moses b. Maimon; Maimonides) [An., Cordova, Mo., Fez, Eg., Cairo 12th–13th centuries]

Mūsā b. Abī al-Faḍāʾil (Moses b. Jekuthiel ha-Rōfē) [An., Eg., 11th–12th centuries]

Mūsā b. Elʿāzār al-ʾIsrāʾīlī (Moses b. Elazar) [It, Oria, M., Qayrawān, Eg. Cairo, 10th century]

Mūsā b. Ifrāʾīm b. Dāʾūd b. Ifrāʾīm b. Yaʿqūb (Ibn Jumayʿ al-ʾIsrāʾīlī al-Ṭabīb) [Eg., Cairo, 14th–15th centuries]

Mūsā b. Isrāʾīl [Iq., Kūfa, 8th century]
A physician, served the Abbasid caliph al-Mahdī (745–95).[364]

Mūsā b. Kūjik (Sharaf al-Dīn) [K., Eg., Sy., 14th century, convert]

Mūsā b. Sayyār [Iq., Baghdad, 10th century]
A Jewish physician.[365]

Mūsā (Abū al-Imrān) b. Yaʿqūb b. Isḥāq al-ʾIsrāʾīlī [Eg., 11th century]

Musallam al-Ṭabīb [Eg., 12th century]
A physician, mentioned in a document (1185), where it was said that his son, Abū al-Barakāt, was marrying Sitt al-ʿAlam b. Nethanel (the fifth).[366]

Muwaffaq al-Dawla Abū al-Faraj ʿAlī b. Abī al-Shujāʿ al-Hamadānī [Ir., Hamadān, 11th–12th centuries]

al-Muwaffaq al-Kohen al-Ṭabīb [Eg., 13th century]
A physician, mentioned in a list of donors, along with Ben bū ʿ[...]ā al-Ṭabīb, Abū al-Riḍā al-ʿAṭṭār and Abū al-Khayr al-ʿAṭṭār.[367]

al-Muwaffaq al-Qaṣīr al-Ṭabīb al-Yahūdī [Sy., Damascus, 13th–14th centuries]
A physician, practised at the big market (*al-sūq al-kabīr*). He was mentioned as the one who fixed the sight problem of his Muslim friend al-Sheikh al-Ṣāliḥ Sharaf al-Dīn Maḥmūd, who was a Ḥadith scholar (c.1300). Fluid was leaking from Sharaf al-Dīn Maḥmūd's eyes; he was blinded in one of them and his sight was weakening in the other. Al-Muwaffaq al-Qaṣīr treated his Muslim friend with medicines mentioned by Ibn al-Bayṭār. He collected all the medicinal drugs Ibn al-Bayṭār mentioned for drying leakages from the eye and prepared a remedy that improved the patient's condition and strengthened his vision.[368]

Nafīs b. Dāʾūd b. ʿAnān al-Tabrīzī [K., Ir., Iq., Baghdad, Eg., Cairo, 14th century, convert]

Naḥman ha-Rōfē [Sy., Aleppo, 11th century]
A physician, active in Aleppo around 1030.[369]

al-Naʿja al-Ṭabīb [Eg., 11th century]
A physician; his grandson, Zikrī b. Musallam b. al-Naʿja al-Ṭabīb, is mentioned in a document.[370]

Najīb al-Dawla [Ir., Tabriz, 13th–14th centuries, convert]
A physician and ophthalmologist, practising in the court of Tabriz (the physician of Ghāzān Khān). He was in touch with the physician Rashīd al-Dīn. In 1305, a number of Jewish physicians in Tabriz, apparently under Najīb al-Dawla's leadership, intended to become Muslims. They were asked to demonstrate their conversion by eating a dish of camel meat cooked in milk, a test attributed to Rashīd al-Dīn.[371] Muslim sources mentioned that during Syria's conquest by the Mongols in 1300, Ibn Taymiyya met up with the high ranks of the Mongol state (in order to relieve the suffering of the inhabitants of Syria). Among these high ranks were al-Najīb al-Kaḥḥāl (the ophthalmologist – probably the same person as Najīb al-Dawla) al-Yahūdī, Saʿd al-Dīn, Rashīd al-Dīn, Faḍl Allāh and Naṣīr al-Dīn al-Ṭūsī.[372]

Najīb Kohen Kamukhī [Eg., Cairo, 13th century]
A physician, appeared in a list of future donors from the time of Abraham Maimonides alongside several other physicians: (anonymous) al-Mawlī al-Muhadhdhab, (anonymous) Awlād al-Raʾīs, (anonymous) al-Gaon al-Munā, Mufaḍḍal al-Mashmiʿa, al-Sheikh Joseph, another al-Sheikh Joseph and his son, Ibn al-Julājilī, R. Yeshūʿā, Abū al-Maʿānī 2, al-Rabīb Kohen, al-Taqī Ibn al-Gadal, Makārim Ibn al-Gadalī and Abū al-Maʿānī.[373]

al-Najīb al-Ṭabīb b. al-Ḥāvēr b. Abū al-Mufaḍḍal [Eg., 13th century]
A physician, appeared in a list of donors and their donations (c.1210), with several other practitioners.[374]

Nathan of Damascus [Sy., Damascus, Crete, Candia, 15th century]

R. Nehorai [Sy., Tiberias, 12th century]
A physician and a pharmacist. He is mentioned in a pilgrim work (1174–87).[375]

Nethanel b. Abraham [Eg., al-Maḥalla, 12th century]
A physician, mentioned in a letter from Mevōrākh b. Nathan b. Samuel, who recommended that the young cantor Abū al-Bayān, during his visit to the Rif, should collect contributions to pay his poll tax.[376]

Nethanel b. Joseph ha-Sar ha-Nikhbād ha-Rōfē [Eg., 12th century]
A physician, mentioned in a memorial list[377] from the twelfth century.

Nethanel b. Moses [Eg., Cairo, 13th century]
A physician, active in Cairo c.1235, was closely associated with the courtiers in Egypt who hired the court physicians.[378]

Nethanel ha-Rōfē [Eg., 12th century]
A physician, his name is mentioned in a memorial list.[379]

R. Nethanel ha-Rōfē b. Abraham [Eg., 14th century]

Nethanel ha-Rōfē b. Joseph b. al-Malī [An., Saragossa, 13th century]
A physician and translator. He translated part of Maimonides' *Mishne Torah* from Arabic to Hebrew. Nethanel testified about himself that he was not very knowledgeable in the Talmud because of his practising medicine, but he dedicated himself to it.[380]

Nethanel ha-Rōfē ha-Sar Nikhbād ha-Yeshiva [Eg., 12th century]
A physician, mentioned in a document from the 1140s.[381]

Nethanel ha-Rōfē Tifēret ha-Rōfēim [Eg., 12th century]
A physician, mentioned in a memorial list.[382]

Nethanel ha-Sar ha-Yaqar ha-Rōfē [Eg., Cairo, 13th century]
A physician, mentioned in a letter (1218) in which he gave the recipients permission to use, as they saw fit, the medical materials which were mentioned from the store of Solomon ha-Levi, who had passed away. The names of the materials and their weights were also mentioned.[383]

Nuʿmān b. Abī al-Riḍā b. Sālim b. Isḥāq [Sy., 13th–14th centuries]
A physician, known for his commentaries on a famous medical book composed of a hundred chapters. He was the teacher of the Muslim ophthalmologist

Ṣalāḥ al-Dīn Ibn Yūsuf al-Ḥamawī.[384] According to Steinschneider, he lived probably around 1280.[385]

Obadia b. Ṣadaqa ha-Rōfē [Eg.]
A physician, mentioned in a document.[386]

Obadia ha-Rōfē [Sy., ?Tripoli, 13th–14th centuries]

Obadia Kahana ha-Rōfē [Eg., Cairo, 16th century]
A physician, served as the head of the Mustaʿarabi Jews in Cairo until 1594–5. His widow is mentioned in the notebook of the treasurer of the *waqf* of the community, where it is recorded that she continued to receive support from the *waqf* treasury after Obadia had died (no later than 1595).[387]

Petahya ha-Levi ha-Rōfē [K., Sy., Damascus, 13th century]

Pinḥas [Sy., Aleppo, 12th–13th centuries]
A physician, mentioned in al-Ḥarīzī's journeys thus: 'There, too, lives the eminent sage and doctor Master Pinḥas, few so great, a man most generous with his estate'.[388]

Rabīb ha-Rōfē [Eg., 11th century]
A physician, mentioned in a letter written by Samuel b. Joseph Yijū to his brothers, Peraḥya and Moses. Rabīb was respected in Sicily and had a personal relationship with the *nagid* of Egypt.[389]

al-Rabīb Kohen [Eg., Cairo, 13th century]
A physician, mentioned in a list of future donors from the period of Abraham Maimonides. Other physicians in the list are (anonymous) al-Mawlī al-Muhadhdhab, (anonymous) Awlād al-Raʾīs, (anonymous) al-Gaon al-Munā, Mufaḍḍal al-Mashmiʿa, al-Sheikh Joseph, another al-Sheikh Joseph and his son, Ibn al-Julājilī, R. Yeshūʿā, Abū al-Maʿānī 2, Najīb Kohen Kamukhī, al-Taqī Ibn al-Gadal, Makārim Ibn al-Gadalī and Abū al-Maʿānī.[390]

Raḍī b. Elijah b. Zechariah (the judge) [Eg., Cairo, 12th–13th centuries]

Rashīd [Eg., 13th century]
A man called Rashīd, who was apparently a physician, received wine as a gift from Solomon b. Elijah.[391]

Rashīd al-Dīn al-Ṭabīb Faḍl Allāh b. al-Dawla, Abū al-Khayr b. ʿAlī Abū al-Hamadānī [Ir., Tabriz, 13th–14th centuries]

Rashīd Ṭabīb [Eg., 13th century]
A physician, mentioned in a document probably written by Emanuel b. Yechiel (mid-13th century). Also mentioned are Abū al-Rabīʿ ʿAṭṭār, al-Rashīd b. al-ʿAjamī ʿAṭṭār, al-Thiqa Ṭabīb and Menahem Ṭabīb.[392]

Saʿd (ʿIzz al-Dawla) b. Manṣūr b. Kammūna [Iq., Baghdad, 13th century]
A philosopher and physician (d. 1284). He is mainly known for his philosophical Arabic writings. He wrote many scientific treatises on medicine, chemistry, philosophy and religion. A book he wrote about eye diseases was quoted by the Egyptian ophthalmologist Ṣadaqa al-Shādhilī (14th century).[393] Saʿd was a fervent advocate of Judaism and condemned his contemporaries who had abandoned it, led by many different motives. He also presented a critical approach towards Islam in his works, which led to a rise against him, from the Muslim side, and a call to execute him. He was saved thanks to the governor of Baghdad, who smuggled him to Hilla, where his son worked as a government official.[394] It is said that he converted to Islam in 1280.[395]

Saʿd al-Dawla b. Ṣafī b. Hibat Allāh b. Muhadhdhib al-Dawla al-Abharī [Ir., Abhar, 13th century]
A physician from Abhar, western Iran (d. 1291). In Persian and Arabic sources, he is mostly referred to as 'Saʿd al-Dawla, the Jew'.[396] He first worked as an agent (*dallāl*) in the markets of Mosul, from where he moved to Baghdad and served as the financial supervisor of the ʿAḍudī hospital. He was dismissed from his job but later on was appointed the deputy to the Mongolian military governor of the city, and in 1287 he became its financial administrator. He lost this job as well because of complaints. Shortly afterwards he was appointed the personal physician of Arghūn Khān, the ruler of the Īl-Khānate dynasty (r. 1284–91), in the dynasty's capital, Tabriz. Saʿd al-Dawla found favour in Arghūn's eyes, both as a physician and as a person; this eventually led to his appointment as a *wazīr*, in charge of whole Īl-Khānate empire. In this capacity he ruled over large areas, and made sure to appoint, as was customary, those once closely associated with him to key positions in the administration. Among these was his relative Abū Manṣūr Muhadhdhab al-Dawla, who

was also a physician.[397] His appointment, and appointing his Jewish relatives to key positions ruling over the Muslim community, together with his success in raising funds, created opposition and hatred towards him among the Mongolian elite and the population in general. These elements took advantage of Arghūn's approaching death and Saʿd al-Dawla was executed on 10 March 1291, following accusations of poisoning Arghūn. Arghūn died five days later. After his murder there were anti-Jewish commotions in some of the cities, which ended only after the authorities intervened.[398]

Saʿadya [K., Eg., 14th–15th centuries]

Saʿadya 2 [Eg., 12th century]
A physician, mentioned in a memorial list as the brother of Japheth.[399]

Saʿadya b. Mevōrākh [Eg., 11th century]

Saʿadya ha-Rōfē Darʿī [K., Eg., Alexandria, 11th century]

Ṣadaqa [K., Eg., Cairo, 15th century]
A respected Karaite physician, mentioned with regard to a quarrel which took place between the Rabbanites and the Karaites in 1465, during which the Rabbinic Jews turned to the Muslim authorities with a complaint against the Karaites. At the end both the Karaites and the Rabbinic Jews had to pay a thousand Ashrafī dinars. The fine was eventually cancelled following the efforts of representatives from both groups in front of the Muslim seniors. The physician Ṣadaqa was the representative for the Karaites, so it seems his status was high among the authorities. He was sent to the emir Qānim (d. 1466), in order to be the advocate on their behalf to the sultan.[400]

Ṣadaqa al-ʾIsrāʾīlī [Sy., Damascus, 12th–13th centuries]

Ṣadaqa al-Ṭabīb [Eg., 12th–13th centuries]
A physician, mentioned in a document (c.1180–1203). In the same document are also mentioned the son of Abū Saʿd al-ʿAṭṭār 2 and al-Sadīd al-Ṭabīb.[401]

Ṣadaqa b. ʿAbd al-Qāhir [Eg., Cairo, 14th century]
A physician, in 1356 he made a copy of the book *Kitāb al-Irshād li-Maṣāliḥ al-Anfus wa-l-Ajsād* by Abū al-Makārim Abū al-Hibat-Allāh b. Zayn b. Ḥasan b. Ephraim b. Yaʿqūb b. Ismāʿīl Ibn Jumayʿ al-ʾIsrāʾīlī.[402]

Ṣadaqa b. Abraham ha-Kohen [Eg., Cairo, 15th century]

A physician, mentioned in a bill (c.1409) kept in the community archive in Cairo. Also mentioned are the physicians David b. Jacob and Moses b. Yerushalayim ha-Kohen.[403] In the bill it is mentioned that following a debt he had to the Cairo community, the *parnāsim* sold David a third of his ownership rights over land that the community had, and in the margins of the bill it was added that Ṣedaqa, Moses and others had arrived at David's house and received from him a mortgage which they had deposited with him.[404]

Ṣadaqa (al-Faḍl) b. Munajjā b. Ṣadaqa al-Sāmirī al-Ṭabīb (Ibn al-Shāʿir) [S., Sy., Damascus, Ḥarrān, 13th century]

A Samaritan physician (d. 1232),[405] according to Max Meyerhof 'the best of the Samaritan physicians'.[406] He was the physician of the Ayyubid sultan al-Ashraf Mūsā b. al-ʿĀdil b. Ayyūb, who ruled Ḥarrān, Baalbek and Damascus (d. 1237), and received from him a fixed monthly allowance and various grants. Ṣadaqa served the sultan until he died; he left many properties, and over ten thousand books and manuscripts. He did not have any children.[407] Ṣadaqa wrote many medical books (for example a commentary on Hippocrates and answers to questions asked by Asʿad al-Dīn (Ibn Ṣabra) al-Maḥallī al-Mutaṭabbib (Jacob b. Isaac)). He also wrote about philosophy, a commentary on the Homesh and Arabic poems.[408]

Ṣadaqa ha-Rōfē [Eg., 12th century]

Ṣadaqa ha-Rōfē is mentioned in a memorial list, he had two sons: Elijah and Aaron.[409]

al-Sadīd [Eg., Minyat Ziftā, 13th century]

A physician, known only by his honorific title (the sound). He was mentioned in a letter to Abraham b. David, the grandson of Abraham Maimonides, in which a struggle was described between him and the physician al-Muhadhdhab over a key position in the community. The two were supported by different groups in the town. Al-Muhadhdhab and his supporters stopped going to the synagogue.[410]

al-Sadīd al-Dimyāṭī al-Ṭabīb al-Yahūdī [K. Eg., Cairo, 13th–14th century]

al-Sadīd al-Ṭabīb [Eg., 12th–13th centuries]

Saʿīd al-Dawla Abū al-Fakhr [K, Eg., 13th century]

Samuel [Eg., Cairo, 12th century]
A physician, the recipient of a letter written by Isaac b. Ṣadaqa from Tripoli (1136). In the letter Isaac thanks Samuel for paying a ransom when he was held captive by the Normans in Tunisia.[411]

Samuel b. Elazar ha- Rōfē [Eg., Alexandria, Qūṣ, 13th century]
A physician from Alexandria, he was active in Qūṣ around 1231, as we learn from the colophon of a book that he copied there that year.[412]

Samuel b. Jacob b. Japheth b. Moses [K., Eg., 15th century]
A Karaite physician, he completed copying the book *al-Murshid* by Samuel b. Moses (Samuel b. Solomon al-Maghribī) in 1435, a year after it had been written. In a private letter that was written around 1400, al-Muwaffaq Yaʿqūb al-Iksandrī and his son Samuel are mentioned – most probably this is Samuel b. Jacob, who was at the time still young, and therefore did not receive the honorary title a physician deserved.[413]

Samuel b. Japheth al-Rashīd [Eg., 13th century]
A physician, mentioned in a document (1225).[414]

Samuel b. Saʿdūn [Eg., 15th century]
A physician, wrote a response to the book by Samuel b. Solomon al-Maghribī (around 1434) which dealt with legal subjects.[415]

Samuel b. Solomon al-Maghribī [K., Eg., Cairo, 14th–15th centuries]
A physician and *dayyān*, called by some sources Samuel b. Moses, wrote a number of essays on religious subjects and was criticised by Samuel b. Saʿdūn, who was also a physician. In 1434, he completed a book called *al-Murshid* ('The Guide', i.e. to religious laws). This book is essentially a collection of materials but is distinct because of the clear organisation of the material and is also important because it preserves forgotten Karaite writings that are included in it. Samuel was the last Karaite to write a complete book of laws (legal codes), of this type, in Arabic.[416] Ashtor referred to this physician, but under the name: Samuel b. Moses b. Yeshūʿā al-Maghribī. He is also men-

tioned as Samuel b. Moses b. Yeshūʿā b. Mordechai b. Amram b. Solomon b. Amram. In addition to this essay, Samuel wrote an article on death, *piyyutim*, and a book dealing with the history of the Temple Mount from the binding of Isaac to the time of the author and also the future to come.[417]

Samuel ha-Kohen [K., Eg., Cairo, 15th century]
A Karaite (according to Ashtor) physician, mentioned in a *maqāma* by Moses Abraham b. Saʿadya, who said that Samuel wrote beautiful songs on Biblical phrases. Ashtor claimed that he should not be identified with Samuel b. Jacob b. Japheth b. Moses.[418]

Samuel ha-Kohen ha-Rōfē [Eg., 11th–12th centuries]
A physician, probably from Alexandria, mentioned in the *dīwān* of Moses b. Abraham b. Saʿadya ha-Rōfē Darʿī, a Karaite physician from Alexandria. Also included in Moses Darʿī's circle of friends (i.e., mentioned in his *dīwān*) are Moses ha-Rōfē b. Isaac ha-Rōfē, Isaac ha-Rōfē, Moses ha-Levi, Elijah b. Samuel and Samuel b. Elijah al-Sinnī.[419]

Samuel ha-Levi b. Solomon [Eg., 13th century]
A physician, mentioned in a letter (1211) whose writers ask Samuel to help them cancel the decree by Abraham Maimonides that forbids saying *piyyutim* in prayer. Scholars disagree regarding the source of the letter, but it is reasonable to assume that it came from the Alexandria community.[420]

R. Samuel ha-Levi ha-Zāqēn (R. Samuel b. Ḥakīm) [Eg., Cairo, EY, Jerusalem, 16th century]
A physician, practised medicine in Cairo and purchased property in Jerusalem. In the first half of the sixteenth century, he immigrated to Eretz-Israel and was among the rabbis of Jerusalem.[421]

Samuel ha-Nagid b. Hananiah (Abū Manṣūr) [Eg., Cairo, 12th century]

Samuel ha-Rōfē [EY, Jerusalem, 16th century]
A physician, the authorised representative of Jacob ha-Rōfē 2, together with Moses ha-Rōfē 3. The three are mentioned in a document of the Muslim court, from 8 January 1550.[422]

Samuel ha-Rōfē 2 [Sy., Tyre, 13th century]
A physician, mentioned in a chronicle by the Templar of Tyre from which we learn that Samuel lived in the city (1283). He was probably respected within the Jewish community.[423]

Samuel ha-Rōfē Ibn al-ʿAmmānī [Eg., Alexandria, 12th–13th centuries]

Samuel Rakaḥ (Rakakh/Rabakh) [Eg., 14th–15th centuries]
A physician, his son Jacob is mentioned by Meshullam of Volterra (who visited Egypt in 1481), in a list of *dayyānim* of the *nagid* as Solomon b. R. Joseph. Meshullam described Samuel as physician to the sultan and his close associates, an honourable man, very wealthy and active in charity. His son, who sat in the court of the *nagid*, was thirty-five years old. Meshullam wrote highly of both of them.[424]

Samuel Sar ha-Sarīm [Eg., Cairo, 13th century]
A physician. A letter of condolence was sent to him.[425]

Ṣanīʿat al-Malik Abū aṭ-Ṭāhir Ismāʿīl [Eg., Cairo, 13th century]

Ṣaqr (Shaqīr/Shuqayr) al-Ṭabīb [Eg., Cairo, 10th–11th centuries]
A physician, was appointed as the physician of caliph al-Ḥākim bi-Amr Allāh in 1007, replacing the Christian physician Ibn al-Nasṭās al-Naṣrānī (d. 1006). With Ṣaqr's appointment, the caliph heaped wealth and honour upon him: he ordered him to be put on a mule, gave him three mules packed with goods and splendid clothes, and provided him with a furnished and well-equipped house whose value was estimated at 4,000 dinars; the value of all the caliph's gifts to the physicians was estimated at about 10,000 dinars. Ibn Saʿīd described in detail the way in which Ṣaqr was appointed the personal physician of the caliph and the way in which he was informed about it. He also described how all the gifts and possessions granted to him caused the physician to stutter. Interestingly, some of the property was confiscated Christian property. Ṣaqr died in 1009.[426]

R. Sar Shālōm ha-Rōfē b. Abraham b. Jacob [Eg., 14th century]

Seth b. Japheth [Sy., Aleppo, Iq., Ir., 13th century]

A physician and a scribe, wrote an important book on Hebrew grammar and another that contains commentaries, Biblical *midrashim* and *haftarot*. He also wrote an abstract of this book of which a number of manuscripts have been preserved as well as the preface in Arabic, in which Seth b. Japheth mentioned he wrote the abbreviated version (1285) for his two sons: Japheth, who is called al-Najīb Abū al-Muḥāsan, and Moses, who is called al-Shāms ʿAbd al-Laṭīf. We learn from the author that he was from Aleppo and that he also sat in Babylon or Iran.[427]

Shabbetay ha-Rōfē [Eg., Minyat Ziftā, 13th century]

Shabbetay ha-Rōfē's son, Abraham b. Shabbetay ha-Rōfē ha-Sōfer, is mentioned in a colophon of a commentary of R. Hananel. Therefore, Shabbetay was probably active around 1250, in the area of Minyat Ziftā.[428]

Shabbetay ha-Rōfē 2 [Constantine (Algeria) or Constantinople, 12th–13th centuries]

R. Elijah Shabbetay b. ha-Rōfē ha-Sōfer is mentioned in a document. It appears the physician was Shabbetay and not Elijah, and he was a physician and a scribe. He lived in 'Qūnsṭanṭīnā', which is probably Constantine in Algeria, but possibly Constantinople.[429]

Shaḥāda b. Abraham [EY, Jerusalem, 16th century]

A physician, lived in the Jewish neighbourhood in Jerusalem and practised medicine, even before he had completed his professional training. On 25 March 1577, the Muslim *qadi* forbade him to practise surgery and ophthalmology until he learnt the theory of surgery. In later documents (1581–3), Shaḥāda is called al-Kaḥḥāl (the ophthalmologist) and by that time had probably received his formal certification.[430]

al-Sheikh Joseph [Eg., Cairo, 13th century]

Shelah ha-Levi b. Yeshūʿā ha-Levi ha-Rōfē [Eg., 13th century]

A physician, mentioned in a few documents, including a *ketubah* (Jewish marriage agreement) written in Fusṭāṭ in 1289.[431]

Shihāb al-Dīn Aḥmad (Sulaymān) al-Maghribī al-Ishbīlī [Eg., 13th–14th centuries, convert]

Solomon b. Jacob [EY, Jerusalem, 16th century]
A Jewish physician from Jerusalem. He was mentioned in a document (1563) regarding renting his store, which was located next to the Chain Gate, to a Muslim.[432]

Solomon ha-Levi [Eg., 12th century]
A physician, was also a book dealer and a copyist.[433]

Solomon ha-Levi ha-Rōfē b. Abraham ha-Levi [Eg., 13th century]
A physician, mentioned in a document from the thirteenth century.[434]

Solomon ha-Rōfē [Ag., ?14th century]
A physician, signed a note found in the Geniza, probably from the fourteenth century.[435]

Solomon ha-Rōfē 2 [Eg., Cairo, 13th century]
A physician, mentioned in a letter written by his wife and addressed to Solomon the Scribe. Solomon the Scribe left his home to free himself from paying taxes. Solomon ha-Rōfē was asked to intervene in his name.[436]

Solomon ha-Rōfē b. ʿAlī [Eg., 11th century]

Solomon ha-Rōfē b. Rabīʿ [Ma., Qayrawān, 11th century]
A physician, mentioned in a document (1041) where his daughter, Surūra, is claiming alimony from her husband Surūr. Solomon was probably active in Qayrawān, Tunisia. He came from a prominent family of merchants and scholars, which originated from M'Sila (Algeria today). He or his family was named 'al-Jāsūs'.[437]

Solomon ha-Sar ha-Nikhbād ha-Talmīd ha-Rōfē b. Daniel ha-Sar ha-Nikhbād [Eg., Alexandria, 13th century]
A physician, apparently active in Alexandria; he died before 1253.[438]

Solomon (Sulaymān) ha-Sar ha-Rōfē b. [...] ha-Rōfē [Eg., 13th century]
A physician, appeared as one of the witnesses in the testimony of the death of the physician Ibrāhīm al-Mutaṭabbib b. Mukhtār (Ibn al-Yām).[439]

R. Solomon Luria [EY, Jerusalem, 16th century]
A physician, from Lublin, a Torah scholar and a Kabbalist. Around 1520,

when he was about eighty years old, he immigrated to Eretz-Israel and settled in Jerusalem.[440]

Solomon Qāmīs [EY, Safed, 16th century]
A physician, originally from Portugal. He left Portugal and at some point arrived at Safed and from there he continued to Cyprus where he lived for over a decade. He was apparently expelled from Famagusta, Cyprus, by order of the governor in the summer of 1568, together with other Jews.[441]

Solomon Rōfē [Eg., 16th century]
Solomon's son, Abraham b. Solomon Rōfē, appeared in a letter that was sent to Egypt in 1573.[442]

Sukra ('Abd al-Qāhir) al-Yahūdī al-Ḥalabī [Sy., Aleppo, 12th century]

Sulaymān b. ʿAlī [EY, Jerusalem, 16th century]
A physician, lived in the Jewish quarter of Jerusalem. On 4 December 1564, the *qadi* of Jerusalem ordered him to leave the neighbourhood because of inappropriate behaviour.[443]

Sulaymān b. Mūsā al-Yahūdī al-Mutaṭabbib [Eg., Cairo]
A physician at a hospital, was active in Cairo.[444]

Sulaymān Ḥakīm [Eg., Cairo, 13th century]
A physician, was 'Head of the Physicians' in Cairo in the first half of the thirteenth century. He was mentioned in a letter sent from Fusṭāṭ to the *nāsī* Solomon b. Jesse, who was sojourning in Bilbays. The author of the letter wrote that he had become ill and was treated by the chief physician Sulaymān, who was the son-in-law of R. Menahem, the former chief judge of Cairo.[445]

Tābit al-Ṭabīb [Eg., 11th–12th centuries]
A physician, known from a letter he wrote to his daughter Umm al-ʿIzz.[446]

Ṭāhir al-Ṭabīb [Eg., 12th century]
A physician, mentioned in a list of books (c.1157).[447]

al-Taqī b. al-Gadal [Eg., Cairo, 13th century]
A physician, appeared in a list of future donors from the time of Abraham Maimonides alongside several other physicians: (anonymous) al-Mawlī al-

Muhadhdhab, (anonymous) Awlād al-Raʾīs, (anonymous) al-Gaon al-Munā, Mufaḍḍal al-Mashmiʿa, al-Sheikh Joseph, another al-Sheikh Joseph and his son, Ibn al-Julājilī, R. Yeshūʿā, Abū al-Maʿānī 2, Najīb Kohen Kamukhī, al-Rabīb Kohen, Makārim Ibn al-Gadalī and Abū al-Maʿānī.[448]

al-Thiqa (al-Sheikh) al-Ṭabīb, b. al-Sheikh Dāʾūd [Eg., Cairo, 13th century]

A physician and a merchant in the Sūq al-ʿAṭṭārīn.[449] He was mentioned in a document probably written by Emanuel b. Yechiel, along with Abū al-Rabīʿ ʿAṭṭār, al-Rashīd b. al-ʿAjamī ʿAṭṭār, Rashīd Ṭabīb and Menahem Ṭabīb.[450] He might be the recipient of a letter sent to Fusṭāṭ, where apparently he was a permanent resident.[451]

Tiqva ha-Levi ha-Rōfē ha-Sar ha-Nikhbād [Eg., 12th–13th centuries]

Tiqva ha-Rōfē b. Sar Shālōm [Eg., 13th century]

A physician, mentioned in a document with his brother, Berākhōt ha-Rōfē.[452]

Tobias ha-Rōfē b. Japheth [Eg., 12th century]

A physician, wrote a bill of release to women slaves from Cairo (1110).[453]

Yaḥyā Abū Zikrī al-Ṭabīb (Judah b. Moses) [Ma., Qayrawān, 11th century]

A physician and a merchant from Qayrawān, member of a Maghribī family of merchants and scholars (active mainly 1040–90). Judah was mentioned in several letters written by his partner, a Venetian merchant. Other letters sent to him asking for assistance in resolving disputes indicate that he was a man of some standing in the Jewish community. His title, 'al-Ṭabīb', implies he probably practised medicine to some extent.[454]

Yaḥyā b. ʿAbbās al-Maghribī (Judah b. Abūn) [Ma., Fez, Iq., Baghdad, 11th–12th centuries]

Yaḥyā b. Joseph b. Solomon [EY, Jerusalem, 16th century]

A physician, certified by the court of the Ottoman sultan in Constantinople. He specialised in medicine and the intuitive physiognomy theory. On 29 October 1564, following his request, he was permitted to practise medicine in Jerusalem, and also received a fixed salary from the state treasury.[455]

Yaḥyā b. al-Ṣāʾigh [An., Granada, 13th–14th centuries]

A physician, serving in Granada, at the court of Abū al-Ḥajjāj (r. 1273–1302), the son of Ibn al-Aḥmar. According to Ibn Khaldūn, Abū al-Ḥajjāj blamed his administrator Khālid for the attempt to poison him and his physician Yaḥyā b. al-Ṣāʾigh for cooperating with him. Khālid was executed, and Yaḥyā was imprisoned and was slaughtered while he was in prison.[456]

Yaḥyā b. Sulaymān al-ʾIsrāʾīlī al-Ṭabīb al-Ḥakīm (Zechariah b. Solomon) [Ye., Dhamār, 15th century]

A physician, active in Dhamār (Yemen).[457] According to Yosef Tobi, Zechariah was the only one among the Yemenite Jewish learned men who was called 'al-Ṭabīb', and from this it can be deduced that he was known as a physician outside of the Jewish community. Zechariah is the author of *Kitāb al-Wajīz* ('Summary Book'), and according to Tobi this is the only book in the Yemenite literature that can be considered an actual medical treatise. The book contains detailed schematic information on different kinds of diseases and their cures. The influence of Maimonides' medical books is very prominent as well. Alongside these influences, there is also an influence of folk medicine, i.e., natural remedies made out of various plants. Also mentioned are treatments that are not part of rational medicine and include healing amulets bearing words, signs and mystical drawings. There are only a limited number of copies of the book that were preserved in manuscript. According to an ancient document held by R. Yaḥyā Qafiḥ,[458] he (Yaḥyā) noted the three parts of the book: (1) *Tarkīb al-Insān, Taʿrīf al-Mizāj alladhī li-l-Marḍā wa-ʿAlāmātihim wa-l-Faṣādāt* (dealing with the composition of the human body and its tempers, signs of disease and phlebotomy), (2) *Sharḥ al-Adwiya al-Qarība wa-Jamīʿ Ṭabāʿihā wa-Tabyīn mā ʿAsara min Alfāḍhā wa-Tabdīl mā Ghufila minha wa-Qānūn al-Sharbāt* (a list of various medicines, their substitutes and effects) and (3) *Tarsīl al-Aʿḍāʾ bi-Adwiyatiha al-Makhṣūṣa min al-Dimāgh ilā al-Qadam wa-Sabab al-Alam wa-ʿAlāmātihi* (a list of organs and their medicines – forty chapters).[459]

Yaḥyā ha-Kohen ha-Rōfē b. Mevōrākh [Eg., 12th century]

A physician, the son of the brother of Menahem ha-Kohen ha-Rōfē b. Zadok, active at the beginning of the twelfth century.[460]

Yaʿqūb (Abū Yūsuf) ʿImrān al-Mutaṭabbib [Eg., 12th–13th centuries]
A physician, mentioned in a Geniza document from the 12th–13th centuries.[461]

Yaʿqūb b. Ghanāʾim (Abū Yūsuf) al-Sāmirī (Muwaffaq al-Dīn) [S., Sy., Damascus, 13th century, convert]
A Samaritan physician, born and raised in Damascus, he excelled in medicine and science, and was one of the greatest physicians of his time. His writings were clear and precise. He wrote *Sharḥ Kulliyāt al-Qānūn* (a commentary upon the principles of Ibn Sīnā's *al-Qānūn*) and allayed the doubts and distrust of Najm al-Dīn b. al-Munāfiḥ[462] in relation to the book. He also wrote a book called *al-Madkhal ilā al-Manṭiq al-Ṭabīʿī wa-l-Illāhī* ('An Introduction to the Logic of Natural Sciences and Metaphysics). Yaʿqūb died in 1282.[463] His honorific title 'Muwaffaq al-Dīn' implies that he converted to Islam.[464]

Yaʿqūb b. Isḥāq [Eg., 11th century]

Yedūthūn [Eg., Cairo, 13th century]
A physician, was active in Fusṭāṭ as part of a group of friends that included cantors, *parnāsim* and physicians. He was mentioned in a letter written by a cantor from Alexandria named Berākhōt to the physician and poet Yedūthūn in Fusṭāṭ. The letter conveys the activities of a group of friends that the two belonged to.[465] He is probably identical with Yedūthūn ha-Levi ha-Rōfē b. Levi ha-Levi, who is mentioned in a colophon from the twelfth century,[466] or with Abū Sahl Yedūthūn ha-Levi (Yedūthūn ha-Levi ha-Rōfē b. Levi ha-Levi).[467]

Yeshūʿā [Eg., Alexandria, 15th century]
A physician, his son Joseph is mentioned in a document from Alexandria (1442): 'Joseph b. Yeshūʿā ha-Rōfē, may his soul rest in Paradise'.[468]

R. Yeshūʿā [Eg., 13th century]
A physician, appeared in a list of future donors dated to the time of Abraham Maimonides. Other physicians that appeared in the list are (anonymous) al-Mawlī al-Muhadhdhab, (anonymous) Awlād al-Raʾīs, (anonymous) al-Gaon al-Munā, Mufaḍḍal al-Mashmiʿa, al-Sheikh Joseph, another al-Sheikh

Joseph and his son, Ibn al-Julājilī, Abū al-Maʿānī 2, Najīb Kohen Kamukhī, al-Rabīb Kohen, al-Taqī Ibn al-Gadal, Makārim Ibn al-Gadalī and Abū al-Maʿānī.[469]

R. Yeshūʿā b. Menahem [Sy., Damascus, 14th century]
A physician, mentioned in a letter sent from Hebron to Joshua and the Cairo community. A Maghribi of Hebron, Jacob the Poet b. Isaac b. David, asked the governor to grant him permanent assistance, as did the physician in Damascus who sent eight dirhams to him every month.[470]

Yeshūʿā ha-Levi ha-Rōfē [Eg., 12th century]
A physician, mentioned in a memorial list from the twelfth century.[471]

Yeshūʿā ha-Levi ha-Rōfē 2 [Eg., 13th century]
A physician, mentioned in a document from the thirteenth century.[472]

Yeshūʿā ha-Levi ha-Rōfē b. Elijah [Eg., 13th century]
A physician, mentioned in a Geniza document.[473]

Yeshūʿā ha-Levi ha-Rōfē b. Hai ha-Levi [Eg., 13th century]
A physician, mentioned in a document from Cairo (c.1230).[474]

Yeshūʿā ha-Rōfē b. Aaron al-ʿAmmānī [Eg., 11th–12th centuries]

Yeshūʿā ha-Rōfē b. Aaron ha-Rōfē Ibn al-ʿAmmānī [Eg., Alexandria/Cairo, 13th century]

Yeshūʿā ha-Rōfē b. Judah [Eg., 13th century]
A physician, mentioned in a document as buying a female slave (c.1217).[475]

Yūsuf ʿAbd al-Sayyid b. al-Muhadhdhab al-ʾIsrāʾīlī al-Mutaṭabib (Joseph b. al-Dayyān) [Sy., Damascus, Homs, 12th–13th centuries, convert]

Yūsuf b. Abī Saʿīd b. Khalaf al-Sāmirī al-Muhadhdhab al-Ṭabīb (Wazīr al-Amjad) [S., Sy., 12th century]

Yūsuf b. Ibrāhīm [EY, Jerusalem, 16th century]
A Jewish physician, practised in Jerusalem (1552–78). His family came from Alexandria and he and his family had many assets in Jerusalem.[476]

Yūsuf b. Isḥāq Ibn Biklārish [An., Saragossa, Almeria, 12th century]
A physician and authority on *materia medica*. Born in Saragossa, he practised in Almeria and at the court of the Hūdid dynasty of Saragossa. In 1106 he completed what is probably the most important Arabic pharmacological treatise, the *Kitāb al-Mustaʿīnī*.[477] The book was dedicated to al-Mustaʿīn biʾllāh Abū Jaʿfar Aḥmad b. Yūsuf al-Muʾtamin biʾllāh, the fourth Hūdid governor of Saragossa (r. 1085–1110). The work contains information on hundreds of medicaments, and lists of substitute drugs with their properties and methods of use.[478] The introduction is a theoretical explanation of pharmacology which is essentially based on Galen, and indicates that Ibn Biklārish was probably one of the extraordinary medical men of his time.[479] The book itself contains a special table-like section, arranged in five unequal columns. The first two small columns give the names and characteristics of the simple medicines, the third contains their explanation together with their Greek, Syriac, Persian, Latin and Mozarabic synonyms, the fourth their succedanea and the fifth their utility, specific effect and region of application. The covering text on the upper and lower margin contains further details, and above all the sources. The order of the drugs follows the abjad in its Maghribī form. Maimonides apparently made use of the *Kitāb* in his *Glossary of Medicines*, although without mentioning it by name.[480] Of other writings of Ibn Biklārish, only one work on dietetics is known by its title: in the introduction to the *Mustaʿīnī* it is quoted twice as *Risālat al-Tabyīn wa ʾl-Tartīb*.[481] The existence of fragments of the book in the Cairo Geniza can teach us about the route of the book's rapid distribution from Spain, where it was written, to Egypt, probably through the Maghrib.[482] Dozens of Geniza documents have been identified as belonging to medical books, but none was written by a Spanish Jewish author, in Judaeo-Arabic, and tabulated. It seems that it was transliterated from a manuscript written in Arabic, apparently from one of the earliest known versions of the book.[483]

Yūsuf b. al-Kazan [An., Almeria, 12th century]
A physician, one of the notables in Almeria, Spain. He was the addressee of a letter from Ḥalfon b. Nethanel.[484]

Yūsuf b. Nūḥ [K., 14th century]
An influential Karaite physician who was given prominence in Ibn al-Hītī's chronicle.[485]

Yūsuf al-Kaḥḥāl [Eg., 13th century]
An ophthalmologist, mentioned in a list of donors (c.1210) which includes several physicians and practitioners.[486]

R. Zadok ha-Rōfē [Sy., Damascus, 12th century]
A physician, mentioned as one of the notable Jews by Benjamin of Tudela, in his description of Damascus.[487] He was probably the father of Menahem ha-Kohen ha-Rōfē b. Zadok, who was probably active in Aleppo at the end of the eleventh century.[488]

Zakī al-Ḥakīm [Eg., Cairo, 16th century]
A physician, one of the representatives of the Mustaʿarabi Jews who stood in front of the Radbaz (Rabbi David b. Zimra, 1479–1573/1589), for a discussion following a dispute that broke out in 1527 between them and the Maghribis in Cairo. Beside him are mentioned 'Ḥakīm' ʿAbd al-Wāḥid ha-Kohen and ʿAbd al-ʿAzīz ha-Ḥazzān.[489]

Zayn al-Dīn Khiḍr al-ʾIsrāʾīlī al-Zuwaylī [Eg., Cairo, 15th century, convert]
A Jewish physician who converted to Islam and was the head physician of the Qalāwūn hospital.[490]

Zechariah (al-Raʾīs) the Alexandrian [Eg., Alexandria, EY., Ashkelon, 12th century]

Anonymous physicians
In this section I present Jewish practitioners on whom we have some biographical details. However, there is no name! It is possible that some of them are presented under the names above, but we have not been able to match

them. They are arranged by century, and within each century approximately west to east geographically.

Anonymous – a physician to Aḥmad b. Ṭūlūn [Eg., 9th century]
A physician, mentioned by al-Masʿūdī as serving the ruler of Egypt and Syria Aḥmad b. Ṭūlūn (r. 868–84). The Jewish physician was allowed to participate in the rulers' official meetings.[491]

Anonymous – a physician, captive in Europe [Eg., 11th century]
A letter describes the redemption of captives from the land of Edom (Europe). The letter was sent from Alexandria. Among the captives were a physician and his wife.[492]

Anonymous – a female physician [Eg., 11th century]
Mubārak b. al-Ṭabība and Farij b. al-Ṭabība are mentioned in a document among dozens receiving alms.[493] Awlād Ibn al-Ṭabība is mentioned in another document.[494] Al-Ṭabība is mentioned in a third document dealing with a household receiving bread.[495] This might be a female physician.[496]

Anonymous – a physician, father of Faḍl b. Ṣāliḥ [Eg., 11th–12th centuries]
Faḍl b. Ṣāliḥ, who is mentioned as one of the most important commanders in the Fatimid army, was the son of a Jewish physician.[497]

Anonymous – a physician, Miny[at Zi]ftī al-Ṭabīb [Eg., Minyat Ziftā, 11th–12th centuries]
A physician, mentioned in a list of donors.[498]

Anonymous – a physician, father of Hiba (b. al-Kallām) [Eg., ?12th century]
A wound specialist (maybe physician); mentioned in a document is a man named Hiba, who was involved in commerce, and was the son of the wound specialist. Also mentioned are Abū Zikrī al-Ṭabīb 2, Abū Riḍā al-Ṭabīb and another anonymous physician.[499]

Anonymous – a physician from Seleucia [Eg., 12th century]
A physician, left Egypt very poor, and from there moved to Seleucia in Byzantium. He had an Arabic education and got rich from his profession

after he moved to Byzantium.[500] From a letter he wrote (Seleucia, 21 July 1137) to his brother-in-law in Fusṭāṭ, we learn that Seleucia had already fallen to the Byzantines. The physician expressed an expectation that the emperor would also conquer Aleppo and Damascus and asked to receive the medical books that would be found there. According to Goitein, the physician was overly confident in his medical skills but was forced to admit that his prescriptions were not always successful. He sent expensive medicines to Egypt and ordered from there seeds of herbs that were not available in Asia Minor. In his medical profession he relied on books in Arabic, although during his time in Asia Minor, he may have learnt to read also in Greek. It is possible that the physician accompanied the Fatimid army that was defeated by the Venetians on a coast near Jaffa in 1124. Also mentioned are other letters sent by the physician from Rhodes and Chios, which were also held by the Venetians during the same journey. Later on, the physician spent a period of time in Constantinople. Perhaps, as a foreign physician he could not find work in the capital and so he moved to Seleucia, where he succeeded in his profession and became a highly successful and respected citizen. His wife's name was Greek, so it seems that she was born in the area and he married her only after his arrival in Seleucia.[501]

Anonymous – a physician, 'ben ha-Sōfer ha-Dayyān' [Eg., Cairo, 12th century]

'Ben ha-Sōfer ha-Dayyān' is mentioned in a notebook[502] (c.1150) of a Jewish physician, from Cairo, who lent him a book. It reveals that in addition to medicine, he worked as a notary and a *warrāq* (someone who bought, sold and lent books), especially in medical books. I agree with Goitein regarding his statement that there is no doubt that this book is 'Ten Treatises on the Eye' by Ḥunain b. Isḥāq and it is most likely that the 'Dayyān' who borrowed the book practised medicine in order to earn his living.[503]

Anonymous – a physician, name unclear [Eg., 12th century]

A physician whose name is not clear is mentioned in a document; also mentioned are Abū Zikrī al-Ṭabīb 2, Abū Riḍā al-Ṭabīb and a son of a wound specialist (*kallām*).[504]

Anonymous – a physician, ha-Rōfē b. Tamīm ha-Zāqēn [Eg., 12th century]

A physician, mentioned in a legal document (concerning a divorce) written by Ḥalfon ha-Levi b. Manasseh.[505]

Anonymous – a physician, al-Ṭabīb [Eg., 12th century]

A physician, mentioned in advice to doctors: treatment of an illness when it became worse. The document was written between the years 1100 and 1138.[506]

Anonymous – a physician, al-Ṭabīb 2 – list of donors [Eg., 12th century]

A physician, mentioned in a list of donors from the Geniza.[507]

Anonymous – a physician, grandfather of the daughter of Joseph b. ha-Rōfē [Iq., ?Baghdad, 12th century]

A document describes how in 1120, the daughter of Joseph b. ha-Rōfē appeared in public and declared that Elijah (the prophet) appeared to her in a dream and told her about the redemption of Israel.[508] The story aroused enthusiasm among the messianists and destabilised the relative stability among the Jews of Baghdad.[509]

Anonymous – a physician, father of ʿAlī b. Joseph ha-Rōfē [Eg., 12th–13th centuries]

ʿAlī b. Joseph ha-Rōfē is mentioned in a Geniza document.[510]

Anonymous – a physician, father of ben al-Ṭabīb [Eg., 12th–13th centuries]

In the second page of a letter, a greeting is sent to ben al-Ṭabīb.[511]

Anonymous – a physician from the Egyptian periphery [Eg., 12th–13th centuries]

This physician wrote a letter to his uncle (1191), detailing his troubles. His wife had died and he remained to look after his son; he remarried a 'bad' woman whose father was called Ibn Ṣabra.[512] This might be Asʿad al-Dīn (Ibn Ṣabra) al-Maḥallī al-Mutaṭabbib (Jacob b. Isaac), from the Ṣabra family of al-Maḥalla in northern Egypt, a distinguished physician and author of medical literature, mentioned by Ibn Abī Uṣaybiʿa for being a friend of one of his uncles.[513] Ibn Ṣabra raised in his house a girl named Akramiyya and released her (c.1217) when she was adult.[514] His daughter married a physician (probably our anonymous) who came to al-Maḥalla in order to study under As'ad and be cured of a chronic illness he was suffering from. As'ad died in Cairo.[515]

Anonymous – a dead physician's medical library [Eg., 12th–13th centuries]

A document (1223) described an auction of books (mainly medical) of an anonymous person (probably a physician), which was held after his death.[516]

Anonymous – a physician, al-Sheikh al-Muhadhdhab al-Ṭabīb [Eg., 12th–13th centuries]

A physician who appeared in a list of taxpayers or donors to a fund, raised for the redemption of captives etc. Alongside him also appear al-Nafīs al-Sharābī, Abū al-'Izz al-Kaḥḥāl, Abū al-Faraj b. al-Nashādirī, Makārim al-Kaḥḥāl, Abū al-Thanā', Abū Naṣr al-Sadīd and (anonymous) al-Wajīh ('honourable') al-Ṭabīb.[517]

Anonymous – a physician, al-Ṭabīb 3 [Eg., 12th–13th centuries]

A physician, mentioned in a list of expenses of the *waqf*.[518]

Anonymous – a physician, al-Ṭabīb al-Maristān [Eg., 12th–13th centuries]

A physician, practising in a hospital. Appeared in a list of donors together with Abū Isḥāq al-'Aṭṭār.[519]

Anonymous – a physician, al-Wajīh ('honourable') al-Ṭabīb [Eg., 12th–13th centuries]

A physician, appeared in a list of taxpayers or donors for fundraising, redemption of captives, etc. Also, in the list are al-Nafīs al-Sharābī, Abū al-'Izz al-Kaḥḥāl, (anonymous) al-Sheikh al-Muhadhdhab al-Ṭabīb, Abū al-Faraj b. al-Nashādirī, Makārim al-Kaḥḥāl, Abū al-Thanā' and Abū Naṣr al-Sadīd.[520]

Anonymous – a physician [Eg., Alexandria, 13th century]

A document relates a story about a man who went to a physician in Alexandria (c.1212) and the physician gave him a medicine that worked.[521]

Anonymous – a physician, father of Joseph b. ha-Rōfē [Eg., Alexandria, 13th century]
Joseph b. ha-Rōfē was mentioned in a document as one of the people who had gathered together to make a decision about appointing a man to run the community.[522]

Anonymous – a physician from Fusṭāṭ [Eg., Cairo, 13th century]
A physician, requested by a friend to go to the countryside. The friend provided answers to questions asked by the physician about eye diseases.[523]

Anonymous – a physician, the 'collector' [Eg., 13th century]
A physician, mentioned as a 'collector' at the top of a weekly payroll list for communal officials and payments to others.[524]

Anonymous – the physician al-Gaon al-Munā [Eg., 13th century]
A physician who is mentioned in a list of future donors from the period of Abraham Maimonides. Other physicians in the list are (anonymous) al-Mawlī al-Muhadhdhab, (anonymous) Awlād al-Raʾīs, Mufaḍḍal al-Mashmiʿa, al-Sheikh Joseph, another al-Sheikh Joseph and his son, Ibn al-Julājilī, R. Yeshūʿā, Abū al-Maʿānī 2, Najīb Kohen Kamukhī, al-Rabīb Kohen, al-Taqī Ibn al-Gadal, Makārim Ibn al-Gadalī and Abū al-Maʿānī.[525]

Anonymous – a physician, son of al-Sheikh Joseph [Eg., Cairo, 13th century]

Anonymous – a physician visiting with Naḥum al-ʿAṭṭār [Eg., 13th century]
In a commercial letter, a visit by an anonymous physician and Naḥum al-ʿAṭṭār was mentioned.[526]

Anonymous – a physician, 'Awlād al-Raʾīs' [Eg., Cairo, 13th century]
'Awlād al-Raʾīs' appeared as a physician on a list of future donors from the period of Abraham Maimonides. Other physicians in the list are (anonymous) al-Mawlī al-Muhadhdhab, (anonymous) al-Gaon al-Munā, Mufaḍḍal al-Mashmiʿa, al-Sheikh Joseph, another al-Sheikh Joseph and his son, Ibn al-Julājilī, R. Yeshūʿā, Abū al-Maʿānī 2, Najīb Kohen Kamukhī, al-Rabīb Kohen, al-Taqī Ibn al-Gadal, Makārim Ibn al-Gadalī and Abū al-Maʿānī.[527]

Anonymous – b. Aaron ha-Rōfē b. Samuel Ibn al-ʿAmmānī [Eg., 13th century]

Anonymous – a physician, al-Mawlī al-Muhadhdhab [Eg., 13th century]
A physician who is mentioned in a list of future donors from the period of Abraham Maimonides. Other physicians in the list are (anonymous) Awlād al-Raʾīs, (anonymous) al-Gaon al-Munā, Mufaḍḍal al-Mashmiʿa, al-Sheikh Joseph, another al-Sheikh Joseph and his son, Ibn al-Julājilī, R. Yeshūʿā, Abū al-Maʿānī 2, Najīb Kohen Kamukhī, al-Rabīb Kohen, al-Taqī Ibn al-Gadal, Makārim Ibn al-Gadalī and Abū al-Maʿānī.[528]

Anonymous – a physician, ha-Sar ha-Rōfē [Eg., 13th century]
A physician, mentioned in a document (his name was not preserved). On the next page of the document, Benjamin ha-Rōfē is mentioned, and he is apparently the recipient.[529]

Anonymous – Yemenite physician [Ye., 13th century]
A Yemenite physician who was riding a mule in fancy clothes and was accompanied by servants, angered a Yemenite *faqīh* (1240–1). The *faqīh* knocked the physician off the mule, took off his shoes and beat him because the physician, he thought, exceeded the limits of what was allowed and thus lost the protection of Islamic law.[530]

Anonymous – a physician, 'murdered' a Muslim patient [Eg., 13th–14th centuries]
Ibn al-Hājj (d. 1337) wrote about a Jewish physician who 'murdered' his Muslim patient.[531]

Anonymous – a physician from Egypt who was sent to the sultan of Yemen [Eg., Ye., 14th century]
'A skilled physician from the Jews of Egypt' was sent by Sultan al-Ẓāhir Barqūq to the sultan of Yemen (1397), as part of a gift that included thirty Turkish mamluks, beautiful slaves and horses. The Jewish physician died less than a month after arrival.[532]

Anonymous [Eg., Cairo, 15th century]
The Muslim historian Ibn Iyās mentioned a Jewish physician who lived on al-Saliba Street in the southern part of the city.[533]

Anonymous – a physician, castration expert [Eg., Cairo, 15th century]
Ibn Iyās mentioned that in 1474 the sultan wanted to punish a mamluk who slept with male army recruits. At the same time one Jew became known in Cairo as an expert in castration. He castrated many people and they recovered after the operation. The sultan called the Jewish physician and he castrated the mamluk. The operation succeeded and the healthy mamluk lived for many more years.[534]

Anonymous – the physician to Sultan al-Muʾayyad Sheikh [Sy., Eg., Cairo, 15th century]
Sultan al-Muʾayyad Sheikh (r. 1412–21), although he imposed decrees on Jews and Christians, was nevertheless assisted by a Jewish physician in times of trouble. He had been ill for many years with rheumatoid arthritis, and in the last two years of his life the disease worsened, and he suffered severe metabolic disorders. His physicians did not know what to do, and so renowned physicians from abroad were called for. A physician from Iran, a physician from Hama and a Jewish physician from Syria were brought in, and they were accompanied by an Iranian physician who lived in Cairo. All of them treated the sultan for a long time.[535]

Anonymous – the physician to Emir Khāirbek [Sy., Aleppo, 16th century]
A physician, treated Emir Khā'irbek al-Ashrafī in Aleppo at the end of the Mamluk period. He saved the emir after the sultan poisoned him.[536]

3.1.2 Biographies of Jewish pharmacists[537]

ʿAbd al-Bāqī al-ʿAṭṭār [Eg. 11th century]
A pharmacist, partner in commerce with Abū al-Ḥusayn Hārūn b. Yeshūʿā al-Tunisī, he is mentioned for passing a letter from Alexandria to Fusṭāṭ.[538]

ʿAbd al-Ḥaqq [Sy., Damascus, 15th century, convert]
A pharmacist, converted to Islam in 1480–1.[539]

ʿAbdūn al-ʿAṭṭār [Eg., 14th century]
A pharmacist, mentioned in a list of accounts (1387).[540]

Abraham al-ʿAṭṭār [Eg., 12th century]

A pharmacist, appeared in a list of donors (c.1110). The names of the donors are abbreviated. The donation is possibly for a singer at a family event.[541]

Abraham al-ʿAṭṭār b. Ṣadaqa al-Ḥanāwī [Eg., 12th century]

A pharmacist, mentioned in a document from 1159–60.[542]

Abraham ha-Levi [Abū I]sḥāq al-Maḥallī al-ʿAṭṭār [Eg., 12th century]

A pharmacist, mentioned in the Blessing of the Dead in a document written in the hands of Ḥalfon ha-Levi b. Manasseh.[543] From his name it is possible to deduce that he is from the city of al-Maḥalla.

Abū Aḥmar al-ʿAṭṭār [Eg., 13th century]

A pharmacist, Abū al-Afḍal, the son of Abū Aḥmar al-ʿAṭṭār, is mentioned in a document dated October 1244 as someone who borrowed books.[544]

Abū al-ʿAlā (Elazar b. Joseph) [Eg., 11th century]

A pharmacist who was active c.1084.[545]

Abū al-ʿAlā Levi [Eg., 13th century]

A pharmacist, appeared in a list of donors to aid payment of a *jizya* (head tax), alongside Abū ʿImrān Levi ʿAṭṭār, Abū ʿImrān Kohen ʿAṭṭār, Abū al-ʿIzz al-Kaḥḥāl, Abū al-Fakhr Levi ʿAṭṭār and Makārim al-Kaḥḥāl.[546]

Abū al-ʿAlā Musallam al-ʿAṭṭār b. Sahl [Eg., 12th century]

A pharmacist who is mentioned in an engagement agreement from 1146.[547]

Abū ʿAlī al-ʿAṭṭār [Eg., 13th century]

A pharmacist, his son is mentioned in a document alongside the son of Abū al-Fakhr al-ʿAṭṭār 3 and Abū al-Rabīʿ al-ʿAṭṭār.[548]

Abū ʿAlī al-ʿAṭṭār (Rabbana Japheth) [Eg., 12th century]

A pharmacist, mentioned in an engagement agreement of his son, Abū Manṣūr Ṣemaḥ, with Sitt al-Khāṣṣa (1146).[549]

Abū al-Barakāt al-ʿAṭṭār [Eg., 12th century]

A pharmacist, mentioned in a document written by Joseph b. Samuel ha-Levi (1180–1212). Abū al-Barakāt was not alive when this document was written.[550]

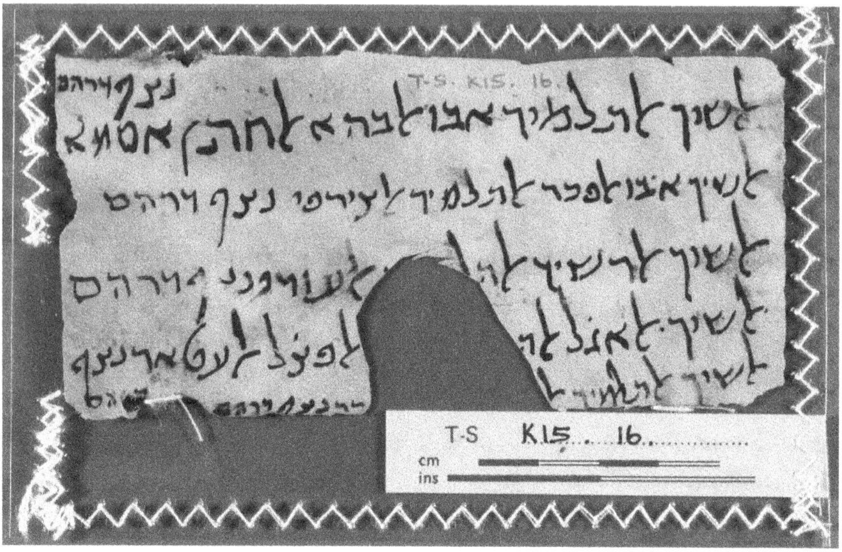

Figure 2 Part of a list of pledges to charity made at a wedding, mentioning Abū Faḍl al-ʿAṭṭār (11th–12th centuries) (TS K 15.16).

Abū Faḍl al-ʿAṭṭār [Eg., 11th–12th centuries]

A pharmacist, mentioned in a document alongside Abū Saʿīd al-ʿAṭṭār,[551] and also mentioned in another document, a list of pledges to charity made at a wedding (see Figure 2).[552]

Abū al-Faḍl al-ʿAṭṭār b. Abū al-Ḥasan [Eg., 13th century]

A pharmacist, mentioned in a legal document concerning a loan from 1292 (see Figure 3).[553]

Abū al-Fakhr al-ʿAṭṭār [Eg., 12th century]

Abū al-Fakhr al-ʿAṭṭār 2 [Eg., 12th century]

A pharmacist, mentioned in a list of donors (1178) written by Mevōrākh b. Nathan. Also mentioned are Makārim al-ʿAṭṭār, Hiba al-ʿAṭṭār 2, Abū Saʿd al-ʿAṭṭār 2, Dāʾūd al-ʿAṭṭār and Abū al-Majd al-Ṭabīb.[554]

Abū al-Fakhr al-ʿAṭṭār 3 [Eg., 13th century]

A pharmacist, his son is mentioned in a document alongside the son of Abū ʿAlī al-ʿAṭṭār and Abū al-Rabīʿ al-ʿAṭṭār.[555]

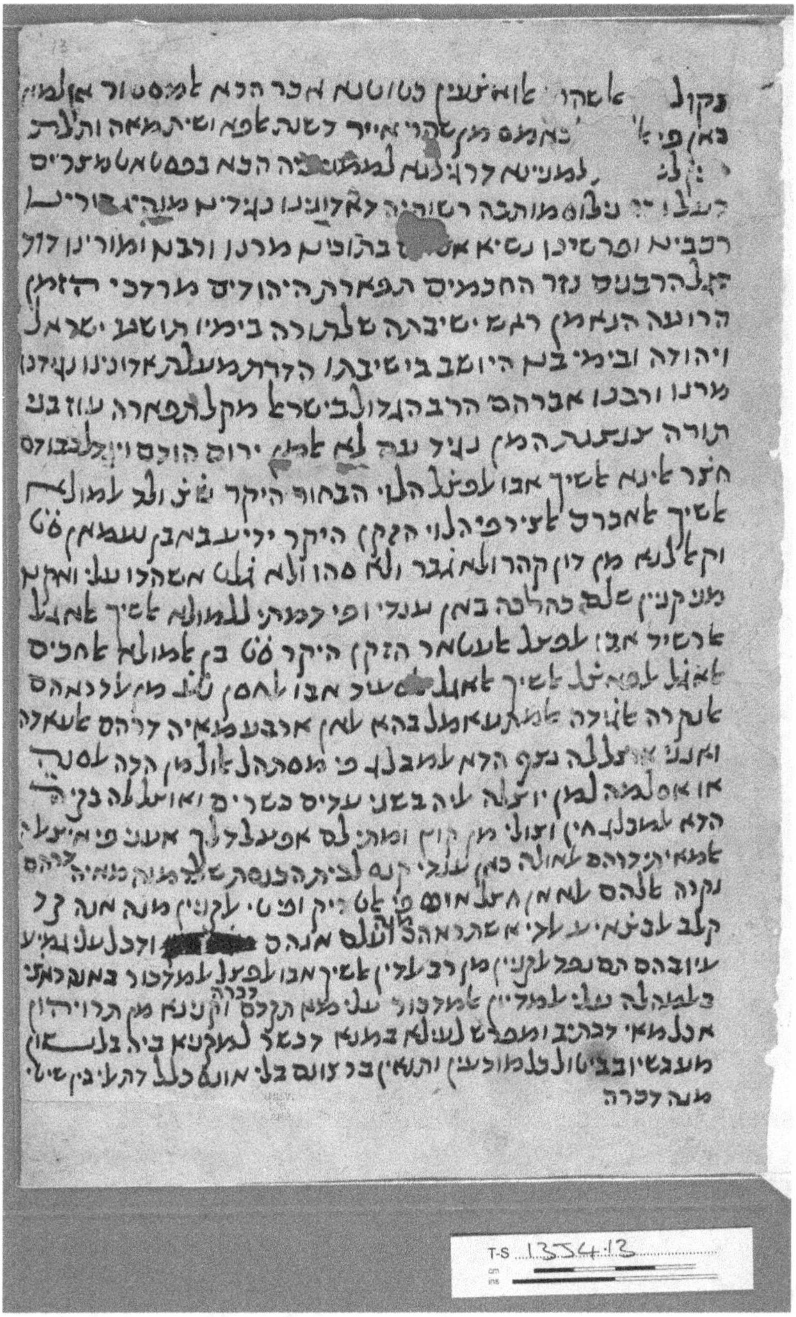

Figure 3 Legal document concerning a loan from Abū al-Faḍl al-ʿAṭṭār b. Abū al-Ḥasan (1292) (TS 13J4.13).

Abū al-Fakhr Levi ʿAṭṭār [Eg., 13th century]
A pharmacist, appeared in a list of donors assisting the payment of a *jizya* (head tax), alongside Abū ʿImrān Levi ʿAṭṭār, Abū ʿImrān Kohen ʿAṭṭār, Abū al-ʿIzz al-Kaḥḥāl, Abū al-ʿAlā Levi and Makārim al-Kaḥḥāl.[556]

Abū al-Faraj al-ʿAṭṭār b. Abū al-Ḥasan al-ʿAṭṭār [Eg., Alexandria, 13th century]

Abū al-Futūḥ al-ʿAṭṭār [Eg., 12th century]
A pharmacist, mentioned in a document, probably from the twelfth century.[557]

Abū al-Ḥasan ʿAṭṭār [Eg., 13th century]
A pharmacist, mentioned in a document alongside Abū ʿImrān, Mufaḍḍ(al) Ṭabīb, Makārim Ṭabīb and Abū al-ʿIzz Ṭabīb.[558]

Abū al-Ḥasan al-ʿAṭṭār [Eg., 13th century]
The son of Abū al-Ḥasan, Joseph b. Abū al-Ḥasan al-ʿAṭṭār (a pharmacist) is mentioned in a Geniza document.[559]

Abū al-Ḥasan al-ʿAṭṭār 2 [Eg., 12th century]
A pharmacist, appeared in a list of donors from c.1180. It is possible that the document was written by the judge Samuel b. Saʿadya ha-Levi. Alongside him also appear Abū al-Faḍāʾil al-Ṭabīb and al-Sheikh Abū al-Faḍāʾil al-Ṭabīb.[560]

Abū al-Ḥasan al-ʿAṭṭār 3 [Eg., 13th century]

Abū al-Ḥasan al-ʿAṭṭār 4 [Eg., 12th century]
A pharmacist, mentioned as working in the 'great market'. Lost his mother in December 1125.[561]

Abū al-Ḥasan al-ʿAṭṭār b. Abū al-Fakhr [Eg., 13th century]

Abū al-Ḥasan b. Mūsā al-Fāṣid (the phlebotomist) al-ʿAṭṭār [Eg., Cairo, 12th century]
A pharmacist, appeared in a list of contributors alongside twenty persons including Abū Isḥāq al-ʿAṭṭār.[562]

Abū al-Ḥasan ha-Levi al-ʿAṭṭār (b. al-Dimyāṭī) [Eg., 12th century]
Mentioned in a document from 1192–3.[563] Might be Abū al-Ḥasan b. Mūsā al-Fāṣid (the phlebotomist) al-ʿAṭṭār.

Abū ʿImrān ʿAṭṭār [Eg., 13th century]

Three pharmacists named Abū ʿImrān are mentioned in a document, alongside Abū al-Ḥasan ʿAṭṭār, Mufaḍḍ(al) Ṭabīb, Makārim Ṭabīb and Abū al-ʿIzz Ṭabīb.[564]

Abū ʿImrān Kohen ʿAṭṭār [Eg., 13th century]

A pharmacist, appeared in a list of donors to aid payment of a *jizya* (head tax) alongside Abū ʿImrān Levi ʿAṭṭār, Abū al-Fakhr Levi ʿAṭṭār, Abū al-ʿIzz al-Kaḥḥāl, Abū al-ʿAlā Levi and Makārim al-Kaḥḥāl.[565]

Abū ʿImrān Levi ʿAṭṭār [Eg., 13th century]

A pharmacist, appeared in a list of donors to aid payment of a *jizya* (head tax) alongside Abū ʿImrān Kohen ʿAṭṭār, Abū al-Fakhr Levi ʿAṭṭār, Abū al-ʿIzz al-Kaḥḥāl, Abū al-ʿAlā Levi and Makārim al-Kaḥḥāl.[566]

Abū Isḥāq al-ʿAṭṭār [Eg., 12th century]

A pharmacist, appeared in a list of donors alongside al-Ṭabīb al-Maristān, and in a list of contributors alongside twenty other persons including Abū al-Ḥasan b. Mūsā al-Fāṣid (the phlebotomist) al-ʿAṭṭār.[567]

Abū Isḥāq al-Maḥallī al-ʿAṭṭār (Abraham b. Sasson) [Eg., 12th century]

A pharmacist, mentioned on a bill dated 1126 and written by Ḥalfon ha-Levi b. Manasseh (active 1100–38).[568]

Abū al-ʿIzz al-ʿAṭṭār [Eg., 13th century]

A pharmacist, mentioned in a letter[569] sent from Abū al-Faraj to Abū ʿImrān in which he announced the arrival of two Jews from Minyat Ziftā.[570]

Abū al-Khayr al-ʿAṭṭār [Eg., 13th century]

A pharmacist, mentioned in a list of donors; also mentioned in the same list are Ben bū ʿ[...]ā al-Ṭabīb, Abū al-Riḍā al-ʿAṭṭār and al-Muwaffaq al-Kohen al-Ṭabīb.[571]

Abū al-Majd al-Ṭabīb [Eg., Cairo, 12th century]

A pharmacist, mentioned in a list of donors (1178), written by Mevōrākh b. Nathan. Also mentioned are Makārim al-ʿAṭṭār, Abū al-Fakhr al-ʿAṭṭār 2, Hiba al-ʿAṭṭār 2, Abū Saʿd al-ʿAṭṭār 2 and Dāʾūd al-ʿAṭṭār.[572]

Abū al-Makārim al-Levi al-ʿAṭṭār b. Nāfiʿ [Eg., Cairo, 12th century]
A pharmacist and an important merchant, active in Cairo around 1180–1.[573]

Abū al-Manṣūr al-ʿAṭṭār [Eg., 13th century]
A pharmacist, mentioned in an inheritance list from the thirteenth century.[574]

Abū al-Manṣūr (Ablmanṣūr) al-ʿAṭṭār [Eg., 13th century]
A pharmacist, mentioned in a document.[575]

Abū al-Munā al-ʿAṭṭār[576] [Eg., 11th–12th centuries]
A pharmacist, appeared in a list of donors headed by the *nagid* Mevōrākh b. Saʿadya (d. 1111). Also appearing in the list are Abū Naṣr al-ʿAṭṭār 2, Ibrāhīm ha-Rōfē, Abū al-Faḍl al-Ṭabīb 2, Salāma al-ʿAṭṭār, (anonymous) ʿAṭṭār and Abū al-Surūr al-Sharābī.[577]

Abū al-Munā al-ʿAṭṭār (Jacob b. David ha-Parnās)[578] [Eg., Cairo, 12th century]
A pharmacist, mentioned in a manuscript written by Ḥalfon ha-Levi b. Manasseh (1126), receiving a loan of 57 dinars for his business through the mediation of a banker.[579]

Abū al-Munā b. Abī Naṣr b. Ḥaffāẓ (al-Kohen al-ʿAṭṭār al-Harunī al-ʾIsrāʾīlī) [K., Eg., 13th century]
A Karaite pharmacist, wrote (1259–60) an instruction manual for pharmacies called *Minhāj al-Dukkān wa-Dustūr al-Aʿyān fī Aʿmāl wa Tarākīb al-Adwiya al-Nāfiʿa a lil-Insān* ('The Management of the Shop and the Rule for the Notables on the Preparation and Composition of Medicines Beneficial to Man').[580] Among its twenty-five chapters, we find ones on simples, substitute drugs, weights and measures. The other chapters, the formulary proper, deal with compound medicines according to their methods of preparation. The manual includes explanations of medicine preparation and advice concerning the preservation of materials.[581] In his introduction, Abū al-Munā stated that he was composing this work because none of the preceding formularies were suitable for pharmacists; rather they had been written by physicians for physicians, and were not as useful in a pharmacy setting as in a hospital one. The book was highly successful and widely used during the Middle Ages and continued to be in use by 'traditional druggists' in Cairo

and other Middle Eastern markets until the twentieth century, and even to the present day.[582]

Abū al-Munajjā al-ʿAṭṭār [Eg., Cairo, 12th–13th centuries]
A pharmacist, mentioned in a bill from Fusṭāṭ. He had two sons, one named Saʿadya; the other's name is unknown. In 1231 he was no longer among the living.[583]

Abū Naṣr al-ʿAṭṭār [Eg., 11th century]
A pharmacist, appeared in a list of donors for a circumcision alongside Ṣadaqa al-ʿAṭṭār.[584]

Abū Naṣr al-ʿAṭṭār 2 [Eg., 11th–12th centuries]
A pharmacist, appeared in a list of donors headed by the *nagid* Mevōrākh b. Saʿadya (d. 1111) alongside Abū al-Munā al-ʿAṭṭār, Ibrāhīm ha-Rōfē the physician, Abū al-Faḍl al-Ṭabīb 2, Salāma al-ʿAṭṭār, (anonymous) ʿAṭṭār and Abū al-Surūr al-Sharābī.[585]

Abū Naṣr al-ʿAṭṭār 3 [Eg., Cairo, 12th century]
A pharmacist, appeared in a document in which Nethanel ha-Levi (Head of the Jews, 1163–9) is mentioned.[586]

Abū Naṣr al-ʿAṭṭār (Ibn Khalaf) [Eg., 12th century]
A pharmacist, mentioned in a document from 1242–3.[587]

Abū Naṣr al-ʿAṭṭār b. Zubaybāt [Eg., 12th century]
A pharmacist, mentioned in a document written by Ḥalfon ha-Levi b. Manasseh.[588]

Abū al-Rabīʿ ʿAṭṭār [Eg., 13th century]
A pharmacist, the brother of Abū Naṣr b. Dāʾūd, mentioned in document probably written by Emanuel b. Yechiel. Also mentioned are al-Rashīd b. al-ʿAjamī ʿAṭṭār, Rashīd Ṭabīb, al-Thiqa Ṭabīb and Menahem Ṭabīb.[589] Abū al-Rabīʿ is also mentioned in a document alongside the son of Abū al-Fakhr al-ʿAṭṭār 3 and the son of Abū ʿAlī al-ʿAṭṭār.[590]

Abū al-Riḍā al-ʿAṭṭār [Eg., 13th century]
A pharmacist, mentioned in a list of donors alongside Abū al-Khayr al-ʿAṭṭār, Ben bū ʿ[...]ā al-Ṭabīb and al-Muwaffaq al-Kohen al-Ṭabīb.[591]

Abū Saʿd al-ʿAṭṭār [Eg., Cairo, 12th–13th centuries]

Abū Saʿd al-ʿAṭṭār 2 [Eg., Cairo, 12th–13th centuries]

Abū Saʿd al-Ḥarīrī [Eg., 12th–13th centuries]
A pharmacist; his son, Faḍāʾil, is mentioned in a document.[592]

Abū Saʿīd [Eg., Cairo, 12th century]
A pharmacist, mentioned in a document alongside Aaron ha-Rōfē b. Yeshūʿā ha-Rōfē Ibn al-ʿAmmānī.[593]

Abū Saʿīd (al-Sheikh al-Muhadhdhab) [Eg., 13th century]
A pharmacist, mentioned in a document (1223) as one of the purchasers of a medical book in a public auction held after the death of an anonymous man who was probably a physician.[594]

Abū Saʿīd al-ʿAṭṭār [Eg., 11th–12th centuries]
A pharmacist, appeared in a list of donors alongside Abū al-Munā al-Sharābī and Abū al-Faḍl al-Ṭabīb,[595] and in another document alongside Abū Faḍl al-ʿAṭṭār.[596]

Abū al-Surūr al-ʿAṭṭār (Peraḥya ha-Zaqēn ha-Talmid) [Eg., 12th century]
A pharmacist, mentioned in a document written by Ḥalfon ha-Levi b. Manasseh.[597]

Abū al-Surūr b. Binyām ha-Levi [Eg., 12th century]
A pharmacist, in 1124 married Sitt al-Ahl. He was the co-owner of Joseph Lebdi's house together with Sitt al-Ahl's niece. He was mentioned in a letter from the court clerk Ḥalfon ha-Levi b. Manasseh to Abraham b. Bundār in which Ḥalfon thanked Abraham and the 'leader of the communities' for red silk from India, which he received from them as a present and was delivered to him by Abū al-Surūr b. Binyām ha-Levi.[598]

ʿAlī ha-Busmī [Eg., 11th century]

Banīn b. Daʾūd [Eg., Cairo, 12th century]
A pharmacist, mentioned in a list of debts of three retailers to a deceased drugs wholesaler (Banīn b. Daʾūd). The list consists of pharmacist's scales, pots of Kabul myrobalan and syrup of honey and vinegar.[599]

Baqāʾ al-ʿAṭṭār [Eg., 12th century]
A pharmacist, mentioned in a list of donors, apparently for the redemption of captives; he donated half a dinar. The document was written by Maimonides, apparently in 1171–2.[600]

Benyām al-Rashīdī al-ʿAṭṭār [Eg., Alexandria, 12th century]
A pharmacist, mentioned in a letter[601] sent by Abū al-Ḥasan al-Iskandarānī to Abū Saʿīd al-ʿAfṣī in Cairo.[602]

Dāʾūd al-ʿAṭṭār [Eg., Cairo, 12th century]
A pharmacist, his son is mentioned in a document.[603] Dāʾūd is also mentioned in a list of donors from 1178, written by Mevōrākh b. Nathan, alongside Makārim al-ʿAṭṭār, Abū al-Fakhr al-ʿAṭṭār 2, Hiba al-ʿAṭṭār 2, Abū Saʿd al-ʿAṭṭār 2 and Abū al-Majd al-Ṭabīb.[604]

Dāʾūd al-ʿAṭṭār b. Abū al-Faḍl ha-Kohen [Eg., 12th–13th centuries]
A pharmacist, mentioned in a Geniza document.[605]

al-Dimashqī [Eg., Cairo]
A pharmacist, mentioned in a document including many simples.[606]

Elazar the pharmacist [Eg.]
A pharmacist, probably from Egypt, wrote a Bible commentary.[607]

Ephraim al-ʿAṭṭār [Eg., Alexandria, 11th century]
A pharmacist, mentioned in a letter[608] sent to Naharay b. Nissīm.[609]

Ephraim b. Shemarya [Eg., Cairo, 11th century]
A pharmacist, mentioned in a letter (c.1020),[610] which was sent to him by Josiah Gaon.[611]

Faraḥ b. Abū al-ʿAlā [Eg., Cairo, 12th century]
A pharmacist and a merchant, mentioned in a contract (1139) that dealt with the partnership between himself and Sayyid al-Ahl b. Hiba. In the contract,[612] Sayyid reserved for himself the right to sell on his own account a popular medicine (*qirṭās taḥyīj*) for making women plump (the ideal of female beauty at the time), tooth powder, eye powder and arsenic. This privilege was a compensation for him being the shop manager (buying the

materials for these medicines would be on his account). In the contract it was agreed that each partner would receive a daily salary of 1–2 dirhams.[613]

Hārūn b. Khulayf b. Hārūn [Eg., 11th century]
A pharmacist, mentioned to have purchased a house from Khulayf b. ʿUbayd.[614]

Hiba al-ʿAṭṭār [Eg., 13th century]
A pharmacist, mentioned in a list of contributors and their contributions dated c.1230 (see Figure 4).[615]

Hiba al-ʿAṭṭār 2 [Eg., 12th century]
A pharmacist, mentioned in a list of donors from 1178, written by Mevōrākh b. Nathan. Also mentioned are Makārim al-ʿAṭṭār, Abū al-Fakhr al-ʿAṭṭār 2, Abū Saʿd al-ʿAṭṭār 2, Dāʾūd al-ʿAṭṭār and Abū al-Majd al-Ṭabīb.[616]

Ḥusayn al-ʿAṭṭār [Eg., 12th century]
A pharmacist, mentioned in the Blessing of the Dead in a document probably written by Ḥalfon ha-Levi b. Manasseh.[617]

Ibrāhīm al-ʿAṭṭār [Eg., 13th century]
A pharmacist, appeared in a list of forty-five donors dated c.1235, alongside Manṣūr al-ʿAṭṭār.[618]

al-ʾIsrāʾīlī al-Ṣaydalānī [Eg., Cairo]
A pharmacist, mentioned in an Arabic Geniza document together with al-Yahūdī al-ʿAṭṭār.[619]

Joseph al-ʿAṭṭār [Eg., 12th–13th centuries]
A pharmacist; Joseph's son, Munajjā b. Joseph al-ʿAṭṭār, is mentioned in a document.[620]

Joseph b. Elazar al-ʿAṭṭār [Eg., 12th century]
A pharmacist, mentioned in a legal document (1132) dealing with a partnership in a pharmacy between him and Ṣadaqa ha-Kohen b. Maṣlīaḥ.[621]

Joshua Jacob al-ʿAṭṭār [Eg. 13th century]
A pharmacist, mentioned in a list of donors.[622]

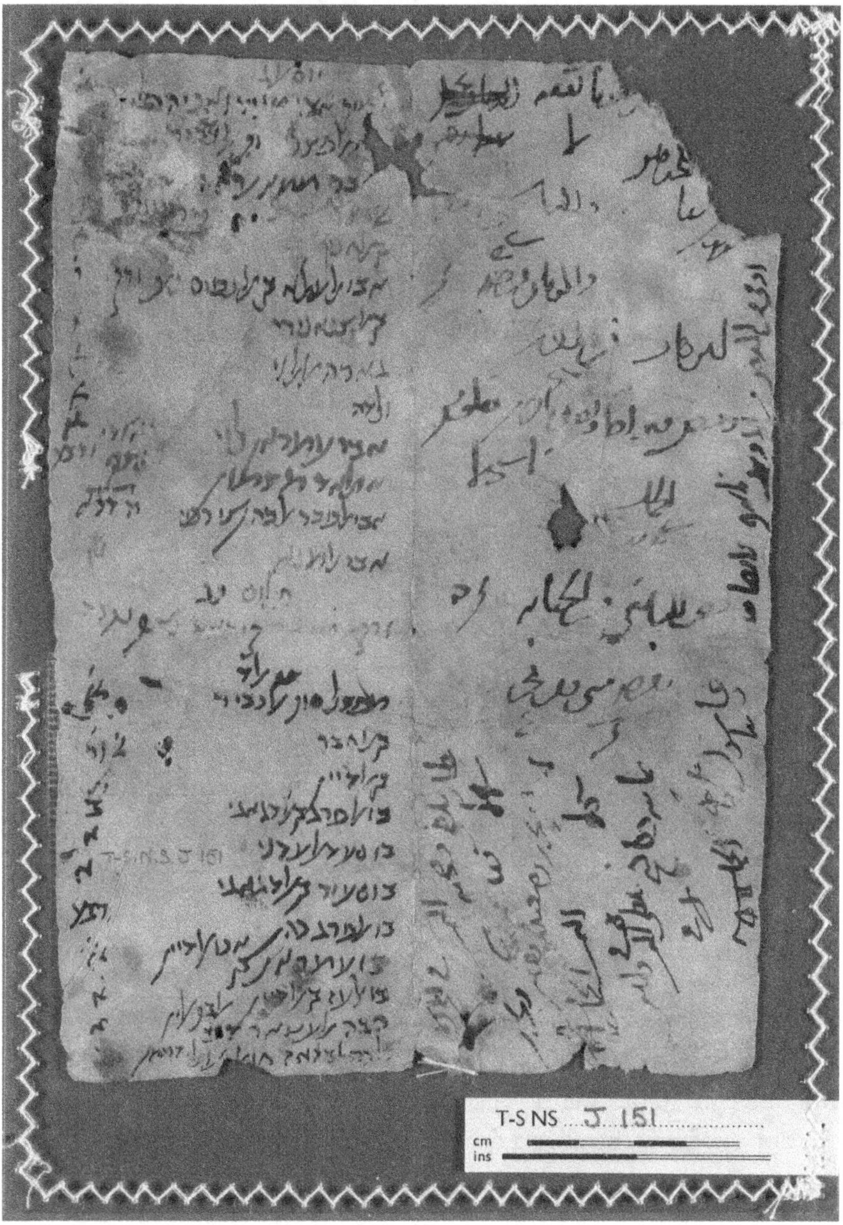

Figure 4 List of contributors and their contributions (1230), including the pharmacist Hiba al-ʿAṭṭār (TS NS J 151).

al-Levi al-ʿAṭṭār ha-Zāqēn [Eg., 13th century]
A pharmacist, mentioned in a document from 1221.[623]

Makārim al-ʿAṭṭār [Eg., 12th century]
A pharmacist, mentioned in a list of donors (1178) written by Mevōrākh b. Nathan. Also mentioned are Abū al-Fakhr al-ʿAṭṭār 2, Hiba al-ʿAṭṭār 2, Abū Saʿd al-ʿAṭṭār 2, Dāʾūd al-ʿAṭṭār and Abū al-Majd al-Ṭabīb.[624]

Makīn ʿAṭṭār [Eg., 13th century]
A pharmacist, mentioned in a list of donors (1231–65). Also mentioned in the list is Mūsā ʿAṭṭār.[625]

Manṣūr al-ʿAṭṭār [Eg., 13th century]
A pharmacist, appeared in a list of forty-five donors (c.1235). Also mentioned in the list is Ibrāhīm al-ʿAṭṭār.[626]

Moses b. Yaḥyā ha-Bassāmi [Ma., 11th century]
A perfumer, active in the Maghrib, mentioned in a letter sent from the Jewish community in Sicily to the Jewish communities in Qayrawān and al-Mahdiyya (see Figure 5).[627]

Munajjā al-ʿAṭṭār b. Abū Saʿd al-ʿAṭṭār [Eg., Cairo, 12th–13th centuries]

Mūsā ʿAṭṭār [Eg., 13th century]
A pharmacist, mentioned in a list of donors (1231–65). Also mentioned in the list is Makīn ʿAṭṭār.[628]

Mūsā al-ʿAṭṭār [Eg., Cairo, 13th century]
A pharmacist; his son, Abū al-Ḥasan, in mentioned in a list of donors, apparently from the thirteenth century.[629]

Musallam al-ʿAṭṭār [Eg., 12th century]
A pharmacist, mentioned in a document from the twelfth century.[630]

Naḥum al-ʿAṭṭār [Eg., 13th century]
A pharmacist, mentioned in a commerce-related letter; also mentioned is a visit from an anonymous physician (see anonymous – visited with Naḥum al-ʿAṭṭār).[631]

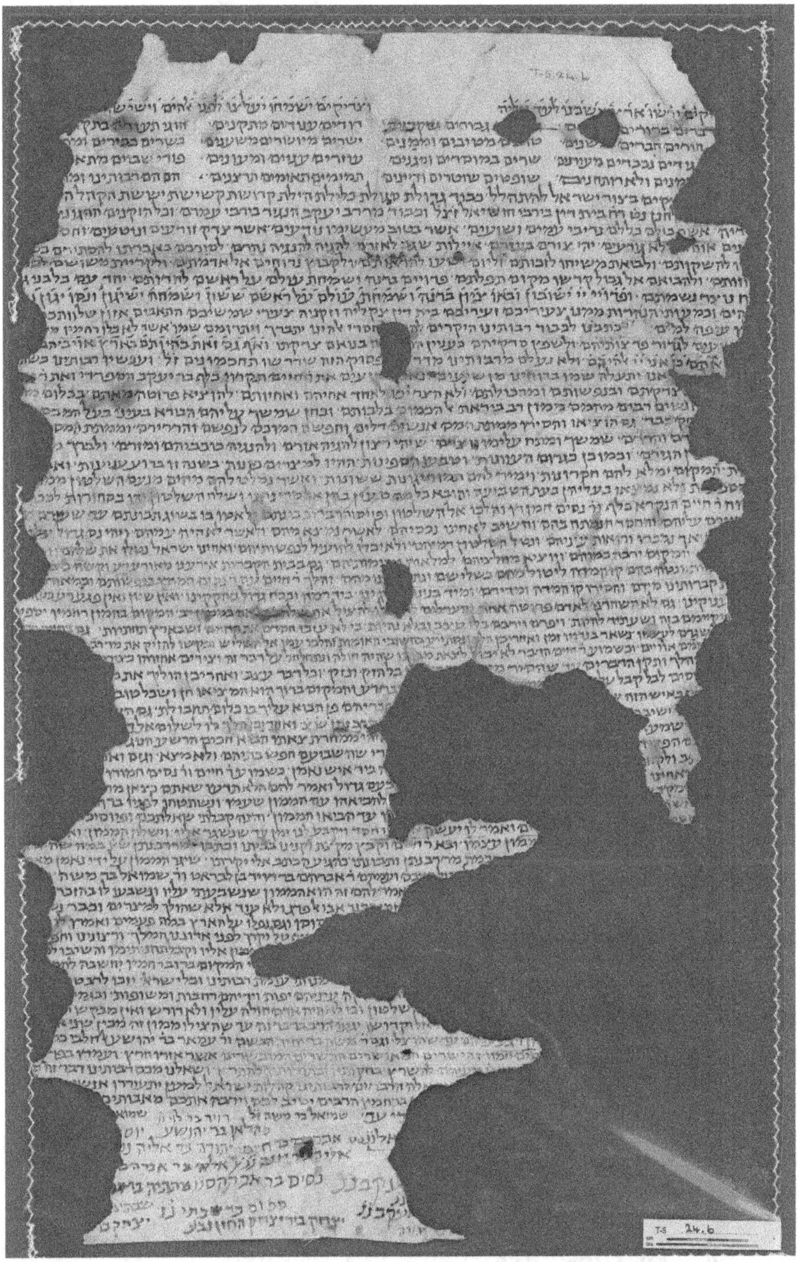

Figure 5 Part of a letter (1030) from the Jewish community in Sicily, its court and elders (probably the principal community in Palermo), to the Jewish communities in Qayrawān and al-Mahdiyya. The letter mentions the perfumer Moses b. Yaḥyā ha-Bassāmi among other individuals (TS 24.6).

al-Rashīd b. al-ʿAjamī ʿAṭṭār [Eg., 13th century]
A pharmacist, mentioned in a document probably written by Emanuel b. Yechiel. Also mentioned are Abū al-Rabīʿ ʿAṭṭār, Rashīd Ṭabīb, al-Thiqa Ṭabīb and Menahem Ṭabīb.[632]

Ṣadaqa al-ʿAṭṭār [Eg., 11th century]
A pharmacist, mentioned in a list of donors, along with Abū Naṣr al-ʿAṭṭār.[633]

Ṣadaqa ha-Kohen b. Maṣlīaḥ [Eg., 12th century]
A pharmacist, mentioned in a legal document (1132) dealing with a partnership in a pharmacy between him and Joseph b. Elazar al-ʿAṭṭār.[634]

Sahlān b. Abraham [Eg., Cairo, 11th century]
A pharmacist, active in Cairo in the eleventh century.[635]

Salāma al-ʿAṭṭār [Eg., 11th–12th centuries]
A pharmacist, appeared in a list of donors (c.1100) headed by the *nagid* Mevōrākh b. Saʿadya (d. 1111). Also in the list appeared Abū al-Munā al-ʿAṭṭār, Ibrāhīm ha-Rōfē, Abū Naṣr al-ʿAṭṭār 2,. Abū al-Faḍl al-Ṭabīb 2, (anonymous) ʿAṭṭār and Abū al-Surūr al-Sharābī.[636]

Salāma al-ʿAṭṭār (Solomon ha-Zāqēn) [Eg., 12th century]
A pharmacist, mentioned in a document written by Ḥalfon ha-Levi b. Manasseh between 1129 and 1139. Solomon had a daughter named Sitt al-Banāt.[637]

Samuel b. Saʿadya ha-Levi [Eg., Cairo, 12th century]
A *dayyān* and a scribe in the court of Maimonides. He was active between 1165 and 1203. When he was younger, apparently, he worked as a pharmacist; we learn this from a single document in his handwriting that listed various medical materials, their price and the person who purchased them.[638]

Sayyid al-Ahl al-ʿAṭṭār[639] [Eg., 12th century]
A pharmacist, mentioned in a list written by Ḥalfon ha-Levi b. Manasseh.[640]

Sayyid al-Ahl b. Hiba[641] [Eg., Cairo, 12th century]
A pharmacist and a merchant, mentioned in a contract (1139) that dealt with the partnership between himself and Faraḥ b. Abū al-ʿAlā. In the contract,[642] Sayyid reserved for himself the right to sell on his own account a popular

medicine (*qirṭās taḥyīj*) for making women plump (the ideal of female beauty at the time), tooth powder, eye powder and arsenic. This privilege was a compensation for him being the shop manager (buying the materials for these medicines would be on his account). In the contract it was agreed that each partner would receive a daily salary of 1–2 dirhams.[643]

Shamlā al-ʿAṭṭār [Sy., Damascus, 15th century]
A pharmacist from Damascus, whose daughter converted to Islam.[644]

Sulaymān al-ʿAṭṭār [Eg., 13th century]
A pharmacist, mentioned in a list of donors, apparently from the thirteenth century.[645]

al-Yahūdī al-ʿAṭṭār [Eg., Cairo]
A pharmacist, mentioned in an Arabic Geniza document together with al-ʾIsrāʾīlī al-Ṣaydalānī.[646]

Yazīd ha-Bassām [Eg., Cairo, 10th century]
A pharmacist who is mentioned for selling a house to a woman.[647] He was probably active during the tenth century.

Yūsuf b. Abū al-Faraj b. Abū al-Barakāt al-Ṭabīb [Eg., Alexandria, 13th century]

Anonymous pharmacists
Like the anonymous physicians in Section 3.1.1, the anonymous pharmacists listed here are arranged by century, and within each century approximately west to east geographically.

Anonymous – a pharmacist [Eg., 11th–12th centuries]
'Al-ʿAṭṭār' is mentioned in a bill that was apparently written by Hillel b. ʿAlī (1065–1108).[648]

Anonymous – a pharmacist, father of Abū Saʿīd b. al-ʿAṭṭār [Eg., Cairo, 12th century]
The pharmacist's son – Abū Saʿīd b. al-ʿAṭṭār, who is known as Ben al-ʿAfṣī – is mentioned in a letter sent to him.[649] Under the name Abū Saʿīd al-ʿAfṣī, he is also the addressee of a letter[650] sent by Abū al-Ḥasan al-Iskandarānī in

which another pharmacist is mentioned – Benyām al-Rashīdī al-ʿAṭṭār.[651] From another letter sent to him concerning business matters regarding commodities such as *tamar hindī* (tamarind) and *jullanār* (pomegranate flowers) we learn that he was either a merchant of medicinal substances or a pharmacist himself.[652]

Anonymous – a pharmacist, father of Ben Raja ʿAṭṭār [Eg., Cairo, 12th century]

Mentioned in a document along with Abū al-Faraj b. al-Kallām.[653]

Anonymous – ʿAṭṭār [Eg., 12th century]

A pharmacist, active around 1100. He appeared in a list of donors headed by the *nagid* Mevōrākh b. Saʿadya (d. 1111). Also appearing in the list are Abū al-Munā al-ʿAṭṭār, Ibrāhīm ha-Rōfē, Abū Naṣr al-ʿAṭṭār 2, Abū al-Faḍl al-Ṭabīb 2, Salāma al-ʿAṭṭār and Abū al-Surūr al-Sharābī.[654]

Anonymous – ʿAṭṭār 2 [Eg., 12th century]

A pharmacist, appeared in a Geniza document.[655]

Anonymous – a pharmacist, father of Abū al-Karam [Eg., 12th–13th centuries]

In a document written by Joseph b. Samuel ha-Levi, a pharmacist who is no longer alive is mentioned.[656]

Anonymous – al-ʿAṭṭār ha-Levi b. Saʿ(adya) [Eg., 13th century]

A pharmacist, mentioned in a document from the thirteenth century.[657]

Anonymous – al-ʿAṭṭār al-Ḥakīm [Eg., 13th century]

A pharmacist (and maybe also a physician), mentioned in a list of donors along with Joshua Jacob al-ʿAṭṭār.[658]

3.2 Jewish Pharmacists in the Muslim World

> One need not delve deeply into the writings of the Cairo Geniza in order to discover that a great many of them refer to the professions connected with the processing and sale of drugs, spices, perfumes and potions for medical and culinary uses.[659]

The terminology of the profession of pharmacy is complex:[660] the occupational name ʿAṭṭār, usually translated as 'perfumer' or 'druggist', is among those occurring most commonly in the Geniza.[661] Interestingly, in an anthroponymic study of occupational *laqab*s of the Andalusian *'ulmā'*, Manuela Marín revealed that ʿAṭṭār and Ibn al-ʿAṭṭār were the most frequent; that is, perfumers or druggists who were considered part of the manufacturing activities of Muslim scholars connected with economic activities centred in the urban milieu of tenth- to twelfth-century Andalusia.[662] The *ʿaṭṭārīn* usually operated in a special area of the market called the *sūq al-ʿaṭṭārīn*; the term *murabbaʿat al-ʿaṭṭārīn* is mentioned as well.[663]

Another term, *ṣaydalānī* or *ṣaydanī*, is also translated as 'pharmacist', 'apothecary' or 'druggist'.[664] The word *ṣaydalānī* is traditionally explained as a dealer in sandalwood (*Santalum sp.*), so *ṣaydalānī*, like *ʿaṭṭār*, originally designated a perfumer.[665] The medieval Arabic pharmacists or apothecaries (*ṣaydalānī*)[666] were trained to collect and preserve the various medicaments brought from near or far-off lands.[667] Leigh Chipman found in the Muslim Arabic sources of the Mamluk period seventy-five reports of men bearing the professional *nisba* al-ʿAṭṭār but did not find anyone carrying the *nisba* al-Ṣaydalānī.[668] Similarly, out of the 111 pharmacists found in the Geniza and presented above, only one (al-ʾIsrāʾīlī al-Ṣaydalānī) bears this *nisba*. Therefore, it seems that this term fell out of use for a few centuries and made a comeback in the Early Modern and Modern period, mainly as the basic name for apothecaries' shops.

Unlike our knowledge regarding the Jewish physicians, which is based on both Muslim Arabic sources and the documents from the Cairo Geniza; the information regarding the Jewish pharmacists is based mainly on Jewish sources, that is, fragments of the Cairo Geniza. As Chipman concluded, no pharmacists who were not also physicians appear in Muslim Arabic biographical dictionaries, thus indicating 'a conscious separation between the two professions in the mind of the author'.[669] And indeed, despite the close connection between pharmacy and the art of medicine, the profession of pharmacist was strictly separated from it, reinforcing the testimony of the Geniza.

3.2.1 Jewish pharmacists (apothecaries, perfumers and druggists)

Pharmacy was highly popular within all the fields of the art of healing.[670] A significant number of pharmacists are mentioned in documents found in the Geniza.[671] Therefore, reading Goitein's remarks is meaningful: 'The prominence of the Jews in the professions of druggist and pharmacist during the High Middle Ages – which is paralleled by their equally strong representation in the fields of medicine on the one hand, and in that of the international trade in spices and drugs on the other – calls for comment.' He went on to explain that phenomenon not as the continuation of a pre-Islamic tradition, but as a law of economic history which is still in effect today: minority groups have a chance of being successful in occupations which are not as yet monopolised by the more privileged classes of society.[672] A subsidiary element might have been the fact that the pharmacist's profession was a bookish one. The use of handbooks, classical *materia medica* and medical books was an important part of the work. The Jewish religion too, as it developed in post-Talmudic times, had become very scholarly. Out of 607 practitioners for whom biographical details of their medical activity have been traced in the Cairo Geniza (hardly none in the Muslim Arabic sources), 111 were pharmacists.[673] The vast majority of the pharmacists were active in Egypt in general and Cairo in particular and are from the eleventh to the thirteenth centuries; this is natural, since the information came from the Geniza, and the classical Geniza period, as mentioned above, was in those centuries (see Chart 1). One of the explanations for this small number, which contradicts the statement by Goitein above, might be that the Muslim Arabic sources did not write about pharmacists, because their biographies or deeds were of little interest at that time!

Despite its close connection with the medical arts, the profession of the druggist was strictly separated from them, at least as far as the testimony of the Geniza is concerned. Goitein stated that only in rare cases do we find a man called '*X.* b. *X.*, the physician, the *ʿaṭṭār*' or '*X.* b. *X.*, the phlebotomist, the *ʿaṭṭār*'. He claimed that the first profession attached to the name was that of the father and served as a family name, but by no means indicated that the person concerned exercised the two professions.[675]

Negative views of Jewish practitioners did not overlook the Jewish phar-

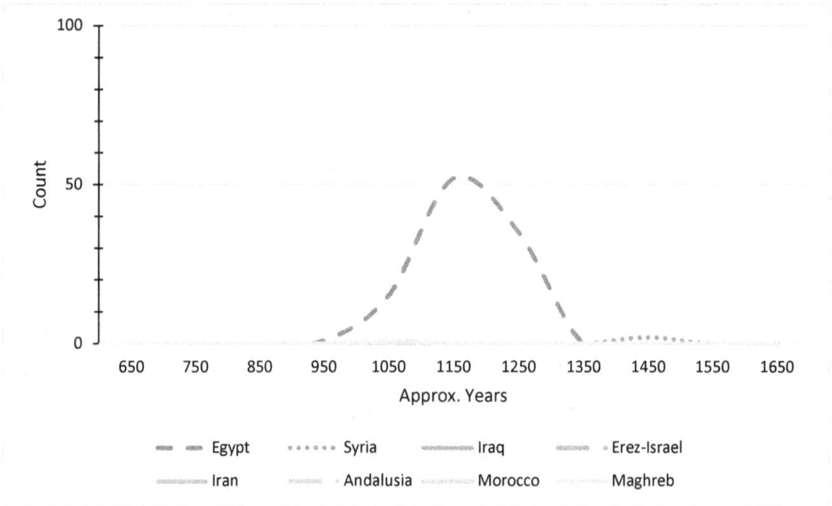

Chart 1 Dispersion of Jewish pharmacists in the Muslim world by year and location.[675]

macists; consider for instance al-Jawbarī's view on the Jewish sellers of drugs or perfume in Syria:

> This [ethnic] group is made up of the worst creatures and the biggest Muslim haters. Externally they show off subservience and poverty as they can't do any harm to a person, especially Muslims; but when they have the opportunity, they insert poison into the food, serving it to a person so that he will on the spot fall asleep, and then they kill him in a hidden place. Such are the doings of their wise men, and the common people deal in counterfeit perfumes and sell them to the Muslims.

He added: 'Jewish pedlars wander around houses, villages and gardens, selling "kinds" of "drugs" that wives insert later to their husbands' food, and stupefy them to do their wishes.'[676]

The centre for the drugs and perfume business in big towns such as Cairo and Alexandria was the Square of the Perfumers, *Murabbaʿat al-ʿAṭṭārīn*, often abbreviated to *Murabbaʿa* or *al-ʿAṭṭārīn*. According to Goitein about a third of the Geniza letters that have an address are directed to the Square of the Perfumers, making the square second only to the synagogue.[677] Drugstores were often used as an address in letters, since they served as a landmark in a neighbourhood. It is important to note, however, that some of the pharmacists worked in hospitals, for example: al-Kohen al-ʿAṭṭār al-Harunī al-ʾIsrāʾīlī.[678]

An idea of the pharmacist's everyday life can be gained from this selection of insights, information and anecdotes:

a. **Charity** plays an important part in religious Jewish tradition and culture, and hundreds of lists of names of contributors of money or products for various purposes such as freeing captured Jews and supporting the poor have been found in the Geniza. These are an exceptionally good source for the study of the socio-economic status of different occupations.[679] According to Cohen, pharmacists, druggists and perfumers were regarded as part of the 'non-poor' (in other words the middle class), and their names appeared on many lists of donors,[680] along with other professionals such as the beadle of a synagogue, cantor, tanner, errand boy (factotum), young man (slave or free man/apprentice/factotum), flax merchant, carpenter, teacher, translator, astrologer, maker or seller of olive oil, meat cook, seller of honey sherbet, butcher, seller of chickens, cheesemaker, milkman, glassmaker, fishmonger, darner, tailor, journeyman, cake master, maker or seller of sugar, silk worker, dyer, dyer of purple, banker/moneychanger, money assayer, goldsmith or silversmith.[681] The engagement of the son of a perfumer to a girl from a prominent family of India traders can teach us about the high socio-economic status of perfumers.[682] From the case of Samuel b. Saʿadya ha-Levi (a. 1165–1203) we can learn about the option of changing occupations and moving up the social and economic ladder. At first, when he was young, Samuel worked as a pharmacist (we learn this from a single document in his handwriting that listed various medical materials, their price and the person who purchased them); however, he served later as a *dayyān* and a scribe in the court of Maimonides.[683]
b. **Legal aspects:** Drugstores and pharmacies appeared in documents dealing with economic and legal aspects of commercial and industrial partnerships, more than any other occupation. I present here a few examples only. From among many such documents dating back to 1126, one deals with the dissolution of a partnership in a perfumery, *dukkān al-ʿiṭr*, which was

shared by two partners (interestingly enough, neither of their names have an epithet related to such activity); in another document, Abū al-Munā al-ʿAṭṭār Jacob b. David ha-Parnās received a loan of 57 dinars for his perfumery business through the mediation of a banker; other documents teach us that loans were given and received by *ʿaṭṭārs* and *sharābīs*.[684]

c. **Real estate:** There is much evidence in the Geniza that pharmacists were active in real estate. Here are some examples that were studied by Goitein and Kahn: a certain *ʿaṭṭār* rented a place, in (New) Cairo, for eight years (1150), making renovations worth 40 dinars (the equivalent of eight annual rents of 5 dinars); a perfumer rented part of a communal building for a period of at least four years in order to use it for storing rose water (1180–4); another *ʿaṭṭār* paid a lady (presumably Muslim) 28 dirhams for the monthly rent for his store (1334); and a Jewish pharmacist bought from three Christian ladies one-quarter of a house (paying 70 dinars), as he already possessed the other three-quarters of it, thus acquiring full ownership; a *sharābī* sold to an *ʿaṭṭār* (before a Jewish court) one-eighth of a house, which he shared in common with Christians and a fellow Jew (1179). In another document an estate was left by a Jewish *ʿaṭṭār*, and his two sisters certified that they had received their shares – namely the stock of drugs, the storage room and the goods found in it;[685] a complete (but old and partly neglected) house, bordering on one Christian and two Muslim properties, was acquired by a Jewish *ʿaṭṭār* in December 1088, in the presence of a Muslim notary.[686]

d. **Druggists' shop contents:** From legal documents such as wills and partnership agreements that were studied by Goitein we may get an idea of the contents of the druggist's shop.[687] A list of debts of three retailers to one deceased druggists' wholesaler consists of: pharmacist's scales, pots of Kabul myrobalan and syrup of honey and vinegar.[688] Dozens of lists of medicinal substances, which are remnants and evidence of the trade in and use of these drugs, were found in the Geniza and studied,[689] as well as the uses of the substances found in them.[690]

It is important to note here that based on my study of dozens of practical prescriptions found in the Geniza (including one that was written by Maimonides, and a few others whose author was identified as a physician), I suggest that it was the physician, not the pharmacist, who was responsible for writing prescriptions.

Rarely do historical sources provide us with specific information regarding drugs. Therefore, it is worth mentioning Ibn al-Qifṭī's story about Mūsā b. El'āzār al-'Isrā'īlī (Moses b. Elazar) (10th century) who was described as a knowledgeable physician and pharmacist; for instance he specifies in detail a drug he invented: *sharāb al-uṣūl*, which supposedly treated constipation, prevented bad odours and abdominal pain associated with the menstrual cycle in women, and cleaned the uterus of waste, which was considered a cause of miscarriage. It also benefited the renal system, cleaning the kidneys of stones and other waste created in them; guided medicine to the core of the infected organs; and dissolved yellow bile from the intestines, causing it to be excreted through urine.[691]

3.2.2 Related professions: potion makers

Besides pharmacists, the Geniza documents contain information about professions related to pharmacy, that is, producers of drugs.

The *sharābī* (potion maker and seller) is a person that prepares and/or sells medical potions, light beverages and wines. This is another occupation frequently occurring in the Geniza. The *ṭabbākh sharāb*, preparer of potions, presumably produced *sharāb* wholesale and supplied them to *sharābī* retailers.[692] According to Cohen, preparers or sellers of potions[693] were among the non-poor (comfortably off) in the Jewish community.[694] Here are some examples:

a. al-Nafīs al-Sharābī appeared in a list of taxpayers or benefactors to a fund, raised for the redemption of captives and so on.[695]
b. Abū al-Surūr al-Sharābī headed a list of donors from 1110.[696]
c. Abū al-'Izz al-Sharābī was mentioned in a list of donors from c.1210.[697]
d. Abū al-Barakāt al-Ṭabīb, who operated in Fusṭāṭ in the mid-twelfth century, and lived in a store at the end of Wax Manufacturers Street, was mentioned as 'Barakāt b. al-Sharābī' in a list of donors.[698]

In some documents, physicians practising in a *sharābī*'s shop are mentioned;[699] for example Abū al-Faraj b. Ma'mar al-Sharābī (Nethanel ha-Levi

b. Amram), whose store is mentioned in Geniza documents (11th century). The store was probably large, since it was used to keep imported metals and as the clinic of Abū al-Ghālib (a Christian physician) as well as a Jewish practitioner named R. Amram b. Saʿīd b. Mūsā.[700] An order to a *sharābī* teaches us about the use of charge accounts: a child or a servant was sent to a store with a message indicating the commodities and quantities desired. After a number of such notes had accumulated in the store the potion maker would send them back with the account. Thirty orders, sent by the prominent India trader Abū Zikrī Kohen to two different *sharābī*s, contained many items which were found in the Geniza.[701]

3.2.3 Commercial aspects of drugs

The Fatimid caliphate was formed, besides other political aspects, thanks to economic prosperity in the Maghrib (north Africa) and Egypt, in contrast to the demise of the Abbasid caliphate, which suffered economic collapse in Iraq. Egypt was a centre of intensive commercial activity, peopled by big merchants, small traders, various middlemen and others. This process was accompanied by a major migration of talented and skilled men, merchants and administrators alike, from Iraq to Egypt. The new court that was established in Cairo, its administration and the new bourgeois socio-economic class created an increasing demand for luxury products such as perfume, silk, gemstones, spices and drugs. And indeed, Egypt became the main transit market between the Indian Ocean and the Mediterranean world. The trade with India (mainly by Muslims and Jews), and in 'Indian' products including drugs, yielded enormous profits. Geniza sources of the eleventh and twelfth centuries mention profits of 100 per cent. The amounts of products and the size of the shipments to Egypt mentioned in Geniza sources are astonishing! Our knowledge of the commercial activity of the period between the eleventh and the thirteenth centuries is based mainly on the Cairo Geniza documents. The Geniza's merchants were well acquainted with the trading routes and they operated in the main centres of trade: Aden, Oman, Cairo-Fusṭāṭ, Alexandria, Qayrawān and Sicily. Traders of various religious and ethnic groups cooperated in these commercial activities; the predominant groups included the Tustaris, Radhanites, Kārimīs, Maghribis, Amalfitans and Venetian merchants.[702]

The trade in medicinal substances from India, Iran, the Levant, north Africa and other areas was only a fraction of this multifaceted activity, which included spices, textiles, tools and so on. Extensive information on this aspect of medieval mercantile activity can be gathered from documents published by various scholars.[703] Albert Dietrich published an early example: an order sent from Aden in southwest Arabia to the capital of Egypt which reflects the international trade in drugs rather than the profession of druggist. The Adenese merchant had entrusted a business friend travelling to Fusṭāṭ with 14 pounds of cardamom and asked him to order for him Western drugs from two perfumers. The drugs ordered are arranged in two sections, one containing those items the writer knew to be available, and one listing those of which he was not sure. He purposely does not indicate quantities or prices, leaving the choice to the experience and trustworthiness of his correspondent, who would buy in accordance with the fluctuating market situation.[704]

On a local scale, there are many documents dealing with trade in drugs. Among other examples is an order from a druggist that was sent from Alexandria (or Rosetta) to Fusṭāṭ, containing drugs needed by the sender for local consumers. Letters from small towns in the Egyptian Rif frequently contain orders of drugs which reveal their writers to be *ʿaṭṭār*s.[705]

Very often, patients bought their medicines from the pharmacists at the marketplace. These drug sellers probably relied for their sales not only on a prescription written by a physician, but also on their own diagnoses, suggesting methods of treatment, or even on their customers' self-medication. The market police were in charge of protecting the customers' wallets, ensuring that expensive materials were not adulterated with cheaper substitutes. The drug sellers were monitored by an official known as the *muḥtasib*, who was well versed in religious matters, and whose duties included inspecting and assaying drugs.[706]

An interesting account is a partnership contract (1139) between the pharmacists Faraḥ b. Abū al-ʿAlā and Sayyid al-Ahl b. Hiba. Sayyid reserved for himself the right to sell autonomously a popular medicine for making women plump (the ideal of female beauty at the time), tooth powder, eye powder and arsenic (buying the materials for these medicines would be on his account). This privilege would be a recompense for being the shop manager. In the contract it was agreed that each partner would receive a daily salary of 1–2 dirhams.[707]

Every hospital contained a stock of ready-made drugs and medicines that could be given on the spot to urgent cases and patients in a critical condition. Based on medieval Muslim Arabic sources, Ahmed Ragab suggested that 'although the medications themselves may not have been different from others produced in the market, their immediate availability gave the *bīmāristān* a significant edge'.[708]

3.3 Dynasties of Jewish Practitioners

3.3.1 Introduction

A dynasty is a sequence of successive rulers or leaders, or a series of family members who are distinguished by their success, wealth or occupation. In general, families, and sometimes ethnic groups, tended to stick to certain types of professions.[709] The Jewish tradition strongly suggests that fathers should teach their sons an occupation, and according to Goitein, this means either that the father teaches him his own profession, or that he pays for his son's tuition in another craft from someone else. Since there were no vocational schools in the Muslim world of the medieval period, the teaching was done by specialists, and the communication was mainly verbal. Therefore, we have only a few records of the way such teaching was conducted.[710]

Preceding the emergence of physician dynasties in Jewish culture, there were dynasties of rabbis who served as community leaders. The latter is a known phenomenon in Jewish social culture. However, in early Jewish history, rabbis did not function as community leaders, rather they ran Talmudic academies and courts of justice (*yeshivot*). Later on, in the Geonic period (from the eighth century), the office of *rosh yeshiva* (head of a Talmudic college and a court of justice) was considered a 'family patrimony'.[711] Among the reasons for this process, as noted by Avraham Grossman, are the changes that occurred in the Muslim society within which the Jews lived. In the early Islamic period, based on the ancient tribal laws, the leader was chosen by the members of the tribe, and therefore, inheritance of leadership was far from their perception. However, over the years, and mainly during the Abbasid period, dynasties of rulers became common. By then, many of the Jews of that period had moved to the big cities and Muslim capitals, and quite a few of them were close to the rulers' courts. Influenced economically and culturally by these rulers, the principle of inheritance infiltrated Jewish society's religious and secular leadership.[712]

Dynasties of scholars and other occupations were a normal and known custom in the Muslim world among families of all religions. The main target was to preserve the socio-economic status of the family through cooperation within the family, with respect to business and education; in Marín's words, regarding Muslim society, 'kinship appears as a crucial element in the reproduction of *'ulmā'* as an elite group'.[713] Among the many examples, I will mention only a few: the Nuʿmān, a distinguished family of tenth-century Fatimid *qadis*;[714] the Subkī family, which was prominent in the intellectual life of Cairo and Damascus for six generations or more in the thirteenth and fourteenth centuries;[715] and the Banū Jamāʿa family, a dynasty of Shāfi'ite jurists in the Mamluk period.[716] Having a scholar or specialist as a father, grandfather or other close relative could be of enormous advantage to an individual seeking to carve out an academic or professional career, leading to creating networks of personal, intellectual, business or professional relationships through which a reputation was established.[717] Other interesting cases were portrayed by Avraham Elmakias in his work on the naval commanders of early Islam. In it he presented what he called 'the succeeding son phenomenon'. The examples are actual 'dynasties' of Muslim naval commanders.[718]

Geniza studies indicates that not only heads of *yeshivot*, judges and government officials, but also members of powerful merchant houses, religious dignitaries and scholars, tended to perpetuate themselves by raising their offspring in the same profession or by adopting someone of similar status. This trend was common practice among physicians as well.[719] According to the Hippocratic oath, the student of medicine or the novice physician should regard his teachers with respect equal to that which he has for his parents, and therefore, should pass on medical expertise and knowledge to his teachers' sons as well as to his own.

Indeed, frequently throughout the history of medicine, the father was also the teacher, and the 'art' of medicine was considered an endowment to be handed down.[720] Miri Shefer suggested that 'although medical careers were open to many; it is clear that those with family "in business", so to speak, would be likely to have a smoother path than those without such advantages. Having a successful physician as a relative made it easier to find good teachers either within the family or outside, and to start building connections.'[721] The emergence of dynasties of Jewish physicians was probably encouraged by the tendency to tutor their offspring privately in medical knowledge. Peter Pormann and Emilie Savage-Smith claimed that when dealing with medical education, 'many physicians handed down medical knowledge to their own offspring, thereby creating some famous lineages'.[722] While the transmission of medical knowledge prevailed among Muslim families, it was even more common in Jewish and Christian families. As *dhimmīs*, or *ahl al-Dhimma*, their options for receiving medical instruction from Muslims were more limited.[723]

In Christian Spain, Jews, who were prevented from accessing universities or medical schools, studied Arabic and Hebrew medical texts independently, and in most cases within the family.[724] Similarly, in Muslim Spain (Andalusia, al-Andalus), as there were no hospitals at the time, medical training often remained 'within the family'.[725] The situation in the eastern Muslim territories was better, especially during the Fatimid and Ayyubid periods. In most cases the study of medicine during these periods was inter-religious. Jewish students studied with Muslim and Christian teachers, and famous Jewish physicians taught students of other religions.[726] Examples of this occurrence can be found in the biographical dictionaries of physicians by Ibn al-Qifṭī (1172–1248) and Ibn Abī Uṣaybiʿa (1203–70).[727] In addition, medical knowledge was also transmitted in established hospitals.[728] It seems, therefore, that the transmission of medical knowledge within the Jewish family facilitated the medical profession, and indeed, this method appeared to be the primary channel for the transmission of medical knowledge among Jews in medieval Christian Europe, as well.[729]

As mentioned before, physicians in the Islamic world could acquire their medical knowledge through private tutoring, apprenticeship, hospital training, self-teaching and familial tuition.[730] After that, they were tested and received official graduation diplomas from the governing body, affording the physician recognition as qualified to work in his field.[731] As mentioned above, renowned physicians would often serve in a hospital, not necessarily for the financial benefits, but for the sake of the admiration the position generated, and in order to train new young doctors.[732]

So far, forty-nine separate dynasties of Jewish medical practitioners who

Table 3 Dynasties of Jewish practitioners in the Fatimid, Ayyubid and Mamluk periods[734]

No.	*Name*	*Generations*	*Places*	*Centuries*	*Positions held*	*Remarks; regime*
1	Moses b. Elazar	4	Tunisia, Cairo	10th–11th	Court physicians, Head of the Jews/ chief administrators	Fatimid
2	Ḥasday	3–5	Cordova, Saragossa	10th–12th	Court physicians, diplomats	Umayyad
3	Moses Ben Maimon – Maimonides	6 (Fatimid-Ayyubid)[a] generationsincluding Mamluk period	Cairo, Damascus	11th–15th	Court physicians, hospitals, Head of the Jews, judges	Fatimid-Ayyubid, Mamluk
4	Isaac ha-Kohen ha- Rōfē b. Furāt	2	Cairo, Ramle	11th	Court physicians, probably Head of the Jews	Fatimid
5	Ephraim b. al-Zaffān	?	Cairo	11th	Court physicians, traders/merchants	Fatimid
6	ʿAlī ha-Busmī	2	Egypt	11th	Physician, pharmacist	Fatimid
7	Abraham ha-Rōfē	2	Egypt	11th	Physicians	Fatimid
8	Moses Darʿī	3	Alexandria	11th–12th	Karaites; physicians	Fatimid-Ayyubid
9	Ibn Qamniʾel	2/3	Andalusia, Seville, Saragossa, Marrakesh	11th–12th	Physicians	Various including Almoravid
10	Yaḥyā b. ʿAbbās al-Maghribī	2	Baghdad	11th–12th	Court physicians	Fatimid-Ayyubid
11	Saʿadya b. Mevōrākh	3	Cairo	11th–12th	Court physicians, Head of the Jews	Fatimid
12	Moses b. Jekuthiel	4	Andalusia, Cairo	11th–12th	Physicians, traders/merchants, community leaders	Fatimid-Ayyubid
13	Salāma b. Mubārak	2	Cairo	11th–12th	Physicians	Fatimid
14	Aaron ha-Rōfē al-ʿAmmānī	8	Amman, Alexandria	11th–13th	Court physician, communal leaders, judges	Fatimid-Ayyubid

15	Muwaffaq al-Dawla Abū al-Faraj ʿAlī b. Abī al-Shujāʿ al-Hamadānī	3	Hamadān, Tabriz	11th–14th	Court physicians, hospitals	Mongol (Īl-Khānate)
16	ʿAlī ha-Rōfē	2	Egypt	11th	Physician, pharmacist	Fatimid
17	Moses b. Nethanel ha-Levi (Abū Saʿd)	2	Cairo	12th	Possibly court physicians, hospitals, Head of the Jews	Fatimid-Ayyubid
18	Abū al-Faḍl b. al-Nāqid	2	Cairo	12th	Ophthalmologists	Converted to Islam (son); Fatimid- Ayyubid
19	Abū Manṣūr (Isaac)	3	Cairo	12th	Physicians	Fatimid- Ayyubid
20	Samuel b. Hananiah (Abū Manṣūr)	2	Cairo	12th	Court physician, Head of the Jews	Fatimid
21	Zechariah the Alexandrian	3	Alexandria, Jerusalem, Cairo	12th–13th	Court physicians/communal leaders, judges; traders/merchants	Fatimid-Ayyubid
22	Ṣadaqa al-ʾIsrāʾīlī	2	Damascus (primarily)	12th–13th (until 1239)	Court physician(s), hospitals	Fatimid-Ayyubid
23	Abū al-Barakāt b. al-Sharābī	4[b]	Cairo, Alexandria	12th–13th	Physicians	Fatimid- Ayyubid
24	Abū Saʿd al-ʿAṭṭār	2	Cairo	12th–13th	Pharmacists	Ayyubid
25	Sukra al-Yahūdī al-Ḥalabī	3	Aleppo, Damascus	12th–13th	Court physicians – Zengi and Saladin	Zengid, Ayyubid, Mamluk; descendants converted to Islam
26	Abū al-Barakāt Ibn Shaʿya	2[c]	Cairo	Probably Ayyubid period	Karaites; court (?) physician	Ayyubid, possibly very early Mamluk
27	Khalaf al-Sāmirī	3	Damascus, Baalbek	12th–13th	Samaritans; court physicians, hospitals	Fatimid-Ayyubid
28	Abū al-Bayān	2	Cairo	12th–13th	Karaites; court physicians, hospitals	Fatimid-Ayyubid
29	al-Sadīd al-Ṭabīb	2	Cairo	12th–13th	Physician, pharmacist	Fatimid-Ayyubid

Table 3 continued

No.	*Name*	*Generations*	*Places*	*Centuries*	*Positions held*	*Remarks; regime*
30	Ibn Jumayʿ	2+	Cairo, Alexandria	12th–15th	Physicians	Ayyubid, Mamluk
31	Petahya ha-Levi	2	Damascus	13th	Karaites; physicians	Ayyubid
32	al-Sheikh Joseph	2	Cairo	13th	Physicians	Ayyubid
33	Abū al-Fakhr al-ʿAṭṭār	2	Cairo	13th	Pharmacists	Ayyubid
34	Tiqva ha-Levi	2	Cairo	13th	Physicians, possibly communal leaders	Ayyubid
35	Abū al-Ḥasan al- Aṭṭār 3	2	Egypt, Alexandria	13th	Pharmacists	Ayyubid
36	Maḥāsin (Obadia ha-Dayyān)	3	[al-Bīra] (Birecik)]	13th–14th	*Ḥakīms/mutatabbib*, philosopher, *dayyān*	Mamluk periphery
37	Ibn al-Kirmānī	2	Cairo	13th–14th (1260–1324)	Karaites; ophthalmologist	Mamluk
38	ʿAbd al-Sayyid b. Isḥāq	3–4	Damascus	13th–14th	Physicians, hospitals, *dayyāns*	Mamluk; converted to Islam
39	Shihāb al-Dīn Aḥmad al-Maghribī	2–3	(Maghrib), Cairo, (?Damascus)	13th–14th	Court physicians, 'Head of Physicians' (as Muslims), hospitals, high state bureaucrats	Ayyubid, Mamluk; converted to Islam
40	Ibn Ṣaghīr	2*	Cairo	13th–14th	Karaites; court physicians (mostly as Muslims), 'Head of Physicians' (as Muslims)	Ayyubid, Mamluk; converted
41	Ibn Kūjik	2[d]	Cairo	14th	Karaites; court and distinguished physicians	Mamluk; converted to Islam
42	Saʿadya	3	Maghrib, Cairo, Alexandria	14th–15th	Karaites; physicians	Mamluk
43	Jacob ha-Rōfē	3	Cairo	14th	Physicians, communal leaders	Mamluk
44	Obadia ha-Rōfē	2	Tripoli	14th	Physicians	Mamluk

45	Nafīs b. Daʾūd b. ʿAnān al-Tabrīzī	3	Cairo	14th–15th (1354–1413)	Karaites; court physicians (as Muslims); 'Head of the Physicians'; state secretary	Mamluk; converted to Islam
46	ʿAbd Allāh b. Daʾūd b. Abī al-Faḍl al-Daʾūdī	3	?Cairo	14th–15th (c.1300–1428)	Karaites; court/distinguished physicians	Mamluk; converted to Islam
47	David b. Jacob	2	Egypt	14th–15th	Physicians	Mamluk
48	Joseph from Damascus	2	Damascus, Candia, Crete	15th	Physicians	Mamluk
49	Joseph b. Abraham Sakandarī	3	Andalusia, Alexandria, Cairo	15th–16th	Physicians, communal leaders, judges	Mamluk

a Six generations refers to the Maimonidean physicians in the Fatimid-Ayyubid period. Considering the family of Moses Maimonides' wife, whose father and great-grandfather were physicians, as well as her son Abraham, and possibly her grandson David, we can count nine generations.
b Four generations of practitioners; the founder of the dynasty was a *sharabī* (preparer or seller of potions).
c This family might be the forebear of the Ibn Ṣaghīr/Ibn Kūjik dynasties, see below.
d Part of a long dynasty that was related to the Ibn Ṣaghīr and probably the Ibn Shaʿya dynasties, as discussed in Mazor and Lev, 'The Phenomenon'.

were active in the medieval Muslim world have been traced; the vast majority of them were active in Egypt and Syria between the tenth and the early sixteenth centuries, while the rest were from other parts of the Muslim world, mainly Andalusia, Iran, Iraq and Azerbaijan. Examples of Jewish medical dynasties are also to be found in lists of contributors, where, for instance, in one list, three or more physicians belonging to the same family live in one house and the same is noted of two ophthalmologists, father and son.[734]

I did not consider two brothers practising medicine as a dynasty, although we have some examples of this phenomenon: Berākhōt ha-Rōfē b. Sar Shālōm and Tiqva ha-Rōfē b. Sar Shālōm (13th century),[735] and Abū al-ʿIzz al-Ṭabīb and Abū al-Mufaḍḍal al-Muhadhdhab (also 13th century).[736] I decided to present the biographies of the dynasties' members together, for the sake of making the connection between them clearer to the reader. Headings of each biography of a physician that was part of a dynasty have been retained in Section 3.1.1, and likewise with pharmacists in Section 3.1.2; these can be found in alphabetical order.

The dynasties and the detailed biographies of each member are presented below. The main pieces of geographical, chronological and professional information have been gathered and presented in Table 3.

3.3.2 Biographies and family trees[737]

In order to better understand the dynasties of practitioners that are presented below, a family tree was built for each one of them. In this book, I have chosen to present family trees only for dynasties consisting of three generations or more), representing different kinds of dynasties, periods, patterns and geographical location. A few trees have been presented in previous publications.[738] A short introduction has been written for the more interesting, complicated or important dynasties.

Dynasty 1 – Moses b. Elazar

The dynasty of Moses b. Elazar is the earliest known dynasty of Jewish practitioners; it includes four generations of court physicians, viziers and chief leaders of the Jewish community. This family filled these offices in Tunisia and later in Egypt, from the mid-tenth to the mid-eleventh centuries. This dynasty and its features embodied the golden age of the Jews, particularly of

Jewish physicians, in medieval Egypt and Syria: the passing of the medical profession through several generations, serving as court physicians to the caliphs, serving as chief leaders of the Jewish community, and serving as chief administrators, or *wazīrs*, in charge of the state treasury. It is especially the last office that was entrusted to the hands of this Jewish dynasty, which made them the most powerful of all known dynasties of Jewish physicians in medieval Egypt and Syria.[739]

DYNASTY 1

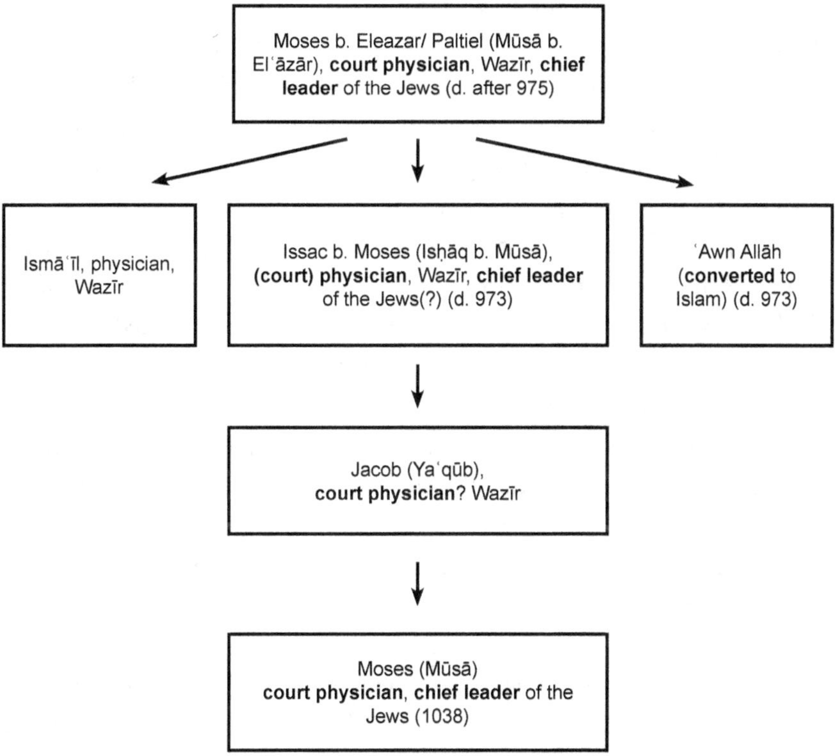

Mūsā b. Elʿāzār al-ʾIsrāʾīlī (Moses b. Elazar) [It, Oria, M., Qayrawān, Eg., Cairo, 10th century]

A physician known for his expertise in medicine, and considered the best Jew at his profession in Cairo. Moses was originally from the town of Oria, southern Italy. In 925, Fatimid corps led by Abū Aḥmad Jaʿfar b. ʿAbīd invaded Oria and captured Moses, who was released at Qayrawān (present-day Tunisia).[740] According to some scholars, in Qayrawān he became a disciple of the famous Jewish court physician and medical writer Isḥāq b. Sulaymān al-ʾIsrāʾīlī (Isaac b. Solomon); also known as Isaac Israeli. Later he served two Fatimid caliphs: al-Manṣūr bi-Ilāh (r. 946–53) and al-Muʿizz li-Dīn Allāh (r. 953–75). He arrived in Egypt after it was conquered by the Fatimids in 969, with al-Muʿizz li-Dīn Allāh. Having served at the Fatimid court for such a long time, Moses became one of the most influential figures in Fatimid Cairo. The caliph, who trusted and valued him, appointed him as his personal physician.[741] Moses made up many pharmaceutical compounds for the caliph, including a tamarind-based beverage. The methods for producing these compounds were mentioned by the physician al-Tamīmī al-Muqaddasī.[742] Ibn al-Qifṭī depicted Moses as a knowledgeable physician and pharmacist. It is also mentioned that Moses invented *sharāb al-uṣūl*, which supposedly treats constipation, prevents bad odours and abdominal pain associated with the menstrual cycle, and cleans the uterus of waste, which was considered a cause for miscarriage. Ibn al-Qifṭī specified that it also benefits the renal system, cleaning the kidneys of waste and stones created in them; guides medicine to the core of the infected organs; and dissolves yellow bile (originally '*al-māʾ al-aṣfar*') from the intestines, causing it to be excreted through urine.[743] Moses is mentioned as an excellent royal physician in a letter from al-Muʿizz to his famous general Jawhar, saying that Moses had made an excellent theriac for Jawhar's sickness.[744] He attended to the caliph during the illness from which he died. He was also the physician to the caliph al-ʿAzīz bi-Allah (r. 975–96).[745] Moreover, he was probably the founder of a dynasty of court physicians who also supposedly were the supreme leaders of the Jewish community until the year 1039 (see below).[746] His sons, Isḥāq b. Mūsā b. Elʿāzār and Ismāʿīl b. Mūsā b. Elʿāzār, his grandson Yaʿqūb b. Isḥāq and his great-grandson Mūsā b. Yaʿqūb all served the caliph, some of them as physicians.

Among his writings are a paper on coughs, and two books dedicated to Caliph al-Muʿizz: *al-Kitāb al Muʿizzī fī al-Ṭabīkh* and *Kitāb al-Qarābādhīn*, which according to Goitein was lost, but descriptions of medical conditions and recipes for medicine included in it are mentioned in other books.[747] Al-Maqrīzī detailed the events of the year 974–5, during the era of Caliph al-Muʿizz. He mentioned the professionals and specified Moses b. Elazar as al-Muʿizz's physician several times. It is also said that when the caliph became ill, his physician Moses b. Elazar suggested drinking a beverage made of *al-burullusī* watermelon.[748] At first, they were only able to find one watermelon of that kind in Egypt and they bought it for five dinars. Afterwards, they found eighteen more and purchased them for eighteen dinars. Moses b. Elazar attended al-Muʿizz during his illness for thirty-eight days until he died.[749]

Bernard Lewis convincingly argued that Mūsā b. Elʿāzār is in fact Palṭiel b. Shephatiah (Shefaṭya).[750] The enigmatic figure of Palṭiel is mentioned in an eleventh-century Jewish family chronicle known as the Aḥimaʿaṣ scroll. Lewis based his argument mainly on the fact that Palṭiel is mentioned in this chronicle as a counsellor of al-Muʿizz who originally was taken captive from Oria in 925 during the Fatimid raids on southern Italy. Since Muslim Arabic sources mention this fact as well, it is clear enough to assume that Palṭiel is identical to Moses.[751] Most scholars accept Lewis's view.[752] The Aḥimaʿaṣ chronicle (scroll) mentioned also that Palṭiel was appointed 'master of al-Muʿizz's house and domain', that is, in the position of a *wazīr*.[753] Interestingly enough, this detail with regard to Moses' son Isaac (Isḥāq) was mentioned also by Ibn Abī Uṣaybiʿa and especially by al-Maqrīzī.[754] One might deduce that the senior position of Moses in the Fatimid court was inherited and even strengthened by his son Isaac. Indeed, Moses seems to have held power in the Fatimid court which extended his official executive profession as the chief physician of the caliph. Moses was probably a close friend of the converted Jew and *wazīr* of the Fatimid Caliph, Yaʿqūb Ibn Killis.[755] If we are to identify Moses b. Elazar with Palṭiel, then we can say with certainty, according to the Aḥimaʿaṣ chronicle, that he was the caliph's viceroy.[756] In addition, it seems that Palṭiel/Moses also filled the position of Head of the Jews, since he is mentioned in Aḥimaʿaṣ chronicle several times as *nagid*.[757] According to H. Z. Hirschberg, Moses b. Elazar, or Palṭiel, was the leader of the Maghrib Jewry also before he moved to Egypt, after the Fatimid conquest of this land in 969.[758]

Thanks to his high position, Moses managed to establish a four-generation dynasty of court physicians, statesmen and probably Jewish leaders too: his sons, his grandson and his great-grandson (see below).

Isḥāq b. Mūsā b. Elʿāzār (Abū Yaʿqūb al-Ṭabīb) (al-Mutaṭabbib) [Ma., Mahdiyya, Eg., Cairo, 10th century]

A physician, came to Egypt from the former capital city of the Fatimid caliphate, al-Mahdiyya, Tunis, together with his father, Mūsā b. Elʿāzār al-ʾIsrāʾīlī (Moses b. Elazar), his brother ʿAwn Allāh b. Mūsā, who was a Muslim, and the Fatimid caliph al-Muʿizz li-Dīn Allāh.[759] Ibn Abī Uṣaybiʿa mentioned him with the epithet 'al-Mutaṭabbib'.[760] Hence, it seems very plausible that Isaac, together with his father, served al-Muʿizz as personal physicians. However, the main responsibility of Isaac was being the chief administrator of the caliphate. Ibn Abī Uṣaybiʿa mentioned that 'Isḥāq was of a great ability in al-Muʿizz's court and he was appointed over all of al-Muʿizz's government'.[761] Al-Maqrīzī details more, mentioning that 'Isḥāq was the director of the state, the supervisor over all the matters/issues (*umūr*) of al-Muʿizz and his treasury, from small to large, the one who permits and forbids'. In other words, Isaac was in the position of the Wazīr.[762] It seems that he also inherited this position from his father, but he concentrated even more power in his hands. According to some scholars, Isaac might also have succeeded his father's position as Head of the Jews.[763] According to the Muslim Arabic sources, Isaac died in Cairo in 973, while his father was still alive. His Muslim brother, ʿAwn Allāh, died a day earlier. Caliph al-Muʿizz is said to be saddened by the death of the talented Isaac.[764] When Isaac died al-Muʿizz appointed his brother Ismāʿīl b. Mūsā in his place. The sources specify that Moses and his son Isaac served Caliph al-Muʿizz li-Dīn Allāh as his personal physicians in his palace, as the chief administrators of the al-Muʿizz caliphate, and possibly also as court physicians.[765]

Ismāʿīl b. Mūsā b. Elʿāzār [Ma., Mahdiyya, Eg., Cairo, 10th century]

The brother of Isḥāq b. Mūsā b. Elʿāzār and the son of Moses b. Elazar, the known physicians of the Fatimid caliph al-Muʿizz. He and Isaac's son, Jacob (Yaʿqūb), were appointed as successors to their brother and father respectively as the chief administrators of al-Muʿizz's caliphate, and possibly also as a court physician after Isaac's death in 973. They seemed to fill the high position of *wazīr*/chief administrator for two years only, since after al-Muʿizz's death (975), this office was transferred to another person.[766] According to Steinschneider, Ismāʿīl was a physician, like the rest of the members of this family.[767]

Yaʿqūb b. Isḥāq [Eg., 11th century]

A physician, the son of Isḥāq b. Mūsā b. Elʿāzār and the grandson of Mūsā b. Elʿāzār al-ʾIsrāʾīlī. As discussed above, the family practised medicine during the time of the Fatimid caliph al-Muʿizz; when Isḥāq, Yaʿqūb's father, died in 973 he was appointed as court physician. Yaʿqūb was probably also the chief leader of the Jews.[768]

Mūsā (Abū al-Imrān) b. Yaʿqūb b. Isḥāq al-ʾIsrāʾīlī [Eg., 11th century]

The great-grandson of Mūsā b. Elʿāzār al-ʾIsrāʾīlī (?Palṭiel). He was a court physician and probably also served as the supreme leader of the Jews.[769] In a legal document (1038), considering a Muslim's complaint regarding the foundation of a new synagogue, he is mentioned as 'the just sheikh Abū al-Imrān Mūsā b. Yaʿqūb b. Isḥāq the Israelite, physician to the exalted Majesty and Chief of the Jewish community, Rabbanite, Karaite and Samaritan'.[770] Shulamit Sela suggested that the titles in the document refer to Moses' grandfather, court physician Isḥāq al-ʾIsrāʾīlī.[771] Mazor and Lev argued that 'this evidence is instructive, since it indicates that the combined position of court physician and head of the Jewish community were held by Moses, and in fact, were preserved in this dynasty for four generations'.[772]

Dynasty 2 – Ḥasday

A dynasty of descendants of Ḥasday b. Shaprūṭ. The information regarding the conversion of the various members of the family is incomplete and even contradictory, and therefore, there are differences of opinion among the researchers. In any case, most of the family members were deeply assimilated in the Arabic culture. According to Sarah Stroumsa, it was a long and progressive process, that was stretched over a few generations, in which even the converted members of the family kept some of their Jewish identity.[773]

Ḥasday b. Shaprūṭ [An., Cordova, 10th century]

A scholar, physician, and trusted adviser at the court of the Umayyad caliphs ʿAbd al-Raḥmān III (912–61) and al-Ḥakam II (905–75) in Cordova, the patron of the first Jewish intellectuals and poets in Andalusia. Ḥasday was a scion of a well-established family. His father, Isaac, had moved the family from its home in Jaén to Cordova, the capital of the caliphate, and there founded a synagogue. Isaac hired Menahem b. Sarūq, a philologist and poet, as secretary,

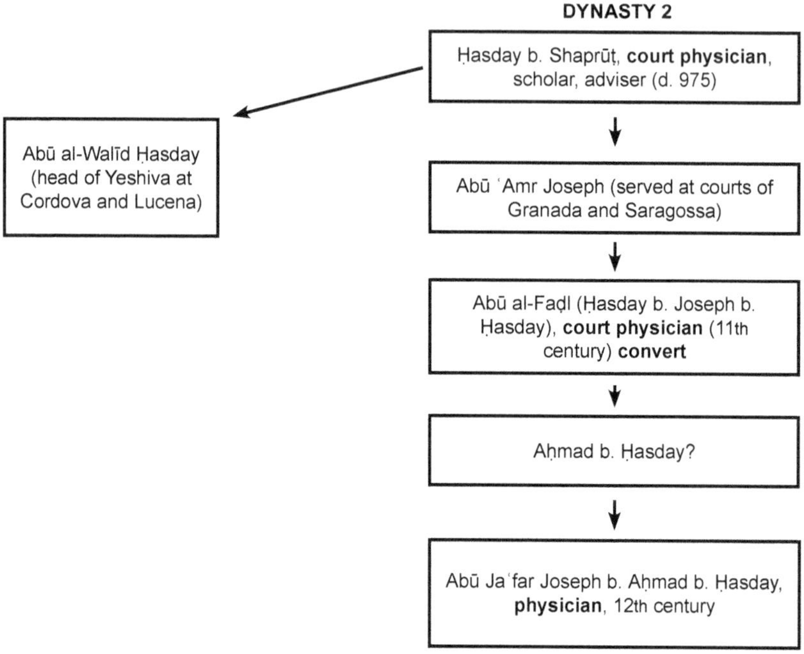

and became one of the first representatives of Andalusian Jewish culture. After the death of his father, Ḥasday continued his work and soon became the most distinguished Jew in Andalusia, enjoying great wealth and social status.[774] In about 940 he was appointed as a physician to the caliph ʿAbd al-Raḥmān III, who had declared an independent Muslim Iberian caliphate in 929. Ḥasday, with his engaging manners, knowledge, character and extraordinary ability, gained his master's confidence to such a degree that he became the caliph's confidant and faithful counsellor. Without bearing the title of *wazīr* he was in reality minister of foreign affairs; he had also control of the customs and ship-dues in the port of Cordova. Ibn Abī Uṣaybiʿa wrote of him:

> Ḥasday b. Isaac was among the foremost Jewish scholars versed in their law. He opened to his coreligionists in Andalusia the gates of knowledge of the religious law, of chronology, etc. Before his time, they had to apply to the Jews of Baghdad on legal questions, and on matters referring to the calendar and the dates of the festivals.[775]

In his capacity as a trusted courtier, Ḥasday undertook a number of diplomatic missions for ʿAbd al-Raḥmān III. In the late 940s, he played a significant role in the negotiations between the caliph and the Byzantine emperor Constantine VII Porphyrogennetos that led to the exchange of delegations between Constantinople and Cordova. The Byzantine delegation brought a gift copy of the Greek manuscript of Dioscorides' pharmacopoeia, *De Materia Medica*, which was and remained – up to the sixteenth century – one of the standard reference works in pharmacology. Ḥasday collaborated in translating this important work into Arabic after it was first translated from Greek to Latin with the aid of the monk Nicholas. In particular, he identified the many medicinal plants mentioned and provided their Arabic names.[776] According to Ibn Abī Uṣaybiʿa, he was the first physician in Iberia to re-create the legendary compound theriac (*tiriyāq al-fārūq*).[777] The caliph assigned Ḥasday important functions and privileges, including oversight of the customs bureau. He also appointed him *nāsī* (president) of the Jewish communities in Andalusia. As such, Ḥasday represented his coreligionists at court as their spokesman, defender and patron, promoting their welfare and appointing the spiritual leaders of the various communities.[778] Ḥasday also played an important role in the caliph's negotiations with the Holy Roman Emperor Otto I. He employed his diplomatic and medical skills to achieve another success; he persuaded Queen Toda of Navarre and her grandson Sancho I (the Fat), the deposed king of León, to come to Cordova to receive treatment for his obesity and with the assistance of the caliph to recover his throne.[779] As *nāsī* of Andalusian Jewry, Ḥasday was also named 'Rish Cala' or Abū Yūsuf;[780] he carried on an extensive correspondence with Jewish communities in other countries. He also wrote to Constantine VII and Empress Helena, urging them to provide for the welfare and protection of the Jews of Byzantium, who had been persecuted under the previous emperor, Romanos Lekapenos. In the same letter he alluded to the land of the Khazars, showing his personal interest in that Jewish kingdom, an interest fired by reports of the Lost Tribes of Israel. Travellers and merchants coming from the East to Andalusia had reported that the majority of the Khazars, and even their king, were Jewish. Ḥasday instructed his secretary, Menahem b. Sarūq, to write a letter in Hebrew to Joseph, the Khazar king. The body of the letter described the Umayyad caliphate and the Jewish communities of Andalusia, and enquiries about Joseph's realm, its history and language, and its practice of Judaism and messianic expectations. As chief patron of Jewish culture in

Andalusia, Ḥasday encouraged Biblical, Talmudic, grammatical and philological studies, as well as Hebrew. His court was brightened by the literary sessions of a brilliant circle of scholars and poets.[781] Ḥasday sent expensive presents to the academies of Sura and Pumbedita, and corresponded with Dosa, the son of Saadia Gaon. He was also instrumental in transferring the centre of Jewish science from Babylonia to Spain, by appointing Moses b. Enoch, who had been stranded at Cordova, director of a school, and thereby detaching Judaism from its dependence on the East, to the great joy of the caliph.[782] When Ibn Shaprūṭ died around 975, Cordova had become the Jewish cultural centre that he had sought, and he had become the model of the Sephardi Jewish courtier and patron of scholarship and the arts.[783]

Abū al-Faḍl (Ḥasday b. Joseph b. Ḥasday) [An., Saragossa, 11th century, convert]

A very knowledgeable physician, poet and scholar; member of one of the most important and well-known Jewish families in Andalusia.[784] He worked as a physician for the Almoravid ruler, and according to the Muslim sources he converted to Islam after he fell in love with a Muslim girl.[785] He was a scholar in various fields: general and life sciences, languages, poetry, mathematics, engineering astrology, music, culture.[786] Ibn Abī Uṣaybiʿa pompously called him a descendant of the prophet Moses. He related further that Ḥasday was an excellent poet, an orator, a clever logician and physician, and was well versed in mathematics and astronomy.[787] Al-Muqtadir b. Hūd[788] praised Abū al-Faḍl Ḥasday and wrote: 'The *wazīr* and clerk Abū al-Faḍal is one of a kind in his virtues, he is compassionate, the source of nobility; as the people said: Abū al-Faḍal has compassion and nobility and there no one like him among the public.'[789] The *wazīr* Abū al-ʿAmr b. al-Faraj sent Abū al-Faḍl a request for a drug named *al-dayyākhīlūn*[790] and promised him to pay a decent amount of money; in response Abū al-Faḍl wrote the recipe in verses of song; however, he asked Abū al-ʿAmr to trust his medical knowledge and experience and wrote that the requested drug was not the right one for his medical problem. He then suggested the *wazīr* use absinthe instead.[791]

Abū Jaʿfar Joseph b. Aḥmad b. Ḥasday [An., Saragossa, 12th century]

A physician, native of Saragossa, born to a father, Abū al-Faḍl (Ḥasday b. Joseph b. Ḥasday), who converted to Islam. He practised in Moorish Spain, and later moved to Egypt, where the *wazīr* al-Maʾmūn became his patron. Joseph wrote commentaries on Hippocrates' writings: *al-Sharḥ al-Maʾmūnī* (probably at the request of al-Maʾmūn), *Kitāb al-Imān* (on the oath of Hippocrates) and *Sharḥ al-Fuṣūl* (on his *Aphorisms*). Among his other known works are *Fāwāʾid* (useful observations and extracts from the commentary of ʿAlī Ibn Riḍwān on the *Glaukon* of Galen) and *al-Qawl ʿalā Awwal al-Ṣināʿāt al-Ṣaghīra* (study of book one of the *Mikrotechne* of Galen).[792]

Dynasty 3 – Moses Ben Maimon – Maimonides

The most instructive medical dynasty (named after one of the foremost medieval Jewish figures – Moses Maimonides), during the course of which the medical profession passed through three different political regimes in Egypt and Syria: Fatimid, Ayyubid and Mamluk. Combining Jewish sources, namely from the Cairo Geniza, with data extracted from contemporary Muslim Arabic sources enables us to construct a rich narrative about this dynasty, which was prominent in the Jewish political and religious arenas. The Maimonideans held the office of Head of the Jews, in a unique aspect: it was conveyed from father to son for nearly 250 years – from 1171 until around 1415,[793] several members of the family served as physicians.[794] The Maimonidean family were part of the golden age of dynasties of Jewish physicians, during the Fatimid and Ayyubid periods, in which dynasties of court physicians almost constantly occupied the office of Head of the Jews as well. The medical profession in the Maimonidean dynasty, including the dynasty of Maimonides' wife, lasted (with interruptions) for nine generations. Interestingly enough, there is no indication in the sources that any pressure was brought to bear on them to convert to Islam in order to maintain their high offices.[795]

R. Mishael ha-Rōfē [Eg., Cairo, 11th century]

A physician, grandfather of Mishael b. Josiah (Isaiah) ha-Levi ha-Rōfē ha-Sar, a physician. We know this since the Hebrew title 'ha-Rōfē' is written next to both of their names.[796]

Abū al-Maḥāsin al-Sheikh al-Thiqa (Mishael b. Josiah (Isaiah) ha-Levi ha-Rōfē ha-Sar) (b. Daniel, ha-Bāḥūr ha-Ṭōv) [Eg., Cairo, 11th century]

A physician and a government official, Moses Maimonides' father-in-law.

Mentioned in a genealogical list of this family preserved in the Geniza.[797] He is also mentioned in a bill (12th–13th century), saying that when it was written he was no longer alive;[798] and in other documents.[799]

Mūsā b. ʿAbd Allāh al-ʾIsrāʾīlī al-Qurṭubī (Moses b. Maimon; Maimonides) [An., Cordova, Mo., Fez, Eg., Cairo, 12th–13th centuries]
A physician, one of the most important Jewish scholars and Halakhics. Maimonides (1138–1204), was born at Cordova, emigrated to Fez, and later on settled in Egypt (1166). He studied medicine, perhaps in Spain and certainly in Fez. He lived in Fusṭāṭ.[800] According to contemporary sources he may have served the last Fatimid caliphs, and they may have even recommended him as a physician to one of the Crusader kings, but Maimonides refused to treat him. After the rise of the Ayyubids (1171) he served in the sultanate court. According to Ibn Abī Uṣaybiʿa (who was a colleague of his son Abraham Maimonides) he served as a physician to Saladin (although some scholars doubt it)[801] in the years before 1182, when Saladin left Egypt. Joel Kraemer suggests that it is reasonable to suppose he was Saladin's physician during the years in which he served as the Head of the Jews, 1171–3. It was Maimonides' patron, the *wazīr* al-Qāḍī al-Fāḍil, who gave him a salary as a court physician, with the rise of the Ayyubids. Maimonides cooperated with other court physicians since he was not yet experienced enough to give treatment by himself. Maimonides was certainly the physician of Saladin's son, al-Malik al-Afḍal (r. 1193–6). He governed from Damascus, though for two years, from January 1199 to December 1200, he stayed in Egypt. These were the years when, apparently, Maimonides served this ruler at the same time as his second tenure as the Head of the Jews.[802] Maimonides wrote ten essays on medical topics:[803] 'Medical Aphorisms of Moses', 'The Art of Curing', 'Commentary on the Aphorisms of Hippocrates', 'Treatise on Haemorrhoids', 'Treatise on Cohabitation', 'Treatise on Asthma', 'Treatise on Poisons and Their Antidotes', 'Regimen of Health' and 'Glossary of Drug Names'. His offspring took over his position as the Head of the Jews, and some of them are known to have been physicians.[804]

Abraham b. Maimon (Maimonides) [Eg. Cairo, 12th–13th centuries]
The son of Moses b. Maimon (Maimonides). Like his father, Abraham (1186–1237) was a famous physician, a Halakhist and the *nagid* of the Jewish

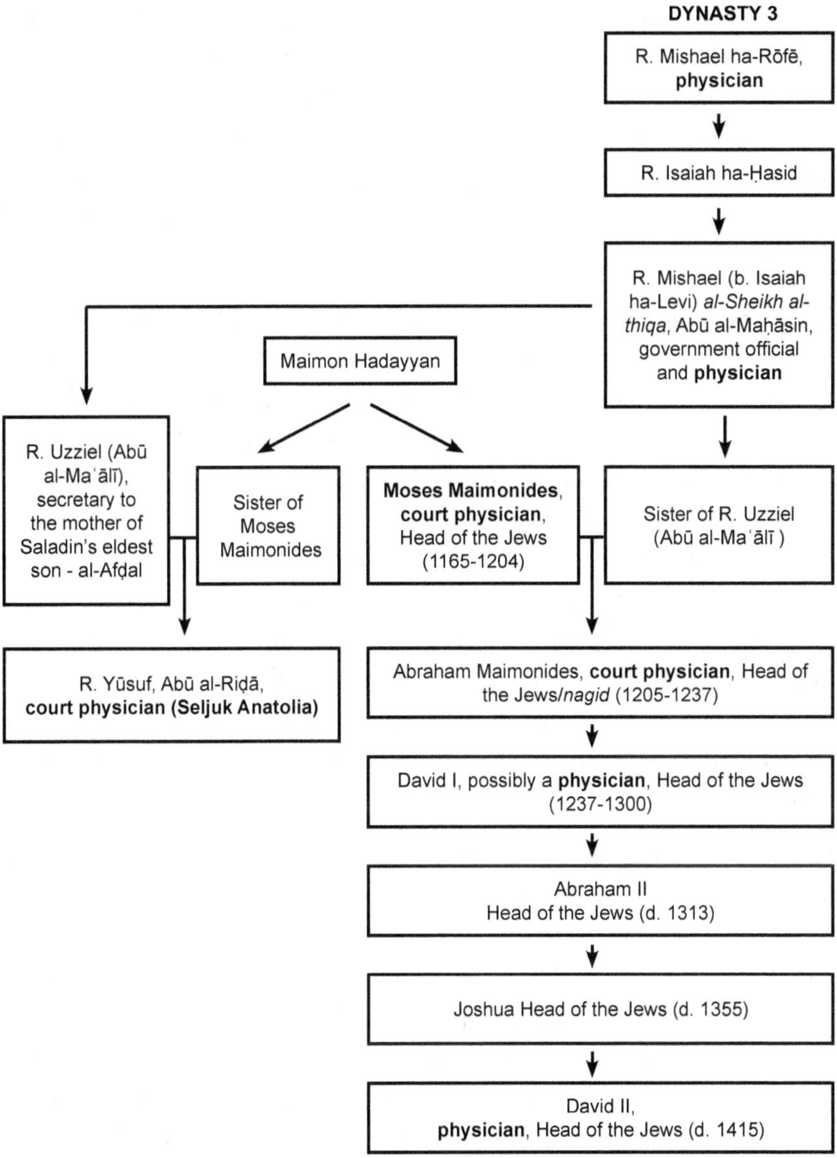

community in Egypt and Syria (1205–37). He was the court physician of al-Malik al-Kāmil Muḥammad b. Abī Bakr b. Ayyūb (1218–38).[805] Ibn Abī Uṣaybiʿa met him during his work in the Cairo hospital between 1234 and 1235 and said of him: 'I have found a tall sheikh with a lean body, with good relations, soft spoken and an excellent physician'.[806] According to Zinger, writing about Goitein's legacy, he was a merchant-physician-scholar-poet.[807] In his capacity as the *nagid*, Abraham Maimonides was highly influential, heavily involved in community affairs and an arbiter in Halakhic matters, regulations and laws. Abraham had connections with the community leaders including R. Isaac b. Ḥalfōn and Judah ha-Melammēd b. Aaron ha-Rōfē Ibn al-ʿAmmānī.[808] Abraham was known for his pietism and his liturgical and devotional reforms.[809]

David b. Abraham b. Moses b. Maimon [Eg., Cairo, 13th century]
Maimonides' grandson, a *nagid*, and probably also a physician who was active in Cairo.[810] He lived between 1222 and 1300 and for many decades led the Jewish community in Egypt. David held the title 'Head of the Yeshiva of the Torah' and was often in contact with Rabbinical scholars in Spain, Damascus and Italy and spent much time defending Maimonides' doctrines.[811] He wrote sermons on the weekly Torah portion 'Midrash Rabbi David' and commentary on *Pirkei Avot* (although Maimonides' legacy does not appear in it and it is uncertain that he actually wrote it). At the end of his life he was forced to move to Acre where he fought to defend Maimonides' name and path. He died in Egypt and his bones were transferred and reburied next to his grandfather in Tiberias, where his grave was discovered in the twentieth century.[812]

David b. Joshua Maimon (al-Maimūnī) [Eg., Cairo, Sy., Aleppo, Damascus, 14th–15th centuries]
A physician (d. c.1415), the last son in the Maimon family who served as *nagid*. He wrote on Biblical weights and measurements, a commentary on *Mishne Torah* as well as a philosophy book. David was also a physician who gave free medical services to the needy. During the 1370s he was forced to leave Egypt and lived for a number of years in Aleppo and Damascus. At the beginning of the 15th century he returned to Egypt and became the *nagid*.[813]

Dynasty 4 – Isaac ha-Kohen ha-Rōfē b. Furāt
A father-and-son dynasty about which we learnt only from Geniza sources. Both father and son were physicians who served the Fatimid rulers and practised at Ramle as well as in Cairo in the eleventh century.

Isaac ha-Kohen ha-Rōfē b. Furāt [Eg., Cairo, EY, Ramle, 11th century]
A physician, born in Fusṭāṭ and active around 1029 in Ramle.[814] He perished, it seems, in a court intrigue. Isaac was the father of Abraham b. Isaac ha-Kohen b. Furāt.

Abraham b. Isaac ha-Kohen b. Furāt [Eg., Cairo, EY, Ramle, 11th century]
A physician and a public figure active in Fusṭāṭ,[815] His father, Isaac ha-Kohen ha-Rōfē b. Furāt, was also a physician who was active in Ramle.[816] He resided in Ramle for about twenty years, until the middle of the eleventh century.[817] He served as the physician to the Fatimid ruler in Ramle, and as head of the dysentery department in the hospital there,[818] where he was asked by Solomon b. Judah, the *gaon* (head of the yeshiva) of Jerusalem, once to intervene with the Muslim chief justice of Palestine, once to make a request to the governor, and once to act in intra-Jewish affairs.[819] He was called the 'great benefactor and protector of the community', and was flattered in a letter as an 'outstanding scholar of Jewish studies'.[820] On his arrival in Cairo he was appointed as a court physician and became an important figure in the relationship between the Jewish community in Egypt and Eretz-Israel and the Fatimid government (he was probably the Head of the Jews). He was especially close to the *qadi* al-Yazūrī, who later became the Fatimid *wazīr*, and he even moved together with him to Egypt. He was involved in the selection and appointment of *geonim* as well as appointments in the Jewish community in Fusṭāṭ.[821]

Dynasty 5 – Ephraim b. al-Zaffān
A dynasty of Jewish physicians and merchants, on which we have information mainly on one member, who was considered the most prominent student of the famous Muslim physician ʿAlī Ibn Riḍwān. Interestingly, he studied with a well-known Muslim physician, and was in turn the teacher of a Jewish physician (Salāma b. Raḥmūn), a member of another medical dynasty (no. 13). The information regarding these practitioners was extracted both from Muslim Arabic sources and from documents found in the Cairo Geniza.

Ephraim b. al-Ḥasan b. Isḥāq b. Ibrāhīm b. Yaʿqūb Abū Kathīr al-Zaffān (Ephraim b. al-Zaffān) [Eg., Cairo, 11th century]

A physician (d. 1068), considered the most prominent student of the famous Muslim physician ʿAlī Ibn Riḍwān from Giza; Salāma b. Raḥmūn was his student. He served several caliphs and used the high salary he earned from them to build a comprehensive library which included mainly medical works. Approximately 10,000 of his books were sold to the *wazīr* al-Afḍal and an additional 20,000 books remained in his heir's possession when he died. He had his own ex-libris, and Ibn Abī Uṣaybiʿa mentioned seeing books bearing it two centuries later.[822] Al-Zaffān wrote a number of medical writings, among them *Taʿālīq wa-Majarayāt* ('Cases and Their Expansions'); an advice book for his student Sheikh Abū al-Qāsim ('Recommendations for the Composition of Medicines'); *al-Tadhkira al-Ṭibbiya fī Maṣlaḥat al-Aḥwāl al-Badaniyya* ('Knowledge Needed for the Treatment of Physical Conditions'); and an essay on white phlegm (*balgham*).[823] The al-Zaffān family is mentioned several times in the Geniza as a family of merchants and physicians.[824]

Dynasty 6 – ʿAlī ha-Busmī

An interesting father-and-son medical dynasty from the classical Geniza period: the father was a pharmacist or perfume maker, and the son was a physician. There are only two Geniza fragments from which we know about this small dynasty.

ʿAlī ha-Busmī [Eg., 11th century]

A perfumer, mentioned in a document written by Ephraim b. Shemarya, who was active in 1007–55. His son, Solomon, is apparently Solomon ha-Rōfē b. ʿAlī.[825]

Solomon ha-Rōfē b. ʿAlī [Eg., 11th century]

A physician, the recipient of a letter from 1039 written by Solomon b. Judah, the head of Yeshivat Gaon Jacob in Ramle (in the years 1027–51).[826]

Dynasty 7 – Abraham ha-Rōfē

A father-and-son medical dynasty, about which we have learnt from only one Geniza fragment.

Abraham ha-Rōfē [Eg., 11th century] and Isaac ha-Kohen ha-Rōfē [Eg., 11th century]

Abraham's son Isaac ha-Kohen ha-Rōfē is mentioned in a document, possibly from the eleventh century. It seems that both of them were physicians.[827]

Dynasty 8 – Moses Darʿī

A three-generation Karaite medical dynasty.

DYNASTY 8

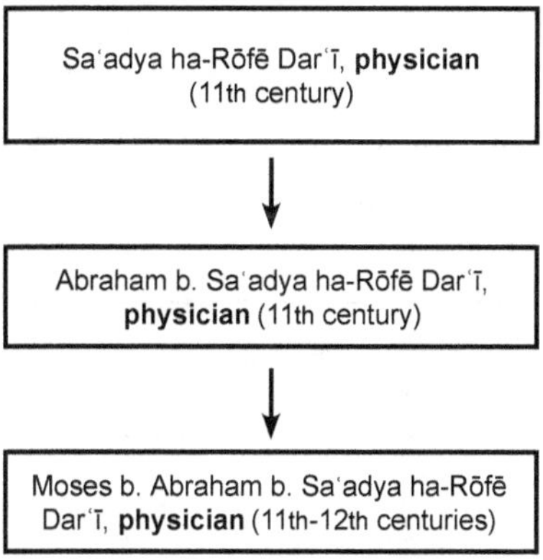

Saʿadya ha-Rōfē Darʿī [K., Eg., Alexandria, 11th century]

A Karaite physician, the family arrived originally from Spain and settled in Morocco in the town of Darʿa. Abraham his son and Moses his grandson were both physicians.[828]

Abraham b. Saʿadya ha-Rōfē Darʿī [K, Eg., Alexandria, 11th century]

A Karaite physician from Spanish and Moroccan origin. Abraham son, Moses as well as his father, Saʿadya, practised medicine.[829]

Moses b. Abraham b. Saʿadya ha-Rōfē Darʿī [K., Eg., Alexandria, 11th–12th centuries]

A Karaite physician, considered among the most gifted poets of Middle Ages Karaism. In a *dīwān* (collection of essays) he wrote, poems, prayers, praise, condemnations, complaints, lamentations, satires and riddles are included. The final version of a collection of his poems is dated to 1163. Moses worked in the profession regardless of the prohibitions made by ʿAnan b. David regarding the practice of medicine, which he found to be irreconcilable with trust in God's healing power.[830] Moses married and had several children, two of whom died during his lifetime. Included in Moses' circle of friends were Moses ha-Rōfē b. Isaac ha-Rōfē of the Tarifi family, for whose wedding Dar'ī dedicated a wedding song. In addition, mentioned in Moses' *dīwān* are a few of his contemporaries, among them Isaac ha-Rōfē, Moses ha-Levi, Samuel ha-Kohen ha-Rōfē, Elijah b. Samuel and Samuel b. Elijah al-Sinnī.[831]

Dynasty 9 – Ibn Qamni'el

Three physicians, who were all also community leaders and intellectuals, active mainly in Andalusia, are presented here. They are connected to the same distinguished family; however, we could not establish the exact relationship between these historical figures.

DYNASTY 9

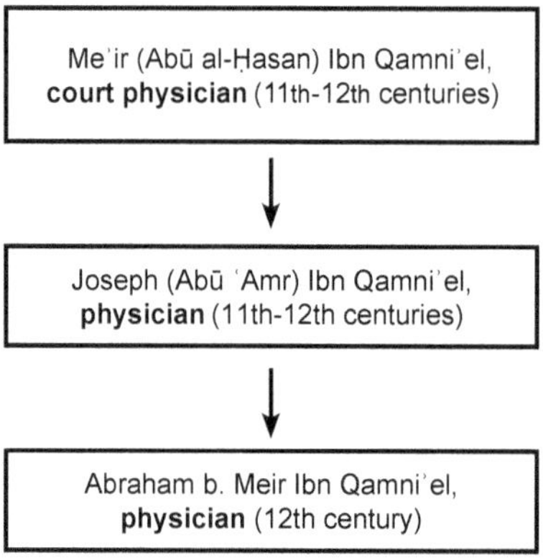

Me'ir (Abū al-Ḥasan) Ibn Qamni'el [An., Saragossa, Seville, Ma., Marrakesh, 11th–12th centuries]

A Jewish poet and physician; born in Saragossa as a member of one of the most important Jewish families. Another Jewish physician, Abū Ibrāhīm b. Muwaril, told Joseph b. 'Aqnīn of the effort of Me'ir to convince the Almoravid ruler that the Biblical book Song of Songs was holy, against other Jewish physicians that claimed that it was a secular book of love songs.[832] The little information about his life came mainly from poems dedicated to him by Judah ha-Levi, who gave him the title *wazīr*. One poem begins with a harsh satire of the leading families of Seville Jewry that juxtaposes their ignorance with Ibn Qamni'el's wisdom and praises his family. Another poem by ha-Levi indicates that he moved to

Morocco and rose in the Almoravid court, facts confirmed by Maimonides in his *Treatise on Asthma.*[833] Thanks to Maimonides, it is known that Ibn Qamniʾel was a court physician to Sultan Yūsuf b. Tāshufīn (r. 1061–1106) in Marrakesh. He is named as one of the four court physicians, who included Solomon b. al-Muʿallim of Seville, who was also a friend of Judah ha-Levi, and due to an error in preparing a dosage of theriac brought about the sultan's death.[834] In addition to the poems mentioned above, Ibn Qamniʾel was the recipient of three other poems by Judah ha-Levi. These compositions record for example his ceremonial appointment to a high post.[835]

Joseph (Abū ʿAmr) Ibn Qamniʾel [An., 11th–12th centuries]
A physician, a member of a distinguished family from Seville and probably related to one of its most distinguished members, Meʾir Ibn Qamniʾel. He seems to have practised medicine. Three poems dedicated to Joseph by Moses b. Ezra are the only source of information about him. Moses b. Ezra also wrote a poem on the occasion of Joseph's wedding, which took place when Joseph returned from a trip to Portugal. The praises of Joseph utilise conventional motifs (such as wisdom and generosity) and extol his medical knowledge and power to cure 'with his hand or his mouth' with different images. The poem alludes to the difference in age between the young Joseph and the now mature Ibn Ezra.[836]

Abraham b. Meʾir Ibn Qamniʾel [An., Ma., 12th century]
A Jewish physician from time of the Almoravid emir ʿAlī b. Yūsuf b. Tāshufīn (r. 1106–42). Abraham guarded the Jewish community, helped the Jewish people to keep their status and solved their problems, as was testified by a poet of his time, Moses b. Ezra. Abraham and another fellow physician, Abū Ayyūb al-Yahūdī (al-ʾIsrāʾīlī) (Solomon b. al-Muʿallim), were in charge of collecting the *jizya* tax from the members of the Jewish community. Another member of Abraham's family, Joseph (Abū ʿAmr) b. Qamniʾel (11th century) was also a physician. Meʾir (Abū al-Ḥasan) Ibn Qamniʾel, a physician himself, was probably the father of Abraham.[837]

Dynasty 10 – Yaḥyā b. ʿAbbās al-Maghribī
A two-generation dynasty of the twelfth century; it is an example of the phenomenon of immigration that characterised the Jews in this period: the

father came from Fez, and therefore was called al-Maghribī, and the son, who was a physician and mathematician, converted to Islam in Baghdad (1163). The conversion of Abū Naṣr Samawʾal b. Yaḥyā al-Maghribī is interesting as well and will be dealt with below.

Yaḥyā b. ʿAbbās al-Maghribī (Judah b. Abūn) [Ma., Fez, Iq., Baghdad, 11th–12th centuries]

A physician and a poet from Fez (d. 1138). His son was the physician Abū Naṣr Samawʾal b. Judah b. ʿAbbās al-Maghribī. Judah immigrated to Baghdad before Samawʾal was born. His father encouraged him to study medicine, and so he did, becoming an expert in the field as well as in engineering and mathematics.[838] Ḥaddād mentioned in his book a number of famous Jews who lived in Aleppo when Benjamin of Tudela passed there, among them the poet Judah b. Ayyūb b. ʿAbbās al-Fāsī al-Maghribī.[839]

Abū Naṣr Samawʾal b. Yaḥyā al-Maghribī (Samuel b. Judah b. ʿAbbās al-Maghribī) [Ir., Iq., Baghdad, 12th century, convert]

A physician and a mathematician, converted to Islam 1163, and died in 1170 or 1175. According to al-ʿUmarī and Ibn Abī Uṣaybiʿa, Samawʾal lived and worked for a while in Baghdad and in Diyarbakır (present day southern Turkey), and later moved to Iran.[840] Ibn al-Qifṭī mentioned that Samawʾal originated from Andalusia, and he moved to the East with his father, who pushed and encouraged him to study medicine. Indeed, Samawʾal became a well-known physician and a scholar of the sciences, engineering and mathematics.[841] At the end of the twelfth century he reached Azerbaijan and settled in the then capital, Marāgha. He served the court of Bahlawān and the princes of the kingdom. Among the emirs he served were Shams al-Dīn Aldajiz (1136–72) and his son Maḥmūd (r. 1172–85). He had several children, some of whom became physicians as well. He died and was buried around 1175 at Marāgha.[842] ʿAbd al-Laṭīf al-Baghdādī (1162–1231) wrote that Samawʾal was expert in the fusion of fractures, and that he wrote a few medical books.[843] Ibn Abī Uṣaybiʿa asserted that he wrote eight books and Steinschneider added four more to the list; the books were on medicine, engineering, mathematics and gemstones.[844] In any case he was the author of works on science (mainly mathematics) and of a polemical attack on the Jews and Judaism, *Ifḥām al-Yahūd* ('Silencing the Jews'),[845] authored following his conversion, as well as an autobiographical account of his conversion. Samawʾal refrained from converting for a long time out of respect for his father (a well-known poet, Judah b. Abūn, a friend of Judah ha-Levi). In his autobiography he described his conversion as the product of a process of study and intellectual analysis which took place over a considerable period of time. He eventually became a Muslim shortly before his father's death. Samawʾal's conversion was one of several important people at the time: besides Samawʾal, we know also of the physician and philosopher Abū al-Barakāt Hibat Allāh, who converted at the end of his life, and of Isaac the son of Abraham b. Ezra. As all three were acquainted, there have been suggestions that Hibat Allāh may have acted to influence the other two to convert, or that all these converts were part of a circle of intellectuals with shared interests and paths to Islam.[846] Stroumsa argues persuasively that this supposition is unfounded, and that the conversions were independent.[847]

Dynasty 11 – Saʿadya b. Mevōrākh

An early three-generation medical dynasty composed of four physicians known so far; the members of this family also served as court physicians and Jewish leaders.

DYNASTY 11

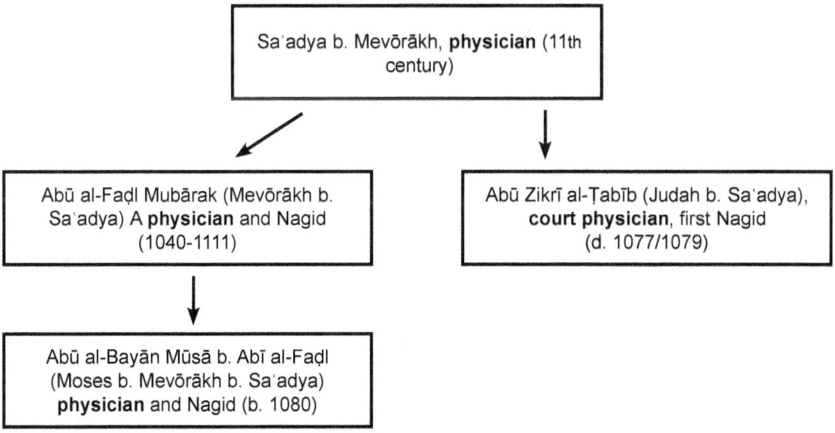

Saʿadya b. Mevōrākh [Eg., 11th century]

A physician. His two sons, Mevōrākh Abū al-Faḍl b. Saʿadya and Judah b. Saʿadya, and his grandson, Moses b. Mevōrākh (all three of them *nagids*), practised medicine during the Fatimid period under the rules of al-Mustanṣir biʾllāh, al-Mustaʿlī and al-Āmir (r. 1036–1129).[848] In a memorial list the names Mevōrākh, his son Saʿadya and his son Judah ha-Nagid are mentioned. These might be Saʿadya, his father and his son.[849]

Abū al-Faḍl Mubārak (Mevōrākh b. Saʿadya) [Eg., Cairo, Alexandria, 11th–12th centuries]

A physician and *nagid* (1040–1111), the son of the physician Saʿadya b. Mevōrākh. Some scholars regarded Mevōrākh as the real founder of the office of the *nagid*.[850] He was an influential physician, belonging to a family that practised medicine at the court of the Fatimid caliph, mainly in the time of the caliphs al-Mustanṣir biʾllāh, al-Mustaʿlī and al-Āmir (r. 1036–1129).[851] Mevōrākh's brother, Judah b. Saʿadya, and his son, Moses b. Mevōrākh, who is also known as Abū al-Bayān, were physicians as well. Another son of his was Nethanel, who is also known as Abū al-Barakāt. Mevōrākh was appointed *Raʾīs al-Yahūd* (Head of the Jews) for the years 1078–82, apparently after his brother Judah b. Saʿadya.[852] He was removed from his duty by David b. Daniel b. Azariah and was forced to escape to Alexandria. He attained the position again in 1094 (until 1111), among other things thanks to his relationship with the Fatimid *wazīr* al-Afḍal b. Badr al-Jamālī. The decline of the Palestinian Halakhic leadership (*geonim*) helped him gain power in his position, which included appointing judges in Egypt and representing the Jews in Egypt in the Fatimid court. Mevōrākh introduced considerable innovations in the fields of family law and the standardisation of ritual in synagogues.[853]

Abū Zikrī al-Ṭabīb (Judah b. Saʿadya) [Eg., 11th century]

A physician, the eldest of Saʿadya b. Mevōrākh's five sons (d. 1077/1079). Like his father, he served as a physician in the Fatimid court. He was first mentioned in the Geniza in a document dating from 1043. He had two titles, 'Head of the Assembly', which was given to him by one of the leaders in Iraq after the Sura and Pumbedita academies had been closed, and 'Exalted Member', given to him by the Jerusalem yeshiva. In the years 1062–4, Judah became the first Egyptian to bear the title *nagid*, which was probably given to him by the *gaon* of Jerusalem, Elijah ha-Kohen b. Solomon.[854] He was mentioned in a few business letters (c.1045–55), some of which were written by Barhūn b. Mūsā Ṭāhratī, a merchant from Tripoli, and sent to Naharay b. Nissīm, who was his relative and younger associate, sojourning either in Alexandria or in Fusṭāṭ at that time.[855] The writer sends his regards to Abū Zikrī al-Ṭabīb and to his brother;[856] according to Gil, Abū Zikrī is identical with Judah b. Saʿadya.[857] He was mentioned in a poem written by Solomon ha-Kohen b. Joseph as an 'elder of splendour' in the court of the Fatimid ruler Badr al-Jamālī. Judah's brother, Mevōrākh, continued to serve as the ruler's personal physician. Moreover, he and his son, Moses b. Mevōrākh, served as the *Raʾīs al-Yahūd* (Head of the Jews).[858] The Muslim physician ʿAlī Ibn Riḍwān, who was Ephraim b. al-Zaffān's teacher, addressed two of his treatises to Judah.[859]

Abū al-Bayān Mūsā b. Abī al-Faḍl (Moses b. Mevōrākh b. Saʿadya) [Eg., Cairo, 11th–12th centuries]

A physician and a *nagid* in Cairo, born around 1080. He was the grandson of Saʿadya b. Mevōrākh and the firstborn of the physician Mevōrākh Abū al-Faḍl b. Saʿadya. He belonged to a family that practised medicine during the Fatimid period, during the time of the caliphs al-Mustanṣir biʾllāh, al-Mustaʿlī and al-Āmir.[860] Moses replaced his father as *Raʾīs al-Yahūd* after he died (1111), but the position did not pass to his sons in turn. Rather it went to Maṣlīaḥ ha-Kohen ha-Gaon b. Solomon in 1127, probably because Moses' sons were too young. The circumstances for him leaving his job are unclear. He may have died or been removed from it because of intrigues in the court.[861] He was an important minister in the caliphate court and helped the Jewish community of the time to deal with Muslim decrees.[862]

Dynasty 12 – Moses b. Jekuthiel

A four-generation medical dynasty of physicians (some of whom were also merchants). Its origin was Andalusia; however, most of the family members practised at Cairo.

Mūsā b. Abī al-Faḍāʾil (Moses b. Jekuthiel ha-Rōfē) [An., Eg., 11th–12th centuries]

A physician,[863] and the father of Jekuthiel b. Moses (merchant's representative).[864] Moses left Spain and immigrated to Egypt after his father, also named Jekuthiel, was executed in 1039.[865] He was called 'the Spaniard'.[866] Moses was identified as a physician in another document, which mentions 'R. Moses ha-Rōfē'.[867] His grandson, Abū al-Faḍāʾil Jekuthiel, was also a physician, as can be learnt from another document (1175).[868]

DYNASTY 12

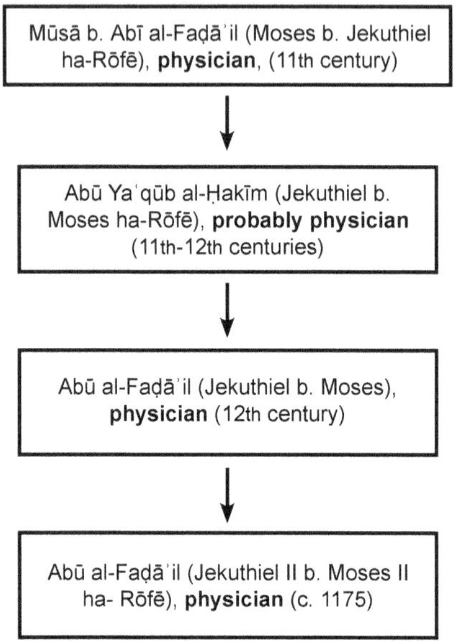

Abū Yaʿqūb al-Ḥakīm (Jekuthiel b. Moses ha-Rōfē) [Eg., Cairo, 11th–12th centuries]

A prominent representative of the merchants in Fusṭāṭ. It is not proven that he was a physician, but it can be reasonably assumed that he studied medicine and practised it a little.[869] Jekuthiel took part in Mediterranean trade and in trade with India, and was known as a tough merchant. He was a familiar figure in Fusṭāṭ and was active in the court.[870] Jekuthiel was a hard bargainer in business, as well as in his personal life as portrayed by Zinger's writing about his tough divorce.[871] His son also acted as a representative of the merchants, whereas his grandson, Abū al-Faḍāʾil Jekuthiel II b. Moses II ha-Rōfē, went back to medicine, his great-grandfather Moses' profession.[872]

Abū al-Faḍāʾil (Jekuthiel b. Moses) [Eg., Cairo, 12th century]

A physician, grandson of the physician Moses b. Jekuthiel. He is mentioned in a document (1175).[873]

Abū al-Faḍāʾil (Jekuthiel II b. Moses II ha- Rōfē) [Eg., 12th century]

A physician, who was active around 1175. His grandfather, Jekuthiel b. Moses, was a representative of the merchants in Fusṭāṭ. His father, Moses, was a *kātib* (senior clerk) and also a superintendent of the merchants (probably the same title as his grandfather). It is told that he sold his slave, Fayrūz (meaning turquoise), who was raised in his house, for only 12 dinars. The low price shows that the slave was probably a boy when he was sold.[874]

Dynasty 13 – Salāma b. Mubārak

A two-generation Egyptian Jewish medical dynasty; the father was considered in his time to be one of the best physicians in Egypt.

Abū al-Khayr Salāma b. Mubārak b. Raḥmūn b. Mūsā al-Ṭabīb (Salāma b. Raḥmūn) [Eg., Cairo, 11th–12th centuries]

A physician, considered one of the best in Egypt. He studied medicine, for a long time, under the guidance of Ephraim b. al-Zaffān and was his best student. At the same time, he studied philosophy with the learned Fatimid prince al-Mubashshir b. Fātik, who was also a collector of scientific manuscripts. According to Ibn Abī Uṣaybiʿa, Salāma's practice was based on *Ṣināʿat al-Ṭibb* ('The Medical Profession') by the Jewish physician Ephraim b. al-Zaffān, and he also taught medicine. A distinguished physician from Spain, Abū al-Ṣalt Umayya b. ʿAbd al-ʿAzīz al-Andalusī, witnessed the esteem in which Salāma was held, and when he arrived in Cairo (1096), he praised his medical and philosophical erudition. Moreover, Salāma was mentioned by Abū al-Ṣalt in a letter he wrote during a visit to Egypt (1116), where he described the physicians in the area and referred to Salāma as 'one of the smartest and wisest' among the Egyptian physicians. Salāma wrote several metaphysical and medical books which have been lost. Two of these were on the reason for the scarcity of rain in Egypt, and on why the women of Cairo become obese in middle age. Salāma's son, Mubārak b. Salāma b. Mubārak b. Raḥmūn b. Abū al-Khayr, was also a physician.[875]

Mubārak b. Salāma b. Mubārak b. Raḥmūn b. Abū al-Khayr [Eg., 12th century]

A physician and the son of the physician Salāma b. Raḥmūn; wrote a book on anthrax. Ibn Abī Uṣaybiʿa mentioned he was born and educated in Egypt, where he lived.[876]

Dynasty 14 – Aaron ha-Rōfē al-ʿAmmānī

The Ibn al-ʿAmmānī family was a unique dynasty of physicians, judges (*dayyānim*) and cantors, originally from Amman (present-day Jordan). Members of this medical family were very active also as leaders of the Jewish community, mainly in Alexandria. This dynasty's occupation was medicine (possibly with interruptions) for at least eight generations, and it endured consecutively for about two hundred years, at least six generations, in a father-son line. Nine members of this family served as physicians (some of them court physicians), communal leaders and cantors.

The 'last' generation of physicians of the Ibn al-ʿAmmānī dynasty had married into another powerful dynasty of leaders and court physicians – that of Zechariah of Alexandria (dynasty 21). Judah's son, Hibat Allāh (Nethanel), married the cousin of Solomon (and the court physician Abū Zikrī), the son of Elijah ha-Dayyān b. Zechariah. Hibat Allāh Ibn al-ʿAmmānī's wife was, in fact, the niece (sister's daughter) of Elijah, the prominent judge (*dayyān*) in the court of Abraham Maimonides.[877] A similar phenomenon of marriage between two dynasties of important physicians is the Maimonidean family: Moses Maimonides married a woman from a distinguished dynasty of physicians.

Interestingly, the data about the al-ʿAmmānīs is found only in Jewish sources. Their prominent role in the Jewish community explains the abundant material in Jewish sources. The fact that none of the members were mentioned in Muslim sources should not surprise us, since there is no hint in Muslim sources of other distinguished dynasties of Jewish court physicians.[878]

Aaron ha-Rōfē al-ʿAmmānī [Sy. Amman, Eg., Alexandria, 11th century]

The first known physician of the Ibn al-ʿAmmānī family of physicians. Aaron probably lived in Amman. He was the father of Ṣadaqa, and the grandfather of Aaron. We learn about this lineage thanks to his grandson, who is mentioned in a Geniza document from Alexandria (1089) by the name Aaron b. Zedaqa b. Aaron ha-Rōfē al-ʿAmmānī. He is the first member of his family named al-ʿAmmānī, meaning 'of Amman'. Since he was named al-ʿAmmānī and not 'Ibn al-ʿAmmānī', he was the one who migrated from Amman to Egypt and the founder of the al-ʿAmmānī dynasty in Egypt.[879]

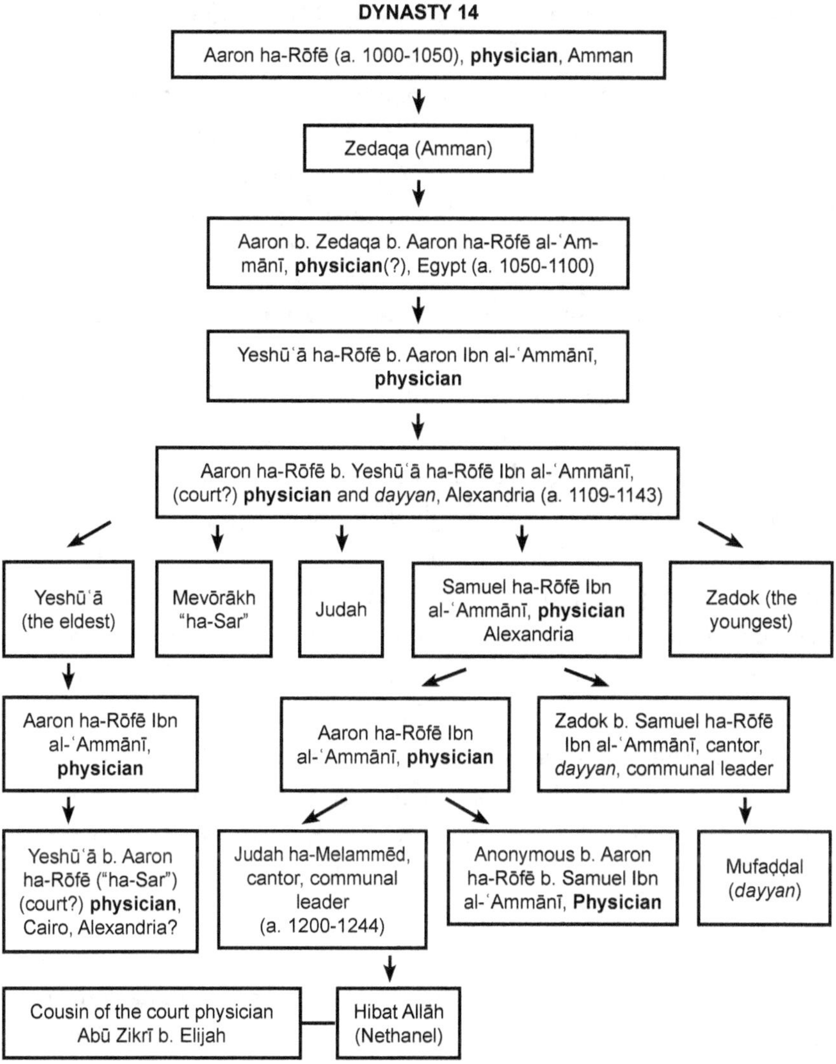

Aaron b. Zedaqa b. Aaron ha-Rōfē al-ʿAmmānī [Eg., Alexandria, 11th century]

A physician, presumably active in Alexandria (1089).[880] Father of Yeshūʿā ha-Rōfē b. Aaron al-ʿAmmānī and grandfather of Aaron ha-Rōfē b. Yeshūʿā ha-Rōfē Ibn al-ʿAmmānī. Yeshūʿā signed a guardianship bill in 1065, which also mentions Abraham b. Moses ha-Rōfē.[881]

Yeshūʿā ha-Rōfē b. Aaron al-ʿAmmānī [Eg., 11th–12th centuries]

A physician, we learn about him as a young doctor (or medical student) in Cairo, when he was applying for an appointment at a hospital in his native city, Alexandria. In this letter, his cousin Judah gives him some practical advice on how to achieve this goal.[882] Yeshūʿā's son, Aaron, signed a bill in 1109, after Yeshūʿā's death.[883] Yeshūʿā signed a guardianship bill in 1056, which also mentions Abraham b. Moses ha-Rōfē.[884]

Aaron ha-Rōfē b. Yeshūʿā ha-Rōfē Ibn al-ʿAmmānī [Eg., Alexandria, 12th century]

A physician and a judge who was active in Alexandria (1109–43).[885] It might be that Aaron was a court physician, since the famous poet Judah ha-Levi praised his medical abilities and used in this context the Hebrew title '*ha-Sar*' (the notable) and mentioned his *misra* (high office). As a judge (*dayyān*), Aaron was a permanent member of the Alexandria court.[886] In addition, he was a writer of *payṭan*, liturgical poetry, some of which survived and was found in the Cairo Geniza. In addition to his role as community leader and physician, Aaron was a book dealer. In a letter from Alexandria written in his own handwriting, he enquires of a certain perfumer from Fusṭāṭ about seven parchment volumes that he sent to him, which included Biblical commentary, three volumes of the handbook of the Greek pharmacologist Dioscorides, two volumes of Jewish law and a volume on the writings of a tenth-century Hebrew poet.[887] Aaron was the leader of the community of Alexandria in the mid-twelfth century).[888] However, though Aaron expected his five sons to inherit his position as supreme communal leaders, as one can deduce from Judah ha-Levi's poems of praise to him,[889] Goitein noted that 'none of the five sons of Aaron Ibn al-ʿAmmānī, the most prominent Jewish judge of Alexandria during the 12th century, functioned as a Dayyān in that city after their father's death'.[890] Nevertheless, it seems that the sons played a role in the community's leadership, even if they did not bear an official title such as *dayyān*, equivalent to the status of their father and to other members of this dynasty.[891] Thanks to one of Judah ha-Levi's poems we know that Yeshūʿā was the eldest son, and after him came Mevōrākh, Judah, Samuel and Zadok, the youngest. Mevōrākh is mentioned with the epithet '*ha-Sar*', which might indicate high office in the service of the Muslim rulers.[892] Among his sons, Samuel was a physician in Alexandria.[893]

Samuel ha-Rōfē Ibn al-ʿAmmānī [Eg., Alexandria, 12th–13th centuries]
A physician from the al-ʿAmmānī dynasty of physicians. He was active in Alexandria. His son Zadok was the cantor of Alexandria, as well as a judge and a prominent community leader. He signed a document from 1214 regarding importing cheese from Sicily, in which he confirmed that the two merchants made a declaration regarding the amount of cheese, and about it being kosher, and asked for permission to sell it in the villages.[894]

Aaron ha-Rōfē b. Samuel Ibn al-ʿAmmānī [Eg., Alexandria/Cairo, 13th century]
A physician; his son signed as 'Judah ha-Melammēd b. Aaron ha-Rōfē Ibn al-ʿAmmānī' in several documents.[895] Judah ha-Melammēd was another prominent member of this dynasty who was active during almost the whole first half of the thirteenth century in Alexandria. He was not officially a physician, but he had some knowledge of medicine and considered himself qualified to give medical consultation. This knowledge was probably given to him by his family. Judah earned his living in Alexandria by being, *inter alia*, a *melammēd* (teacher of young boys) and a *ḥazzān* (cantor). He was involved with local politics and took an active part in the local legal system.[896]

(Anonymous) b. Aaron ha-Rōfē b. Samuel Ibn al-ʿAmmānī [Eg., 13th century]
A physician of the dynasty of Ibn al-ʿAmmānī, brother of Judah ha-Melammēd b. Aaron ha-Rōfē Ibn al-ʿAmmānī. From a letter of Judah al-ʿAmmānī, written to the *nagid* Abraham Maimonides (1217), we infer that they both were physicians; he mentioned the successful treatment of Muslim patients by his brother.[897]

Aaron ha-Rōfē b. Yeshūʿā Ibn al-ʿAmmānī [Eg., Alexandria/Cairo, 13th century]
Aaron's son, Yeshūʿā ha-Rōfē b. Aaron ha-Rōfē, is the addressee of a letter from 1217, sent to him at Cairo from Alexandria by his cousin and brother-in-law, Judah Ibn al-ʿAmmānī. Judah's father was Aaron ha-Rōfē b. Samuel.[898]

Yeshūʿā ha-Rōfē b. Aaron ha-Rōfē Ibn al-ʿAmmānī [Eg., Alexandria/ Cairo, 13th century]

One of the last known physicians from the Ibn al-ʿAmmānī dynasty of physicians. He was active in Cairo/Alexandria. Yeshūʿā is the addressee of a letter sent from Alexandria by his cousin and brother-in-law Judah ha-Melammēd (1217). As mentioned above, the letter might be interpreted in two ways. According to Goitein, Yeshūʿā was a young doctor or a medical student in Cairo at that time, who was striving to get an appointment in a hospital in his native city, Alexandria (that seems to be the more reasonable interpretation). His cousin Judah ha-Melammēd gave him in this letter some practical advice in order to achieve this goal.[899] According to Frenkel, in this letter, Judah made use of Yeshūʿā ha-Rōfē b. Aaron, his cousin who served as a court physician in Cairo, to help Judah's brother receive a licence for practising medicine.[900] Thus, if we accept this interpretation we have two physicians of Ibn al-ʿAmmānī's dynasty in this generation, one of whom is even a court physician in Cairo. From a second letter of Judah al-ʿAmmānī, written to the *nagid* Abraham Maimonides in 1217, we infer that a brother of his was indeed a physician. Judah mentioned the successful treatment of Muslim patients by his brother.[901]

Dynasty 15 – Muwaffaq al-Dawla Abū al-Faraj ʿAlī b. Abī al-Shujāʿ al-Hamadānī

A three-generation dynasty of Jewish physicians and pharmacists who were active at Hamadān and Tabriz,[902] Iran (or Azerbaijan). The best-known figure of this dynasty is Rashīd al-Dīn al-Ṭabīb Faḍl Allāh b. al-Dawla, Abū al-Khayr b. ʿAlī Abū al-Hamadānī (1247–1318). Born Jewish in Hamadān, he converted to Islam and became a philosopher and one of the greatest statesmen and historians of medieval Iran.

Muwaffaq al-Dawla Abū al-Faraj ʿAlī b. Abī al-Shujāʿ al-Hamadānī [Ir., Hamdān, 11th–12th centuries]

The grandfather of the famous Rashīd al-Dīn al-Hamadānī. Ibn al-Fuwaṭī, the Muslim historian who lived in the Īl-Khānate court and who knew Rashīd al-Dīn personally and worked with him, described Muwaffaq as 'a physician

DYNASTY 15

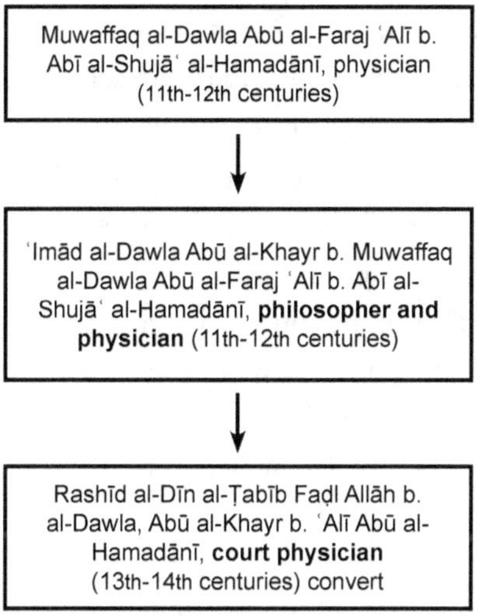

and a man of culture and letters being one of the philosophers of the world and of the well-bred individuals of the time'.[903]

ʿImād al-Dawla Abū al-Khayr b. Muwaffaq al-Dawla Abū al-Faraj ʿAlī b. Abī al-Shujāʿ al-Hamadānī [Ir., Tabriz, 13th century]

A physician (or pharmacist according to some sources), father of Rashīd al-Dīn al-Ṭabīb Faḍl Allāh b. ʿImad al-Dawla. Ibn al-Fuwaṭī described him as *al-ḥakīm wa-l-ṭabīb* (a philosopher and physician).[904]

Rashīd al-Dīn al-Ṭabīb Faḍl Allāh b. al-Dawla, Abū al-Khayr b. ʿAlī Abū al-Hamadānī [Ir., Tabriz, 13th–14th centuries, convert]

A physician (1247–1318), philosopher and one of the greatest statesmen and historians of medieval Iran. He was born Jewish in Hamadān as the son of a family of practitioners.[905] He started out as physician to Abāqa (r. 1265–82) and Gaykhātū (r. 1291–5) in the court of the Īl-Khānate in Tabriz. Up until his conversion to Islam, he was a loyal member of the Jewish community, in which he was educated and learnt Hebrew and Jewish traditions and customs. In 1298 he was appointed by Ghāzān Khān (d. 1304) a *wazīr*,[906] or the deputy to the grand *wazīr* Ṣadr al-Dīn al-Zinjānī,[907] and remained in office under the rulers Öljeitü [r. 1304–16] and Abū Saʿīd Khan. Under Abū Saʿīd's reign, following a plot by his adversary Jalāl al-Dīn b. al-Ḥazzān, who accused him of murdering

Abū Saʿīd's father, Rashīd al-Dīn was executed at the age of seventy-one, near Tabriz, in 1318.[908] He was famous for his medical writings in Iran, the medical knowledge he transferred from China to the Muslim world and to the West,[909] the establishment of hospitals, colleges and libraries, his care for students and the founding of a neighbourhood for that purpose, called Rashīdiyya. This fame made the Mongol courts in Tabriz and Sulṭāniyya some of the most important centres of learning in the East and in the Muslim world. It is known that a number of Jewish officials in the court at Tabriz, including Jalāl al-Dīn and the ophthalmologist Najīb al-Dawla, were in contact with Rashīd al-Dīn.[910] In his writings, he transmitted historical, cultural and religious knowledge about the Arabs, Iranians, Turks, Franks, Mongols and Jews.[911]

Dynasty 16 – ʿAlī ha-Rōfē

A two-generation Egyptian Jewish medical dynasty of physicians.

ʿAlī ha-Rōfē [Eg., Cairo, 12th century]

A physician, active in Cairo, died before 1182.[912]

Abū Manṣūr al-Mutaṭabbib (Shemarya b. ʿAlī ha-Rōfē) [Eg., Cairo, 12th century]

Son of ʿAlī ha-Rōfē, also a physician.[913]

Dynasty 17 – Moses b. Nethanel ha-Levi (Abū Saʿd)

Three biographies of a two-generation dynasty of physicians that practised at Cairo (father and two sons). At least the father Moses worked at a hospital, and all three of them were probably heads of the Jewish community in Egypt. The most interesting figure is Abū Zikrī Yaḥyā, also named in Hebrew Sar Shālōm, or Zūṭā.

Moses (Abū Saʿd) b. Nethanel ha-Levi [Eg., Cairo, 12th century]

A physician at the government hospital.[914] Moses was a contemporary of the physician Samuel ha-Nagid b. Hananiah (Abū Manṣūr)[915] and tried to take his place as the head of the Jewish community. The appointment was in fact given to a physician who was praised but his name is not recorded. In the same document, another person is being condemned, perhaps a physician as well. Sela suggested another option – identifying the first as Abū Manṣūr

DYNASTY 17

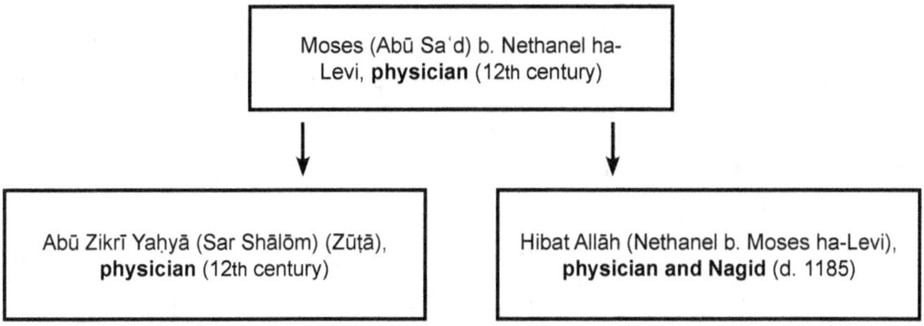

and the second as Moses.[916] Samuel ha-Nagid b. Hananiah (Abū Manṣūr's successor) was Moses' son ha-Gaon Nethanel ha-Levi (Hibat Allāh Nethanel b. Moses ha-Levi), who was also a physician.[917]

Hibat Allāh (Nethanel b. Moses ha-Levi) [Eg., Cairo, 12th century]
A physician and a *nagid* (d. 1185). It is said that as a child, his father, Moses b. Nethanel ha-Levi, who was also a physician, gave him 25 dinars in order for him to stop associating with superficial friends and to devote himself to his studies. Nethanel indeed studied medicine intensively, but also studied Hebrew, Arabic and religion. Because of his studies he seldom left his house and had complained about being away from his friends. As he got older, he became known as a physician and was appointed, in 1160, by the Fatimid caliph al-ʿĀḍid (r. 1160–71) as Head of the Jews after Samuel ha-Nagid b. Hananiah (Abū Manṣūr) (1140–59), and filled this office for several years between 1160 and 1169. He received a lot of property from the last Fatimid caliph, which helped him survive the Fatimid downfall and the rise of the Ayyubid dynasty.[918] He belonged to the family of *geonim* of the Palestinian Academy, ha-Levi, who were bitter enemies of the leadership of the Maimonideans, Moses and his son Abraham.[919]

Abū Zikrī Yaḥyā (Sar Shālōm) (Zūṭā) [Eg., Cairo, 12th century]
A famous figure who was apparently a physician. His deeds and achievements are described in the 'Zūṭā scroll', which describes the Jewish community sometime during the second half of the twelfth century. The scroll was apparently written in 1196, probably by Abraham b. Hillel, who might be Hillel b. Nissīm or Hillel ha-Ḥavēr. It seems that the events narrated

in it predate 1196, since the author noted that his father told him about Zūṭā's actions. In the scroll it is told that Zūṭā bought the office of Head of the Jews after the death of the *nagid* Samuel ben Hananiah, promising to pay the government 200 dinars a year by charging a fixed percentage of the incomes of the Jewish public servants. This was authorised by the new ruler of Egypt, probably meaning Saladin. Zūṭā held this authorisation for four years until Maimonides was able to dismiss him from the office. The document described the arrival of Maimonides in Cairo and his dismissal of Zūṭā thanks to the reputation he had. It was probably impossible for Maimonides to have had this kind of influence on public issues before 1175. Another important rabbi is mentioned in the scroll, Isaac b. Shoshan ha-Dayyān, who saved the Jews from the damage Zūṭā had caused and was a member of the court headed by Maimonides.[920] In an additional document,[921] related to the story, an ordinance appeared which opposed the demand by Abū Zikrī, the Head of the Jews, to receive a fixed percentage from the income of the judge and rabbi of the city of Al-Maḥalla.[922] He claimed to be a learned physician.[923] According to Mordechai Friedman, 'Zūṭā' was the name used for a whole family: Zūṭā and his sons is the way Moses b. Nethanel ha-Levi and his two sons Hibat Allāh Nethanel b. Moses ha-Levi and Sar Shālōm Abū Zikrī were referred to.[924]

Dynasty 18 – Abū al-Faḍl b. al-Nāqid

A short medical dynasty of a father and a son (both were probably ophthalmologists), who practised in Cairo in the twelfth century. The son, Abū al-Faraj b. Abū al-Faḍāʾil b. al-Nāqid, converted to Islam.

Abū al-Faḍl (Abū al-Faḍāʾil) b. al-Nāqid b. Obadia, al-Ṭabīb al-Muhadhdhab (Mevōrākh ha-Kohen) [Eg., Cairo, 12th century]

A famous physician (d. 1188), born in Cairo. At the beginning of his career he practised internal medicine but later, according to Ibn Abī Uṣaybiʿa, specialised in ophthalmology. Although he had a room to study medicine, he had little time to learn and train, since most of his time and energy was devoted to the treatment of patients. As a result, he instructed his students during treatments, or while riding from place to place. His services were in high demand because of his fame and abilities and he became very wealthy.[925] He wrote a number of books, including *Mujarrabātī fī al-Ṭibb* ('My Experience in Medicine'). His son Abū al-Faraj b. Abū al-Faḍā'il b. al-Nāqid converted to Islam and was also a physician and ophthalmologist.[926] His name appeared in two documents: the purchase of a sixth of two shops in the lamp manufacturers' street in Fusṭāṭ from his deceased brother's sons (1143), and another document that illuminates the details of a deal in which Abū al-Faḍl sold the same property to a family member, Sitt al-Sada, who was the daughter of the physician Abū Naṣr al-Ṭabīb b. al-Tinnīsī, and the widow of the merchant Abū al-Barakāt b. Joseph Lebdī, who was active in India.[927]

Abū al-Faraj b. Abū al-Faḍā'il b. al-Nāqid [Eg., Cairo, 12th century, convert]
A respected ophthalmologist and a convert to Islam. The son of Abū al-Faḍl (Abū al-Faḍā'il) b. al-Nāqid al-Ṭabīb al-Muhadhdhab, who was also a physician.[928]

Dynasty 19 – Abū Manṣūr (Isaac)
A dynasty of two physicians that practised in Cairo in the twelfth century, a grandfather and his grandson.

DYNASTY 19

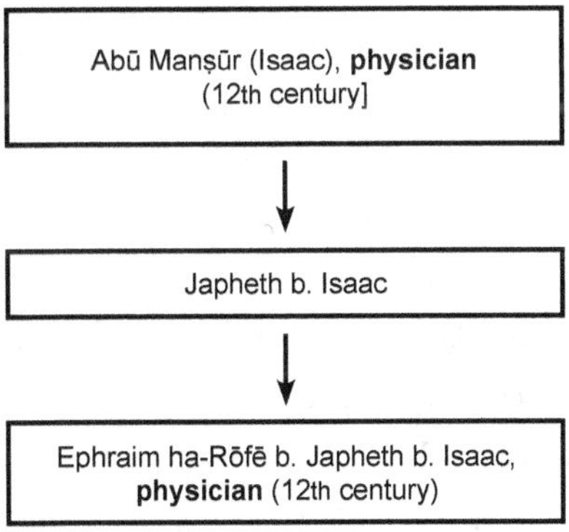

Abū Manṣūr (Isaac) [Eg., Cairo, 12th century] and Ephraim ha-Rōfē b. Japheth b. Isaac [Eg., Cairo, 12th century]
A physician and his grandson. The latter, 'Ephraim ha-Rōfē b. Japheth b. Isaac Abū Manṣūr al-Ṭabīb', is mentioned in a list of people who dedicated a Torah scroll to the Babylonian synagogue in Fusṭāṭ, from 1183.[929]

DYNASTY 20

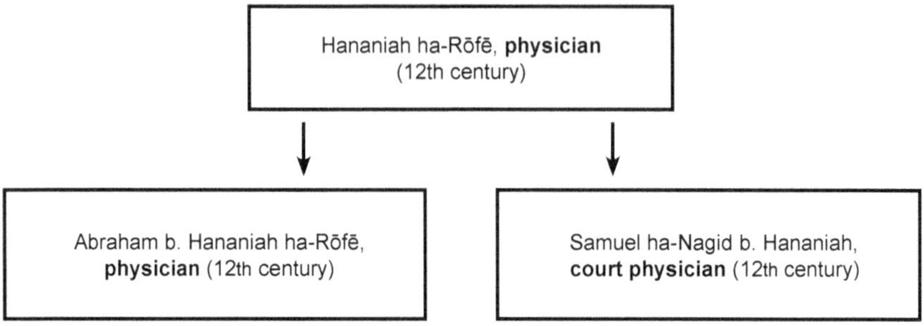

Dynasty 20 – Samuel b. Hananiah (Abū Manṣūr)

A two-generation dynasty, a father and his two sons. One son Samuel ha-Nagid b. Hananiah was a court physician and leader of the Jewish community.

Hananiah ha-Rōfē [Eg. 12th century]

A physician, the father of Samuel ha-Nagid b. Hananiah. Hananiah had another son by the name Abraham b. Hananiah,[930] who was also a physician.[931] They belonged to a noble family that traced back to the House of David.[932]

Samuel ha-Nagid b. Hananiah (Abū Manṣūr) [Eg., Cairo, 12th century]

A physician and the leader of the Jewish community in Fusṭāṭ between the years 1140 and 1159. He served under the Fatimid caliph al-Ḥāfiz li-Dīn Allāh (r. 1130–49). We learn from Muslim Arabic chronicles, that during a military rebellion against al-Ḥāfiz's son, the soldiers demanded that the caliph turn in his son. The caliph eventually decided to put his son to death, and asked two physicians, one of whom was Samuel, to prepare a poisonous potion. Samuel refused, claiming he did not know how to concoct such potions, whereas the second physician, Ibn Qarqa, undertook the task. After putting his son to death (1134), and taking control of the rebellion, the caliph executed Ibn Qarqa and nationalised his property. He gave Samuel many honours and appointed him Head of the Jews (*Raʾīs al-Yahūd*).[933] From a recently published document, we learn that Samuel was appointed as the *nagid* of the Jews of Egypt after the execution of the previous Head of the Jews, Maṣlīaḥ Gaon. Another document sheds light on Samuel's skills as a physician. Amram b. Isaac's wife was very ill, but Nagid Samuel apparently misdiagnosed her illness, and the drugs he prescribed for her only worsened her condition. Amram nevertheless pinned his hopes on him and asked him to prescribe other drugs after describing her illness in more detail. From this we can also learn that in this case the medical diagnosis was made from a distance, and the physician was not present.[934]

Abraham b. Hananiah ha-Rōfē [Eg., 11th–12th centuries]
A physician, the son of Hananiah ha-Rōfē.[935]

Dynasty 21 – Zechariah the Alexandrian
An influential family in the Jewish community of Alexandria, and at the courts of the Ayyubid princes. Members of this family lived and practised in Egypt (Alexandria and Cairo), and in Eretz-Israel (Ashkelon and Jerusalem). Letters they wrote to each other were found in the Geniza and are the main source of our knowledge regarding their lives and activities.[936]

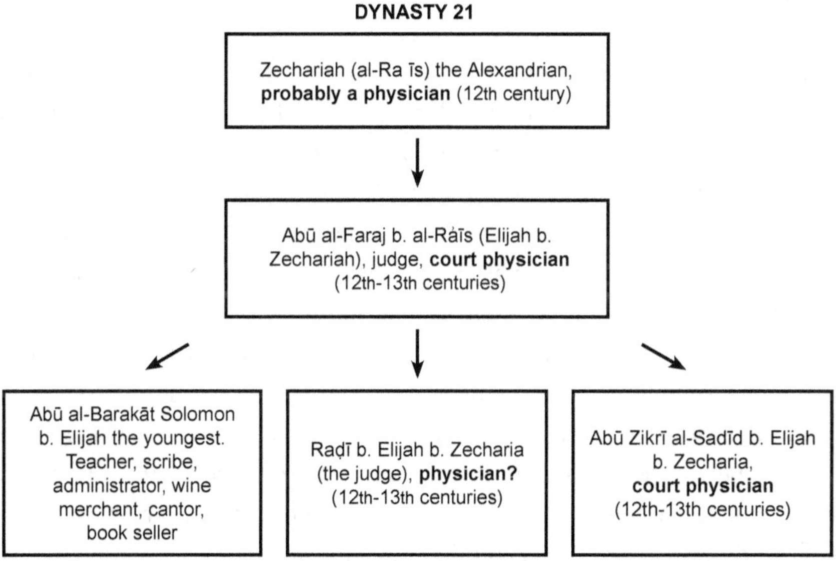

Zechariah (al-Raʾīs) the Alexandrian [Eg., Alexandria, EY, Ashkelon, 12th century]
Probably a physician, father of Elijah b. Zechariah ha-Dayyān.[937] It is possible that he originated from Alexandria, immigrated and settled in Eretz-Israel (perhaps Ashkelon). It seems that he is the founder of a medical dynasty which was active in Eretz-Israel and Egypt and served the Ayyubid rulers.[938]

Abū al-Faraj b. al-Raʾīs (Elijah b. Zechariah) [Eg., Alexandria, Cairo, EY, Jerusalem, 12th–13th centuries]
A prominent judge and physician (1160–1242) in the court of Abraham Maimonides. His family came from Egypt and he operated in and lived for a long time in Jerusalem during the occupation of the city by Saladin. It is possible that he served under the Ayyubid sultan al-Malik al-Kāmil. According to Goitein, Elijah was a court physician in the service of the Ayyubid sultan al-Malik al-ʿAzīz in Cairo (r. 1193–8); later he retired and became a judge. Two of Elijah's sons, Abū Zikrī al-Sadīd b. Elijah and Raḍī b. Elijah b. Zechariah (the Judge), were physicians. Abū Zikrī also served at al-ʿAzīz's court, specialising in ophthalmology.[939]

Abū Zikrī al-Sadīd b. Elijah b. Zechariah [Eg., Alexandria, EY, Jerusalem, 12th–13th centuries]
A physician, the eldest son of the judge and retired physician Elijah b. Zechariah, named after his grandfather. Abū Zikrī was an ophthalmologist who attended the sultan al-Malik al-ʿAzīz, the son of and successor to Saladin (r. 1193–8). Abū Zikrī also attended other royal figures such as al-Malik al-Muʿaẓẓam ʿIsā, the son of al-Malik al-ʿĀdil, who was the brother of Saladin. He was probably among the physicians who accompanied the court's armed forces. In a letter the young Abū Zikrī (aged twenty) described the condolences he received from all the Muslim Ayyubid leaders after the death of his brother Raḍī.[940] In a different letter to his father, Abū Zikrī proposed his help with getting a stipend from the sultan al-Malik al-Kāmil (r. 1218–38), due to Abū Zikrī's connections to the army of al-Malik al-Muʿaẓẓam ʿIsā, the brother of al-Kāmil.[941] While Aryeh Motzkin described Abū Zikrī as a liberal intellectual and an individualist who rebelled against his father, according to Goitein, based on Geniza documents, Abū Zikrī is described differently. Abū Zikrī, like his brother Solomon and his father, worked at the service of Alexandria's community. In a document (c. 1230), he is mentioned at the top of the list of donors who donated bread for the poor. In one of his letters to his father from Alexandria, Abū Zikrī writes about the Jewish community leader (the *nāsī*) who takes bribes and steals carpets and books from the synagogue, and suggested that his father should take his place as *nāsī*. Interestingly, like his father and brother, Abū Zikrī was also a merchant.[942]

He was married, but his wife's name is not mentioned and it is unclear if he had children.[943] In 1196,[944] Abū Zikrī and his father stayed in Jerusalem.[945] Around the year 1219 he served the Ayyubid sultan al-Muẓaffar.[946] Another source revealed that he served in the army of the Ayyubid prince al-Malik al-Muʿaẓẓam ʿIsā in 1220.[947] He was probably influential although he could not free himself at will from military service.[948] Motzkin claimed that he was often mentioned in different documents: visiting Jerusalem at least twice (once with his wife and once on his own), occasionally ill, being depressed by his loneliness.[949] Abū Zikrī was the addressee of a letter written by his father concerning significant changes in the Jewish and Muslim communities in Alexandria.[950] In another letter, Abū Zikrī expressed his longing for his home and family, since his military service had caused a long absence. Abū Zikrī was the addressee of another letter in which his brother-in-law expressed the sadness of his wife because of his absence.[951] His brother Solomon put together an inventory of the wine collection owned by him, his brother and their father.[952] In another letter to his father, an incident is mentioned, in which Abū Zikrī took without paying a medical book belonging to orphans. The father was asked to demand from his son the return of the book or to pay for it.[953]

Raḍī b. Elijah b. Zechariah (the Judge) [Eg., Cairo, 12th–13th centuries]
A physician, son of Abū al-Faraj b. al-Raʾīs (Elijah b. Zechariah), and brother of Abū Zikrī al-Sadīd b. Elijah, both of them physicians.[954]

Dynasty 22 – Ṣadaqa al-ʾIsrāʾīlī
A dynasty of two generations of physicians, a father and son, both active in Damascus in the twelfth and thirteenth centuries. The son, Imrān b. Ṣadaqa al-ʾIsrāʾīlī al-Ḥakīm Awḥad al-Dīn al-ʾIsrāʾīlī, was considered a very good physician, and practised at the court of the Ayyubid sultan in Syria and Egypt.

Ṣadaqa al-ʾIsrāʾīlī [Sy., Damascus, 12th–13th centuries]
A physician, famous according to Ibn Abī Uṣaybiʿa. The father of Imrān b. Ṣadaqa al-ʾIsrāʾīlī al-Ḥakīm Awḥad al-Dīn al-ʾIsrāʾīlī.[955]

ʿImrān b. Ṣadaqa al-ʾIsrāʾīlī al-Ḥakīm Awḥad al-Dīn al-ʾIsrāʾīlī (Moses b. Ṣadāqā) [Sy., Damascus, Homs, 12th–13th centuries]

A physician, born in Damascus (1165) to a famous physician father. According to Meyerhof, he was the most important Jewish physician after Maimonides.[956] ʿImrān excelled in his medical knowledge and the quality of his treatment and was popular and requested among the rulers, who trusted him to treat and cure their illnesses. He received in return much money and many other benefits. ʿImrān was not closely associated with any ruler, and did not accompany any of their journeys, but he attended whenever any ruler called for him and provided the best treatment. ʿImrān was called by the ruler of Homs, al-Malik al-ʿĀdil, to treat him,[957] and be among his escorts and serve as his personal physician, but he refused. Al-Naṣīr Dāʾūd[958] called for him, during his stay in Karak (Jordan), in order to cure him. ʿImrān treated him until he was cured, and in return, the king gave him an honorary degree, dressed him in a robe, and gave him a monthly salary of 1,500 Nāṣirī dirhams, all in order for him to serve him. The physician stayed in Hama for a while when he was treating the sultan.[959] Despite his previous refusal, ʿImrān became the court physician of al-Malik al-ʿĀdil. He would come to serve the sultan (his family and wives) in the private sections of the sultan's palace in the Cairo fortress, and he did so also in the time of al-Malik al-Muʿaẓẓam ʿIsā (who ruled Damascus and Eretz-Israel). For this, he received a salary and an allowance. Additionally, he worked in the public hospital al-Bīmāristān al-Kabīr, and treated patients there.

ʿImrān had many books that were not found elsewhere.[960] Ibn Abī Uṣaybiʿa mentioned that ʿImrān told him that he had bought many books from the inheritance of his colleague, a Christian physician who converted to Islam, al-Muwaffaq Asʿad b. Iliyās b. al-Maṭrān, who was Saladin's physician. Ibn al-Muṭrān's library included thousands of volumes, and it was offered for sale for a sum of 3,000 dirhams. ʿImrān bought most of the books. He reached an agreement, according to which he would purchase each book for one dirham.[961]

A known Muslim physician, named Raḍī al-Dīn al-Raḥbī, told Ibn Abī Uṣaybiʿa that he had never taught medicine to anyone among the Ahl al-Dhimma except for two: ʿImrān al-ʾIsrāʾīlī and Ibrāhīm b. Khalaf al-Sāmirī, and even this was done only after the two had pushed him and worked hard for it. And indeed, they both were deserving and became respectable physicians. ʿImrān, at some point, was the teacher of Ibn Abī Uṣaybiʿa.[962]

ʿImrān worked in the Nūrī hospital (established in 1154 in Damascus). Ibn Abī Uṣaybiʿa, who also worked in the hospital for a while, wrote about ʿImrān and his friend, the Muslim physician ʿAbd al-Raḥīm al-Dakhwār, that their collaboration was very beneficial in treating patients.[963] He praised ʿImrān especially for his diagnoses and therapeutic abilities[964] and said, 'He treated many diseases and patients with chronic illnesses who had lost their passion for life, and whom other physicians had lost hope to cure. He used strange drugs and gave them wonderful and admirable treatment.'[965]

Al-Ḥarīzī dedicated several poems to him, praising his personality and medical activity.[966] He is also praised in the poems by Moses b. Abraham b. Saʿadya ha-Rōfē Darʿī.[967] ʿImrān died in Homs, in 1239.[968]

Dynasty 23 – Abū al-Barakāt b. al-Sharābī

A three-generation dynasty, including two brothers. The head of the family was presumably a *sharabī* (preparer or seller of potions). Hence, we might have here a case of 'evolution' of the profession, in which the descendants of a *sharabī* became physicians.

Abū al-Barakāt al-Ṭabīb b. al-Sharābī [Eg., Cairo, 12th century]

A Cairene physician, lived in a store at the end of Wax Manufacturers Street.[969] He is mentioned in a document from 1143.[970] He is also the recipient of a letter written by Japheth, in which he was informed of bad news that had occurred.[971] Additionally, he was mentioned as 'Barakāt b. al-Sharābī' in a list of donors dated to the first half of the twelfth century.[972]

Abū al-Ḥasan [Eg., 12th–13th centuries]

A physician, appeared in a family letter addressed to Abū al-Faraj b. Abū al-Barakāt, a physician from Fusṭāṭ, and the brother of Abū al-Ḥasan, written by his son Joseph from Alexandria.[973] From the letter we learn that the brother of the addressee is a physician, possibly the same Abū al-Ḥasan mentioned in the address.

Abū al-Faraj b. Abū al-Barakāt [Eg., Cairo, 12th–13th centuries]

A physician, father of Joseph (Yūsuf). He received in Cairo a letter from his

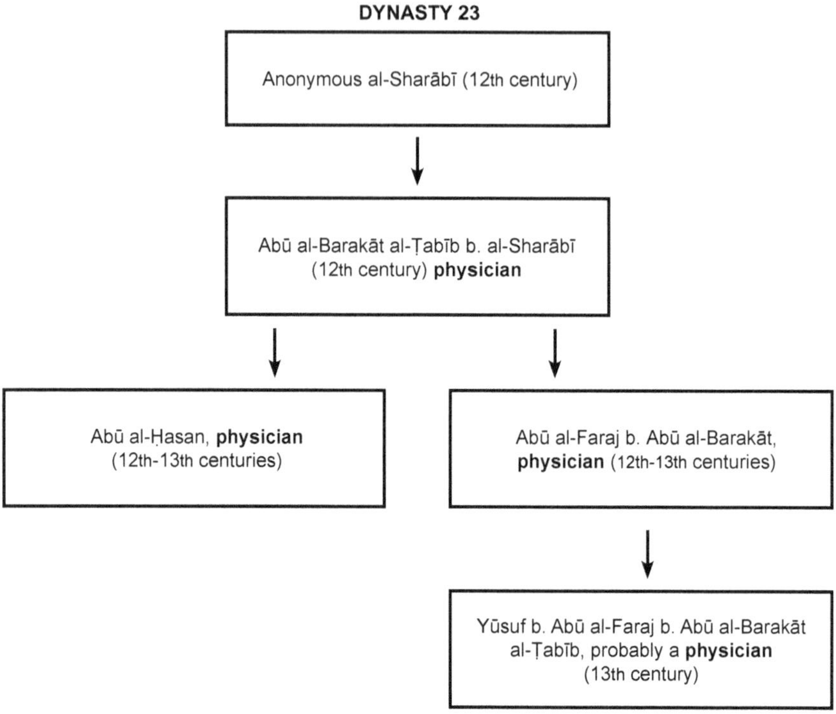

son, sent from Alexandria. His name appeared in another letter from his son, who lived in Alexandria.[974]

Yūsuf b. Abū al-Faraj b. Abū al-Barakāt al-Ṭabīb [Eg., Alexandria, 13th century]
Probably a physician, mentioned in several letters he sent from Alexandria to his father in Cairo.[975]

Dynasty 24 – Abū Saʿd al-ʿAṭṭār
Abū Saʿd al-ʿAṭṭār [Eg., Cairo, 12th–13th centuries]
A pharmacist. His son, Munajjā al-ʿAṭṭār, was mentioned in a bill (1218), but in that year Abū Saʿd was no longer alive. On the second page of the document, there is another bill from the same year, in which Abraham ha-Rōfē b. Simḥā is mentioned.[976]

Munajjā al-ʿAṭṭār b. Abū Saʿd al-ʿAṭṭār [Eg., Cairo, 12th–13th centuries]
A pharmacist, mentioned in a bill (1218).[977] He is also mentioned in a list of

donors written by Samuel b. Saʿadya ha-Levi (a. 1165–1203) and by his son, Joseph b. Samuel (a. c.1180–1212).[978]

Dynasty 25 – Sukra al-Yahūdī al-Ḥalabī

A dynasty of court physicians that was active in Aleppo during the second half of the twelfth and the first half of the thirteenth centuries. Members of this dynasty converted to Islam and continued to fill important positions in the Mamluk period, not necessarily as physicians.

All the information about this dynasty derives only from Muslim Arabic sources. Sukra and ʿAfīf remained Jews, since they were mentioned explicitly as Jews, with the epithet Yahūdī, usually used for non-converted Jews (as opposed to the more ambiguous *nisba* 'al-ʾIsrāʾīlī').[979] In addition, had one of them converted, the Muslim sources would have definitely underscored this act for the glorification of Islam. It seems that the conversion of this dynasty took part in the late Ayyubid period, or even more plausibly, in the early Mamluk period, when the pressures to convert intensified.

Interestingly, a physician from Damascus who lived in the second half of the thirteenth century, named ʿAfīf b. ʿImrān (Amram), was mentioned by Steinschneider as a possible member of this dynasty.[980]

Ibn Faḍl Allāh al-ʿUmarī (1301–49), the prominent bureaucrat in the Mamluk sultanate, in his encyclopedia for scribes wrote that Sukra's descendants converted to Islam and then achieved powerful administrative positions in the chanceries of several districts.[981] They served the sultans Nūr al-Dīn Zengī and his successor Saladin in the second half of the twelfth century. The third generation of this dynasty, in the thirteenth century, maintained the family's medical profession in Aleppo, though they may already have converted to Islam.[982]

Sukra (ʿAbd al-Qāhir) al-Yahūdī al-Ḥalabī [Sy., Aleppo, 12th century]

A physician, according to the sources he had good manners and his advice was good 'like sugar'. Ibn Abī Uṣaybiʿa described him as 'sheikh', a devoted person, an honest man from the Jews of Aleppo, knowledgeable and experienced with ways of treatment and healing. Sukra served the ruler Nūr al-Dīn Zengī[983] and treated his mistress (who was staying at Aleppo fortress) when she became ill, and cured her in spite of her being cared for previously by the

DYNASTY 25

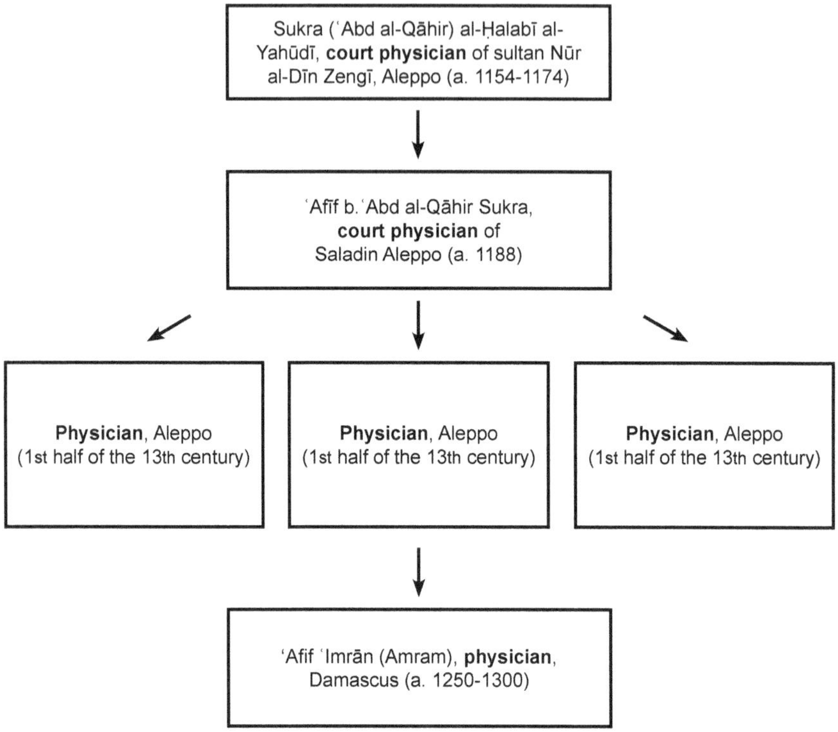

best physicians. Sukra noticed that she ate sparsely and was moody since she wasn't accustomed to the food given to her outside of her country. He asked her about her origins and about her eating and drinking habits, and ordered food and beverages he recommended to be prepared for her. He repeated this treatment for several days and cured her. When she woke and regained her strength, the mistress gave him a plate full of jewellery. Sukra asked her to write a letter to the sultan, telling him about his treatment, and so she did. In her letter she specified that without Sukra's treatment, she would have died, and that all the other physicians sent to her by the sultan could not cure her, and that she regained her health and strength thanks to him. Sukra was invited to Damascus and the Sultan gifted him with five *faddāns*[984] in the village of Ṣamaʿ and five *faddāns* in the village of Anadān, assigned to his ownership. As a result, Sukra became wealthy and he and his sons lived comfortably.[985] Sukra is the father of the physician ʿAfīf, who fathered physicians himself, and so they are part of a dynasty. Al-ʿUmarī (1301–49) mentioned that Sukra's offspring became Muslim and received powerful administrative positions in the chanceries of different districts.[986]

ʿAfīf b. ʿAbd al-Qāhir[987] Sukra al-Yahūdī al-Ḥalabī al-Ṭabīb [Sy., Aleppo, 12th century, ?convert]

A knowledgeable physician known for his treatment and diagnostic skills. ʿAfīf had sons who also practised medicine, all of them residents of Aleppo. Among his writings is an article on *al-qūlanj* (intestinal pain and spasms) which he wrote for Saladin.[988] Ibn al-ʿAdīm (d. 1262) wrote in his history of Aleppo that one of Saladin's physicians in Damascus, ʿAfīf b. Sukra,[989] recommended the use of wine to Saladin. Then, Saladin became ill with colic and his illness became severe.[990] ʿAfīf revisited him and allegedly they had a secret dialogue in which ʿAfīf offered wine again, and received this answer:

> O physician, I had thought you intelligent, but our Prophet, may God grant him blessings and peace, says that God has not placed a cure for my nation in that which He has forbidden to it. Now what is to guarantee that I will not die after drinking it and so meet God with wine in my belly? I swear by God that even if one of the angels told me that your cure lay in wine I would not use it'.[991]

Daniel Nicolae suggested that one of the literary intentions of this story is to provide an entertaining etymology for the name Ibn Sukra (literally 'the son of the one who causes drunkenness').[992] Ibn Abī Uṣaybiʿa did not mention anything about the incident reported by Ibn al-ʿAdīm. Therefore, Nicolae suggested that it was a literary fantasy which stresses the piety of Saladin.[993] Ibn Abī Uṣaybiʿa added that ʿAfīf b. Sukra had 'children and family members most of whom practice medicine'.[994] Ibn Faḍl Allāh al-ʿUmarī added that these descendants of Sukra converted to Islam.[995] According to Anne-Mare Eddé he died around 1188.[996]

Dynasty 26 – Abū al-Barakāt Ibn Shaʿya

A dynasty of Karaite physicians that lasted for many generations, during the Fatimid, Ayyubid and Mamluk periods. In the Mamluk period, the court physicians of this dynasty were Muslims. It might be that this family was only a part of a much bigger dynasty of physicians; that is, that the members of the Ibn Ṣaghīr dynasty of physicians (dynasty 40) were in fact descendants of the Ibn Shaʿyā family. Abū al-Barakāt belonged to the notable family of Ibn Shaʿyā (= Isaiah), mentioned in both Muslim Arabic historical sources and Geniza documents from the eleventh century. This was an eminent family of great traders, bankers, government officials and agents. The family also included important physicians; for example, a possible member was a certain Dāniyāl (Daniel) Ibn Shaʿyā, the author of a celebrated treatise on ophthalmology.[997] If this is the case, we have a complex dynasty of distinguished physicians and other dignitaries, which existed throughout the Fatimid, Ayyubid and Mamluk periods, including the families of Ibn Shaʿyā, Ibn Ṣaghīr and Ibn Kūjik (dynasty 41). The complete and complex relations between the branches of these families, however, are impossible to trace at this time.[998]

DYNASTY 26

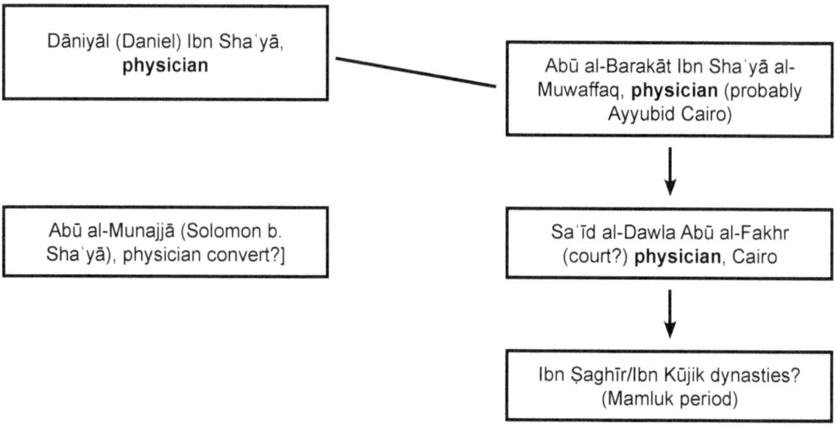

Dāniyāl (Daniel) Ibn Shaʿyā [K, Eg., 11th century]

A physician, probably a member of the famous family of Ibn Shaʿyā (= Josiah, Isaiah) mentioned in both Muslim Arabic historical sources and Geniza documents from the eleventh century. This was a distinguished family of great traders, bankers, government officials and agents. The family also included important physicians such as Abū al-Barakāt Ibn Shaʿyā al-Muwaffaq. Dāniyāl (Daniel) Ibn Shaʿyā is the author of a famous treatise on ophthalmology (recommended in a Geniza letter as worthy of being memorised).[999] Yu Hoki suggested that ‘although the presence of *Dāniyāl ibn*

Shuʿyā in Arabic medical history has not been evaluated, it is possible that his work was one of the most popular ophthalmologic books and a considerable number of copies were circulating at least among ophthalmologists of the Jewish community of Fusṭāṭ'.[1000]

Abū al-Barakāt Ibn Shaʿyā al-Muwaffaq [K, Eg., 12th–13th centuries]
A Karaite physician who was active in Egypt, probably during the Ayyubid period, even though Ibn Abī Uṣaybiʿa does not mention when Abū al-Barakāt lived. Ramaḍān holds that it is reasonable to assume that this historian referred to his contemporary, otherwise he would have mentioned that he served the Fatimid.[1001] Ibn Abī Uṣaybiʿa wrote a short biographical entry on this Jewish physician as follows:

> This physician was called al-Muwaffaq, he was a famous sheikh. He had a great deal of experience in therapy and his abilities in healing were commendable. He lived 86 years and died in Cairo. He left behind a son named Saʿīd al-Dawla Abū al-Fakhr who was also a physician and lived in Cairo.[1002]

Abū al-Barakāt belonged to the famous family of Ibn Shaʿyā (= Josiah, Isaiah) mentioned in both Muslim Arabic historical sources and Geniza documents from the eleventh century. This was a distinguished family of great traders, bankers, government officials and agents. The family also included important physicians. One who might belong to this family was a certain Dāniyāl (Daniel) Ibn Shaʿyā, the author of a famous treatise on ophthalmology.[1003]

Abū al-Munajjā (Solomon b. Shaʿyā) [Eg., 11th–12th centuries, ?convert]
A physician; a prominent member of this family was an influential banker and administrator, in charge of agriculture under the Fatimid ruler's deputy, al-Afḍal. According to the Muslim chronicler Ibn Duqmāq (d. 1407), al-Munajjā was one of the ancestors of the Ibn Ṣaghīr dynasty, which included several court physicians in the Mamluk period, most of whom converted to Islam and became physicians of kings and sultans.[1004]

Saʿīd al-Dawla Abū al-Fakhr [K., Eg., 13th century]
A physician, son of Abū al-Barakāt Ibn Shaʿyā, who was also a physician.[1005]

Dynasty 27 – Khalaf al-Sāmirī

A dynasty of Samaritan physicians from the twelfth and thirteenth centuries. So far, we have information regarding three of them. All of them were mentioned only by Muslim Arabic sources. Some of them were court physicians, others were *wazīrs* and one converted to Islam.

DYNASTY 27

Yūsuf b. Abī Sa῾īd b. Khalaf al-Sāmirī al-Muhadhdhab al-Ṭabīb, **court physician**, Wazīr, consultant (12th century)

Ibrāhīm b. Khalaf al-Sāmirī, **court physician** (12th century)

Amīn al-Dawla Abū al-Ḥasan b. Ghazāl b. Abī Sa῾īd al-Sāmirī, **physician, convert**, Wazīr (13th century)

Yūsuf b. Abī Sa῾īd b. Khalaf al-Sāmirī al-Muhadhdhab al-Ṭabīb (Wazīr al-Amjad) [S., Sy., 12th century]

A Samaritan physician from Damascus (a contemporary of Maimonides). He studied medicine at the Al-Ṣalāḥiyya institute, and from the physicians Ibrāhīm b. Faraj b. Mārūth, al-Muhadhdhab b. al-Naqqāsh, Ismā῾īl b. Abū al-Waqqār and ῾Alī Abī al-Yamān al-Kindī.[1006] He became known for offering a successful treatment to Sitt al-Shām b. Ayyūb – the wife of the governor of Homs, and Saladin and Sayf al-Dīn's sister – who was afflicted with dysentery. He treated her using camphor together with roasted seeds and a potion concocted from pomegranates and sandalwood.[1007] He served the Ayyubid emir of Baalbek, Farrukh Shāh, and after he died (1179) he served his successor, al-Amjad Bahrām Shāh. The latter also appointed him a consultant and later on a *wazīr*. Yūsuf became rich in his position and started receiving criticism from the Samaritan community for giving away jobs to his friends. Eventually, they told the sultan about his doings, and he arrested him and confiscated his property. In the end, he returned to his homeland, Damascus, and died in 1227. According to Ashtor, based on Ibn Abī Uṣaybi῾a, Yūsuf was murdered because he angered the Muslims by appointing his protégés.[1008] He is probably related to Ibrāhīm b. Khalaf.[1009]

Ibrāhīm b. Khalaf al-Sāmirī (the Samaritan) [S., Eg., Damascus, 12th–13th centuries]

A medical student, who along with another Jewish student, ʿImrān b. Ṣadaqa al-ʾIsrāʾīlī, was permitted to enter the lectures ofRaḍī al-Dīn al-Raḥbī, who taught medicine in Damascus in the middle of the twelfth century. In principle, apart from these two, al-Raḥbī did not teach non-Muslims. He was probably a relative of Yūsuf b. Abī Saʿīd b. Khalaf,[1010] and he served Saladin.[1011]

Amīn al-Dawla Abū al-Ḥasan b. Ghazāl b. Abī Saʿīd al-Sāmirī (Wazīr al-Ṣāliḥ, and Sharaf al-Milla ('the Glory of the Nation')) [S., Sy., Baalbek, 13th century, convert]

A Samaritan physician; his uncle on his father's side wasYūsuf b. Abī Saʿīd b. Khalaf al-Sāmirī al-Muhadhdhab al-Ṭabīb. He also served as the court physician of the prince of Baalbek, al-Amjad Bahrām Shāh. During that period, he wrote a five-volume medical book. He converted to Islam (1237) and became the *wazīr* of the ruler of Damascus, al-Malik al-Ṣāliḥ (d. 1250). As a *wazīr*, he performed very well, was capable of carrying out policies and was highly influential. He built many structures, renewed schools and scholarly institutions and amassed great power and wealth. Ibn Abī Uṣaybiʿa, who was his pupil and even dedicated to him his book *Ḥikāyāt al-Aṭibbāʾ* ('The Tales of Physicians'), described him as extremely clever, well mannered, very knowledgeable and someone who possessed a full and precise ability in medicine in its various aspects. Abū al-Ḥasan was interested in collecting books on various scientific subjects and many of the authors carried on a correspondence with him. For example, he ordered ten writers to write the history of Damascus in ten volumes, a project they worked on for two years. Ibn Abī Uṣaybiʿa noted that during his lifetime, Abū al-Ḥasan managed to amass great wealth, a fact that was anathema in the eyes of many high-ranking officials in the kingdom. Abū al-Muẓaffar recounted that after Abū al-Ḥasan died, it turned out that he owned a lot of money and many precious stones, worth about 3,000 dinars, and he also had about 10,000 valuable books.[1012]

Abū al-Ḥasan got tangled in the inner quarrels of the Ayyubid dynasty between al-Ṣāliḥ Ismāʿīl, the ruler of Damascus, and al-Ẓāhir, who at the time ruled Egypt. When al-Malik al-Ṣāliḥ came to power, Abū al-Ḥasan was dispossessed of all his belongings and status and imprisoned in the Egypt Citadel for five years. After his release he was executed in Egypt by the Mamluks, who replaced the Ayyubid dynasty in 1250.[1013]

Abū al-Ḥasan's writings include *Al-Nahj al-Wāḍiḥ fī al-Ṭibb* (a collection of articles dealing with a classification of the medical profession and its rules), *al-Adawiya al-Mufrada wa-Quwwāhā* ('The Book of Singular Medicines and Their Efficiency'), *Al-Adawiya Al-Murakkaba wa-Manāfiʿhā* ('The Book of Compound Medicines and Their Benefits') and *Tadbīr al-Aṣiḥḥāʾ* (on the treatment of diseases, their causes and symptoms).[1014]

Dynasty 28 – Abū al-Bayān

A Karaite physician and probably his grandson, highly distinguished practitioners that practised medicine in Egypt in the twelfth and thirteenth centuries, treating the Ayyubid rulers at their courts and working also in hospitals. Both members of the dynasty were highly esteemed, and besides honour, they received presents and financial support from the Muslim rulers and courts. Both 'grandfather' and 'grandson' were authors of medical books and were mentioned mainly by the Muslim Arabic sources. Interestingly, more than a dozen parts of the medical book *al-Dustūr al-Bimāristānī fī 'l-Adwiya 'l-Murakkaba*[1015] written by the 'grandson' were found in the Geniza.[1016]

Abū al-Bayān b. al-Mudawwar al-Sadīd [K., Eg., 12th century]

A physician (lived probably 1101–84) known for the quality of his medical treatment and his wide knowledge of medicine. He was part of the Karaite congregation and served the last rulers of the Fatimid dynasty and kept his position during the time of Saladin (r. 1171–93), who kept paying him a monthly allowance of 24 Egyptian dinars, even when he was old and unfit for service. He lived for eighty-three years, during which he taught many students, including Zayn al-Ḥassāb. Many emirs and rulers, local and foreign, turned to him for advice. His most famous writing was possibly titled 'On Medical Experience' but it was lost and has not been found.[1017] It is probable that he was the grandfather of the physician Abū al-Faḍl Dāʾūd b. Sulaymān b. Abū al-Bayān al-ʾIsrāʾīlī al-Sadīd (David b. Solomon), who was known as 'Sadīd al-Dīn'.[1018]

Abū al-Faḍl Dā'ūd b. Sulaymān b. Abū al-Bayān al-'Isrā'īlī al-Sadīd (David b. Solomon) [K., Eg., Cairo, 12th–13th centuries]

A Karaite physician (1161–1236), student of Ibn Jumayʿ and Ibn al-Nāqid (an ophthalmologist). He was appointed as a physician at the Nāṣirī hospital in Cairo, which was established by Saladin in 1181. Ibn Abī Uṣaybiʿa, who worked with him in the hospital, noted that he was knowledgeable in the theory and practice of medicine, as well as complex and simple medicines, and excelled at diagnosing illnesses in patients. He wrote the hospital's rule book *al-Dustūr al-Bimāristānī fī 'l-Adwiya 'l-Murakkaba*,[1019] which included all of the prevalent medicines in hospitals and pharmacies in the area. Additionally, he wrote a book of notes on Galen's book of pains. He served the Ayyubid ruler al-Malik al-ʿĀdil and became the most prominent Egyptian physician of his time. He apparently carried on a correspondence with al-Kohen al-ʿAṭṭār, a correspondence that includes various prescription drugs.[1020] He might have been the son or the grandson of Abū al-Bayān b. al-Mudawwar al-Sadīd.

Dynasty 29 – al-Sadīd al-Ṭabīb

A unique example of a small dynasty for which we have found information only on a physician father and his pharmacist son. In most cases of that period, and in Arabic medicine, the normal 'evolutionary line' was from pharmacists to physicians. They both practised at Cairo during the twelfth and thirteenth centuries, and both were mentioned only by a Jewish source, the Cairo Geniza, in two different lists of donors.

al-Sadīd al-Ṭabīb [Eg., 12th–13th centuries]

A physician, mentioned in a list of donors (1180–1203); also mentioned are his son, Abū Saʿd al-ʿAṭṭār 2, and Ṣadaqa al-Ṭabīb.[1021]

Abū Saʿd al-ʿAṭṭār 2 [Eg., Cairo, 12th–13th centuries]

A pharmacist, mentioned in a list of donors (1180–1203), alongside his father, al-Sadīd al-Ṭabīb, and Ṣadaqa al-Ṭabīb.[1022] He might be identical with Abū Saʿd al-ʿAṭṭār, who is mentioned in a list of donors from 1178 written by Mevōrākh b. Nathan, alongside Makārim al-ʿAṭṭār, Abū al-Fakhr al-ʿAṭṭār 2, Hiba al-ʿAṭṭār 2, Dā'ūd al-ʿAṭṭār and Abū al-Majd al-Ṭabīb. Additionally, Munajjā al-ʿAṭṭār may be his son.[1023]

*Dynasty 30 – Ibn Jumay*ʿ

A dynasty of physicians, of whom we have managed to gather information about only three. The information is both from Muslim Arabic sources and from a Jewish source, the Cairo Geniza. The father, Abū al-ʿAshāʾir Hibat-Allāh b. Zayn b. Ḥasan b. Ifrāʾīm b. Yaʿqūb b. Ismāʿīl Ibn Jumayʿ al-ʾIsrāʾīlī, known as 'al-Sheikh al-Muwaffaq Shams al-Riʾāsa', and in Hebrew as Nethanel b. Samuel, was a highly esteemed physician, serving Saladin and other Muslim dignitaries. We have found only a few biographical details on his son, and his medical activity. The third physician, Mūsā b. Ifrāʾīm b. Dāʾūd b. Ifrāʾīm b. Yaʿqūb, was active at the Mamluk period, and thanks to his name and some biographical details we managed to reveal his relation as part of the dynasty. I suspect that there are a few other links in the chain of this medical dynasty; however, we have not been able to trace them, neither in the Muslim Arabic sources nor in the Cairo Geniza.

DYNASTY 30

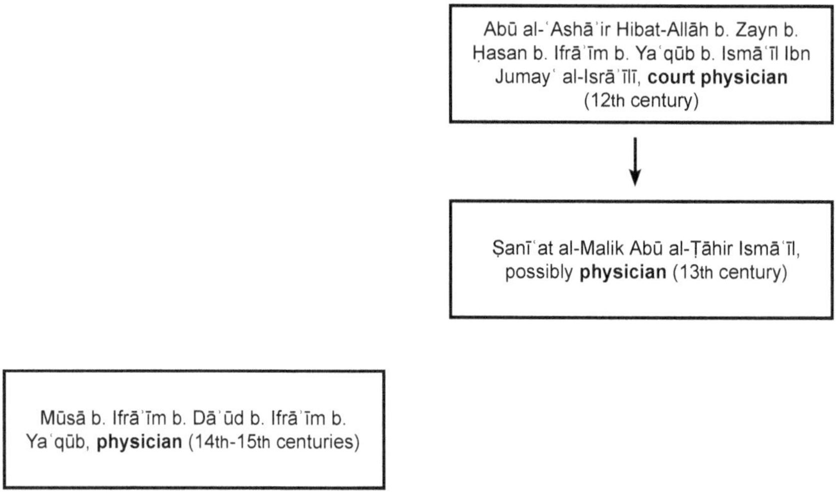

Abū al-ʿAshāʾir Hibat-Allāh b. Zayn b. Ḥasan b. Ifrāʾīm b. Yaʿqūb b. Ismāʿīl Ibn Jumayʿ al-ʾIsrāʾīlī (Nethanel b. Samuel) [Eg., Cairo, 12th century]

A well-known physician, known as 'al-Sheikh al-Muwaffaq Shams al-Riʾāsa'. He was born and raised in Fusṭāṭ.[1024] Ibn Jumayʿ served under Saladin and later on his successor.[1025] He became famous after he managed to bring back to life a man considered dead that happened to pass by on a stretcher near the clinic. Ibn Jumayʿ noticed that the supposedly dead man's legs were stretched out and not dangling as would be expected. He was a teacher for students of all religions and took part in discussions about the standards of medicine.[1026] Ibn Abī Uṣaybiʿa mentioned that he had a clinic in the Sūq al-Qanādīl (Market of Lamps) in Fusṭāṭ. Later on, he moved to Cairo, to the Zawīla neighbourhood, close to the al-ʿAshūriyya and al-Quṭubiyya al-Jadīda schools. It is also mentioned that he had a group that was studying medicine. He died in 1198.

Ibn Jumayʿ wrote several essays on medicine, on the climate of Alexandria, and on first aid: *Kitāb al-Irshād li-Maṣāliḥ al-Nafs wa-l-Ajsād* (directions for the improvement of souls and bodies, 4 volumes); *Kitāb al-Taṣrīḥ bi-l-Maknūn fī Tankīḥ al-Qānūn* (criticism of Ibn Sīnā's al-Qānūn), *Maqāla fī al-Līmūn wa-Sharābihi wa-Manāfiʿihi* (on the benefits of lemons and their consumption), and a treatise on colic, titled *al-Risāla al-Sayfiyya fī al-Adwiya al-Mulūkiyya*. In his essay *al-Maqāla al-Salāḥiyya fī Iḥyāʾ al-Ṣināʿa al-Ṭibbiya* (on how to revive medicine)[1027] Ibn Jumayʿ deals with the reasons for the decline in the medical profession. The reasons, as he saw them, were the lack of access to the inner organs, which makes it hard to identify illnesses; physicians not practising anatomy; and deviations from the teachings of Hippocrates and Galen in many commentaries and summaries. In order to revive medicine, kings should give care to the teachers and students of medicine, one should only learn from Hippocrates and Galen, medical students should be trained in hospitals, and physicians should be examined before practising medicine and supervised when doing medical work.[1028] Nicolae claimed that Ibn Jumayʿ's medical writings were thoroughly secular, and his religious ideas appear to have been completely disconnected from his medical world, which was mainly influenced by Galenic ideals.[1029] Some of his books were dedicated to the Fatimid *wazīr* ʿAbd al-Raḥīm b. ʿAlī al-Baysānī, who supported some of the non-Muslim physicians and was their patron.[1030] Al-Maqrīzī wrote that Ibn Jumayʿ was a *kātib* (senior clerk) of the *wazīr* Qarāqūsh (Asad al-Dīn Saʿīd Qarāqūsh b. ʿAbd Allāh al-Asadī, also called 'Bahāʾ al-Dīn'), who was at first the *zimām al-qaṣr* (palace director) for Saladin and later on was appointed his deputy.[1031] In the same place, al-Maqrīzī mentioned that it was Ibn Jumayʿ al-Yahūdī al-Ṭabīb, Qarāqūsh's secretary, who sold his house in the Zuwayla neighbourhood to the wife of the emir Ayāzkūj (who was, like Qarāqūsh, a supporter of Saladin). She founded in this house a Ḥanafī school named after her, al-ʿAshūriyya.[1032] Ibn Jumayʿ is even mentioned as serving as the 'Head of the Physicians' in Cairo.[1033]

Nicolae suggested that Ibn Jumayʿ's uniqueness was because he 'saw his duty as a physician not only in systematising the knowledge of his predecessors, but also in adding to what they had said'.[1034] He added that Ibn Jumayʿ's attitude towards Muslim physicians was positive; however, it was negative towards Christian physicians. In his treatise to Saladin, Ibn Jumayʿ expressed the notion that Christians were intellectually lazy and hence opposed to medical progress.[1035] Ibn Jumayʿ is apparently mentioned as 'al-Sheikh al-Muwaffaq' in many documents from the Geniza,[1036] one of which is a deathbed declaration of Abū al-Faraj (Ibn al-Kallām), a rich Jewish merchant and a trustee of the court, dated to 1182. From that document we learn that he owed money to some of his associates (including Maimonides, Qāḍī Ibn Sanāʾ al-Mulk, Ibn Ṣawla and a certain Abū al-Khayr of Haifa). The largest sum, more than four dinars, was paid by al-Sheikh al-Muwaffaq, for Abū al-Faraj's poll tax. He is probably mentioned in a letter sent to a young physician who is looking for a position in a hospital in Alexandria. In the letter, the physician's cousin, who wrote the letter, advises the young physician to show his recommendation letter to prominent figures in Alexandria, among them to Ibn Jumayʿ.[1037]

Ṣanīʿat al-Malik Abū al-Ṭāhir Ismāʿīl [Eg., Cairo, 13th century]

Might be a physician, the son of al-Muwaffaq Ibn Jumayʿ, and was probably a student of his father. He gathered his father's medical lectures into a book he entitled *Kitāb al-Irshād li-Maṣāliḥ al-Anfus wa al-Ajsād* ('Guidance for the Welfare of Souls and Bodies').[1038]

Mūsā b. Ifrāʾīm b. Dāʾūd b. Ifrāʾīm b. Yaʿqūb (Ibn Jumayʿ al-ʾIsrāʾīlī al-Ṭabīb) [Eg., Cairo, 14th–15th centuries]

A physician, worked at the hospital of Saladin in Cairo; a colophon at the end of Ibn Sīnā's book *al-Qānūn fi-l-Ṭibb* tells us that the book was copied around 1397.[1039] His name and other biographical details leave very little doubt that he belonged to the Ibn Jumayʿ family, a dynasty of prominent Jewish physicians that continued from Saladin's times to (at least) Mamluk Egypt at the beginning of the fifteenth century.

Dynasty 31 – Petahya ha-Levi

Petahya ha-Levi ha-Rōfē [K., Sy., Damascus, 13th century] and Jekuthiel ha-Levi b. Petahya [K., Sy., Damascus, 13th century]

Two physicians, apparently Karaites, mentioned in a document from Damascus. One is perhaps Jekuthiel ha-Levi b. Petahya and the other is Jekuthiel's father, Petahya ha-Levi ha-Rōfē.[1040]

Dynasty 32 – al-Sheikh Joseph

al-Sheikh Joseph [Eg., Cairo, 13th century] and Anonymous – a physician, son of al-Sheikh Joseph [Eg., Cairo, 13th century]

'Al-Sheikh Joseph and his son (*wa-waladuhu*)', both physicians, are mentioned in a list of future donors from the period of Abraham Maimonides. Other physicians in the list include al-Mawlī al-Muhadhdhab, Awlād al-Ra᾿īs, al-Gaon al-Munā, Mufaḍḍal al-Mashmiʿa, Ibn al-Julājilī, R. Yeshūʿā, Abū al-Maʿānī 2, Najīb Kohen Kamukhī, al-Rabīb Kohen, al-Taqī Ibn al-Gadal, Makārim Ibn al-Gadalī and Abū al-Maʿānī.[1041] It is possible that the name of the son was Abū al-ʿAlā, if the Joseph mentioned here is the same Joseph who is mentioned in a note written by Abraham Maimonides, in which he warns that the physician is wanted by the law authorities in Fusṭāṭ.[1042]

Dynasty 33 – Abū al-Fakhr al-ʿAṭṭār

Abū al-Fakhr al-ʿAṭṭār [Eg., 12th century] and Abū al-Ḥasan al-ʿAṭṭār b. Abū al-Fakhr [Eg., 13th century]

Two pharmacists, Abū al-Fakhr al-ʿAṭṭār and his son Abū al-Ḥasan al-ʿAṭṭār b. Abū al-Fakhr, are mentioned in a Geniza document.[1043]

Dynasty 34 – Tiqva ha-Levi

Tiqva ha-Levi ha-Rōfē ha-Sar ha-Nikhbād [Eg., 12th–13th centuries] and Elazar b. Tiqva ha-Levi ha-Sar ha-Nikhbād ha-Rōfē [Eg., 12th–13th centuries]

Tiqva ha-Levi was a physician, mentioned in a document (1228) with his son, Elazar b. Tiqva ha-Levi, in which it is mentioned that the judge Elijah served as Elazar's representative in his marriage to Yāmūn the widow, daughter of Elijah b. Joseph al-Dalātī. Tiqva was no longer alive.[1044]

Dynasty 35 – Abū al-Ḥasan al-ʿAṭṭār 3

Abū al-Ḥasan al-ʿAṭṭār 3 [Eg., 13th century] and Abū al-Faraj al-ʿAṭṭār b. Abū al-Ḥasan al-ʿAṭṭār [Eg., Alexandria, 13th century]

Two pharmacists, father and son. The son, Abū al-Faraj al-ʿAṭṭār b. Abū al-Ḥasan, was the addressee of a letter addressed to him in Alexandria, written by Elijah b. Zechariah and dated to the beginning of the thirteenth century.[1045]

Dynasty 36 – Maḥāsin (Obadia ha-Dayyān)

A dynasty of three physicians, grandfather, son and grandson. All were probably practising in the fourteenth century at al-Bīra, Iraq.

DYNASTY 36

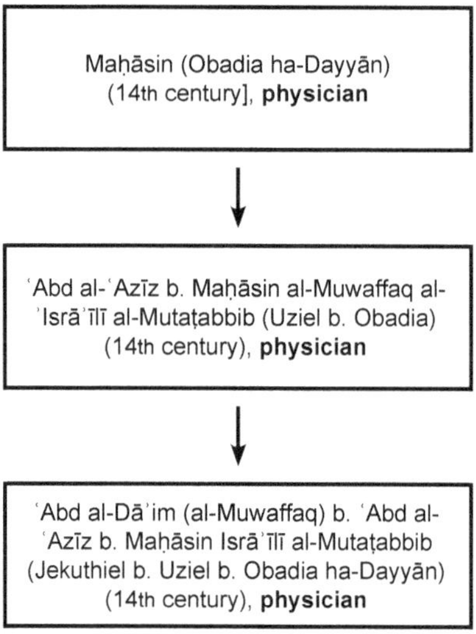

Maḥāsin (Obadia ha-Dayyān) [Iq., al-Bīra, 14th century] and ʿAbd al-ʿAzīz b. Maḥāsin al-Muwaffaq al-ʾIsrāʾīlī al-Mutaṭabbib (Uziel b. Obadia) [Iq., al-Bīra, 14th century]

The grandson of Maḥāsin (Obadia ha-Dayyān), Jekuthiel b. Uziel b. Obadia ha-Dayyān (in Arabic ʿAbd al-Dāʾim b. ʿAbd al-ʿAzīz b. Maḥāsin al-Muwaffaq al-ʾIsrāʾīlī al-Mutaṭabbib), wrote a philosophical book in al-Bīra (Birecik) at the beginning of the fourteenth century. He added the epithet 'Ḥakīm' to his father's and grandfather's names, implying that they were physicians like him.[1046]

ʿAbd al-Dāʾim (al-Muwaffaq) b. ʿAbd al-ʿAzīz b. Maḥāsin ʾIsrāʾīlī al-Mutaṭabbib (Jekuthiel b. Uziel b. Obadia ha-Dayyān) [Eg., Iq., al-Bīra, 14th century]
A physician, lived in al-Bīra (Birecik); his father and grandfather were physicians. He wrote a philosophical book in Arabic, in which he mainly followed Ibn Sīnā's (d. 1037) logic, and the commentary about its writing by Naṣīr al-Dīn al-Ṭūsī. The book, *Kitāb al-ʿIlmayn* ('The Book on the Two Wisdoms') is written as questions and answers and deals with 'natural wisdom' and 'divine wisdom'. At the end of the treatise, the author mentioned that he had finished writing it on 8 September 1315, adding that he stood with the philosophers' method and had written the book in that spirit, and that he declared himself to be a Jew.[1047]

Dynasty 37 – Ibn al-Kirmānī
A short dynasty of two Karaite physicians; father and son, who practised medicine in Cairo in the Mamluk period.

Abū al-Fakhr b. Abī al-Faḍl b. Abī Naṣr b. Abī al-Fakhr al-Yahūdī (Aaron ha-Levi Ibn al-Kirmānī, al-Kaḥḥāl) [K., Eg., Cairo, 13th–14th centuries]
A physician and ophthalmologist from a family of Karaite physicians, mentioned in business documents of the Karaite community in Cairo. He purchased a house in 1260, sold half of it six years afterwards, and after his death, in 1324, his two sons redistributed the inheritance of the remaining half of the house.[1048]

Abū al-Bishr b. Aaron ha-Levi al-Kirmānī al-Ḥakīm [K, Eg., Cairo, 14th century]
A Karaite physician, son of Aaron ha-Levi Ibn al-Kirmānī, who was also a physician. His name appeared in a memorial list of the Kirmānī family. After the death of Aaron ha-Levi in 1324, Abū al-Bishr decided that his part would be owned by his wife. In the document selling his portion of the house he is called al-Sheikh al-Rashīd Abū al-Bishr, and in the lineage of this family he is called Abū al-Bishr al-Ḥakīm.[1049]

Dynasty 38 – ʿAbd al-Sayyid b. Isḥāq

A dynasty of Jewish physicians that was active in Syria in the Mamluk period, during the thirteenth and fourteenth centuries. They were working in hospitals and some of them had positions in the Jewish community. Three members of the dynasty, a father and two sons, converted together to Islam (1302), in an event echoed in the writings of several Muslim Arabic sources.

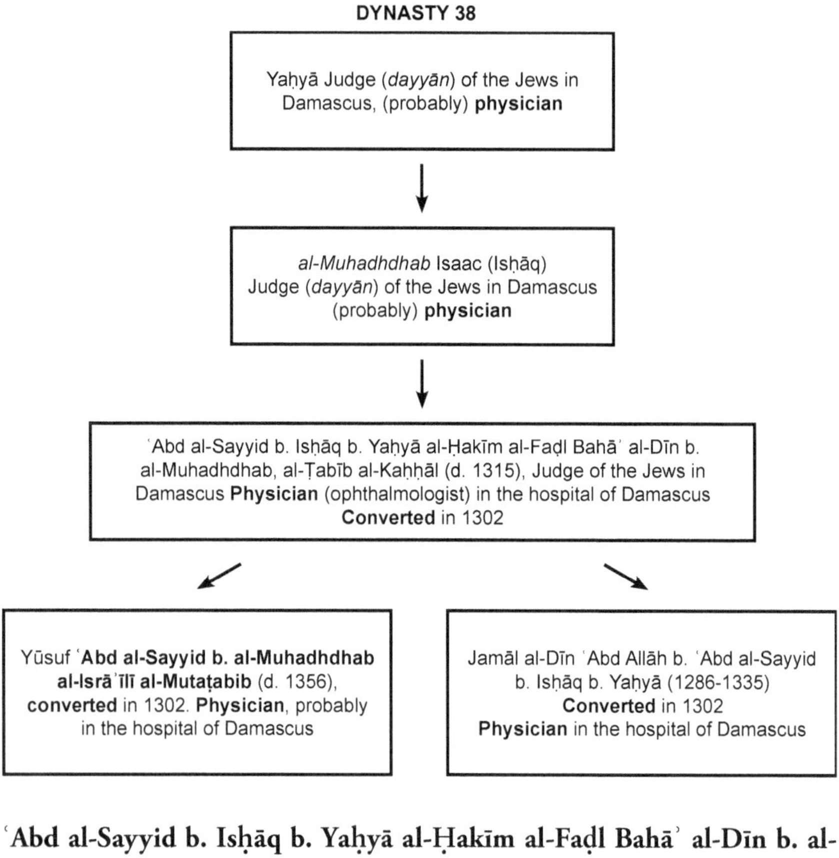

ʿAbd al-Sayyid b. Isḥāq b. Yaḥyā al-Ḥakīm al-Faḍl Bahāʾ al-Dīn b. al-Muhadhdhab, al-Ṭabīb al-Kaḥḥāl [Sy., Damascus, 13th–14th centuries, convert]

A physician and *dayyān*, converted to Islam in 1302. According to the Muslim sources, he was in friendly terms with Ibn Taymiyya (a famous Muslim theologian, 1263–1328) even before he converted to Islam, and maybe he was converted by him.[1050] The sources tell us of intellectual contacts he had with Sufis and Muslim theologians before his conversion to Islam. The day of his conversion together with his family, in July 1302, is mentioned in several Muslim Arabic sources in detail as an especially happy and important day in which the elite took part. According to the sources, ʿAbd al-Sayyid was invited to the palace of justice (*Dār al-ʿAdl*) in the citadel of Damascus, together with his sons. They all converted to Islam and the governor of Damascus bestowed upon them robes of honour. The converted family rode on horseback in a royal parade in Damascus, in order to publicise their conversion. ʿAbd al-Sayyid was appointed by the governor as one of the chief physicians in the public hospital of Damascus, al-Nūrī (*al-Bīmāristān al-Nūrī*). Many other Jews are said to have converted with him and after him. ʿAbd al-Sayyid died in 1315 and was buried on the slopes of Mount Qasioun, west of the city of Damascus.[1051] It is reasonable to assume that ʿAbd al-Sayyid's father was also a physician. This is because of the title *al-Muhadhdhab* (the courteous, the decent) which is given mostly to physicians.[1052] In addition, al-Yūnīnī mentioned that ʿAbd al-Sayyid inherited his position as a *dayyān* from his father and grandfather.[1053] Many times a community leader also serves as a physician, especially of the government. Two of his sons who converted to Islam with him were physicians.

Yūsuf ʿAbd al-Sayyid b. al-Muhadhdhab al-ʾIsrāʾīlī al-Mutaṭabib (Joseph b. al-Dayyān) [Sy. Damascus, Homs, 13th–14th centuries, convert]
A prominent physician in Damascus who converted to Islam with his father ʿAbd al-Sayyid and brother Jamāl al-Dīn ʿAbd Allāh in 1302. He heard and transmitted *ḥadīth* (the oral tradition of Islam) and was talented in the medical profession. He is referred to by the epithet *Raʾīs* (head), conferred upon doctors, and especially on physicians who acted as head of department in the hospital.[1054] It might be possible that like his father and brother, he too used to work in the public al-Nūrī hospital in Damascus. Yūsuf died in 1356.[1055]

Jamāl al-Dīn ʿAbd Allāh b. ʿAbd al-Sayyid b. Isḥāq b. Yaḥyā [Sy. Damascus, 13th–14th centuries, convert]
A physician (1286–1335), working at the al-Nūrī hospital in Damascus. After he had converted to Islam with his father in 1302, when he was about sixteen years old, he was appointed a teacher in a madrasa. Afterwards he studied medicine and became a good and talented physician.[1056]

DYNASTY 39

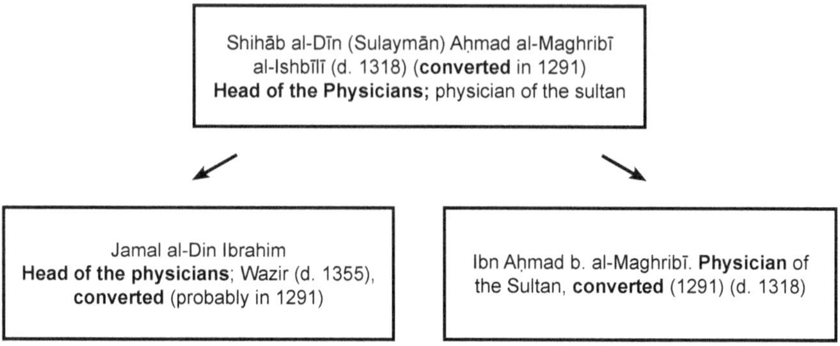

Dynasty 39 – Shihāb al-Dīn Aḥmad al-Maghribī

The Ibn al-Maghribī family included several court physicians of the sultan al-Nāṣir Muḥammad b. Qalāwūn. Shihāb al-Dīn Aḥmad al-Maghribī al-Ishbīlī and his son Jamāl al-Dīn Ibrāhīm occupied the office of the 'Head of the Physicians'. Shihāb al-Dīn Aḥmad was originally a Jew named Sulaymān. It seems that, since he is mentioned by the name al-Maghribī, and not Ibn al-Maghribī, he was the founder of this dynasty in Egypt, arriving in Egypt from elsewhere in north Africa (the Maghrib).[1057] According to Muslim sources, descendants of the Jewish dynasty of Ibn al-Maghribī, filled the office of 'Head of the Physicians' during the late thirteenth and the fourteenth centuries. Similarly, converted descendants of the Jewish dynasty of Ibn Ṣaghīr (dynasty 40) held this office during the late fourteenth and the fifteenth centuries.

Shihāb al-Dīn Aḥmad (Sulaymān) al-Maghribī al-Ishbīlī [Eg., 13th–14th centuries, convert]

A physician, originally named Sulaymān. He was the physician of the sultan al-Nāṣir Muḥammad b. Qalāwūn (d. 1340). He converted to Islam in 1291 during the time of the sultan al-Ashraf Khalīl b. Qalāwūn, and his name was changed from Sulaymān to Aḥmad. He was appointed thereafter the 'Head of the Physicians'. His sons also served as the sultan's physicians. His son Jamāl al-Dīn Ibrāhīm al-Maghribī (d. 1355), who replaced him as the 'Head of the Physicians', was apparently born a Jew, and converted to Islam during his childhood, together with his father. Aḥmad died in 1318.[1058] He excelled in a variety of natural sciences, especially in philosophy, geometry and astronomy/astrology.[1059] He was very wealthy and is said to have left after his death gold worth 30,000 dinars.[1060]

Jamāl al-Dīn Ibrāhīm b. Shihāb al-Dīn Aḥmad (Sulaymān) al-Maghribī [Eg. 14th century, convert]
A physician (d. 1355), served the sultan and worked in the public hospital of Cairo during his father's lifetime. He was appointed as the 'Head of the Physicians', probably after his father's death, in 1318. Jamāl filled this office during most of the third reign of al-Nāṣir Muḥammad and he became one of the sultan's closest associates. In addition, he gained a very distinguished position in the sultanate and received an enormous salary. According to al-Ṣafadī, he was at the level of *wazīr* (chief administrator). Al-ʿUmarī testified that Jamāl gave him good medical advice.[1061]

Ibn Aḥmad b. al-Maghribī [Eg., 13th–14th centuries, convert]
A physician, the son of Shihāb al-Dīn (Sulaymān) Aḥmad al-Maghribī, 'Head of the Physicians' (d. 1318). Al-ʿUmarī mentioned him at the service of the sultan al-Nāṣir Muḥammad, probably as a physician.[1062] His brother Ibrāhīm b. al-Maghribī, was the 'Head of the Physicians', the sultan's personal physician and a *wazīr*. He probably converted to Islam with his father at a young age.

Dynasty 40 – Ibn Ṣaghīr
The dynasties of Ibn Ṣaghīr and Ibn Kūjik (dynasty 41), eminent Karaite families, were the most famous dynasties of court physicians in Mamluk Egypt. The combined information extracted from both Muslim historians and Geniza documents teaches us that members of these families included several important merchants, high government officials, community leaders and court physicians. The founders of these families in Egypt emigrated from Iran, possibly during the eleventh century. Some members of the family kept their original Iranian name (Kūjik, meaning 'small' in Persian), whereas others Arabised it to Ṣaghīr ('small' in Arabic).[1063] Muslim Arabic sources have informed us about descendants of this family (Muslim) such as ʾAlaʾ al-Din ʾUmar b. Muḥammad (d. 1462).[1064]

DYNASTY 40

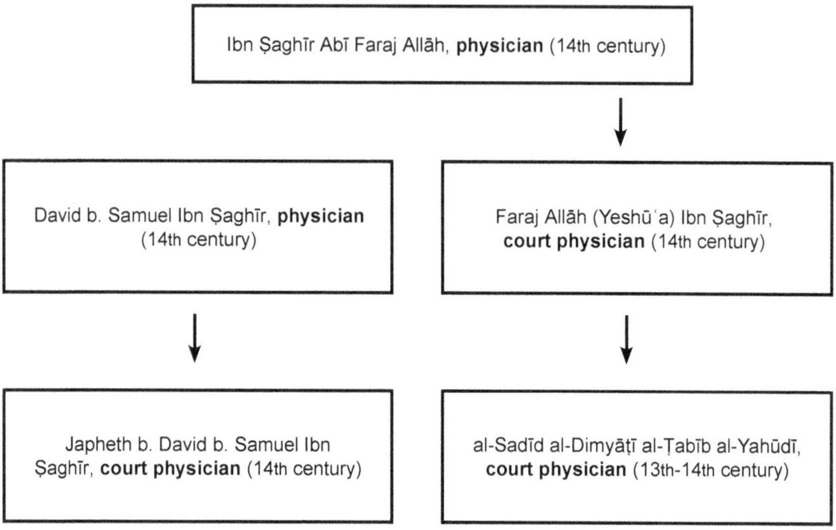

Ibn Ṣaghīr Abī Faraj Allāh [K., Eg., 14th century]
A physician, father and tutor of Faraj Allāh (Yeshūʿā) Ibn Ṣaghīr, the sultan's private physician.[1065]

Faraj Allāh (Yeshūʿa) Ibn Ṣaghīr [K., Eg., Cairo, 13th–14th centuries]
A prominent Karaite physician; studied the medical profession with his father (Ibn Ṣaghīr Abī Faraj Allāh), and with Ibn al-Nafīs (d. 1288)[1066] and other physicians. He specialised in general medicine and ophthalmology and was highly successful in curing patients and was known for his kind and gentle approach to treatment. He served in Cairo at the court of al-Nāṣir Muḥammad b. Qalāwūn (r. 1310–41), from whom he received a high salary and had a very high status in the court. Al-Nāṣir trusted him and appointed him as one of the physicians to the residents of the palace, namely, the sultan's wives, concubines and children. In addition, Faraj Allāh was the most distinguished physician of the household of the high-ranking Mamluk officer (Emir) Baktamur al-Sāqī (d. 1333), who preferred him over any other physician. Faraj Allāh's practice was pleasant and polite and he used to write long and detailed prescriptions.[1067] Alongside him served also the Jewish physician al-Sadīd al-Dimyāṭī, a relative of his, and the 'Head of the Physicians' was Jamāl al-Dīn Ibrāhīm b. Shihāb al-Dīn Aḥmad (Sulaymān) al-Maghribī

(dynasty 39). The information about Faraj Allāh originates from his close associate, the historian Ibn Faḍl Allāh al-ʿUmarī (1301–49). Al-ʿUmarī stressed his strong friendship with Faraj Allāh and mentioned some of his own experiences as one of his patients. However, he ended his description with this sentence: 'If only he had lived longer. My grief for a man like him, who died while still holding his Jewish faith …' One may interpret this statement as an indication of Faraj Allāh's intention to convert, probably due to pressure from the Muslim environment and since, as it seems, most of his family members had converted to Islam by that time.[1068] Faraj Allāh died after 1337.[1069]

David b. Samuel Ibn Ṣaghīr [K., Eg., 13th–14th centuries]
A Karaite physician, father of the physician and scholar Japheth b. David b. Samuel Ibn Ṣaghīr.[1070]

Japheth b. David b. Samuel Ibn Ṣaghīr (al-Ḥakīm al-Ṣafī)[1071] [K., Eg., Cairo, 13th–14th centuries]
A Karaite physician and scholar, mentioned in Ibn al-Hītī's chronicle. It is possible that he is a relative of Mūsā b. Kūjik (dynasty 41) and al-Sadīd al-Dimyāṭī.[1072] Japheth mentioned Israel ha-Dayyān al-Maghribī as his teacher, hence he spent some time in Egypt. His father, David b. Samuel Ibn Ṣaghīr, was also a physician. Firkovich identified this Japheth Ibn Ṣaghīr with the Karaite Ḥākhām Japheth, who mentioned the poet Moses b. Samuel. Jacob Mann agreed with this identification. The poet in turn mentioned Japheth as a *ḥākhām* (scholar) who lived in Cairo and beautifully described him.[1073]

al-Sadīd al-Dimyāṭī al-Ṭabīb al-Yahūdī [K., Eg., Cairo, 13th–14th century]
A prominent Karaite physician (a. c.1339–42),[1074] belonged to the Ibn Kūjik branch of the Ibn Ṣaghīr/Ibn Kūjik ('Small') family.[1075] According to the Muslim Arabic sources he studied under the physician ʿImād al-Dīn al-Nābulsī. He was one of the five physicians in the court of the Mamluk sultan al-Nāṣir Muḥammad b. Qalāwūn (1285–1341), alongside his relative Faraj Allāh Ibn Ṣaghīr (the two might have been related to Mūsā b. Kūjik and Japheth b. David b. Samuel Ibn Ṣaghīr),[1076] and had a respected status. Al-Ṣafadī asserted that the 'Head of the Physicians', Jamāl al-Dīn Ibrāhīm b. Shihāb al-Dīn Aḥmad (Sulaymān) al-Maghribī, would not enter the king's court without

being accompanied by al-Sadīd al-Dimyāṭī,[1077] adding that he saw him in Cairo more than once, and that he had observed his treatments many times. He testified that al-Sadīd al-Dimyāṭī was knowledgeable in the writings of Euclid, mathematics, natural science and other sciences. Al-Ṣafadī was present when al-Sadīd al-Dimyāṭī treated the judge Sharaf al-Dīn and operated on him and added that he heard many effective recommendations from him. Al-Ṣafadī described al-Sadīd al-Dimyāṭī as having a thinly structured body, a bent neck, a hard lean face, as one who did not speak much of other physicians, but was capable in his job and professional, knowledgeable in the natural world and one of the best caregivers of his time.[1078] Al-Dimyāṭī was closely associated with his teacher al-Nafīs as well as with the *qadi* and historian Ibn Wāṣil and the historians Khalīl b. Aybak al-Ṣafadī (1297–1363) and Ibn Faḍl Allāh al-ʿUmarī (1301–49), who provided much of the information we have about him.[1079] Al-Dimyāṭī told Ibn al-Nafīs that he had written a commentary on the scientific and philosophical encyclopedia of Ibn Sīnā, *Kitāb al-Shifāʾ* ('The Book of Healing'). Many of al-Dimyāṭī's patients were members of the political and military elite. Al-Dimyāṭī was also an expert on the poetry of al-Mutanabbī.[1080]

Dynasty 41 – Ibn Kūjik

As mentioned above, the dynasty of Ibn Kūjik belonged to a complex and long-lasting network of medical dynasties of distinguished dignitaries and physicians which were active during the Fatimid, Ayyubid and Mamluk periods. These also included the families of Ibn Shaʿyā (dynasty 26) and Ibn Ṣaghīr (dynasty 40). Unfortunately, we do not have enough details that would enable us to reconstruct a clear and consistent lineage of closed dynasties, and even of the different branches of this dynasty. What is clearer, however, is that from the second half of the fourteenth century, most of the important physicians of the 'Small' dynasty converted to Islam, probably in order to maintain their positions as court physicians.[1081]

Ibn Kūjik [K., Eg., 13th century]

A Jewish physician, one of the famous and dignified Kūjik/Ṣaghīr family of Karaite physicians. The first name of Ibn Kūjik is unknown. Historians of Islam mentioned that he treated some famous Muslim scholars. His son, the physician Mūsā b. Kūjik, converted to Islam and died in 1360.[1082]

DYNASTY 41

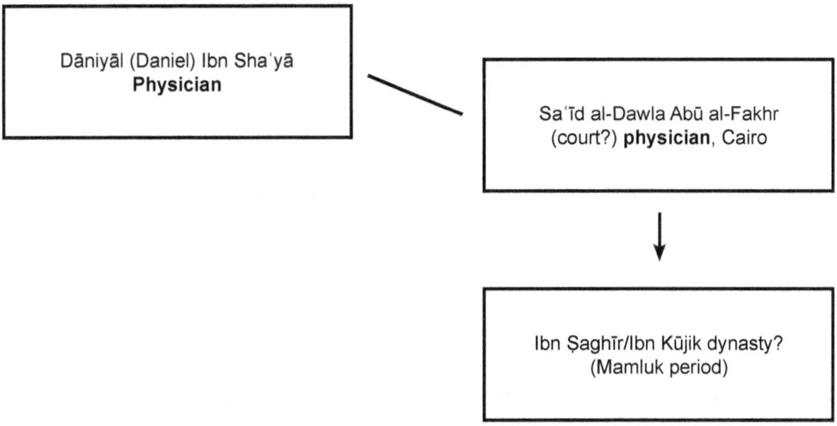

Mūsā b. Kūjik (Sharaf al-Dīn) [K., Eg., Sy., 14th century, convert]

A prominent physician who converted to Islam and died in 1360. His father (Ibn Kūjik) was also a physician. Ibn Kūjik treated some famous Muslim scholars, which apparently influenced his son's conversion to Islam. He might be related to other physicians of the family branches of Ibn Kūjik/Ṣaghīr, such as the court physicians al-Sadīd al-Dimyāṭī and Faraj Allāh Ibn Ṣaghīr, as well as Japheth b. David b. Samuel Ibn Ṣaghīr.[1083]

Dynasty 42 – Saʿadya

A medical dynasty of at least three generations of Karaite physicians of north African origin. They all practised medicine in Egypt, mainly in Alexandria in the fourteenth and fifteenth centuries.

Saʿadya [K, Eg., 14th–15th centuries] and Abraham b. Saʿadya [K, Eg., 15th century]

Saʿadya was a Karaite physician, his family's origin was in the Maghrib. His son Abraham and his grandson Moses were also physicians. We learn of this thanks to a *maqāma* that was written in honour of the head of the Karaites in Cairo.[1084]

Moses b. Abraham b. Saʿadya [K., Eg., Alexandria, Cairo, 15th century]

A Karaite physician, of north African origin. He was born in Alexandria and

DYNASTY 42

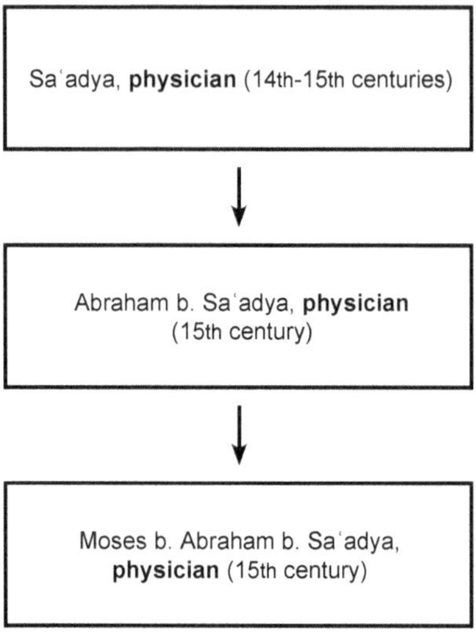

moved to Cairo from there. His father and grandfather were also physicians. Known as al-Ḥakīm al-Iskandrī al-Murabbā al-Maghribī (meaning 'grew up in Alexandria and his roots are in the Maghrib').[1085]

Dynasty 43 – Jacob ha-Rōfē

A dynasty of at least three generations of Jewish physicians that were practising medicine in Mamluk Egypt during the fourteenth century. The source of information is the Cairo Geniza only. The four physicians of the family are all mentioned in a bill of the sale of the house of the daughter Shimr or Shams under the titles ha-Sar ha-Nikhbād ha-Zāqēn ha [...], ha-[...] ha-Rōfē ha-[...] and ha-[...]. Therefore, I presume that they were among the heads of the Jewish community and were apparently senior physicians. The document was published by Ashtor,[1086] and discussed by Goitein.[1087]

R. Jacob ha-Rōfē ha-Sar ha-Nikhbād ha-Zāqēn ha-[...] ha-Rōfē ha-[...] [Eg., 14th century], R. Abraham ha-Rōfē b. Jacob [Eg., 14th century] and R. Nethanel ha-Rōfē b. Abraham [Eg., 14th century]

Jacob was a physician, mentioned in a document from the Geniza, dated 1378: 'R. Jacob ha-Sar ha-Nikhbād ha-Zāqēn ha-[...] ha-Rōfē ha-[...]'. Jacob's son, Abraham, was also a physician. Abraham in turn had two sons who were also physicians: R. Sar Shālōm ha-Rōfē and R. Nethanel ha-Rōfē b. Abraham.[1088]

DYNASTY 43

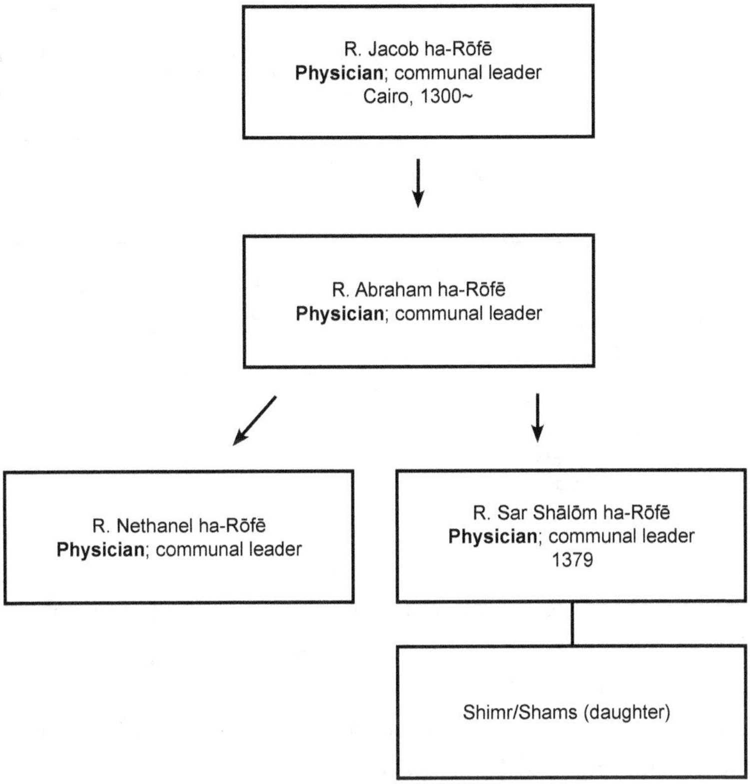

R. Sar Shālōm ha-Rōfē b. Abraham b. Jacob [Eg., 14th century]

A physician, mentioned in the above-mentioned document (1378), had a daughter named Shimr (or 'Shams' according to Goitein and Ashtor). His brother, Nethanel ha-Rōfē b. Abraham, was a physician. Likewise, the father of the two brothers, R. Abraham ha-Rōfē b. Jacob, was a physician, as was Abraham's father, Jacob. So, we have here three generations of physicians.[1089]

Dynasty 44 – Obadia ha-Rōfē

A short dynasty of father and son, physicians who practised medicine in Mamluk Tripoli, in the thirteenth and fourteenth centuries.

Obadia ha-Rōfē [Sy., ?Tripoli, 13th–14th centuries] and Eliezer ha-Rōfē b. Obadia ha-Rōfē [Sy., Tripoli, 14th century]

Obadia ha-Rōfē and his son, Eliezer ha-Rōfē b. Obadia ha-Rōfē, were

DYNASTY 45

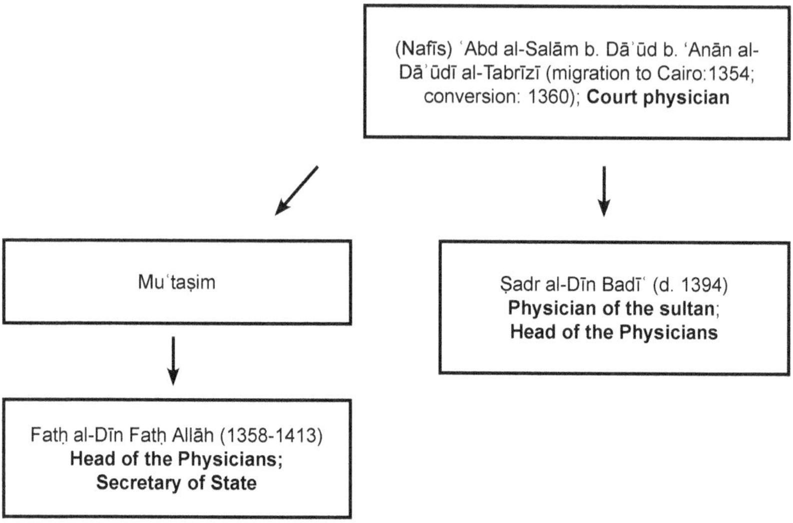

physicians. Obadia's grandson, Solomon, lived in Tripoli, Lebanon, in the second half of the fourteenth century. Solomon copied parts of the Bible from Tanchum of Jerusalem's *Kitāb al-Bayān*; he finished the commentary on Samuel in 1380. Other commentaries concluded in 1382, 1384 and 1385. Solomon is not mentioned as a physician.[1090]

Dynasty 45 – Nafīs b. Daʾūd b. ʿAnān al-Tabrīzī

A Karaite Jewish dynasty, originating from Tabriz, some of whose members held the office of 'Head of the Physicians'. Members of the Nafīs al-Dāʾūdī dynasty were active in the second half of the fourteenth century. The founder of this dynasty in Egypt was a distinguished physician from the House of King David named Nafīs b. Dāʾūd b. ʿAnān al-Dāʾūdī al-Tabrīzī.[1091]

Nafīs b. Dāʾūd b. ʿAnān al-Tabrīzī [K., Ir., Iq., Baghdad, Eg., Cairo, 14th century, convert]

A Karaite physician, originally from Tabriz, who moved with his family to Baghdad. In 1353–4 Nafīs arrived in Cairo with his two sons (Badīʿ and Muʿtaṣim), his slaves and his servants, and he became a leading physician and scholar. Muslim historians testify that the Jews of Cairo rejoiced at his arrival since he was considered the 'Head of the Diaspora' (*Raʾīs al-Jālūt*, *Rosh Gola* in

Hebrew) and he belonged to the sacred lineage of kings Solomon and David. It seems, therefore, that immediately after his arrival, he became the head of the Karaite Jews of Cairo. Nafīs converted to Islam at the initiative and in the presence of Sultan al-Nāṣir Ḥasan, during his second rule (1354–61). Shortly before his conversion, when he arrived in Cairo, Nafīs cured the sultan's deputy, Qublāy, of rheumatism. His family converted with him, together with 'many Jews'. Nafīs attained high position and his son, Badīʿ b. Nafīs b. Dāʾūd b. ʿAnān al-Dāʾūdi al-Tabrīzī, was physician to al-Ẓāhir Barqūq and was also appointed 'Head of the Physicians'. Especially successful was Nafīs's grandson, Fatḥ al-Dīn Fatḥ Allāh b. Nafīs, who also served as 'Head of the Physicians' and later on was appointed the government's secretary. He played a central role in the Mamluk sultanate until he was imprisoned and tortured to death (1413).[1092]

Badīʿ (Ṣadr al-Dīn) b. Nafīs b. Dāʾūd b. ʿAnān al-Dāʾūdi al-Tabrīzī [?K., Ir., Tabriz, Eg., Cairo, 14th century, convert]

A physician, probably converted to Islam with his father, Nafīs b. Dāʾūd b. ʿAnān al-Tabrīzī, who arrived in Cairo from Tabriz in 1354. He inherited the high status of his father among the rulers and became a leading physician and scholar and one of their closest confidants. He was knowledgeable in medicine and Islamic studies and wrote many medical books. Badīʿ was the physician of Sultan al-Ẓāhir Barqūq (r. 1382–9, 1390–9) and was appointed as 'Head of the Physicians' together with ʿAlāʾ al-Dīn Ibn Ṣaghīr, who was also a descendant of a converted Jewish dynasty.[1093] Badīʿ filled this office until his death in 1394.[1094]

Fatḥ Allāh b. Muʿtaṣim b. Nafīs (Fatḥ al-Dīn) [K., Ir., Tabriz, Eg., 14th–15th centuries, convert]

A physician and statesman, born in Tabriz (1358) to a distinguished converted Karaite family. In his childhood he arrived in Egypt with his father, Muʿtaṣim. Like his father, his grandfather Nafīs b. Dāʾūd b. ʿAnān al-Tabrīzī, and his uncle Badīʿ b. Nafīs b. Dāʾūd b. ʿAnān al-Dāʾūdi al-Tabrīzī, Fatḥ al-Dīn Fatḥ Allāh converted to Islam, probably in the middle of the 1360s. He received a good Islamic and medical education. After the death of his uncle Badīʿ and his joint 'Head of the Physicians', ʿAlāʾ al-Dīn Ibn Ṣaghīr, in 1394, Fatḥ Allāh was appointed 'Head of the Physicians'. As the 'Head', Fatḥ Allāh treated Sultan al-Ẓāhir Barqūq, who liked him also because of his vast knowledge of many languages and history. Fatḥ Allāh is said to have filled this office with decency and honesty. About five years later, al-Ẓāhir Barqūq appointed Fatḥ Allāh to the high bureaucratic office of state secretary (*kātib al-Sirr*). Fatḥ Allāh filled this office also during the reigns of the subsequent sultans al-Nāṣir Faraj and al-Mu'ayyad Sheikh, almost without interruption, until he was deposed and arrested in 1413, as a result of court intrigues. Fatḥ Allāh's end was bitter. He was tortured for several months until he was executed in June 1413. The historian al-Maqrīzī was a close friend of Fatḥ Allāh.[1095]

Dynasty 46 – ʿAbd Allāh b. Daʾūd b. Abī al-Faḍl al-Daʾūdī
A dynasty of converted Karaite physicians, also from the descendants of King David, which was founded by Taqī al-Dīn ʿAbd Allāh b. Dāʾūd b. Abī al-Faḍl b. Abī al-Munajjab (or al-Mūnā) b. Abī al-Fityān (or al-Bayān) Dāʾūdī. This physician converted to Islam in the first decade of the Mamluk period.

ʿAbd Allāh (Taqī al-Dīn) b. Dāʾūd b. Abī al-Faḍl b. Abī al-Munajjab (or al-Mūnā) b. Abī al-Fityān (or al-Bayān) al-Dāʾūdi [K., Eg., 14th–15th centuries, convert]
A Karaite physician, claiming descent from King David. ʿAbd Allāh converted in the first decade of the Mamluk period. His son Ibrāhīm and his grandson Jamāl al-Dīn Yūsuf were also distinguished physicians in the service of state

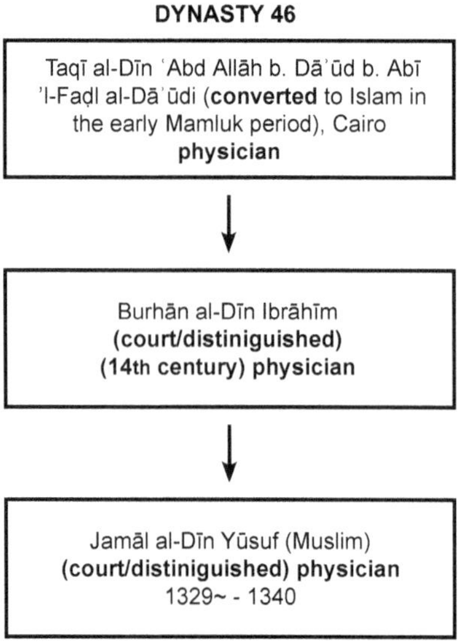

officials, and of this dynasty. Jamāl al-Dīn was probably born Muslim. ʿAbd Allāh was excellent in his medical treatment and had close relations with the members of the state elite.[1096]

Burhān al-Dīn Ibrāhīm [K., Eg., 14th century, probably convert]
A Karaite physician, son of Taqī al-Dīn, converted as a child or born as a Muslim. His son, Jamāl al-Dīn Yūsuf, was a Muslim physician.[1097]

Dynasty 47 – David b. Jacob
A father and son, both of them Jewish physicians who practised medicine in Mamluk Egypt in the fourteenth and fifteenth centuries.

Jacob [Eg., 14th century] and David b. Jacob [Eg., 14th–15th centuries]
David b. Jacob was a physician; mentioned in a bill (c.1409) which had been kept in the Cairo community archive.[1098] The bill states that following the debts owed to the community of Cairo, the Parnāsim sold David a third of the ownership rights over some land which the community had. In the margins of the bill it was added that Ṣedāqā b. Abraham ha-Kohen and Moses b. Yerushalayim ha-Kohen, who were both physicians, and others had arrived at David's house and received from him a mortgage which they had deposited with him. According to Ashtor, David's father, Jacob, was also a physician (he does not offer support of this claim when he discusses his son).[1099]

Dynasty 48 – Joseph from Damascus
A dynasty of three middle-class Jewish physicians, a father and two sons that practised medicine in Mamluk Syria (15th century). The sons were also moneylenders, and in order to make a living they moved to and lived in Candia, Crete.

DYNASTY 48

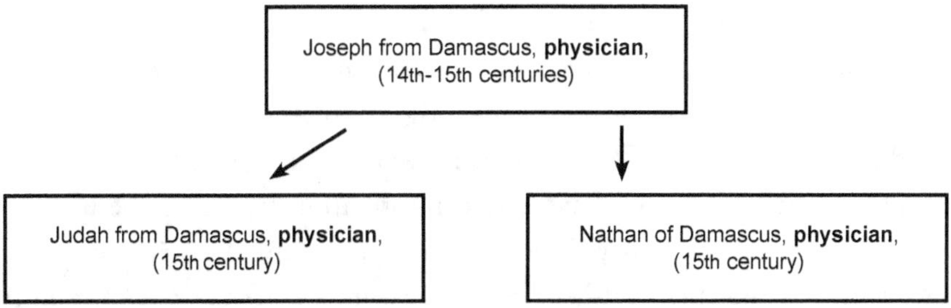

Joseph from Damascus [Sy., Damascus, Crete, Candia, 15th century]
A physician. His two sons, Nathan and Judah, were physicians as well. The father and his sons were active in Crete. The three belonged to the middle class and were not given an annual salary from the government, as other Jewish physicians were.[1100]

Nathan from Damascus [Sy., Damascus, Crete, Candia, 15th century]
Nathan of Damascus was a physician and moneylender who was active in Candia (Crete). He belonged to the middle class and practised private medicine. This is probably the reason why Nathan also worked as a moneylender, a common phenomenon in those days. From Nathan's will, which was written in Candia on 15 March 1429, we learn he was a widower and had no offspring. He had assets which he owned together with his brother Judah, some of which they inherited from their father, Joseph. The two brothers cooperated in professional, legal and business-related matters.[1101] Nathan is mentioned also in some additional documents from Crete: a list of physicians from 1396–7 and various notarial acts from 1423–4.[1102]

Judah from Damascus [Sy. Damascus, Crete, Candia, 15th century]
A surgeon and a moneylender from Damascus, who was active also in Candia (Crete). In Crete, in 1419, Judah was accused of giving a woman, who according to rumour was carrying his baby, a beverage to terminate the pregnancy. The woman died, and Judah was sentenced to permanent exile from Crete. If he returned, his hand would be cut off, and he would be hanged. Judah fled Crete the same year. In May 1421, he was acquitted after appealing the verdict, from Venice where he was staying. He held some property together with Nathan. The two brothers cooperated,[1103] and are mentioned in a notarial document from Crete, dated to 1423–4.[1104]

Dynasty 49 – Joseph b. Abraham Sakandarī
A dynasty of Jewish physicians that practised medicine in Mamluk Cairo (15th–16th centuries). Their primary origin was Andalusia; later on they lived in Alexandria and after that they moved to Cairo (a well-known route at that period). So far, we have traced information regarding the medical activity of three of them (father, son and grandson). It is important to mention that the three of them were active in the *Mustaʿrib* community

(Jews of native Arabic-speaking origin) and also served as leaders and judges.

DYNASTY 49

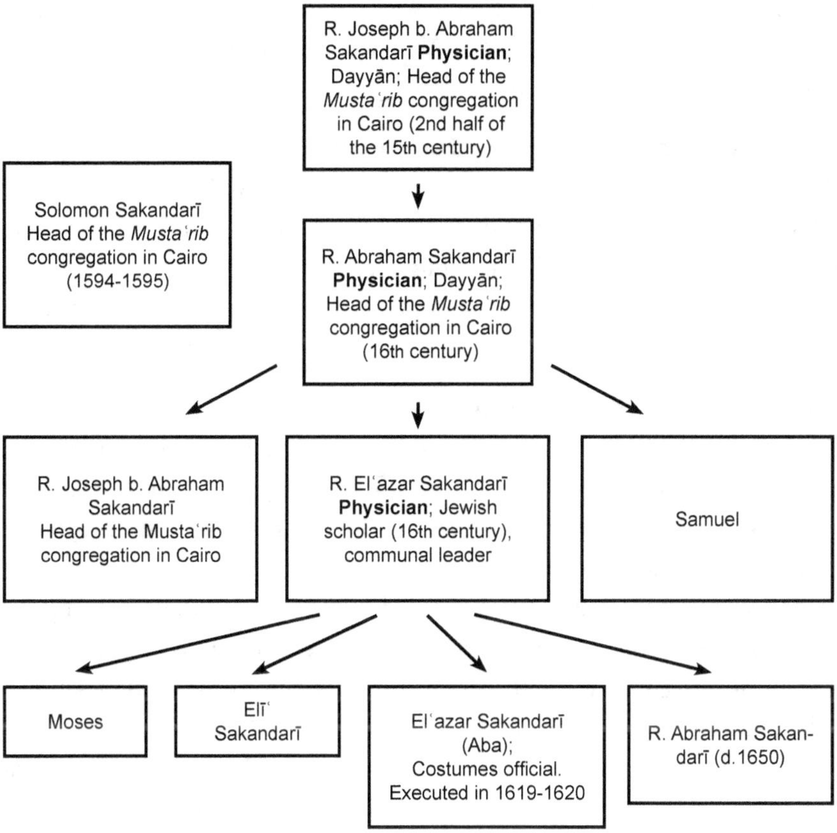

R. Joseph b. Abraham Sakandarī (Iskandarī or Iskandarānī) [An., Eg., Alexandria, Cairo, EY, Jerusalem, Safed, 15th–16th centuries]

R. Joseph left Spain before the expulsion. At first, he lived in Alexandria (the city from which the name of the family derived), and later he moved to Cairo, where he acted as the head of the *Musta'rib* congregation. His son, Abraham, and grandson, Elazar, were also physicians.[1105] In Cairo, Joseph served as a *dayyān* for many years, and due to his efforts, one of the synagogues in Cairo, which had been closed for several decades, was reopened in 1580.[1106]

Towards the end of his life he emigrated to Eretz-Israel and settled in Safed. Joseph wrote a commentary on one of R. Joseph Karo's books. Around the beginning of the sixteenth century, Joseph lived in Jerusalem. He studied there with Obadia of Bartenura. In the second decade of the sixteenth century, Joseph was living in Safed again. Abraham his son succeeded him as a *dayyān* in Cairo. According to the Jewish chronicler Joseph Sambari (probably 1640–1703), both Joseph and Abraham were physicians. His grandson Joseph was only mentioned as a *dayyān*.[1107]

Abraham Sakandarī [Eg., Cairo, 16th century]
A physician and a *dayyān* in Cairo, where he also served as the head of the *Musta ͑rib* congregation, a position he inherited from his father Joseph. He came from a Spanish family that emigrated to Egypt before the expulsion. His father, Joseph, was a physician and a *dayyān* in Cairo, and Abraham's son Elazar was also a physician.[1108]

Elazar Sakandarī [Eg., Cairo, 16th century]
A physician; his father, Abraham, and his grandfather, Joseph, were also physicians. It is possible that he is 'Elazar Sakandarī' mentioned in a bill from the Geniza.[1109] According to the seventeenth-century Jewish historian Joseph Sambari, R. Elazar was great in the wisdom of medicine, and taught non-Jews in this field. In addition, Elazar mediated with the authorities regarding the opening of a synagogue in Cairo that had been closed for decades, thanks to which the synagogue was indeed reopened in 1580. Elazar's brother Joseph inherited their father's position as the head of the *Musta ͑rib* Jews in Cairo. He was not a physician. Elazar had four sons, none of whom was mentioned as being a physician: R. Abraham Sakandarī, who died in 1650; Elazar/Abba Sakandarī, who was a tax collector and administrator and was executed in 1620; ͑Eli Sakandarī; and Moses.[1110]

3.3.3 Medical dynasties among Egyptian Jewish practitioners in the Muslim World

The vast majority of the medieval Jewish dynasties of practitioners in the Muslim world that are presented in this book consisted of physicians; only three were pharmacists and one was mixed (physician and pharmacist).

The position of the medieval Jewish medical dynasties can be assessed by examining the following, among other aspects: the number of generations engaged in the medical profession, patterns of transmission, the existence of distinguished physicians, and the communal leadership among these dynasties. Based on the information we have been able to gather, most of the dynasties lasted for two generations, some lasted for three generations and a few for four generations or more.[1111] In one dynasty, the Maimonidean dynasty (including the dynasty of Maimonides' wife), the profession was held for six generations during the Fatimid-Ayyubid period and continued for no fewer than nine generations including the Mamluk period. In another dynasty, the Ibn al-ʿAmmānī dynasty, the profession lasted for eight generations during the Fatimid-Ayyubid period alone. All in all, we have traced thirty-two dynasties of Jewish medical practitioners from the Fatimid-Ayyubid period. The large number of distinguished physicians who served in Muslim rulers' courts and/or in public hospitals is also instructive. About half of all the dynasties included at least one court physician. Among them, five dynasties included physicians who worked in public hospitals.

The medical profession was transmitted usually through a consecutive line of fathers and sons, although it sometimes 'skipped' a generation, so in a few cases we find it going from grandfather to grandson.[1112] Moreover, the sons' inheritance of their fathers' positions included, in nearly half of the discussed dynasties, inheriting communal leadership as well, either as Head of the Jews – as in the dynasties of Moses b. Elazar and the Maimonideans, or as local leaders, usually taking on the position of *dayyān*, as in the case of the Ibn al-ʿAmmānī dynasty. Thus, six dynasties included physicians who were also chief leaders of the Jews, and four dynasties included individuals who served as community leaders at lower levels. The long-lasting dynasties of Jewish physicians, including court and hospital physicians, together with the prominence of local as well as national communal leadership among these dynasties, reinforce the notion of the high status of Jewish doctors in the Fatimid and Ayyubid periods.

It seems that there is no difference in numbers of dynasties between the Fatimid and the Ayyubid periods; moreover, no significant difference was found in the social and political positions of the Jewish dynasties between these regimes. In both periods there were dynasties of court physicians, physicians who worked in public hospitals, and dynasties of court physicians who were also chief leaders of the Jews, or community leaders at lower levels. These findings strengthen the notion that the general decline in the situation of the Jews in the Ayyubid period had almost no impact on the position of the Jewish physician, nor on the dynasties of Jewish physicians.[1113]

Interestingly, in the Fatimid-Ayyubid period there is only one case of conversion to Islam of a Jewish physician: the son of Abū al-Faḍl b. al-Nāqid, who was part of a medical dynasty of ophthalmologists who practised mainly in Cairo during the second half of the twelfth century. This is instructive, since it is in total contradiction to the situation of the dynasties of Jewish physicians from the Mamluk period: at least seven of the dynasties of Jewish practitioners from that period converted to Islam. All of those converted dynasties included distinguished physicians who served rulers.[1114]

The change in the position of Jewish dynasties of physicians between the Fatimid-Ayyubid period and that of the Mamluk is far more conspicuous. A clear decline in all aspects is discernible. For instance, we see that in the Mamluk period, while members of the Maimonidean dynasty still held the position of Head of the Jews, they did not act additionally as court physicians.[1115] It is especially the pressure on those families to convert to Islam that is typical of this later period. Suffice it to say that a third or more of the known dynasties from the Mamluk period converted to Islam. All of the converted dynasties included distinguished physicians who served Muslim rulers.

There were at least eighteen dynasties of Jewish physicians practising in the Muslim world during the Mamluk period.[1116] Examination of various Muslim Arabic sources reveals that members of most prominent Jewish dynasties of court physicians mentioned in these sources converted to Islam at some time or other. Hence, it seems as though the Mamluk period marks a severe deterioration in the position of the Jewish physicians, compared to former periods. This change was especially embodied in the severe pressure to convert in order to maintain their status quo and positions. Magnificent dynasties of three and four generations who remained Jewish acted as court physicians and Head of the Jews and sometimes also held the highest bureaucratic positions of the state. But this is characteristic mainly of the Fatimid, and also of the Ayyubid, periods.[1117] Indeed, the position of 'Head of the Physicians', which apparently could have been taken up by a Jewish physician such as Ibn Jumayʿ in the Ayyubid period,[1118] was filled during the Mamluk period only by Jews who had converted or belonged to converted Jewish dynasties, such as Ibn Ṣaghīr, Ibn al-Maghribī and Nafīs al-Dā'ūdī.[1119]

However, since Muslim Arabic sources of the Mamluk period generally tend to ignore important *dhimmīs*, the impression might be deceptive. It is not that Jewish dynasties of physicians, and even prominent physicians, disappeared in Syria and Egypt during the fourteenth and fifteenth centuries and the beginning of the sixteenth. Rather, Jewish sources reveal that non-converted dynasties were active during the whole Mamluk period in Cairo and Alexandria, as well as in peripheral areas such as al-Bīra and Tripoli. These dynasties lasted mostly for three generations or more and sometimes included brothers who were doctors. Moreover, there were several dynasties whose members were communal leaders and judges who were also connected to the government. However, there is no clear indication of a dynasty of Jewish court physicians, a phenomenon that was common in the Fatimid-Ayyubid period. In one particular case, the dynasty of Moses b. Elazar (dynasty 1), the triple offices of court physician to the caliph, Head of the Jews and the chief administrator of the caliphate continued, so it seems, over four generations.[1120]

Another phenomenon is intermarriage among members of medical dynasties. This also occurred in Muslim society, where it was common among families of scholars and dynasties of religious-juridical administration.[1121] In this case, a good example is the 'last' generation of physicians of the Ibn al-ʿAmmānī dynasty (dynasty 14), who had married into another powerful dynasty of leaders and court physicians – that of Zechariah the Alexandrian (dynasty 21). Judah's son, Hibat Allāh (Nethanel), married the cousin of Solomon (and the court physician Abū Zikrī), the son of Elijah ha-Dayyān b. Zechariah. Hibat Allāh (Nethanel) Ibn al-ʿAmmānī's wife was, in fact the niece of Elijah, the prominent *dayyān* in the court of Abraham Maimonides. Interestingly enough we can find this phenomenon of marriage between two dynasties of important physicians in the Maimonidean family (dynasty 3) as well: Moses Maimonides married a woman from a distinguished dynasty of physicians.[1122]

In spite of the fragmentary source data that we have regarding Jewish dynasties of physicians, the relatively large number of these dynasties, their high-ranking status and the long duration of many of them all indicate that during the Fatimid-Ayyubid period they were a very prominent phenomenon. It seems that they were more common than Muslim dynasties of physicians and even Christian dynasties, due to certain circumstances that attracted a small minority such as the Jews to specialise in the medical or pharmacological profession.

In order to evaluate the prominence of Jewish medical dynasties, their relatively large number and high position should be examined in comparison to those of Muslim and Christian physicians. Pormann and Savage-Smith mentioned that 'many (Muslim) physicians handed down medical knowledge to their own offspring, thereby creating some famous lineages'.[1123] Thanks to the information gathered from Muslim Arabic sources, we know of several medieval Muslim dynasties of physicians. One of the most prominent ones was the Ibn Zuhr family of scholars and physicians (known in the West as Avenzoar). Members of this dynasty practised first in the Maghrib and then in Andalusia during the eleventh and twelfth centuries, for at least four generations. Some family members were also high-ranking administrators, and others were famous authors of medical books. According to contemporary sources, most of the physicians of this family, including Ibn Zuhr (d. 1130) himself, studied medicine from their fathers.[1124] In this context we should mention another important Muslim dynasty of physicians, that of Ibn Abī al-Ḥawāfir, who was active in Egypt and Syria during the thirteenth and fourteenth centuries.[1125] A four-generation Muslim dynasty of ophthalmologists in Damascus, from the second half of the twelfth to the mid-fourteenth century, is also noteworthy.[1126]

As for Christian dynasties, a famous medical dynasty of Eastern physicians is the Bukhtīshūʿ, an Iranian or Assyrian Nestorian Christian family, who produced distinguished doctors between the seventh to the ninth centuries, over about six generations; and lasted for about 250 years and possibly more. Members of the family held posts as directors of hospitals, authored medical books, and worked at the courts of different rulers in Baghdad.[1127] This dynasty, however, is unique in its length. We know, nevertheless, about Christian dynasties of court physicians of three generations from the Umayyad period (seventh century) onward.[1128] From a later period, we know of the dynasty that was established by a physician of Saladin named Abū Sulaymān Daʾūd Abī al-Munā, and continued through his sons and nephew, who served the Ayyubid and first Mamluk rulers, at the beginning of the fourteenth century. Its members converted to Islam at the beginning of the Mamluk period.[1129]

Notes

1. Talbot and Hammond, *The Medical Practitioners in Medieval England*, p. viii.
2. See Goitein, *A Mediterranean Society*, vol. VI, pp. 271–2.
3. See Netzer, 'Rashīd al-Dīn'.
4. Schimmel, *Islamic Names*, pp. 1–13; Poznański, 'Die jüdischen Artikel in Ibn al-Qifti's Gelehrtenlexikon', p. 52.
5. Mann, *Texts and Studies*, p. 283.
6. Ibid., p. 281.
7. Arad, 'The Community as an Economic Body', p. 61 n. 213.
8. Amar, *The History of Medicine in Jerusalem*, p. 136.
9. Ibid., p. 136.
10. Cohen, 'Jews in the Mamlūk Environment'; Gottheil, 'Dhimmis and Moslems in Egypt', p. 384.
11. Rustow, 'Karaites Real and Imagined', p. 55.
12. Cohen, 'Jews in the Mamlūk Environment'.
13. Ashtor, *The History of the Jews in Egypt and Syria*, vol. II, pp. 86–7.
14. Wiet, *Cairo*, pp. 45–6, 55–6.
15. Arad, 'The Community as an Economic Body', p. 61 n. 213.
16. Steinschneider, 'An Introduction to the Arabic Literature of the Jews I', 11(4), p. 590.
17. Bareket, 'Abraham Ben Hillel'.
18. Gil, *Palestine during the First Muslim Period*, vol. III, pp. 25–6.
19. See Goitein and Friedman, *India Book I*, pp. 52–89 on Abraham generally, p. 68 on his medical knowledge.
20. On his journey back, especially from a material-cultural point of view, see Lambourn, *Abraham's Luggage*.
21. He dealt, among other things, in laws of inheritance, bills and marriages; see for example Goitein and Friedman, *India Book III*.
22. Goitein and Friedman, *India Traders of the Middle Ages*, p. 84.
23. Friedman, 'Maimonides, Zūṭā and the Muqaddams'.
24. Mann, *Texts and Studies*, p. 151.
25. Amar, *The History of Medicine in Jerusalem*, p. 135.
26. Mann, *Texts and Studies*, p. 142.
27. Bodl. MS heb. a. 2, fol. 14.
28. ENA 2592.22.
29. Zeldes and Frenkel, 'The Sicilian Trade', p. 118.

30. TS AS 153.31.
31. Olszowy-Schlanger, *Karaite Marriage Documents from the Cairo Geniza*, no. 56.
32. Gil, *In the Kingdom of Ishmael*, vol. III, p. 29; Simonsohn, *The Jews in Sicily*, no. 147.
33. ENA 2727.28.
34. TS Ar. 54.20; Baker and Polliack, *Arabic and Judaeo-Arabic Manuscripts*, no. 7813.
35. Goitein, *A Mediterranean Society*, vol. III, p. 82 n. 47 (p. 443); ENA 2559.13.
36. Friedenwald, *The Jews and Medicine*, vol. II, p. 634; Alfonso, 'Ibn al-Muʿallim, Solomon'; Roth, *Jews, Visigoths and Muslims*, p. 175.
37. Bos, *Maimonides on Asthma*, pp. 102–5; Alfonso, 'Ibn al-Muʿallim, Solomon'.
38. Alfonso, 'Ibn al-Muʿallim, Solomon'; Friedenwald, *The Jews and Medicine*, p. 634; Roth, 'Medicine', p. 436; al-Khālidī, *al-Yahūd Taḥta Ḥukm al-Muslimīn*, pp. 190–1; Weisz, 'The Jewish Physicians', p. 27.
39. Friedenwald, *The Jews and Medicine*, p. 634; Weisz, 'The Jewish Physicians', p. 27; Alfonso, 'Ibn al-Muʿallim, Solomon'; Roth, *Jews, Visigoths and Muslims*, p. 175.
40. Alfonso, 'Ibn al-Muʿallim, Solomon'; al-Ḥarīzī, *Taḥkemoni*, no. 45.
41. Wasserstein, 'Samauʾal ben Judah'.
42. A Seljuk sultan who ruled in eastern Iraq and died in 1118.
43. Ibn Abī Uṣaybiʿa, *ʿUyūn al-Anbāʾ*, vol. I, pp. 278–80; Ibn al-Qifṭī, *Taʾrīkh al-Ḥukamāʾ*, pp. 343–6; al-Ṣafadī, *Kitāb al-Wāfī bi-l-Wafayāt* (2000), vol. XXVII, p. 178; al-ʿUmarī, *Masālik al-Abṣār*, vol. IX, pp. 247–50; Stillman and Pines, 'Abū al-Barakāt al-Baghdadī'; Steinschneider, 'An Introduction to the Arabic Literature of the Jews II', 13(1), p. 93; also mentioned by Goitein, *A Mediterranean Society*, vol. II, pp. 302, 380; Gil, *Jews in Islamic Countries*, pp. 468–72; Ashtor, *The Jews and the Mediterranean Economy*, p. 151; Poznański, 'Die jüdischen Artikel in Ibn al-Qifti's Gelehrtenlexikon', p. 52.
44. Stillman and Pines, 'Abū al-Barakā t al-Baghdadī'; Steinschneider, 'An Introduction to the Arabic Literature of the Jews II', 13(1), p. 93.
45. Khalīl b. Aybak al-Ṣafadī mentioned that it was an excellent book that contained a treatise on the rising and setting of the stars.
46. al-Bayhaqī, *Tārīkh Ḥukmāʾ al-Islām*, p. 171; al-Ṣafadī, *Kitāb al-Wāfī bi-l-Wafayāt* (2000), vol. XXVII, p. 178; al-ʿUmarī, *Masālik al-Abṣār*, vol. IX, pp. 247–50; Ibn al-Qifṭī, *Taʾrīkh al-Ḥukamāʾ*, p. 343; Gil, *Jews in Islamic Countries*, p. 469.

47. al-Ṣafadī, *Kitāb al-Wāfī bi-l-Wafayāt* (2000), vol. XXVII, p. 178; al-Ghazūlī, *Maṭāli' al-Budūr*, pp. 419–20.
48. Ibn al-Qifṭī, *Ta'rīkh al-Ḥukamā'*, p. 343; for more stories about his healing abilities see Gil, *Jews in Islamic Countries*, p. 469.
49. For more on this author see Kahl, *The Dispensatory of Ibn al-Tilmīḏ*.
50. al-Ṣafadī, *Kitāb al-Wāfī bi-l-Wafayāt* (2000), vol. XXVII, p. 178; al-'Umarī, *Masālik al-Abṣār*, vol. IX, p. 250; Steinschneider, 'An Introduction to the Arabic Literature of the Jews II', 13(1), p. 94; Lewicka, 'Healer, Scholar, Conspirator', p. 129; Gil, *Jews in Islamic Countries*, pp. 469–70; regarding Abū al-Barakāt's worry for his daughters remaining Jewish see Goitein, *A Mediterranean Society*, vol. II, p. 303; el-Leithy, 'Coptic Culture and Conversion', p. 73; Stillman and Pines, 'Abū al-Barakāt al-Baghdadī'.
51. An historian, judge and author who was born in Irbil, Iraq in 1211 and died in Damascus in 1282.
52. According to Gil he was blinded by leprosy but died of it also: *Jews in Islamic Countries*, p. 470.
53. Steinschneider, 'An Introduction to the Arabic Literature of the Jews II', 13(1), p. 94.
54. Gil, *Jews in Islamic Countries*, p. 469.
55. al-Ṣafadī, *Kitāb al-Wāfī bi-l-Wafayāt* (2000), vol. XXVII, p. 178; al-'Umarī, *Masālik al-Abṣār*, vol. IX, pp. 247–50; Ibn al-Qifṭī, *Ta'rīkh al-Ḥukamā'*, p. 343; Steinschneider, 'An Introduction to the Arabic Literature of the Jews II', 13(1), p. 94; Gil, *Jews in Islamic Countries*, p. 470; Stillman and Pines, 'Abū al-Barakāt al-Baghdadī'.
56. Ibn Abī Uṣaybi'a, *'Uyūn al-Anbā'*, vol. II, p. 117; Meyerhof, 'Medieval Jewish Physicians in the Near East', pp. 450–1; Meyerhof, 'Jewish Physicians Contemporaries of Maimonides', p. 392.
57. Ḥaddād, *Riḥlat Ibn Yūna*, p. 122 n. 3.
58. An astronomer and mathematician who lived between 1135 and 1213 and studied in Aleppo and Mosul.
59. Ibn al-Qifṭī, *Ta'rīkh al-Ḥukamā'*, p. 426; see Eddé, 'Les Médecins dans la société syrienne', p. 103.
60. Bodl. MS heb. e. 94, fol. 21.
61. Bodl. MS heb. c. 50, fol. 17.
62. The dating is according to al-Ḥarīzī's life.
63. Yahalom and Blau, *The Wanderings of Judah Alharizi*, p. 122, ll. 556–9.
64. ENA 2591.8.

65. TS Misc. 26.2.
66. This is possibly is Abū 'l-Fakhr al-Ṭabīb; see Goitein and Friedman, *India Traders of the Middle Ages*, p. 101.
67. Goitein and Friedman, *India Traders of the Middle Ages*, p. 101.
68. Zeldes and Frenkel, *The Sicilian Trade*, pp. 109–13.
69. Friedman, 'The Family of Ibn al-Amshāṭī', esp. pp. 277–82.
70. This is possibly Abū 'l-Fakhr Saʿadya b. Abraham; see Goitein and Friedman, *India Traders of the Middle Ages*, p. 101.
71. In the East it was common for a merchant not to be confined to a single product but to sell a variety of commodities, including books.
72. Allony, *The Jewish Library in the Middle Ages*, pp. 161, 164–5, 174, 211.
73. Bodl. MS heb. f. 22, fol. 34.
74. TS 13J20.27. The dating is according to Samuel b. Hananiah.
75. CUL Or. 1080 J138.
76. TS AS 151.5.
77. ʿAbd al-Laṭīf (1162–1231) accused Yūsuf (without mentioning his name) of intentionally causing the death of his patients. And he specifically tells about the circumstances of the death of al-Malik al-Ẓāhir al-Ghāzī, following his last illness, in 1216–17. For more on the topic see Stern, 'A Collection of Treatises by ʿAbd al-Laṭīf al-Baghdādī', pp. 60–1.
78. Ibn al-Qifṭī, *Taʾrīkh al-Ḥukamāʾ*, pp. 392–4; Lasker, 'Ibn Simeon, Judah b. Joseph'; Yahalom and Blau, *The Wanderings of Judah Alharizi*, pp. 33–4; Meyerhof, 'Jewish Physicians Contemporaries of Maimonides', p. 393; Eddé, *Les Médecins dans la société syrienne*, p. 109.
79. Miller, 'Doctors without Borders', p. 113; Yahalom and Blau, *The Wanderings of Judah Alharizi*, pp. 33–4; Meyerhof, 'Jewish Physicians Contemporaries of Maimonides', p. 393; Kraemer, *Maimonides*, pp. 363–4.
80. Yahalom and Blau, *The Wanderings of Judah Alharizi*, pp. 16, 18, 67 (ll. 219 ff.), 69 (ll. 204–10); Kraemer, *Maimonides*, pp. 364–5.
81. Prats, 'Ibn ʿAknīn, Joseph b. Judah Jacob'.
82. Among them Bacher, Baron, Guttmann, Schirmann, Steinschneider, Twersky, Vajda and more.
83. See for example Luṭf, *Yahūd Miṣr al-Ayyūbiya*, p. 96; for details of the chain of errors see Prats, 'Ibn ʿAknīn, Joseph b. Judah Jacob'.
84. Scheindlin, 'Judah (Abū 'l-Ḥasan) ben Samuel ha-Levi'; Gil and Fleischer, *Yehuda ha-Levi and His Circle*; Silman, *Philosopher and Prophet.*
85. Zinger, 'Women, Gender and Law', p. 15.

86. Goitein, *A Mediterranean Society*, vol. V, pp. 448–51 with n. 163; Goitein, 'The Biography of Rabbi Judah ha-Levi'.
87. Scheindlin, 'Judah (Abū 'l-Ḥasan) ben Samuel ha-Levi'; Gil and Fleischer, *Yehuda ha-Levi and His Circle*; Silman, *Philosopher and Prophet*.
88. Gil, *Palestine during the First Muslim Period*, vol. III, p. 320, no. 525.
89. Khan, *Arabic Legal and Administrative Documents*, pp. 249–50, no. 51.
90. Goitein, *A Mediterranean Society*, vol. III, p. 243 n. 138.
91. Rustow, 'At the Limits of Communal Autonomy', p. 150.
92. Ashtor, *The History of the Jews in Egypt and Syria*, vol. I, pp. 130–1; al-Maqrīzī, *Kitāb al-Sulūk*, vol. I, p. 728; Ibn al-Furāt, *Taʾrīkh Ibn al-Furāt*, vol. VIII, p. 18.
93. Gil, *Palestine during the First Muslim Period*, vol. II, pp. 443–5, no. 243.
94. Goitein, *A Mediterranean Society*, vol. II, pp. 263–4, 582 n. 20.
95. ENA 2738.1.
96. ENA NS 77.404.
97. TS AS 146.24.
98. Dated according to the lifetime of Meʾir Abū 'l-Ḥasan Ibn Qamniʾel.
99. Roth, *Jews, Visigoths and Muslims*, p. 115.
100. Steinschneider, *Die Arabische Literatur der Juden*, p. 135.
101. Ibn Abī Uṣaybiʿa, *ʿUyūn al-Anbāʾ*, vol. II, p. 50.
102. Roth, *Jews, Visigoths and Muslims*, p. 94; Friedenwald, *The Jews and Medicine*, vol. II, p. 633; Finkel, 'An Eleventh Century Source', p. 52; al-Andalusī, *Ṭabaqāt al-ʾUmam*, pp. 204–5; Martínez Delgado, 'Ibn Yashūsh, Isaac (Abū Ibrāhīm) Ibn Qasṭār'; Roth, 'Medicine', p. 436.
103. Bruce, *The Taifa of Denia*.
104. Neubauer, 'Sur la lexicographie hébraïque', p. 249.
105. Ashtor, *The Jews of Moslem Spain*, vol. II, p. 293; Martínez Delgado, 'Ibn Yashūsh, Isaac (Abū Ibrāhīm) Ibn Qasṭār'.
106. TS NS J163.
107. Friedenwald, *The Jews and Medicine*, p. 634.
108. Prats, 'Moses ben Joseph ha-Levi'; Sirat, *A History of Jewish Philosophy*, p. 266.
109. Altmann and Avenary, *Moses ben Joseph Ha-Levi*.
110. Gil and Fleischer, *Yehuda ha-Levi and His Circle*, pp. 130–2.
111. Saénz-Badillos, 'Ibn Muhājir, Abraham'.
112. Ashtor, *The Jews of Moslem Spain*, vol. III, p. 172; Saénz-Badillos, 'Ibn Muhājir, Abraham'.

113. TS AS 151.5.
114. On the Geonim and their role in medieval Jewish history see in depth: Brody, *The Geonim of Babylonia.*
115. Goitein, 'The Qayrawan United Appeal', pp. 160–2.
116. Stillman, 'Ibn ʿAtāʾ, Abū Isḥāq Ibrāhīm'; Ben-Sasson, *The Emergence of the Local Jewish Community*, pp. 23, 353.
117. Cohen, *Poverty and Charity*, p. 60 n. 114.
118. Goitein, 'Three Letters from Qayrawan', pp. 166–9, 174–5.
119. Strauss, 'Documents for the Economic and Social History of the Jews', pp. 142–5; Bodl. MS heb. c 28, fol. 47 (2876-47).
120. ENA 2591.6.
121. Probably identical with the biography below.
122. TS AS 151.5.
123. ENA 1290.1.
124. Probably identical with the biography above.
125. TS K15.61.
126. Goitein, *A Mediterranean Society*, vol. V, p. 458 n. 189; Goitein, 'The Biography of Rabbi Judah ha-Levi', p. 50.
127. TS AS 151.5.
128. TS Ar. 51.144.
129. Jadon, 'A Comparison of the Wealth', p. 65.
130. Ibn Abī Uṣaybiʿa, *ʿUyūn al-Anbāʾ*, vol. II, p. 117; Ramaḍān, *al-Yahūd fī Miṣr*, p. 448; Luṭf, *Yahūd Miṣr al-Ayyūbiya*, p. 98; Meyerhof, 'Jewish Physicians Contemporaries of Maimonides', p. 392; Ashtor-Strauss, *Saladin and the Jews*, p. 310.
131. Goitein, *A Mediterranean Society*, vol. II, pp. 151–2, 249–50; Hazan, 'Medical, Administrative and Financial Aspects', p. 109.
132. Goitein and Friedman, *India Book IV/B*, p. 440 n. 94; Frenkel, *The Compassionate and Benevolent*, pp. 626–32.
133. TS AS 146.10.
134. Halper (Dropsie) 467.
135. Ibid.
136. Goitein, *A Mediterranean Society*, vol. I, p. 424 n. 100, vol. III, p. 251 n. 8.
137. It is not clear if he himself is a physician or his father, Abū al-Futūḥ al-Ṭabīb.
138. TS AS 151.5.
139. Fischel, 'Azarbaijan in Jewish History', p. 8.
140. TS 8J6.12.

141. Ashtor, 'The Number of Jews in Mediaeval Egypt', 18 (1–4), p. 15, Appendix B, no. 1.
142. Allony, *The Jewish Library in the Middle Ages*, p. 299.
143. Bodl. MS heb. f. 22, fol. 30.
144. TS K15.91.
145. Steinschneider, *Die Arabische Literatur der Juden*, no. 137; Meyerhof, 'Medieval Jewish Physicians in the Near East', p. 456; Meyerhof, 'Jewish Physicians Contemporaries of Maimonides', p. 397.
146. Ashtor, *The History of the Jews in Egypt and Syria*, vol. I, pp. 170–1.
147. TS AS 151.5.
148. Goitein, 'The Exchange Rate of Gold and Silver Money', pp. 34–5.
149. Ashur, 'Engagement and Betrothal Documents', no. 17.
150. TS AS 153.200.
151. TS AS 146.10.
152. ENA 4020.54.
153. ENA 3846.6-7.
154. Goitein, *A Mediterranean Society*, vol. III, p. 487; Golb et al., 'Legal Documents from the Cairo Genizah', p. 27.
155. Bareket, 'Struggles over Jewish Leadership', pp. 174–5.
156. Strauss, 'Documents for the Economic and Social History of the Jews', pp. 142–5; Bodl. MS heb. c 28, fol. 47 (2876-47).
157. ENA 3846.6-7.
158. Frenkel, *The Compassionate and Benevolent*, pp. 365–72, no. 32.
159. TS NS 324.95.
160. Goitein and Friedman, *India Book I*, pp. 261–72, no. 36; Goitein, *A Mediterranean Society*, vol. IV, pp. 317–18.
161. Ashtor, 'The Number of Jews in Mediaeval Egypt', 19 (1–4), p. 5 n. 288; Goitein and Friedman, *India Book I*, pp. 254–60 n. 35.
162. TS NS 321.40.
163. Steinschneider, 'An Introduction to the Arabic Literature of the Jews I', 11(1), p. 118; see also Goitein, *A Mediterranean Society*, vol. II, pp. 248, 577 n. 37.
164. Goitein, *A Mediterranean Society*, vol. II, pp. 48–9, vol. IV, p. 335 n. 196.
165. Molad-Vaza, 'Clothing in the Mediterranean Jewish Society', pp. 228–31, 331–5; Goitein, *A Mediterranean Society*, vol. IV, pp. 195–6 n. 330, 338 n. 236, 463.
166. Molad-Vaza, 'Clothing in the Mediterranean Jewish Society', pp. 331–5.

167. Allony, *The Jewish Library in the Middle Ages*, p. 241.
168. ENA 2727.17a.
169. Ibn Murād, *Buḥūth*, pp. 93–5.
170. TS 10J7.6.
171. Mann, *The Jews in Egypt and in Palestine*, p. 18.
172. Steinschneider, *Die Arabische Literatur der Juden*, no. 198; Meyerhof; 'Medieval Jewish Physicians in the Near East', p. 458; Meyerhof, 'Jewish Physicians Contemporaries of Maimonides', p. 399.
173. TS NS 321.40.
174. Ashtor, *The History of the Jews in Egypt and Syria*, vol. II, p. 512.
175. Meyerhof, 'Medieval Jewish Physicians in the Near East', p. 458; Meyerhof, 'Jewish Physicians Contemporaries of Maimonides', p. 399.
176. TS 13J16.8.
177. Goitein, *A Mediterranean Society*, vol. V, p. 592 n. 24.
178. Ibid., vol. V, pp. 314–16; Goitein, 'Minority Selfrule and Government Control'.
179. Gil, *Palestine during the First Muslim Period*, vol. II, pp. 420–1.
180. Bodl. MS heb. f. 61, fol. 50.
181. TS AS 151.5.
182. Ibn Abī Uṣaybiʿa, *ʿUyūn al-Anbāʾ*, vol. II, p. 218; Goitein, *A Mediterranean Society*, vol. V, p. 271 nn. 80–1; for al-Asʿad the physician see Goitein, *A Mediterranean Society*, vol. III, pp. 81–2 nn. 46–7 (dated 1217), 465 n. 120; Meyerhof, 'Jewish Physicians Contemporaries of Maimonides', p. 392.
183. Goitein, *A Mediterranean Society*, vol. III, pp. 81–2 n. 47.
184. See in detail Zinger, 'Women, Gender and Law', pp. 280–3; regarding the physician, see 'Anonymous – a physician from the Egyptian periphery' below.
185. Richards, 'A Doctor's Petition', p. 303.
186. TS AS 151.5; TS NS J76.
187. Mazor, 'Asad al-Yahūdī'; Mazor, 'Jewish Court Physicians', pp. 54–60; Lewicka, 'Healer, Scholar, Conspirator', pp. 129–130.
188. Ashtor, *The History of the Jews in Egypt and Syria*, vol. I, p. 346.
189. Goitein, *A Mediterranean Society*, vol. V, p. 111 n. 357.
190. Amar, *The History of Medicine in Jerusalem*, p. 137.
191. Yahalom and Blau, *The Wanderings of Judah Alharizi*, pp. 19, 50, ll. 83–90.
192. CUL Or. 1080 J2.
193. ENA 2728.6.
194. TS 8J15.20; Bodl. MS heb. a. 3, fol. 18; TS 10J17.27.

195. TS NS 32.99.
196. TS K15.92.
197. Yahalom and Blau, *The Wanderings of Judah Alharizi*, p. 66, ll. 183–4.
198. Margoliouth, 'Ibn Al-Hītī's Arabic Chronicle', p. 436.
199. Amar, *The History of Medicine in Jerusalem*, p. 135.
200. Mann, *Texts and Studies*, p. 282.
201. The dating is based on al-Ḥarīzī's life.
202. Yahalom and Blau, *The Wanderings of Judah Alharizi*, pp. 16–17, 69, ll. 204–10, 255–74; Frenkel, 'The Medieval Jewish Community of Aleppo', pp. 69–70.
203. Ashtor, *The History of the Jews in Egypt and Syria*, vol. II, pp. 21–2.
204. TS AS 147.23.
205. TS 20.133; Goitein, *A Mediterranean Society*, vol. I, pp. 301, 475.
206. al-Maqqarī, *Nafḥ al-Ṭīb*, vol. III, pp. 528–9; Friedenwald, *The Jews and Medicine*, vol. II, p. 634; Roth, *Jews, Visigoths and Muslims*, p. 174; Hammer-Purgstall, *Literaturgesch*, VI. p. 482; Steinschneider, *Jewish Literature from the Eighth to the Eighteenth Century*, p. 170; al-Khālidī, *al-Yahūd Taḥta Ḥukm al-Muslimīn*, p. 356.
207. Mann, *Texts and Studies*, p. 266.
208. Mosseri VIII.80.1.
209. Mann, *Texts and Studies*, p. 277.
210. Mann, *The Jews in Egypt and in Palestine*, p. 250; Roth, 'Medicine', p. 435.
211. TS 20.47.
212. Mosseri II.195.
213. Goitein, 'A Maghrebi Living in Cairo', pp. 138–9.
214. A well-known Umayyad military leader and statesman (660–714).
215. Ibn al-Qifṭī, *Taʾrīkh al-Ḥukamāʾ*, p. 317.
216. Ibid., p. 225.
217. An Iranian philosopher and one of the greatest physicians in the Muslim world.
218. Zinger, 'Women, Gender and Law', p. 15.
219. Goitein and Friedman, *India Book IV/A*, mainly p. 86; Goitein and Friedman, *India Book IV/B*, p. 226–34.
220. Gil, *Palestine during the First Muslim Period*, vol. III, p. 454.
221. The dating is based on al-Ḥarīzī's life.
222. Segal, *The Book of Taḥkemonī*, pp. 351–2, gate 46.
223. Yahalom and Blau, *The Wanderings of Judah Alharizi*, pp. 69–70, ll. 201–3, 288–90.

224. Ibid., p. 137, l. 812.
225. Wretched because he was unknown and helpful because he was able to cure the caliph.
226. Ibn Abī Uṣaybiʿa, *ʿUyūn al-Anbāʾ*, vol. II, p. 89; Ibn al-Qifṭī, *Taʾrīkh al-Ḥukamāʾ*, p. 178; Meyerhof, 'Medieval Jewish Physicians in the Near East', p. 442; Ramaḍān, *al-Yahūd fī Miṣr*, p. 436.
227. Friedenwald, *The Jews and Medicine*, p. 633.
228. al-Zarhūnī, *al-Ṭibb*, p. 58.
229. TS AS 99.31; Isaacs, *Medical and Para-medical Manuscripts*, no. 993.
230. TS NS J76.
231. Buchman and Amar, *Practical Medicine of Rabbi Hayyim Vital*; Amar, *The History of Medicine in Jerusalem*, p. 139.
232. Fenton, 'Jonah Ibn Ǧanāḥ's Medical Dictionary', p. 122.
233. Prats, 'Ibn ʿAknīn, Joseph b. Judah Jacob'; Roth, 'Medicine', p. 436; Roth, 'Ibn ʿAknīn, Joseph b. Judah'.
234. Kraemer, *Maimonides*, pp. 116–17, 92.
235. Including Steinschneider, Vajda, Baron, Schirmann, Twersky, Bacher and Guttmann.
236. For a detailed account of the errors, see Prats, 'Ibn ʿAknīn, Joseph b. Judah Jacob'.
237. Halper (Dropsie) 467.
238. Sela, 'The Head of the Rabbanite, Karaite and Samaritan Jews', p. 261.
239. See also ibid., p. 261 n. 18.
240. It is unlikely that a non-Jew would run a bathing house for Jews in a Jewish neighbourhood.
241. Ramaḍān, *al-Yahūd fī Miṣr*, pp. 438–9.
242. Ibn Abī Uṣaybiʿa, *ʿUyūn al-Anbāʾ*, vol. II, pp. 116–17; Jadon, 'A Comparison of the Wealth', p. 65; Kraemer, *Maimonides*, pp. 214–15; Meyerhof, 'Medieval Jewish Physicians in the Near East', p. 446; Ramaḍān, *al-Yahūd fī Miṣr*, p. 444; Ashtor-Strauss, 'Saladin and the Jews', p. 310.
243. Ashtor, *The History of the Jews in Egypt and Syria*, vol. I, p. 310.
244. ENA 2727.15e; Goitein, *A Mediterranean Society*, vol. II, p. 485.
245. Goitein, 'The Social Services of the Jewish Community', p. 13.
246. Bodl. MS heb. c 50, fol. 17.
247. al-Sakhāwī, *al-Ḍawʾ al-Lāmiʿ*, vol. I, pp. 116–17.
248. al-Maqrīzī, *al-Mawāʿiẓ*, vol. II, p. 409.
249. Ramaḍān, *al-Yahūd fī Miṣr*, p. 44; Luṭf, *Yahūd Miṣr al-Ayyūbiya*, p. 93;

Ashtor-Strauss, 'Saladin and the Jews', p. 311; Kedar, 'The Frankish Period'; Wedel, *Kitāb aṭ-Ṭabbāḫ*, p. 147; Ben-Hayyim, *The Literary and Oral Tradition*, vol. I, p. 30; Meyerhof, 'Jewish Physicians Contemporaries of Maimonides', p. 395; Crown, Pummer and Tal, *A Companion to Samaritan Studies*, pp. 6–7.

250. Amar and Serri, *The Land of Israel and Syria*, pp. 18, 135–6.
251. Amar, *The History of Medicine in Jerusalem*, p. 136.
252. al-Khālidī, *al-Yahūd Taḥta Ḥukm al-Muslimīn*, p. 357.
253. Ibn Khaldūn, *Ta'rīkh al-'Alāma*, pt. 1, vol. VII, p. 632.
254. It is not clear why he made this tour: it has been suggested that he was trading in horses or in slaves, and it is not impossible that he was on an official intelligence mission for the Umayyad caliphate of Spain. He was probably chosen for this mission in view of the help which he could expect to receive from the Jewish colonies in Europe.
255. al-Qazwīnī, *'Ajā'ib al-Makhlūqāt.*
256. Miquel, 'Ibrāhīm b. Ya'ḳūb'; al-Khālidī, *al-Yahūd Taḥta Ḥukm al-Muslimīn*, p. 107.
257. al-Bakrī, *Kitāb al-Masālik wa-l-Mamālik.*
258. Ashtor, 'Ibrahim Ibn Ya'qūb'.
259. Ashtor, *The History of the Jews in Egypt and Syria*, vol. II, p. 552.
260. Yahalom and Blau, *The Wanderings of Judah Alharizi*, pp. 31–2, 177, ll. 146–52.
261. Weinberger, 'Moses Dar'ī', pp. 450, 452, 454.
262. Amar, *The History of Medicine in Jerusalem*, p. 135.
263. TS NS J260.
264. Ben-Sasson, *The Emergence of the Local Jewish Community*, p. 381.
265. Lasker, 'Israeli, Isaac ben Solomon'.
266. Miller, 'Doctors without Borders', p. 117.
267. Fenton, 'Jonah Ibn Ǧanāḥ's Medical Dictionary', p. 124.
268. Finkel, 'An Eleventh Century Source', pp. 50–1; Roth, 'Medicine', p. 434; al-Andalusī, *Science in the Medieval World*, p. 80; Ibn Juljul, *Ṭabaqāt al-Aṭibbā'*, pp. 87–8.
269. Miller, 'Doctors without Borders', pp. 117–18.
270. Finkel, 'A Risāla of al-Jāḥiẓ', p. 320.
271. Steinschneider, 'An Introduction to the Arabic Literature of the Jews I', 9(4), p. 610.
272. Ibn Ḥazm al-Andalusī, *Rasā'il Ibn Ḥazm*, vol. I, p. 114; Kozodoy, The Jewish

Physician, p. 104; Roth, *Jews, Visigoths and Muslims*, p. 180; al-Khālidī, *al-Yahūd Taḥta Ḥukm al-Muslimīn*, 356.

273. Lewicka and Freudenthal, 'The Reception and Practice of Rationalist Medicine', p. 98.
274. Ashtor, 'New Data for the History of Levantine Jewries', p. 87.
275. Yahalom and Blau, *The Wanderings of Judah Alharizi*, p. 51, ll. 43–4; Segal, *The Book of Taḥkemonī*, p. 335, gate 46.
276. Goitein and Friedman, *India Book IV/B*, pp. 226–34 nn. 44, 45.
277. Amar, *The History of Medicine in Jerusalem*, p. 137.
278. Ashtor, *The History of the Jews in Egypt and Syria*, vol. I, pp. 276–7.
279. ENA NS 18.17a.
280. Fischel, 'Azarbaijan in Jewish History', p. 17 n. 36.
281. al-Dhahabī, *Dhuyūl al-ʿIbar*, vol. IV, p. 3.
282. al-Jazarī, *Ḥawādith al-Zamān*, vol. III, p. 966.
283. Goitein, *A Mediterranean Society*, vol. II, p. 258, vol. I, pp. 252, 463 n. 134.
284. TS K15.92.
285. Frenkel, *The Compassionate and Benevolent*, pp. 338–9.
286. BL Or. 10794.13.
287. Ashtor, *The History of the Jews in Egypt and Syria*, vol. II, pp. 21–2.
288. Adler, *Jewish Travelers*, p. 199; Ashtor, *The History of the Jews in Egypt and Syria*, vol. II, p. 424.
289. Khan, *Arabic Legal and Administrative Documents*, pp. 249–50, no. 51.
290. Schoenfeld, 'Immigration and Assimilation', pp. 5–6.
291. TS Ar. 30.163.
292. Amar, *The History of Medicine in Jerusalem*, p. 138.
293. Assaf, 'Old Geniza Documents', p. 19.
294. Eisenstein, *Ozar Massaoth*, p. 93; Yaari, *Massa Meshullam mi-Volterra*, p. 57; Cohen, 'Jews in the Mamlūk Environment', p. 436.
295. TS 8.195.
296. Ashtor, *The History of the Jews in Egypt and Syria*, vol. II, p. 87.
297. Cohen, 'Jews in the Mamlūk Environment', p. 436.
298. Bareket, *The Jews of Egypt*, pp. 189–90.
299. Mann, *Texts and Studies*, p. 282.
300. ENA 2592.22.
301. TS AS 164.58.
302. Neubauer, 'Egyptian Fragments', p. 552.

303. Steinschneider, 'An Introduction to the Arabic Literature of the Jews II', 13(2), p. 298.
304. Amar, *The History of Medicine in Jerusalem*, p. 136.
305. Ashtor, 'New Data for the History of Levantine Jewries', p. 76.
306. Yahalom and Blau, *The Wanderings of Judah Alharizi*, p. 71, ll. 294–6; Segal, *The Book of Taḥkemonī*, p. 352, gate 46.
307. Ashtor, *The History of the Jews in Egypt and Syria*, vol. II, pp. 112.
308. RNL Yevr. Ar. II 1378; Arad, 'A Pleasant Voice', p. 26.
309. Ibn al-Fuwāṭī, *Majma' al-Ādāb*, vol. V, pp. 324–5.
310. Amar, *The History of Medicine in Jerusalem*, p. 138.
311. Ashtor, *The History of the Jews in Egypt and Syria*, vol. I, p. 174.
312. Ibn Iyās described the incident and claimed he remained Jewish: Ibn Iyās, *Badā'i' al-Zuhūr*, vol. IV, p. 386. According to el-Leithy he converted to Islam: el-Leithy, 'Coptic Culture and Conversion', p. 38; Ashtor, *The History of the Jews in Egypt and Syria*, vol. II, p. 175.
313. ENA NS 57.8.
314. Ashur, 'Engagement and Betrothal Documents', pp. 202–4.
315. Frenkel, 'The Medieval Jewish Community of Aleppo', p. 51.
316. Halper (Dropsie) 467.
317. Richards, 'A Doctor's Petition', p. 301; Goitein, *A Mediterranean Society*, vol. II, pp. 256–7. For an interesting discussion regarding Makārim's identity see Zinger, 'Women, Gender and Law', p. 283.
318. Strauss, 'Documents for the Economic and Social History of the Jews', pp. 142–5; Bodl. MS Heb. c 28, fol. 47 (2876-47).
319. TS K15.49.
320. TS K15.61.
321. Bodl. MS, heb. c. 13, fol. 6.
322. Goitein, *A Mediterranean Society*, vol. III, p. 243 n. 136.
323. Delgado, 'Ibn Janāḥ'; Tenne, 'Ibn Janāḥ, Jonah'.
324. Delgado, 'Ibn Janāḥ'; Fenton, 'Jonah Ibn Ǧanāḥ's Medical Dictionary', p. 108.
325. Ibn Abī Uṣaybi'a, *'Uyūn al-Anbā'*, vol. II, p. 50; al-Andalusī, *Ṭabaqāt al-'Umam*, p. 204; Roth, *Jews, Visigoths and Muslims*, p. 78; Finkel, 'An Eleventh Century Source', p. 52; al-Andalusi, *Science in the Medieval World*, p. 81.
326. Delgado, 'Ibn Janāḥ'; Assis, 'Jewish Physicians and Medicine', p. 35; Fenton, 'Jonah Ibn Ǧanāḥ's Medical Dictionary', pp. 108, 116; Ibn Abī Uṣaybi'a,

ʿ*Uyūn al-Anbāʾ*, vol. II, p. 50; al-Andalusī, *Ṭabaqāt al-ʾUmam*, p. 204; Roth, 'Medicine', p. 436; Amar and Serri, 'Compilation'; Kozodoy, 'The Jewish Physician in Medieval Iberia', p. 104; Kaḥāla, *Muʿjam al-Muʾallifīn*, vol. III, p. 844.

327. Fenton, 'Jonah Ibn Ǧanāḥ's Medical Dictionary', p. 110.
328. MS Ayia Sofia 3603, fols. 1–90b.
329. Fenton, 'Jonah Ibn Ǧanāḥ's Medical Dictionary', pp. 112–14, 118.
330. Tenne, 'Ibn Janāḥ, Jonah'; Roth, *Jews, Visigoths and Muslims*, p. 78; Delgado, 'Ibn Janāḥ'.
331. Tenne, 'Ibn Janāḥ, Jonah'.
332. al-Andalusī, *Ṭabaqāt al-ʾUmam*, p. 115; Ibn al-Qifṭī, *Taʾrīkh al-Ḥukamāʾ*, p. 324; al-ʿUmarī, *Masālik al-Abṣār*, vol. IX, p. 207.
333. Finkel, 'A Risāla of al-Jāḥiẓ', p. 320, Finkel, 'An Eleventh Century Source', p. 50.
334. Ibn Juljul, *Ṭabaqāt al-Aṭibbāʾ*, pp. 61–2; Ibn Abī Uṣaybiʿa, ʿ*Uyūn al-Anbāʾ*, vol. I, pp. 163–4; al-ʿUmarī, *Masālik al-Abṣār*, vol. IX, p. 207; Ibn al-Qifṭī, *Taʾrīkh al-Ḥukamāʾ*, pp. 324–5; al-Andalusī, *Ṭabaqāt al-ʾUmam*, p. 115.
335. Roth, 'Māsarjawayh', pp. 432–3.
336. Langermann, 'From My Notebooks', pp. 283, 288–9, 291.
337. Langermann, 'Three Singular Treatises'.
338. Fenton, 'Jonah Ibn Ǧanāḥ's Medical Dictionary', p. 122.
339. Yahalom and Blau, *The Wanderings of Judah Alharizi*, p. 72, ll. 312–13, p. 148, ll. 888–91; Segal, *The Book of Taḥkemonī*, p. 353, gate 46.
340. Amar and Lev, *Physicians, Drugs and Remedies*, p. 108; Zonta, 'Mineralogy, Botany and Zoology', pp. 278–9.
341. Ben-Shammai, 'Aldabi, Meir ben Isaac'.
342. Bodl. MS heb. f. 56, fol. 126.
343. ENA 2556.9.
344. TS K3.6.
345. Mann, *Texts and Studies*, p. 277.
346. Goitein and Friedman, *India Book III*, pp. 30, 314.
347. Goitein and Friedman, *India Traders of the Middle Ages*, vol. I, p. 86. According to Goitein, the addressed Moses is Maimonides and not Moses b. Peraḥya.
348. Arad, 'The Community as an Economic Body', p. 61.
349. Ashtor, *The History of the Jews in Egypt and Syria*, vol. II, pp. 27–8.
350. Bodl. MS heb. e. 101, fol. 14.

351. Gil, *Palestine during the First Muslim Period*, vol. III, pp. 25–6.
352. Amar, *The History of Medicine in Jerusalem*, p. 137.
353. Weinberger, 'Moses Darʿī', p. 450, 452, 454.
354. Shohetman, 'New Sources from the Geniza', p. 57.
355. Amar and Lev, *Physicians, Drugs and Remedies*, p. 108.
356. Gil, *The Tustaris*, p. 92.
357. TS K15.61.
358. Halper (Dropsie) 467.
359. Ashtor, *The History of the Jews in Egypt and Syria*, vol. I, pp. 169–70; Meyerhof, 'Medieval Jewish Physicians in the Near East', p. 456; Meyerhof, 'Jewish Physicians Contemporaries of Maimonides', p. 397; Kaḥāla, *Muʿjam al-Muʾallifīn*, vol. III, p. 904.
360. Ashtor, 'Some Features of the Jewish Communities', p. 65.
361. Goitein, *A Mediterranean Society*, vol. V, p. 581.
362. Bodl. MS heb. f. 56, fol. 55.
363. Ibn Abī Uṣaybiʿa, *ʿUyūn al-Anbāʾ*, vol. II, p. 50; al-Andalusī, *Ṭabaqāt al-ʾUmam*, p. 204; Finkel, 'An Eleventh Century Source', p. 52; Kozodoy, 'The Jewish Physician in Medieval Iberia', p. 104; Roth, *Jews, Visigoths and Muslims*, p. 176; Roth, 'Medicine', p. 436; Friedenwald, *The Jews and Medicine*, p. 633.
364. Steinschneider, 'An Introduction to the Arabic Literature of the Jews I', 9(4), p. 611.
365. Micheau, 'Great Figures in Arabic Medicine', p. 179; not mentioned as Jewish by other sources.
366. Bodl. MS heb. f. 56, fol. 54.
367. CUL Or. 1080 J2.
368. al-Yūnīnī, *Early Mamluk Syrian Historiography*, vol. II, p. 237.
369. Halper (CAJS) 354.
370. Goitein, *A Mediterranean Society*, vol. V, p. 590 n. 149.
371. Fischel, 'Azarbaijan in Jewish History', p. 17 n. 36.
372. al-Yūnīnī, *Early Mamluk Syrian Historiography*, vol. II, p. 119.
373. Halper (Dropsie) 467.
374. TS AS 151.5.
375. Mitchell, *Medicine in the Crusades*, p. 40.
376. TS 10J17.19.
377. BL Or. 5535.3.
378. Fenton, 'Jewish–Muslim Relations', p. 357.
379. ENA 2592.14.

380. Yahalom and Blau, *The Wanderings of Judah Alharizi*, p. 12.
381. TS NS 246.26.12.
382. ENA 3150.8.
383. TS Misc.25.8.
384. Meyerhof, 'Jewish Physicians Contemporaries of Maimonides', p. 398.
385. Steinschneider, 'An Introduction to the Arabic Literature of the Jews I', 11(2), p. 308.
386. Mosseri, *Catalogue of the Jacques Mosseri Collection*, p. 149.
387. Hacker, 'On the Character of the Cairo Mustaarib Community', p. 93 n. 20; Arad, 'The Community as an Economic Body', pp. 53, 60–2.
388. Yahalom and Blau, *The Wanderings of Judah Alharizi*, p. 71, ll. 304–5; Segal, *The Book of Taḥkemonī*, p. 352, gate 46.
389. Goitein and Friedman, *India Book III*, pp. 358–62.
390. Halper (Dropsie) 467.
391. Goitein, *A Mediterranean Society*, IV, pp. 255, 445 n. 11.
392. TS K3.6.
393. Fischel, 'Azarbaijan in Jewish History', pp. 12–13; Steinschneider, *Die Arabische Literatur der Juden*, n. 178; Meyerhof, 'Jewish Physicians Contemporaries of Maimonides', p. 397; Meyerhof, 'Medieval Jewish Physicians in the Near East', p. 456.
394. Fischel, 'Azarbaijan in Jewish History', pp. 12–13.
395. Steinschneider, *Die Arabische Literatur der Juden*, n. 178; Meyerhof, 'Medieval Jewish Physicians in the Near East', p. 456; Meyerhof, 'Jewish Physicians Contemporaries of Maimonides', p. 397.
396. Fischel, 'Azarbaijan in Jewish History', p. 6; Amitai, 'Saʿd al-Dawla'.
397. Fischel, 'Azarbaijan in Jewish History', pp. 6–8; Amitai, 'Saʿd al-Dawla'.
398. Amitai, 'Saʿd al-Dawla'; Fischel, 'Azarbaijan in Jewish History', pp. 9–10; Meyerhof, 'Jewish Physicians Contemporaries of Maimonides', pp. 398–9.
399. TS NS 324.7.
400. For the full story see: Ashtor, *The History of the Jews in Egypt and Syria*, vol. II, p. 110.
401. TS K6 149.
402. Ashtor, *The History of the Jews in Egypt and Syria*, vol. I, p. 237.
403. Arad, 'The Community as an Economic Body', p. 61.
404. Ashtor, *The History of the Jews in Egypt and Syria*, vol. II, pp. 27–8.
405. According to Eddé he died c.1223; see Eddé, 'Les Médecins dans la société syrienne', p. 108.

406. Meyerhof, 'Jewish Physicians Contemporaries of Maimonides', p. 395.
407. al-Ghazūlī, *Maṭāliʿ al-Budūr*, p. 421.
408. al-Ṣafadī, *Kitāb al-Wāfī bi-l-Wafayāt* (2000), vol. XVI, pp. 173–5; Meyerhof, 'Jewish Physicians Contemporaries of Maimonides', p. 395; Wedel, 'Transfer of Knowledge', pp. 3.78–3.79.
409. TS Misc. 26.2.
410. Ashtor, 'Some Features of the Jewish Communities', p. 65.
411. TS 10J15.26; Goitein, *A Mediterranean Society*, vol. III, p. 150, vol. IV, pp. 283, 439.
412. TS 8K22.12; Goitein, *A Mediterranean Society*, vol. II, pp. 258–9, 580.
413. Ashtor, *The History of the Jews in Egypt and Syria*, vol. II, p. 557.
414. TS 16.200; Goitein, *A Mediterranean Society*, vol. I, pp. 134, 385.
415. Steinschneider, *Die Arabische Literatur der Juden*, n. 199; Steinschneider, *Die Hebraeischen Übersetzungen des Mittelalters*, p. 947; Meyerhof, 'Medieval Jewish Physicians in the Near East', p. 458; Meyerhof, 'Jewish Physicians Contemporaries of Maimonides', p. 399.
416. Steinschneider, *Die Arabische Literatur der Juden*, n. 199; Meyerhof, 'Medieval Jewish Physicians in the Near East', p. 45; Poznański, 'Recent Karaite Publications', p. 445; Margoliouth, 'Ibn Al-Hītī's Arabic Chronicle', 430; Meyerhof, 'Jewish Physicians Contemporaries of Maimonides', p. 399; Schmidtke and Schirmann, 'Samawʾal al-Maghribi'; Nemoy, 'Samuel ben Moses al-Maghribi'.
417. Ashtor, *The History of the Jews in Egypt and Syria* , vol. II, pp. 557–9.
418. Ashtor, *The History of the Jews in Egypt and Syria*, vol. II, pp. 556–7.
419. Weinberger, 'Moses Darʿī', pp. 450, 452, 454.
420. Friedman, 'A Bitter Protest', pp. 129–30.
421. Amar, *The History of Medicine in Jerusalem*, p. 136.
422. Ibid., p. 137.
423. Mitchell, *Medicine in the Crusades*, p. 40.
424. Adler, *Jewish Travelers*, p. 173; Ashtor, *The History of the Jews in Egypt and Syria*, vol. II, p. 44; Eisenstein, *Ozar Massaoth*, p. 94.
425. TS 8J13.14; Goitein, *A Mediterranean Society*, vol. II, p. 490.
426. al-Maqrīzī, *Ittiʿāẓ al-Ḥunafāʾ*, vol. II, pp. 73, 83; Ibn Saʿīd, *al-Nujūm al-Zāhira*, p. 62; Ramaḍān, *al-Yahūd fī Miṣr*, pp. 434–5.
427. Ashtor, *The History of the Jews in Egypt and Syria*, vol. I, pp. 268–9.
428. TS Misc. 20.183.

429. TS AS 146.9; Goitein, *A Mediterranean Society*, vol. V, pp. 36, 515.
430. Amar, *The History of Medicine in Jerusalem*, p. 138.
431 Ashtor, *The History of the Jews in Egypt and Syria*, vol. I, pp. 236–7.
432. Amar, *The History of Medicine in Jerusalem*, p. 137.
433. Frenkel, 'Book Lists from the Geniza', pp. 339–40.
434. Bodl MS heb. d.65, fol. 8.
435. TS AS 148.199.
436. Mann, *The Jews in Egypt and in Palestine*, vol. I, p. 242, vol. II, p. 309.
437. Goitein, *A Mediterranean Society*, vol. III, pp. 202 n. 195, 469 n. 95; Bareket, *The Jewish Leadership in Fusṭāṭ*, pp. 166–8.
438. Bodl. MS heb. d. 68, fol. 101; Goitein, *A Mediterranean Society*, vol. II, p. 423.
439. ENA 2727.15e; Goitein, *A Mediterranean Society*, vol. II, p. 485.
440. Amar, *The History of Medicine in Jerusalem*, p. 136.
441. Yagur, 'The Jews of Cyprus', pp. 7–8.
442. Steinschneider, 'An Introduction to the Arabic Literature of the Jews I', 11(4), p. 589.
443. Amar, *The History of Medicine in Jerusalem*, pp. 137–8.
444. Isaacs, *Medical and Para-medical Manuscripts*, no. 902.
445. Goitein, *A Mediterranean Society*, vol. V, pp. 103–4 nn. 305–7.
446. ENA 2748.2.
447. Bodl. MS heb. f. 22, fol. 41.
448. Halper (Dropsie) 467.
449. Bodl. MS. heb. c. 13, fol. 6.
450. TS K3.6.
451. Ashtor, 'The Number of Jews in Mediaeval Egypt', 18(1–4), p. 17.
452. TS K15.92.
453. Assaf, 'Slavery and the Slave-Trade among the Jews', p. 271.
454. Wechsler, 'Ibn Sughmar Family'.
455. Amar, *The History of Medicine in Jerusalem*, p. 13.
456. Ibn Khaldūn, *Taʾrīkh al-ʿAlāma*, pt. 1, vol. IV, p. 384.
457. For additional information about Zechariah, see: Tobi, 'Ben Solomon, Zechariah ha-Rofeh'.
458. Yaḥyā Qafiḥ was a Yemenite scholar who was engaged in natural medicine during the first half of the twentieth century.
459. Tobi, 'Ben Solomon, Zechariah ha-Rofeh'.
460. ENA 2556.9.

461. ENA 2738.36.
462. Najm al-Dīn Aḥmad b. al-Faḍl Abū al-ʿAbbās, also known as Ibn al-Munāfiḥ.
463. Ibn Abī Uṣaybiʿa, *ʿUyūn al-Anbāʾ*, vol. II, pp. 272–3; al-Ṣafadī, *Kitāb al-Wāfī bi-l-Wafayāt* (2000), vol. XXVIII, p. 5; Wedel, 'Transfer of Knowledge', p. 3.81; al-ʿUmarī, *Masālik al-Abṣār*, vol. IX, pp. 302–3; Meyerhof, 'Jewish Physicians Contemporaries of Maimonides', pp. 396–7. According to Eddé he died c.1238; see Eddé, 'Les Médecins dans la société syrienne', p. 106.
464. Amar and Lev, *Physicians, Drugs and Remedies*, p. 109.
465. Frenkel, *The Compassionate and Benevolent*, p. 557.
466. LG Misc 99.
467. ENA 2727.17a.
468. Ashtor, *The History of the Jews in Egypt and Syria*, vol. II, p. 112.
469. Halper (Dropsie) 467.
470. Cohen, *Poverty and Charity*, p. 103 n. 123; Ashtor, *The History of the Jews in Egypt and Syria*, vol. I, p. 262.
471. BL Or. 5535.3.
472. TS 8J1.2.
473. TS K15.92.
474. TS Ar. 48.117.
475. RNL Yevr. III B 669.
476. Amar, *The History of Medicine in Jerusalem*, p. 136.
477. Levey, 'The Pharmacology of Ibn Biklārish'; see in detail Burnett, *Ibn Baklarish's Book of Simples.*
478. Dietrich, Ibn Biklāri<u>sh</u>.
479. Levey, 'The Pharmacology of Ibn Biklārish'; Sarton, *Introduction to the History of Science*, vol. II, p. 235.
480. Meyerhof, *Un Glossaire*, p. xxviii.
481. Dietrich, 'Ibn Biklāri<u>sh</u>'; Kozodoy, 'The Jewish Physician in Medieval Iberia', p. 103; Ullmann, *Islamic Medicine*, pp. 201, 275; Ibn Abī Uṣaybiʿa, *ʿUyūn al-Anbāʾ*, vol. II, p. 52; Steinschneider, *Die Arabische Literatur der Juden*, p. 147.
482. TS Ar.44.218.
483. Serry and Lev, 'A Judaeo-Arabic Fragment'.
484. TS 8J18.9.
485. Margoliouth, 'Ibn Al-Hītī's Arabic Chronicle', p. 431.

486. TS AS 151.5.
487. Asher, *The Itinerary of Rabbi Benjamin*, p. 86; Ḥaddād, *Riḥlat Ibn Yūna*, p. 117.
488. ENA 2556.9.
489. Arad, 'The Community as an Economic Body', p. 61 n. 213.
490. al-Maqrīzī, *Kitāb al-Sulūk*, vol. IV, pp. 598, 1041–2; Ashtor, *The History of the Jews*, vol. II, pp. 89–90.
491. Ramaḍān, *al-Yahūd fī Miṣr*, p. 433.
492. Cohen, *Poverty and Charity*, p. 112.
493. TS K15.96; Goitein, *A Mediterranean Society*, vol. II, p. 441.
494. TS K15.66; Goitein, *A Mediterranean Society*, vol. II, p. 440.
495. TS 24.76; Goitein, *A Mediterranean Society*, vol. II, pp. 438–9.
496. Regarding woman physicians, see Goitein, *A Mediterranean Society*, vol. III, pp. 63–4.
497. Gil, *The Tustaris*, p. 10.
498. TS J1.43.
499. TS NS 321.40.
500. Goitein, 'A Letter of Historical Importance', p. 523.
501. De Lange, 'Byzantium in the Cairo Genizah', p. 41; Goitein, 'A Letter from Seleucia', pp. 298, 302–3; Goskar, 'Material Worlds', p. 196.
502. Bodl. MS heb. f. 22, fol. 25b-52b.
503. Goitein, 'The Oldest Documentary Evidence', p. 301.
504. TS NS 321.40.
505. TS AS 155.229.
506. TS NS 224.17; Isaacs, *Medical and Para-medical Manuscripts*, no. 838.
507. ENA 2727.23b.
508. Bodl. MS. heb. f. 56, fols. 13-19.
509. Goitein, 'A Report on Messianic Troubles', pp. 57–8, 65.
510. ENA 2592.18.
511. ENA 2730.2.
512. Zinger, 'Women, Gender and Law', pp. 277–305.
513. Ibn Abī Uṣaybiʿa, *ʿUyūn al-Anbāʾ*, vol. II, p. 218; Goitein, *A Mediterranean Society*, vol. V, p. 271 nn. 80–1; al-Asʿad the physician: Goitein, *A Mediterranean Society*, vol. III, pp. 81–2 nn. 46, 47 (dated 1217), 465 n. 120; Meyerhof, 'Jewish Physicians Contemporaries of Maimonides', p. 392.
514. Goitein, *A Mediterranean Society*, vol. III, pp. 81–2 n. 47.
515. Richards, 'A Doctor's Petition', p. 303.

516. TS 20.44; Goitein, 'The Exchange Rate of Gold and Silver Money', pp. 28–9.
517. Strauss, 'Documents for the Economic and Social History of the Jews', pp. 142–5.
518. TS Ar. 4.7.
519. TS Ar. 39.449.
520. Strauss, 'Documents for the Economic and Social History of the Jews', pp. 142–5.
521. Halper (Dropsie) 467.
522. Frenkel, *The Compassionate and Benevolent*, pp. 536–7.
523. Goitein, *A Mediterranean Society*, vol. V, pp. 95, 532; Goitein's index cards, published in Ashur and Lev, 'Medical Recipes'.
524. Cohen, *Poverty and Charity*, p. 212 n. 75; Goitein, *A Mediterranean Society*, vol. II, p. 451.
525. Halper (Dropsie) 467.
527 TS AS 149.17.
527. Halper (Dropsie) 467.
528. Ibid.
529. ENA 2728.6.
530. Lewicka, 'Healer, Scholar, Conspirator', p. 133.
531. Ibid., p. 16.
532. al-Khazrajī, *al-ʿUqūd al-Luʾluʾiyya*, vol. II, p. 242; Ashtor, *The History of the Jews in Egypt and Syria*, vol. II, pp. 173–4, 243.
533. Ashtor, *The History of the Jews in Egypt and Syria*, vol. II, p. 317, based on Ibn Iyās, *Badāʾiʿ al-Zuhūr*, vol. IV, p. 386.
534. Ashtor, *The History of the Jews in Egypt and Syria*, vol. II, p. 174, based on Ibn Iyās, *Badāʾiʿ al-Zuhūr*, vol. IV, p. 386.
535. Ashtor, *The History of the Jews in Egypt and Syria*, vol. II, p. 174.
536. Ibid.
537. Explanations for the order of the biographies, abbreviations, names, titles and origins are found at the beginning of Chapter 3.
538. Ashtor, 'The Number of Jews in Mediaeval Egypt', 19(1–4), p. 5 n. 288.
539. el-Leithy, 'Coptic Culture and Conversion', pp. 73–4 n. 17.
540. TS Ar. 54.52.
541. Halper (CAJS) 464.
542. TS NS 324.47.
543. TS NS 226.30.

544. Allony, *The Jewish Library in the Middle Ages*, p. 231.
545. CUL Or. 1080 5.16.
546. ENA 2591.6.
547. Goitein and Friedman, *India Book I*, no. 36, p. 262.
548. Goitein, *A Mediterranean Society*, vol. II, pp. 494–5.
549. Goitein and Friedman, *India Book I*, no. 36, pp. 261–6; Goitein, *A Mediterranean Society*, vol. IV, pp. 317–18.
550. TS 13J6.25.
551. TS NS J 315.
552. TS K 15.16.
553. TS 13J4.13.
554. TS K 15.6.
555. Goitein, *A Mediterranean Society*, vol. II, pp. 494–5.
556. ENA 2591.6.
557. TS NS 69.52.
558. TS K15.61.
559. Bodl. MS. heb. c. 13, fol. 6.
560. ENA 2591.8 (see image on p. 000).
561. Goitein, *A Mediterranean Society*, vol. II, p. 140.
562. Ibid., vol. II, p. 485.
563. TS 8J19.30.
564. TS K15.61.
565. ENA 2591.6.
566. ENA 2591.6.
567. Goitein, *A Mediterranean Society*, vol. II, pp. 485, 508, App. C 139.
568. Ibid., vol. II, p. 263.
569. TS Ar. 54.91.
570. Ashtor, 'The Number of Jews in Mediaeval Egypt', 18(1–4), p. 33 n. 173.
571. CUL Or. 1080J2.
572. TS K15.6.
573. TS 12.487.
574. Allony, *The Jewish Library in the Middle Ages*, p. 255.
575. TS K15.9.
576. Probably identical with the biography below.
577. Bodl. MS heb. c. 50, fol. 17.
578. Probably identical with the biography above.
579. Goitein, *A Mediterranean Society*, vol. II, p. 582.

580. Abū al-Munā, *Minhāj al-Dukkān.*
581. Meyerhof, 'Jewish Physicians Contemporaries of Maimonides', p. 397; Chipman, *The World of Pharmacy and Pharmacists*; Chipman and Lev, 'Syrups from the Apothecary's Shop'.
582. Levey, *Early Arabic Pharmacology*, p. 98; personal observations during the market surveys I conducted with Zohr Amar: see Lev and Amar, 'Ethnopharmacological Survey of Traditional Drugs Sold in the Kingdom of Jordan'; Lev and Amar, 'Ethnopharmacological Survey of Traditional Drugs Sold in Israel'.
583. ENA 2558.20.
584. Bodl. MS heb. e. 94, fol. 22.
585. Bodl. MS heb. c. 50, fol. 17.
586. Lev, 'Work in Progress', p. 41.
587. TS 8J6.15.
588. TS NS 323.19.
589. TS K3.6.
590. Goitein, *A Mediterranean Society*, vol. II, pp. 494–5.
591. CUL Or. 1080 J2.
592. TS K6.177.
593. Lev, 'Work in Progress', p. 41.
594. TS 20.44; Goitein, 'The Exchange Rate of Gold and Silver Money', pp. 28–9.
595. Bodl. MS heb. e. 94, fol. 21.
596. TS NS J 315.
597. Bodl. MS heb. e. 94, fol. 19.
598. Goitein and Friedman, *India Book I*, no. 34, pp. 247–9; Goitein, *A Mediterranean Society*, vol. IV, pp. 449 n. 35, 321 n. 90.
599. Goitein, *A Mediterranean Society*, vol. II, pp. 262, 582.
600. TS AS 202.396.
601. Bodl. MS heb. d. 66, fol. 52.
602. Ashtor, 'The Number of Jews in Mediaeval Egypt', 19(1–4), p. 7 n. 307. Al-ʿAfṣī was probably a trader in oak gall, used for medicine as well as tanning and the production of ink: see Lev and Amar, *Practical Materia Medica*, pp. 225–7.
603. TS AS 149.37.
604. TS K15.6.
605. Bodl. MS heb. c. 13, fol. 6.
606. Lev, 'Work in Progress', p. 41.

607. Allony, 'Hebrew Manuscript in New York Libraries', p. 31.
608. TS 8 J 16.22.
609. Ashtor, 'The Number of Jews in Mediaeval Egypt', 19(1–4), p. 9 n. 328.
610. Lev, 'Work in Progress', p. 41.
611. Gil, *Palestine during the First Muslim Period*, vol. II, pp. 77–8.
612. Written by Nathan b. Samuel (probably the secretary of the *nagid* Samuel b. Hananiah).
613. Goitein, *A Mediterranean Society*, vol. I, p. 364.
614. Ibid., vol. III, p. 243 n. 138.
615. TS NS J 151.
616. TS K15.6.
617. TS NS 313.17.
618. Goitein, *A Mediterranean Society*, vol. II, p. 503, Appendix C 117.
619. Lev, 'Work in Progress', p. 41.
620. TS K6.177.
621. Goitein, 'Court Records from the Cairo Geniza', pp. 272–6.
622. ENA 2967.3.
623. Bodl MS Heb. e. 101, fol. 13.
624. TS K15.6.
625. TS NS J 108a.
626. Goitein, *A Mediterranean Society*, vol. II, p. 503, Appendix C 117.
627. Lev, 'Work in Progress', p. 41.
628. TS NS J 108a.
629. Goitein, *A Mediterranean Society*, vol. IV, pp. 338 n. 236, 463 nn. 228–31.
630. TS Ar. 54.21.
631. TS AS 149.17.
632. TS K 3.6.
633. Bodl. MS heb. e. 94, fol. 22.
634. Goitein, 'Court Records from the Cairo Geniza', pp. 272–6.
635. ENA 4100.9(c).
636. Bodl. MS heb. c. 50, fol. 17.
637. ENA 2558.4.
638. Goitein, *A Mediterranean Society*, vol. II, pp. 268–9.
639. Probably identical with the biography below.
640. TS NS 190.127.
641. Probably identical with the biography above.

642. Written by Nathan b. Samuel (probably the secretary of the *nagid* Samuel b. Hananiah).
643. Goitein, *A Mediterranean Society*, vol. I, p. 364.
644. el-Leithy, 'Coptic Culture and Conversion', pp. 73–4.
645. TS NS 225.75.
646. Isaacs, *Medical and Para-medical Manuscripts*, no. 982.
647. Goitein, *A Mediterranean Society*, vol. IV, p. 277.
648. TS NS 338.39.
649. ENA 2727.30.
650. Bodl. MS heb. d. 66, fol. 52.
651. Ashtor, 'The Number of Jews in Mediaeval Egypt', 19(1–4), p. 7 n. 307.
652. TS 8J15.25; for the use of these substances in medicine see Lev and Amar, *Practical Materia Medica*, pp. 301–2 and 248–50 respectively.
653. TS NSJ422.
654. Bodl. MS heb. c. 50, fol.17.
655. TS NS 321.77.
656. TS NS 304.4(a).
657. TS AS 150.30.
658. ENA 2967.3.
659. Goitein, *A Mediterranean Society*, vol. II, p. 261.
660. See in depth Chipman, *The World of Pharmacy and Pharmacists*, pp. 129–30.
661. Goitein, *A Mediterranean Society*, vol. II, p. 263, 271–2.
662. Marín, 'Anthroponymy and Society', pp. 277–8.
663. Goitein, *A Mediterranean Society*, vol. II, p. 263.
664. Marín, 'Anthroponymy and Society', p. 274.
665. Goitein, *A Mediterranean Society*, vol. II, p. 261.
666. See Chipman, 'Islamic Pharmacy in the Mamlūk and Mongol Realms'.
667. Isaacs, *Medical and Para-medical Manuscripts*, p. xi.
668. Chipman, *The World of Pharmacy and Pharmacists*, p. 130.
669. Ibid., p. 129.
670. On pharmacy in the Arab world see Chipman, *The World of Pharmacy and Pharmacists*; Said, *al-Biruni's Book*; Levey, *Early Arabic Pharmacology*; Hamarneh, 'The Rise of Professional Pharmacy in Islam'; Hamarneh, 'The Climax of Medieval Arabic Professional Pharmacy'.
671. Perfumers and druggists were mentioned in forty-seven lists, mainly lists of contributors; see for example Goitein, *A Mediterranean Society*, vol. II, pp. 493–5.

672. Goitein, *A Mediterranean Society*, vol. II, pp. 265–6.
673. In general, the biographical entries are dull, and lack important information such as dates of birth and death; from a methodological point of view, the explanation is that the Geniza documents that supplied us the information were dealing mainly with trade, lists of donors, taxes etc.
674. The graph is based on the available data collected in this research.
675. Goitein, *A Mediterranean Society*, vol. II, pp. 271–2.
676. Höglmeier, *al-Ğawbarī und seine Kašf al-asrār*, pp. 137–8; Ashtor, *The History of the Jews in Egypt and Syria*, vol. I, pp. 341–2.
677. Goitein, *A Mediterranean Society*, vol. II, pp. 263–4, 582 n. 20. For example, a letter to Abū al-Ḥasan b. Saʿīd al-Ṣārīfī Ibn al-Maṣmūdī, ṭabīb al-Murabbaʿa ila al-Maṣṣaṣa.
678. See the biography of Abū al-Munā b. Abī Naṣr b. Ḥaffāẓ.
679. Goitein, *A Mediterranean Society*, vol. II, pp. 261–2.
680. Cohen, *Poverty and Charity*, pp. 60, 63; Cohen, *The Voice of the Poor*, for example pp. 165, 172–4, 176. Perfumers and druggists were mentioned in forty-seven lists, mainly lists of contributors; see for example Goitein, *A Mediterranean Society*, vol. II, pp. 493–5.
681. Cohen, *Poverty and Charity*, pp. 60–3.
682. Goitein, *A Mediterranean Society*, vol. II, p. 263.
683. Ibid., vol. II, pp. 268–9.
684. Ibid., vol. I, pp. 173–9, 364, sec. 11, vol. II, pp. 262–3.
685. Ibid., vol. II, pp. 262–3.
686. Khan, *Arabic Legal and Administrative Documents*, pp. 61–8.
687. Goitein, *A Mediterranean Society*, vol. II, pp. 267–8.
688. Ibid., vol. II, pp. 262, 584 n. 52. The late wholesaler was called Banīn b. Daʾūd; see his biography.
689. Lev, 'Drugs Held and Sold'.
690. Lev and Amar, 'Practice versus Theory'; Lev and Amar, *Practical Materia Medica.*
691. Ibn al-Qifṭī, *Taʾrīkh al-Ḥukamā*, p. 320; Ibn Abī Uṣaybiʿa, *ʿUyūn al-Anbāʾ*, vol. II, p. 86; 122; Meyerhof, 'Medieval Jewish Physicians in the Near East', p. 442; Goitein, 'The Medical Profession', p. 179; Ramaḍān, *al-Yahūd fi Miṣr*, p. 433.
692. Goitein, *A Mediterranean Society*, vol. II, p. 261, vol. V, p. 315.
693. They appear on twenty-five donor lists, for example; In one list Cohen found a physician who probably also made potions (*al-ṭabīb sharābī*); see Cohen,

Poverty and Charity, p. 66.

694. Cohen, *Poverty and Charity*, pp. 64–6.
695. Strauss, 'Documents for the Economic and Social History of the Jews', pp. 142–5.
696. Bodl. MS heb. c. 50, fol.17.
697. TS AS 151.5.
698. Cohen, *Poverty and Charity*, p. 217; Goitein, *A Mediterranean Society*, vol. IV, p. 351 n. 65.
699. Goitein, *A Mediterranean Society*, vol. II, p. 261.
700. Ibid., vol. V, pp. 314–19, 592 nn. 23–4.
701. Ibid., vol. II, pp. 271–2.
702. Ashtor, *The Jews and the Mediterranean Economy*; Ben-Sasson, *The Emergence of the Local Jewish Community*; Gil, 'The Rādhānite Merchants'; Gil, *The Tustaris*; Gil, 'The Jewish Merchants'; Gil, 'Shipping'; Goitein, 'From the Mediterranean to India'; Goitein, *Letters of Medieval Jewish Traders*; Goitein and Friedman, *India Traders of the Middle Ages*; Goitein and Friedman, *India Book I*; Goitein and Friedman, *India Book II*; Goitein and Friedman, *India Book III*; Goitein and Friedman, *India Book IV/A*; Goitein and Friedman, *India Book IV/B*; Margariti, *Aden and the Indian Ocean Trade*; Margariti, 'Maritime Cityscapes'; Stillman, 'The Eleventh Century Merchant House'; Strauss, 'Documents for the Economic and Social History of the Jews'.
703. Fischel, 'The Spice Trade in Mamluk Egypt'; Amar and Lev, *Arabian Drugs*, Amar and Lev, 'Trends in the Use of Perfumes and Incense'; Amar and Lev, 'The Significance of the Genizah's Medical Documents'; Goldberg, *Trade and Institutions*.
704. Dietrich, *Zum Drogenhandel in islamischen Ägypten*.
705. Goitein, *A Mediterranean Society*, vol. II, pp. 270–2.
706. Lévi-Provençal, *Un Manuel hispanique de «ḥisba»*; al-Shayzarī, *Nihāyat al-Rutba fī Ṭalab al-Ḥisba*; Hamarneh, 'Origin and Functions of the Ḥisba System'; Buckley, 'The Muḥtasib'.
707. Goitein, *A Mediterranean Society*, vol. I, p. 364, 11.
708. Ragab, *The Medieval Islamic Hospital*, pp. 187–9.
709. Wasserstein, 'Jewish Élites in al-Andalus', p. 106.
710. Goitein, *Jewish Education in Muslim Countries*, pp. 121–6.
711. Grossman, 'The Relationship between the Social Structure and Spiritual Activity', p. 264.
712. Grossman, 'From Father to Son', pp. 199–200.

713. Marín, 'Biography and Prosopography', p. 8.
714. Gottheil, 'A Distinguished Family'.
715. Berkey, 'al-Subkī and His Women'; Schacht, 'al-Subkī'.
716. Salibi, 'The Banū Jamāʿa'.
717. For more on families of administrators and scholars see, among other publications, Walker, *Fatimid History and Ismaili Doctrine*; Gottschalk, *Die Mādarāʾijjun*.
718. Elmakias, *The Naval Commanders of Early Islam*, p. 19.
719. Goitein, *A Mediterranean Society*, vol. III, p. 14.
720. Guthrie, *Janus in the Doorway*, p. 300.
721. Shefer, 'Physicians in the Mamluk and Ottoman Courts', p. 116.
722. Pormann and Savage-Smith, *Medieval Islamic Medicine*, p. 81.
723. For more about this subject and some examples see Section 4.4.4.
725 Kozodoy, 'The Jewish Physician in Medieval Iberia', p. 115.
725. Stroumsa, *Maimonides in His World*, p. 129.
726. Goitein, *Jewish Education in Muslim Countries*, p. 195; See in detail Section 4.4.4.
727. Ibn al-Qifṭī, *Taʾrīkh al-Ḥukamāʾ*; Ibn Abī Uṣaybiʿa, *Uyūn al-Anbāʾ*.
728. Stroumsa, *Maimonides in His World*, p. 129.
729. Kozodoy came to this conclusion 'from the numerous instances in Christian Iberia of Jewish medical dynasties within a single family', She also noted the phenomenon of fathers teaching their sons-in-law, a phenomenon we know also from the Islamic world, as in the case of Maimonides and his son-in-law mentioned below: see Kozodoy, 'The Jewish Physician in Medieval Iberia', pp. 114–15. For the same conclusion regarding other regions in Europe, see Shatzmiller, *Jews, Medicine, and Medieval Society*, pp. 22–7.
730. Hazan, 'Medical, Administrative and Financial Aspects', pp. iv–v, 90–9; Pormann and Savage-Smith, *Medieval Islamic Medicine*, pp. 81–3; Leiser, 'Medical Education in Islamic Lands'.
731. Karmi, 'State Control of the Physicians in the Middle Ages'.
732. Hazan, 'Medical, Administrative and Financial Aspects', pp. v–vi, 101–9.
733. Part of the information in the table has been presented in earlier publications: Mazor and Lev, 'Dynasties of Jewish Physicians'; Mazor and Lev, 'The Phenomenon'. The dynasties are set in the table in chronological order and named usually according to the information we have on the first generation.
734. Goitein, *A Mediterranean Society*, vol. II, p. 245 n. 21.
735. TS K15.92.

736. TS AS 151.5.
737. Explanations for the order of the biographies, abbreviations, names, titles and origins are found at the beginning of Chapter 3.
738. Mazor and Lev, 'Dynasties of Jewish Physicians'; Mazor and Lev, 'The Phenomenon'.
739. See in detail Mazor and Lev, 'Dynasties of Jewish Physicians', pp. 238–44.
740. Ben-Sasson, *The Emergence of the Local Jewish Community*, pp. 182, 381.
741. Ibid.; Lewis, 'Palṭiel', p. 180; Goitein, *A Mediterranean Society*, vol. II, p. 243.
742. Ibn al-Qifṭī, *Taʾrīkh al-Ḥukamāʾ*, p. 320; Mann, *The Jews in Egypt and in Palestine*, p. 18; Miller, *Doctors without Borders*, pp. 111–12. For al-Tamīmī see Amar and Serri, *The Land of Israel and Syria*.
743. Ibn al-Qifṭī, *Taʾrīkh al-Ḥukamā*, p. 320; Ibn Abī Uṣaybiʿa, *ʿUyūn al-Anbāʾ*, vol. II, p. 86; 122; Meyerhof, *Medieval Jewish Physicians*, p. 442; Goitein, 'The Medical Profession', p. 179; Ramaḍān, *al-Yahūd fī Miṣr*, p. 433.
744. Lewis, 'Palṭiel', p. 180; Goitein, *A Mediterranean Society*, vol. II, p. 243.
745. Hence, he served the three caliphs for half a century: between the years 946 and 996.
746. Bareket, 'Abraham ha-Kohen', p. 3 n. 9: Lewis, 'Palṭiel'; Sela, 'The Head of the Rabbanite, Karaite and Samaritan Jews'; Miller, 'Doctors without Borders', pp. 111–12.
747. Ibn al-Qifṭī, *Taʾrīkh al-Ḥukamā*, p. 320; Ibn Abī Uṣaybiʿa, *ʿUyūn al-Anbāʾ*, vol. II, p. 86; Meyerhof, 'Medieval Jewish Physicians in the Near East', p. 442; Goitein, 'The Medical Profession', p. 179; Ramaḍān, *al-Yahūd fī Miṣr*, p. 433.
748. For more about watermelons in this period see Amar and Lev, 'Watermelon, Chate Melon and Cucumber'.
749. al-Maqrīzī, *Ittiʿāẓ al-Ḥunafāʾ*, vol. I, pp. 144, 216, 228.
750. Cohen and Somekh, 'In the Court of Yaʿqūb Ibn Killis', p. 287; Lewis, 'Palṭiel'; Roth, 'Medicine', p. 435.
751. Lewis, 'Palṭiel', pp. 177–8.
752. See Steinschneider, *Die Arabische Literatur der Juden*, pp. 96–7; Hirschberg, *A History of the Jews*, vol. I, p. 205 n. 1; Sela, 'The Head of the Rabbanite, Karaite and Samaritan Jews', pp. 262–4; Bareket, *Abraham ha-Kohen*, p. 3; Cohen and Somekh, 'In the Court of Yaʿqūb Ibn Killis', p. 287; Goitein, *A Mediterranean Society*, vol. II, p. 575. Roth, 'Medicine', p. 435. For other views regarding the identity of Palṭiel, see David and Bornstein-Makovetsky, 'Paltiel', p. 607.

753. Lewis, 'Palṭiel', p. 177.
754. Ibn Abī Uṣaybiʿa, *ʿUyūn al-Anbāʾ*, vol. II, p. 86; al-Maqrīzī, *Kitāb al-Muqaffā*, vol. II, p. 57.
755. Mann, *The Jews in Egypt and in Syria*, vol. I, pp. 17–18; Lewis, 'Palṭiel', pp. 180–1.
756. Hirschberg, *A History of the Jews*, vol. I, pp. 103–4.
757. Cohen, *Jewish Self-Government*, p. 13.
758. Hirschberg, *A History of the Jews*, vol. I, p. 205.
759. Meyerhof, 'Medieval Jewish Physicians in the Near East', p. 442.
760. Literally meaning 'medical practitioner', it is used in Jewish sources also for physicians with general philosophical erudition. Goitein, *A Mediterranean Society*, vol. II, p. 46.
761. Ibn Abī Uṣaybiʿa, *ʿUyūn al-Anbāʾ*, vol. II, p.86.
762. al-Maqrīzī, *Kitāb al-Muqaffā*, vol. II, p. 57.
763. Sela, 'The Head of the Rabbanite, Karaite and Samaritan Jews', p. 264.
764. Ibn Abī Uṣaybiʿa, *ʿUyūn al-Anbāʾ*, vol. II, p. 86; al-Maqrīzī, *Kitāb al-Muqaffā*, vol. II, p. 57; al-Maqrīzī, *Ittiʿāẓ al-Ḥunafāʾ*, vol. I, p. 146.
765. Ibn al-Qifṭī, *Taʾrīkh al-Ḥukamāʾ*, p. 320; Ibn Abī Uṣaybiʿa, *ʿUyūn al-Anbāʾ*, vol. II, p. 86; Mann, *The Jews in Egypt and in Palestine*, pp. 18, 122; Meyerhof, 'Medieval Jewish Physicians in the Near East', p. 442; Goitein, 'The Medical Profession', p. 179; Ramaḍān, *al-Yahūd fī Miṣr*, pp. 433–4; al-Maqrīzī, *Ittiʿāẓ al-Ḥunafāʾ*, vol. I, p. 146.
766. al-Maqrīzī, *Kitāb al-Muqaffā*, vol. II, p. 57; Ibn Abī Uṣaybiʿa, *ʿUyūn al-Anbāʾ*, vol. II, p. 86; al-Maqrīzī, *Ittiʿāẓ al-Ḥunafāʾ*, vol. I, p. 146.
767. Steinschneider, 'An Introduction to the Arabic Literature of the Jews I', 9(4), p. 610.
768. Mann, *The Jews in Egypt and in Palestine*, p. 18; Ramaḍān, *al-Yahūd fī Miṣr*, pp. 433–4; al-Maqrīzī, *Ittiʿāẓ al-Ḥunafāʾ*, vol. I, p. 146; Bareket, *Abraham ha-Kohen*.
769. Bareket, *Abraham ha-Kohen*, p. 3 n. 9; Lewis, 'Palṭiel'; Sela, 'The Head of the Rabbanite, Karaite and Samaritan Jews', pp. 262–4.
770. Gottheil, 'An Eleventh-Century Document', p. 467.
771. Sela, 'The Head of the Rabbanite, Karaite and Samaritan Jews', pp. 262–4.
772. For detailed discussion see Mazor and Lev, 'Dynasties of Jewish Physicians', pp. 242–3.
773. Stroumsa, 'Between Acculturation and Conversion', pp. 28–9.

774. Cano, 'Ḥasday ibn Shaprūṭ'.
775. Ibn Abī Uṣaybiʿa, *ʿUyūn al-Anbāʾ*, vol. II, p. 50; al-Andalusī, *Ṭabaqāt al-ʾUmam*, pp. 203–4.
776. Ashtor, *The Jews of Moslem Spain*, vol. I, pp. 167; al-Zarhūnī, *al-Ṭibb*, p. 35; Ibn Juljul, *Ṭabaqāt al-Aṭibbāʾ*, p. 22.
777. Cano, 'Ḥasday Ibn Shaprūṭ'; Theriac was probably invented by Andromachus of Crete for the Roman emperor Nero; it was composed of sixty-one ingredients and used to cure many diseases in the time of the Roman Empire. With time, the way to prepare the drug was forgotten, but it is possible that Ḥasday's command of the Latin language enabled him to discover the way to make it again. Al-Khālidī, *al-Yahūd Taḥta Ḥukm al-Muslimīn*, pp. 135–6; Ashtor, *The Jews of Moslem Spain*, vol. I, pp. 161–2.
778. Cano, 'Ḥasday Ibn Shaprūṭ'.
779. Roth, 'Medicine', p. 434; Cano, 'Ḥasday Ibn Shaprūṭ'.
780. Cano, 'Ḥasday Ibn Shaprūṭ'; Ashtor, *The Jews of Moslem Spain*, vol. I, pp. 162–3.
781. Cano, 'Ḥasday Ibn Shaprūṭ'.
782. Ibn Abī Uṣaybiʿa, *ʿUyūn al-Anbāʾ*, vol. II, p. 50; Finkel, 'An Eleventh Century Source', p. 51.
783. Cano, 'Ḥasday Ibn Shaprūṭ'.
784. In 1066 he was in his youth.
785. Friedenwald, *The Jews and Medicine*, p. 633.
786. Ibn Abī Uṣaybiʿa, *ʿUyūn al-Anbāʾ*, vol. II, pp. 50–1; al-Shantarīnī, *al-Dhakhīra*, pp. 458–9; al-Andalusī, *Ṭabaqāt al-ʾUmam*, pp. 204–5.
787. Steinschneider, *Die Arabische Literatur der Juden*, p. 100 n. 3.
788. Abū Jaʿfar b. al-Mustaʿīn biʾllāh Sulaymān b. Muḥammad b. Hūd, the second member of the 'Banū Hūd' family, which ruled Saragossa and Denia in the years 1046–1181.
789. al-Shantarīnī, *al-Dhakhīra*, pp. 458–9.
790. A medical ointment for wounds and pains; among its various ingredients are cotton and fenugreek seeds.
791. al-Shantarīnī, *al-Dhakhīra*, pp. 486–7.
792. Steinschneider, *Die Arabische Literatur der Juden*, pp. 148–9; Friedenwald, *The Jews and Medicine*, pp. 174, 633; Alfonso, 'Ibn Ḥasday, Joseph'; Sarton, *Introduction to the History of Science*, vol. II, pp. 229–30; Roth, *Medicine*, p. 435.
793. Ben-Sasson, 'The Maimonidean Dynasty', pp. 1–2.

794. Most of the data we have, though, concerns the first two members of this dynasty, Moses Maimonides and his son Abraham. See for example Russ-Fishbane, *Judaism, Sufism, and the Pietists of Medieval Egypt.*
795. See in detail Mazor and Lev, 'Dynasties of Jewish Physicians'; Mazor and Lev, 'The Phenomenon'.
796. Freimann, 'The Genealogy of Moses Maimonides' Family', pp. 9–11; Kraemer, *Maimonides*, pp. 230, 538 n. 103.
797. Ibid.
798. ENA 2558.15.
799. TS Ar.53.55; ENA 4011.45.
800. For more about his life see Mazor, 'Maimonides' Apostasy'.
801. See in depth Eddé, *Saladin*, pp. 414–16.
802. Kraemer, *Maimonides*, pp. 445–6.
803. A vast amount of literature has been produced on Maimonides' medical writing; see in detail Caballero-Navas, 'Medicine among Medieval Jews', pp. 325–6.
804. Plenty of articles and books have been written about Maimonides and his various activities and achievements; since it is impossible to mention them all in his biography, we have chosen the most relevant to the current book. See for example Nicolae, 'Jewish Physicians at the Court of Saladin', pp. 14–18.
805. Rustow claimed that he also served as physician to al-Malik al-ʿĀdil (1200–18); see Rustow, 'At the Limits of Communal Autonomy', p. 133.
806. Ibn Abī Uṣaybiʿa, *ʿUyūn al-Anbāʾ*, vol. II, p. 118; Steinschneider, *Die Arabische Literatur der Juden*, n. 159; Meyerhof, 'Jewish Physicians Contemporaries of Maimonides', p. 451; Ramaḍān, *al-Yahūd fī Miṣr*, p. 450; Sarton, *Introduction to the History of Science*, vol. II, p. 376. Regarding his family connections see Ben-Sasson, 'The Maimonidean Dynasty'.
807. Zinger, 'Women, Gender and Law', p. 15.
808. Frenkel, *The Compassionate and Benevolent.*
809. There is extensive research on Abraham's pietist lifestyle and leadership, recently discussed in Russ-Fishbane, *Judaism, Sufism and the Pietists of Medieval Egypt.*
810. Goitein, *A Mediterranean Society*, vol. VI, pp. 28–9.
811. Katsh, 'From the Moscow Manuscript', pp. 140–1.
812. Fenton, 'Maimonides, David ben Abraham'.
813. Bareket, 'David ben Joshua Maimonides'; Goitein, *A Mediterranean Society*, V, p. 473 nn 267–270.

814. Gil, *Palestine during the First Muslim Period*, vol. II, pp. 186–8, no. 100.
815. Bareket, *Abraham ha-Kohen*; Mann, *The Jews in Egypt and in Palestine*, pp. 28, 83, 95, 100, 129, 143, 180, 183; Gil, 'Review of Historical Research', p. 26; Goitein, *A Mediterranean Society*, vol. II, p. 118 n. 102.
816. Goitein, *A Mediterranean Society*, vol. II, p. 243.
817. Gil, 'Review of Historical Research', p. 26.
818. Bareket, *Abraham ha-Kohen*.
819. Goitein, *A Mediterranean Society*, vol. II, pp. 243–4.
820. Goitein, *Palestinian Jewry*, pp. 185–6; Goitein, *A Mediterranean Society*, vol. V, pp. 419–20 n. 27.
821. Bareket, 'Ibn Furāt Abraham'.
822. According to Makdisi, al-Malik al-Afḍal bought from Ephraim 20,000 books in order to prevent their expatriation to Iraq. See in detail Makdisi, *The Rise of Humanism*, p. 333.
823. Ibn Abī Uṣaybiʿa, *ʿUyūn al-Anbāʾ*, vol. II, p. 105–6; al-Ṣafadī, *Wāfī bi-l-Wafayāt* (2000), vol. IX, p. 175; Roth, 'Medicine', p. 435; Roth, *Jews, Visigoths and Muslims*, p. 180; Miller, 'Doctors without Borders', pp. 113, 117; Ramaḍān, *al-Yahūd fī Miṣr*, p. 436–7; Meyerhof, 'Von Alexandrien nach Bagdad'; Meyerhof, 'Medieval Jewish Physicians in the Near East', pp. 442–3.
824. Goitein, *A Mediterranean Society*, vol. III, p. 157 n. 74, vol. V, p. 4.
825. TS AS 151.241.
826. TS 16.261.
827. TS NS 324.67.
828. Yeshaya, 'Darʿī, Moses ben Abraham'; Weinberger, 'Moses Darʿī', pp. 445, 450, 452, 454.
829. Ibid.
830. Ibid.
831. Weinberger, 'Moses Darʿī', p. 450, 452, 454.
832. Roth, *Jews, Visigoths and Muslims*, p. 115.
833. Bos, *Maimonides on Asthma*, pp. 102–5; Alfonso, 'Ibn al-Muʿallim, Solomon'.
834. Roth, *Jews, Visigoths and Muslims*, p. 88. Salvatierra, 'Ibn Qamniʾel, Meʾir'.
835. Schirmann, 'Studies of the Research Institute', pp. 267, 268–9.
836. Friedenwald, *The Jews and Medicine*, p. 634; Salvatierra, 'Ibn Qamniʾel, Meʾir'.
837. al-Khālidī, *al-Yahūd Taḥta Ḥukm al-Muslimīn*, p. 356; Friedenwald, *The Jews and Medicine*, p. 634; Weisz, 'The Jewish Physicians', p. 27.

838. Ibn Abī Uṣaybiʿa, *ʿUyūn al-Anbāʾ*, vol. II, pp. 30–1; al-ʿUmarī, *Masālik al-Abṣār*, p. 264; Ibn al-Qifṭī, *Taʾrīkh al-Ḥukamāʾ*, p. 209.
839. Ḥaddād, *Riḥlat Ibn Yūna*, p. 122 n. 3, where Judah is accidentally mentioned as Judah b. Ayyūb (instead of Abūn).
840. Ibn Abī Uṣaybiʿa, *ʿUyūn al-Anbāʾ*, vol. II, pp. 30–1; al-ʿUmarī, *Masālik al-Abṣār*, pp. 264.
841. Ibn al-Qifṭī, *Taʾrīkh al-Ḥukamāʾ*, p. 209.
842. Fischel, 'Azarbaijan in Jewish History', p. 3; Ibn al-Qifṭī, *Taʾrīkh al-Ḥukamāʾ*, p. 209.
843. al-ʿUmarī, *Masālik al-Abṣār*, p. 264.
844. Ibn Abī Uṣaybiʿa, *ʿUyūn al-Anbāʾ*, vol. II, p. 31; Ibn al-Qifṭī, *Taʾrīkh al-Ḥukamāʾ*, p. 209.
845. Perlmann, 'Samauʾal al-Maghribī'.
846. Wasserstein, 'Samauʾal ben Judah'.
847. Stroumsa, 'On Jewish Intellectuals Who Converted'.
848. Roth, 'Medicine', p. 435; Ramaḍān, *al-Yahūd fī Miṣr*, p. 434; Molad-Vaza, 'Clothing in the Mediterranean Jewish Society', p. 40; Goitein, *A Mediterranean Society*, vol. III, p. 19 n. 21.
849. Greenstone, 'Two Memorial Lists from the Genizah', pp. 47, 54.
850. For example Goitein, 'The Title and Office of the Nagid', p. 117.
851. Ramaḍān, *al-Yahūd fī Miṣr*, p. 434; Goitein, *Palestinian Jewry*, p. 53.
852. Gil, *Palestine during the First Muslim Period*, vol. I, p. 490; Bareket, *Abraham ha-Kohen*, pp. 4, 19; Goitein, *Palestinian Jewry*, p. 53; Cohen, *Jewish Self-Government*, pp. 157–9; Ramaḍān, *al-Yahūd fī Miṣr*, p. 434; Molad-Vaza, 'Clothing in the Mediterranean Jewish Society', p. 40.
853. Rustow, 'Mevorakh ben Saʿadya'; Sela, 'The Head of the Rabbanite, Karaite and Samaritan Jews', p. 260; for more about his activity see Rustow, 'The Diplomatics of Leadership', pp. 324–31.
854. Rustow, 'Judah ben Saʿadya'; for more about his activity see Rustow, 'The Diplomatics of Leadership', pp. 324–31; for more on his career see Cohen, *Jewish Self-Government*, pp. 158–71; Hary and Rustow, 'Karaites at the Rabbinical Court', pp. *25–*26.
855. See for example: Simonsohn, *The Jews in Sicily*, nos 66, 83, 88, 97, 98, 122, 143.
856. Udovitch, 'International Commerce and Society', pp. 239–40, 245.
857. Gil, *In the Kingdom of Ishmael*, vol. III, p. 131 n. 22.
858. Rustow, 'Judah ben Saʿadya'.

859. Miller, 'Doctors without Borders', p. 117.
860. Ramaḍān, *al-Yahūd fī Miṣr*, p. 434; Goitein, *Palestinian Jewry*, p. 53; Goitein, *A Mediterranean Society*, vol. VI, p. 75.
861. Rustow, 'Moses ben Mevorakh'.
862. Ashtor, *The History of the Jews in Egypt and Syria*, vol. I, p. 41, Mann, *The Jews in Egypt and in Palestine*, vol. I, p. 207 ff.
863. Gil, *Palestine during the First Muslim Period*, vol. II, pp. 491–2.
864. Signed as a witness to a marriage agreement (*ketubah*) in 1043.
865. Goitein, *A Mediterranean Society*, vol. III, p. 207.
866. TS 10J6.6.
867. Goitein and Friedman, *India Book I*, pp. 45–6.
868. Bodl. MS. heb. b. 13, fol. 39; regarding Moses b. Jekuthiel and his lineage see for example Goitein and Friedman, *India Book I*, pp. 39–42.
869. Goitein and Friedman, *India Book I*, p. 39, and n. 46 on the possibility of him being a physician; Cohen, *Poverty and Charity*, p. 66 n. 167.
870. Goitein and Friedman, *India Book I*, pp. 39–42, 45–116.
871. Zinger, 'Women, Gender and Law', p. 168.
872. Ibid., p. 41.
873. Bodl. MS. heb. b. 13, fol. 39.
874. Goitein and Friedman. *India Book I*, pp. 41–2.
875. Abū al-Ṣalt, 'al-Risāla al-Miṣriyya', vol. I, pp. 35–7; Ibn al-Qifṭī, *Taʾrīkh al-Ḥukamā*, pp. 209–10; Ibn Abī Uṣaybiʿa, *ʿUyūn al-Anbāʾ*, vol. II, p. 107; Ramaḍān, *al-Yahūd fī Miṣr*, pp. 437–8; Steinschneider, *Die Arabische Literatur der Juden*, n. 143; Meyerhof, 'Medieval Jewish Physicians in the Near East', p. 443; Roth, *Jews, Visigoths and Muslims*, p. 180.
876. Ibn Abī Uṣaybiʿa, *ʿUyūn al-Anbāʾ*, vol. II, p. 107; Ramaḍān, *al-Yahūd fī Miṣr*, p. 438; Steinschneider, *Die Arabische Literatur der Juden*, n. 144; Meyerhof, 'Medieval Jewish Physicians in the Near East', p. 443; Roth, *Jews, Visigoths and Muslims*, p. 180. On his father see Ibn al-Qifṭī, *Taʾrīkh al-Ḥukamāʾ*, pp. 209–10.
877. Frenkel, *The Compassionate and Benevolent*, pp. 143–4, 212.
878. See in detail Mazor and Lev, 'Dynasties of Jewish Physicians', pp. 244–51.
879. Goitein, *A Mediterranean Society*, vol. II, pp. 245, 576 n. 21; TS 16.1.
880. TS 16.1.
881. Gil, *Palestine during the First Muslim Period*, vol. III, pp. 25–6.
882. Frenkel, *The Compassionate and Benevolent*, p. 143. According to Frenkel, however, in this letter Judah made use of Yeshūʿā b. Aaron, his cousin who

served as a court physician in Cairo, to help his *brother* get a licence to practise medicine. Transcription and (Hebrew) translation of the letter is on pp. 410–17. See also Goitein, *A Mediterranean Society*, vol. II, pp. 249–50.

883. ENA 2806.2.
884. Gil, *Palestine during the First Muslim Period*, vol. III, pp. 25–6.
885. Frenkel, *The Compassionate and Benevolent*, p. 97; Goitein, *A Mediterranean Society*, vol. II, p. 576 n. 21.
886. Frenkel, *The Compassionate and Benevolent*, pp. 95, 100–1.
887. Ibid., pp. 95–6; Goitein, *A Mediterranean Society*, vol. II, pp. 258, 264, 580 nn. 96, 99.
888. Bareket, 'Alexandria', p. 18; Frenkel, *The Compassionate and Benevolent*, pp. 163–4.
889. Frenkel, *The Compassionate and Benevolent*, pp. 94–5.
890. Goitein, *A Mediterranean Society*, vol. II, p. 320.
891. Frenkel, *The Compassionate and Benevolent*, pp. 98–101.
892. Brody, 'Ahron Alʿamani und seine Sohne', p. 20; Mann, *The Jews in Egypt and in Palestine*, vol. II, p. 305.
893. Goitein, *A Mediterranean Society*, vol. IV, p. 443 n. 184.
894. Ibid., vol. IV, pp. 251, 443 n. 184; Frenkel, *The Compassionate and Benevolent*, p. 143.
895. Frenkel, *The Compassionate and Benevolent*, pp. 132, 143, 148; for example, Judah's name appeared on a certificate from 1243 indicating a cheese was kosher. More documents handwritten by Judah exist dating from 1207–43; see Zeldes and Frenkel, 'The Sicilian Trade', pp. 136–7.
896. Frenkel, *The Compassionate and Benevolent*, pp. 142–9, 180.
897. For a transcription and (Hebrew) translation of this letter see Frenkel, *The Compassionate and Benevolent*, pp. 365–72; see also Goitein, *A Mediterranean Society*, vol. I, pp. 24–7, vol. II, p. 576 n. 21.
898. Goitein, *A Mediterranean Society*, vol. II, p. 576 n. 21; Mann, *The Jews in Egypt and in Palestine*, vol. II, p. 305.
899. Goitein, *A Mediterranean Society*, vol. II, pp. 249–50, 576 n. 21.
900. Frenkel, *The Compassionate and Benevolent*, p. 143.
901. Frenkel, *The Compassionate and Benevolent* ,pp. 365–72; Goitein, *A Mediterranean Society*, vol. I, pp. 24–7, vol. II, p. 576 n. 21.
902. Netzer, 'The Fate of the Jewish Community of Tabriz'.
903. Netzer, 'Rashīd al-Dīn', p. 122.
904. Ibid.

905. Moreen, 'Rashīd al-Dīn Ṭabīb'; Fischel, 'Azarbaijan in Jewish History', pp. 16, 18; for more about his life and Jewish origin see: Netzer, 'Rashīd al-Dīn'; Morgan, 'Rashīd al-Dīn Ṭabīb'.
906. According to Fischel, 'Azarbaijan in Jewish History', p. 13.
907. According to Moreen, 'Rashīd al-Dīn Ṭabīb'.
908. Moreen, 'Rashīd al-Dīn Ṭabīb'; Fischel, 'Azarbaijan in Jewish History', pp. 16–18.
909. Klein-Franke and Zhu, 'Rashīd al-Dīn'; for more see Krawulsky, *The Mongol Īlkhāns*.
910. Fischel, 'Azarbaijan in Jewish History', pp. 14, 17 n. 36.
911. Chipman, 'The ʿAllāma and the Ṭabīb'.
912. TS 16.176.
913. Ibid.
914. Sela, 'The Head of the Rabbanite, Karaite and Samaritan Jews', p. 261. Based on Goitein, *A Mediterranean Society*, vol. II, p. 33.
915. Physician and leader of the Jews in Fusṭāṭ between 1140 and 1159.
916. Sela, 'The Head of the Rabbanite, Karaite and Samaritan Jews' pp. 260–1.
917. Goitein, *A Mediterranean Society*, vol. II, pp. 32, 528 n. 46.
918. Fenton, 'Jewish–Muslim Relations'; Goitein, *A Mediterranean Society*, vol. II, pp. 32, 247–8, 528 n. 46, vol. IV, p. 313; Luṭf, *Yahūd Miṣr al-Ayyūbiya*, p. 92; Ramaḍān, *al-Yahūd fī Miṣr*, pp. 440–1; Meyerhof, 'Medieval Jewish Physicians in the Near East', p. 446; Friedman, 'Maimonides, Zūṭā and the Muqaddams', p. 475 n. 8; Bareket, 'Nethanel ben Moses ha-Levi'.
919. Kraemer, *Maimonides*, pp. 220–2, 267–8.
920. Sela, 'The Head of the Rabbanite, Karaite and Samaritan Jews', pp. 260–1; Goitein, 'A New Autograph by Maimonides', pp. 191–2; Neubauer, 'Egyptian Fragments', pp. 541–4.
921. TS 13J25.16.
922. Goitein, 'A New Autograph by Maimonides', pp. 191–2.
923. Goitein, *A Mediterranean Society*, vol. II, p. 244; see Neubauer, 'Egyptian Fragments', p. 548.
924. Friedman, 'Maimonides, Zūṭā and the Muqaddams'.
925. Ibn Abī Uṣaybiʿa, who praised Abū al-Faḍl's generous character, noted that his income from one day of work was more than 300 black dirhams; see Ibn Abī Uṣaybiʿa, *ʿUyūn al-Anbāʾ*, vol. II, p. 115–16.
926. Steinschneider, *Die Arabische Literatur der Juden*, n. 151; Meyerhof, 'Medieval Jewish Physicians in the Near East', p. 445; Ramaḍān, *al-Yahūd fī Miṣr*,

p. 445; al-Ṣafadī, *Kitāb al-Wāfī bi-l-Wafayāt* (2000), vol. XXIV, p. 14; Luṭf, *Yahūd Miṣr al-Ayyūbiya*, p. 93.

927. See Goitein, *A Mediterranean Society*, vol. I, p. 250, vol. III, p. 327 n. 58, vol. IV, pp. 286, 317–18; Goitein and Friedman, *India Book 1*, p. 258; Ashtor, 'The Number of Jews in Mediaeval Egypt', 19(1–4), p. 5 n. 288.
928. Ibn Abī Uṣaybiʿa, *ʿUyūn al-Anbāʾ*, vol. II, pp. 115–16; Meyerhof, 'Medieval Jewish Physicians in the Near East', p. 445.
929. Bodl. MS heb. f. 56, fol. 50.
930. Mentioned as physician: ENA 2735.1.
931. Bodl. MS heb. f. 56, fol. 122.
932. Goitein, *A Mediterranean Society*, vol. II, p. 244; Ashtor, *The History of the Jews in Egypt and Syria*, vol. I, p. 41.
933. al-Maqrīzī, *Ittiʿāẓ al-Ḥunafāʾ*, vol. III, pp. 153–5; Roth, 'Medicine', p. 441; Bareket, 'Samuel (Abū Mansur) ben Hananiah'; Mann, *The Jews in Egypt and in Palestine*, vol. II, pp. 281–4.
934. Goitein and Friedman, *India Book IV/B*, pp. 431–41, no. 79; Goitein and Friedman, *India Book IV/A*, pp. 227 ff.
935. Bodl. MS heb. f. 56, fol. 122; Bodl. MS heb. f. 61, fol. 42.
936. Goitein, *Palestinian Jewry*, p. 327.
937. Motzkin, 'Elijah ben Zechariah', p. 339.
938. Goitein, *Palestinian Jewry*, p. 327.
939. Goitein, 'Meeting in Jerusalem', pp. 46–7; Goitein, *A Mediterranean Society*, vol. III, p. 245 nn. 158, 159, vol. V, pp. 174, 305; Goitein, *Palestinian Jewry*, pp. 321–7; Motzkin, 'A Thirteenth-Century Jewish Physician', p. 344; Amar and Lev, *Physicians, Drugs and Remedies*, p. 105; Ramaḍān, *al-Yahūd fī Miṣr*, p, 449; Luṭf, *Yahūd Miṣr al-Ayyūbiya*, p. 93.
940. Goitein, *Palestinian Jewry*, pp. 321–6, 262–75.
941. Goitein, *A Mediterranean Society*, vol. II, p. 380; Goitein, *Palestinian Jewry*, p. 322. Goitein suggests that Abū Zikrī might have served al-Malik al-Kāmil as a physician; also mentioned in Ramaḍān, *al-Yahūd fī Miṣr*, p. 449. For more information regarding the private and professional life of Abū Zikrī (studied from his letters), see Rustow, 'Formal and Informal Patronage', pp. 363, 369–70.
942. Goitein, *A Mediterranean Society*, vol. II, pp. 207, 318, 491–2.
943. Motzkin, 'The Arabic Correspondence of Judge Elijah', p. 32–3.
944. Although according to Motzkin, 'The Arabic Correspondence of Judge Elijah', p. 32, Abū Zikrī was born in 1197.

945. Goitein, *Palestinian Jewry*, pp. 321–6; Amar and Lev, *Physicians, Drugs and Remedies*, p. 105.
946. Goitein, 'Meeting in Jerusalem', p. 47.
947. Goitein, *A Mediterranean Society*, vol. II, p. 380 n. 31.
948. Ibid., vol. II, p. 380.
949. Motzkin, 'The Arabic Correspondence of Judge Elijah', p. 33.
950. Goitein, *A Mediterranean Society*, vol. I, p. 64 n. 3.
951. Motzkin, 'A Thirteenth-Century Jewish Physician', pp. 344–9; Goitein, *A Mediterranean Society*, vol. III, p. 264 nn. 88–9.
952. Goitein, *A Mediterranean Society*, vol. IV, p. 259 nn. 36–7.
953. Ibid., vol. III, p. 494.
954. Goitein, 'Meeting in Jerusalem', pp. 46–7; Goitein, *A Mediterranean Society*, vol. III, p. 245 nn. 158, 159, vol. V, pp. 174, 305; Goitein, *Palestinian Jewry*, pp. 326–7; Motzkin, 'A Thirteenth-Century Jewish Physician', p. 344; Amar and Lev, *Physicians, Drugs and Remedies*, p. 105; Ramaḍān, *al-Yahūd fī Miṣr*, p, 449; Luṭf, *Yahūd Miṣr al-Ayyūbiya*, p. 93.
955. Ibn Abī Uṣaybiʿa, *ʿUyūn al-Anbāʾ*, vol. II, pp. 213–14.
956. Steinschneider, 'An Introduction to the Arabic Literature of the Jews II', 13(1), p. 93 n. 1; Meyerhof, 'Medieval Jewish Physicians in the Near East', p. 453.
957. Ruled Egypt and Syria (1143–1218).
958. The fifth Ayyubid ruler in Damascus and ruler of Karak (1206–58).
959. Yahalom and Blau, *The Wanderings of Judah Alharizi*, p. 35.
960. Ibn Abī Uṣaybiʿa, *ʿUyūn al-Anbāʾ*, vol. II, pp. 213–14.
961. Ibid., vol. II, p. 179.
962. Ibid., vol. II, p. 193; Steinschneider, 'An Introduction to the Arabic Literature of the Jews II', 13(1), p. 93.
963. Ibn Abī Uṣaybiʿa, *ʿUyūn al-Anbāʾ*, vol. II, p. 214.
964. Miller, 'Doctors without Borders', p. 113.
965. al-Ṣafadī, *Kitāb al-Wāfī bi-l-Wafayāt* (2000), vol. XXIII, pp. 57–8.
966. Yahalom and Blau, *The Wanderings of Judah Alharizi*, p. 58, ll. 74–80, p. 83, ll. 118–21, p. 217, ll. 366–7, p. 234, ll. 665–8.
967. Meyerhoff, 'Medieval Jewish Physicians in the Near East', p. 453.
968. al-Ṣafadī, *Kitāb al-Wāfī bi-l-Wafayāt* (2000), vol. XXIII, pp. 57–8; Eddé, 'Les Médecins dans la société syrienne', p. 104.
969. Goitein, *A Mediterranean Society*, vol. IV, p. 351 n. 65.
970. Mosseri VII.9.5.
971. TS 10J7.16.

972. TS AS 145.9.
973. Frenkel, *The Compassionate and Benevolent*, doc. 3, pp. 248–51; see also Goitein, *A Mediterranean Society*, vol. IV, p. 238.
974. Ibid.
975. Ibid.
976. TS 13J3.27.
977. Goitein, *A Mediterranean Society*, vol. II, p. 579.
978. TS K6 149.
979. Wasserstein, 'What's in a Name?', pp. 145–6.
980. Steinschneider, 'An Introduction to the Arabic Literature of the Jews I', 11(3), p. 489. This ʿAfīf lived in Damascus (and not in Aleppo as mentioned). He is not explicitly mentioned as a Jew, though according to his name and his friendship with the Sufi Ibn Hūd, who was known for his relations with the Jews of Damascus, it is plausible to assume that he was a Jew. On Ibn Hūd see Goldziher, 'Ibn Hūd', p. 220.
981. al-ʿUmarī, *Masālik al-Abṣār*, vol. IX, pp. 277.
982. Mazor and Lev, 'The Phenomenon'.
983. The reference is to al-Malik al-ʿĀdil Maḥmūd Nūr al-Dīn Zengī (also known as al-Shahīd) (1118–74).
984. A unit of area. One *faddan* equals about 4,200 square metres.
985. Ibn Abī Uṣaybiʿa, *ʿUyūn al-Anbāʾ*, vol. II, pp. 163–4; al-Ṣafadī, *Kitāb al-Wāfī bi-l-Wafayāt* (2000), vol. XV, pp. 180–1; al-ʿUmarī, *Masālik al-Abṣār*, vol. IX, pp. 277–8.
986. al-ʿUmarī, *Masālik al-Abṣār*, vol. IX, p. 277.
987. Ibn Abī Uṣaybiʿa mentions him by the name ʿAfīf b. ʿAbd al-Qāhir Sukra (*ʿUyūn al-Anbāʾ*, vol. II, p. 164). Al-Ṣafadī distorted this name to ʿAfīf b. ʿAbd al-Qādir b. Sukra (*Wāfī bi-l-wafayāt*, vol. XX, p. 233), from which we might mistakenly assume that he was Sukra's grandson. However, since Sukra treated Nūr al-Dīn's mistress between 1154 and 1174, and since ʿAfīf composed a medical treatise for Saladin in 1188, he must have been Sukra's son.
988. Ibn Abī Uṣaybiʿa, *ʿUyūn al-Anbāʾ*, vol. II, p. 164; al-Ṣafadī, *Kitāb al-Wāfī bi-l-Wafayāt* (2000), vol. XX, p. 59.
989. Steinschneider, *Die Arabische Literatur der Juden*, p. 194; Ashtor-Strauss, *Saladin and the Jews*, pp. 311–12; Ibn Abī Uṣaybiʿa, *ʿUyūn al-Anbāʾ*. vol. II, p. 164.
990. According to Ibn Abī Uṣaybiʿa, ʿAfīf ibn Sukra dedicated his treatise on colic to Saladin in 1188.

991. Steinschneider, *Die Arabische Literatur der Juden*, p. 194; see in detail Nicolae, 'A Medieval Court Physician at Work', p. 67.
992. See Steinschneider, *Die Arabische Literatur der Juden*, p. 194; Ashtor-Strauss, *Saladin and the Jews*, p. 311.
993. Nicolae, 'A Medieval Court Physician at Work', p. 67.
994. Ibn Abī Uṣaybiʿa, *ʿUyūn al-Anbāʾ*, vol. II, p. 164.
995. al-ʿUmarī, *Masālik al-Abṣār*, vol. IX, p. 277.
996. Eddé, 'Les Médecins dans la société syrienne', p. 103.
997. Goitein, *A Mediterranean Society*, vol. III, pp. 9–11.
998. For a detailed discussion of the physicians of the Ibn Ṣaghīr/Ibn Kūjik dynasty, see Mazor, 'Jewish Court Physicians'; Mazor and Lev, 'The Phenomenon'.
999. For more about this physician and his writing see Hoki, 'Dāniyāl ibn Shuʿyā's Ophthalmologic Question-and-Answer Textbook'; Goitein, *A Mediterranean Society*, vol. III, pp. 9-10.
1000. Hoki, 'Dāniyāl ibn Shuʿyā's Ophthalmologic Question-and-Answer Textbook', pp. 71–2.
1001. Ramaḍān, *al-Yahūd fī Miṣr*, p. 451.
1002. Luṭf, *Yahūd Miṣr al-Ayyūbiya*, p. 96; Ibn Abī Uṣaybiʿa, *ʿUyūn al-Anbāʾ*, vol. II, p. 118; Meyerhof, 'Medieval Jewish Physicians in the Near East', pp. 450–1.
1003. For more about this physician and his writing see Hoki, 'Dāniyāl ibn Shuʿyā's Ophthalmologic Question-and-Answer Textbook'.
1004. Bareket, 'Abu 'l-Munajja'; Goitein, *A Mediterranean Society*, vol. II, pp. 356–8, vol. III, pp. 9–11; Mann, *The Jews in Egypt and in Palestine*, vol. I, pp. 215–17, vol. II, pp. 264–9, 382.
1005. Ibn Abī Uṣaybiʿa, *ʿUyūn al-Anbāʾ*, vol. II, p. 118; Ramaḍān, *al-Yahūd fī Miṣr*, p. 451.
1006. Meyerhof, 'Jewish Physicians Contemporaries of Maimonides', p. 395; Ibn Abī Uṣaybiʿa, *ʿUyūn al-Anbāʾ*, vol. II, pp. 233–4; al-Ṣafadī, *Kitāb al-Wāfī bi-l-Wafayāt* (2000), vol. XXIX, p. 89.
1007. Meyerhof, 'Jewish Physicians Contemporaries of Maimonides', pp. 395–6; al-ʿUmarī, *Masālik al-Abṣār*, vol. IX, pp. 290–1; Ibn Abī Uṣaybiʿa, *ʿUyūn al-Anbāʾ*, vol. II, pp. 233–4; Wedel, 'Transfer of Knowledge', pp. 3.79–3.80.
1008. Meyerhof, 'Jewish Physicians Contemporaries of Maimonides', p. 396; al-Ṣafadī, *Kitāb al-Wāfī bi-l-Wafayāt* (2000), vol. XXIX, p. 89; al-ʿUmarī, *Masālik al-Abṣār*, vol. XIX, pp. 290–1; Ashtor, *The Jews and the Mediterranean Economy*, pp. 152–3.

1009. Meyerhof, 'Jewish Physicians Contemporaries of Maimonides', p. 396.
1010. Ibid., p. 396; Steinschneider, 'An Introduction to the Arabic Literature of the Jews II', 13(1), p. 93.
1011. Jadon, 'A Comparison of the Wealth', p. 66.
1012. He appeared in Ibn Abī Uṣaybiʿa's writing as Al-Ṣāḥib Amīn al-Dawla: see *ʿUyūn al-Anbāʾ*, vol. II, pp. 234–5. See also al-Ṣafadī, *Kitāb al-Wāfī bi-l-Wafayāt* (2000), vol. XII, pp. 65–6; al-ʿUmarī, *Masālik al-Abṣār*, vol. IX, p. 292; Meyerhof, 'Jewish Physicians Contemporaries of Maimonides', p. 396; Wedel, 'Transfer of Knowledge', pp. 3.80–3.81.
1013. al-Ṣafadī, *Kitāb al-Wāfī bi-l-Wafayāt* (2000), vol. XII, pp. 65–6; al-ʿUmarī, *Masālik al-Abṣār*, vol. IX, pp. 291–2; Meyerhof, 'Jewish Physicians Contemporaries of Maimonides', p. 396; Eddé, 'Les Médecins dans la société syrienne', p. 103.
1014. al-Ṣafadī, *Kitāb al-Wāfī bi-l-Wafayāt* (2000), vol. XII, p. 66.
1015. Sbath, 'Le Formulaire des hôpitaux'.
1016. Lev, Chipman and Niessen, 'A Hospital Handbook for the Community'.
1017. Ashtor-Strauss, 'Saladin and the Jews', p. 311 n. 21, notes that the year of al-Bayān's death and the period of his retirement as reported by Ibn Abī Uṣaybiʿa are not necessarily reconcilable. Ibn Abī Uṣaybiʿa, *ʿUyūn al-Anbāʾ*, vol. II, p. 115; al-Ṣafadī, *Kitāb al-Wāfī bi-l-Wafayāt* (2000), vol. XV, p. 80; Nicolae, 'Jewish Physicians at the Court of Saladin', p. 19; Ramaḍān, *al-Yahūd fī Miṣr*, p. 442; Luṭf, *Yahūd Miṣr al-Ayyūbiya*, pp. 91–2; Steinschneider, *Die Arabische Literatur der Juden*, n. 153; Meyerhof, 'Medieval Jewish Physicians in the Near East', p. 445; Jadon, 'A Comparison of the Wealth', p. 67.
1018. Ramaḍān, *al-Yahūd fī Miṣr*, p. 442 n. 1, no. 26, p. 94.
1019. Sbath, 'Le Formulaire des hôpitaux'; Lev, Chipman and Niessen, 'A Hospital Handbook for the Community'.
1020. Ibn Abī Uṣaybiʿa, *ʿUyūn al-Anbāʾ*, vol. II, p. 118–19; Meyerhof, 'Jewish Physicians Contemporaries of Maimonides', pp. 393–4; Ramaḍān, *al-Yahūd fī Miṣr*, p. 449–50; Steinschneider, *Die Arabische Literatur der Juden*, n. 154; Meyerhof, 'Medieval Jewish Physicians in the Near East', p. 452.
1021. TS K6 149.
1022. Ibid.
1023. TS K15.6.
1024. Miller, 'Doctors without Borders', p. 113; Kaḥāla, *Muʿjam al-Muʾallifīn*, vol. IV, p. 56. See detailed biography in Nicolae, 'Jewish Physicians at the Court of Saladin', pp. 8–14.

1025. For more about Ibn Jumayʿ's life, see Nicolae, 'A Medieval Court Physician at Work', pp. 31–43; Eddé, *Saladin*, p. 414. For Jewish physicians practising in Muslim courts in general, and Ibn Jumayʿ's religion in particular, see Nicolae, 'A Medieval Court Physician at Work', pp. 54–74.
1026. Ibn Abī Uṣaybiʿa, *ʿUyūn al-Anbāʾ*, vol. II, pp. 112–15; Steinschneider, *Die Arabische Literatur der Juden*, n. 145; Meyerhof, 'Medieval Jewish Physicians in the Near East', pp. 444–5; Jadon, 'A Comparison of the Wealth', p. 65; Miller, 'Doctors without Borders', p. 113; Mazor and Lev, 'A mosaic of medieval historical sources'.
1027. For an English translation see Ibn Jumayʿ, *Treatise to Ṣalāḥ ad-Dīn*.
1028. Ibn Abī Uṣaybiʿa, *ʿUyūn al-Anbāʾ*, vol. II, pp. 112–15; Ramaḍān, *al-Yahūd fī Miṣr*, pp. 442–4; Jadon, 'A Comparison of the Wealth', pp. 74–5; Miller, 'Doctors without Borders', pp. 112; 117, 118; Ashtor-Strauss, 'Saladin and the Jews', p. 310.
1029. Nicolae, 'A Medieval Court Physician at Work', p. 73.
1030. Miller, 'Doctors without Borders', p. 113; for a detailed discussion regarding Ibn Jumayʿ's writings, see Nicolae, 'A Medieval Court Physician at Work', pp. 43–53.
1031. Luṭf, *Yahūd Miṣr al-Ayyūbiya*, p. 80; Goitein, *A Mediterranean Society*, vol. I, pp. 121–2 n. 44; Jadon, 'A Comparison of the Wealth', pp. 70–1.
1032. al-Maqrīzī, *al-Mawāʿiẓ*, vol. II, p. 368; Lev, *Saladin in Egypt*, p. 127; Ashtor, *The History of the Jews in Egypt and Syria*, vol. I, pp. 242–3.
1033. al-Dhahabī, *Taʾrīkh al-Islām*, vol. XLVIII, p. 299.
1034. Nicolae, 'Jewish Physicians at the Court of Saladin', p. 42.
1035. See in detail Nicolae, 'A Medieval Court Physician at Work', p. 62.
1036. Bodl. MS heb. f. 56, fol. 45.
1037. See Goitein, *A Mediterranean Society*, vol. II, pp. 249–51 with n. 42.
1038. Nicolae, 'A Medieval Court Physician at Work', pp. 40–51; Nicolae, 'Jewish Physicians at the Court of Saladin', p. 12; see also Ashtor, *The History of the Jews in Egypt and Syria*, vol. I, p. 237.
1039. Behrens-Abouseif, *The Book in Mamluk Egypt and Syria*, p. 148.
1040. TS 13J8.25.
1041. Halper (Dropsie) 467.
1042. Isaacs, *Medical and Para-medical Manuscripts*, no. 1081.
1043. Bodl. MS heb. c.13, fol. 6.
1044. Motzkin, 'The Arabic Correspondence of Judge Elijah', p. 19 n. 5; Ashtor, 'The Number of Jews in Mediaeval Egypt', 19(1–4), p. 19.

1045. Wien, N: H 85 (PER H 85); Goitein, *A Mediterranean Society*, vol. III, pp. 160–1, 461.

1046. Ashtor, *The History of the Jews in Egypt and Syria*, vol. I, p. 277; Steinschneider, *Die Arabische Literatur der Juden*, p. 245 n. 187; Meyerhof, 'Jewish Physicians Contemporaries of Maimonides', p. 399.

1047. Ibid.

1048. They are mentioned in the Kirmānī family tree; see Mann, *Texts and Studies*, p. 261.

1049. Goitein, *A Mediterranean Society*, vol. IV, p. 100 nn. 101–3; Richards, 'Arabic Documents', p. 111; Mann, *Texts and Studies*, p. 261.

1050. Ibn Kathīr, *al-Bidāya wa-l-Nihāya*, vol. XIV, p. 86.

1051. al-Yūnīnī, *Early Mamluk Syrian Historiography*, vol. II, p. 255 (English translation vol. I, pp. 206–7); Ibn Ḥajar al-ʿAsqalānī, *al-Durar al-Kāmina*, vol. II, p. 476; al-Ṣafadī, *Aʿyān al-ʿAṣr*, vol. III, p. 65; Ibn Kathīr, *al-Bidāya wa-l-Nihāya*, vol. XIV, p. 86; Ashtor, *The History of the Jews in Egypt and Syria*, vol. I, p. 288; el-Leithy, 'Coptic Culture and Conversion', pp. 173–4.

1052. See Goitein, *A Mediterranean Society*, vol. II, pp. 247, 421, 577; Goitein and Friedman, *India Traders of the Middle Ages*, vol. I, pp. 84–5 n. 94; Ashtor, *The History of the Jews in Egypt and Syria*, vol. II, p. 333.

1053. al-Yūnīnī, *Early Mamluk Syrian Historiography*, vol. II, p. 255 (English translation vol. I, p. 207).

1054. Goitein, *A Mediterranean Society*, vol. II, p. 246, vol. IV, pp. 453 n. 59, 640 n. 283.

1055. Ibn Ḥajar al-ʿAsqalānī, *al-Durar al-Kāmina*, vol. V, p. 237; al-Dhahabī, *Dhuyūl al-ʿIbar*, vol. IV, p. 173.

1056. al-Jazarī, *Ḥawādith al-Zamān*, vol. III, p. 821; Ashtor, *The History of the Jews in Egypt and Syria*, vol. I, p. 289.

1057. See Mazor and Lev, 'Dynasties of Jewish Physicians'.

1058. Mazor, 'Jewish Court Physicians', p. 61.

1059. al-Maqrīzī, *Kitāb al-Sulūk*, vol. II, pp. 187–8.

1060. Ashtor, *The History of the Jews in Egypt and Syria*, vol. I, pp. 282–3.

1061. al-Ṣafadī, *Kitāb al-Wāfī bi-l-Wafayāt* (2008–10), vol. V, pp. 314–17; al-Ṣafadī, *Aʿyān al-ʿAṣr*, vol. I, pp. 54–6; al-ʿUmarī, *Masālik al-Abṣār*, vol. IX, p. 361; Ibn Ḥajar al-ʿAsqalānī, *al-Durar al-Kāmina*, vol. I, p. 17. According to al-Jazarī, Ibrāhīm served (also?) as the 'Head of the Physicians' in Damascus; see al-Jazarī, *Ḥawādith al-Zamān*, vol. II, p. 168.

1062. al-ʿUmarī, *Masālik al-Abṣār*, vol. IX, p. 361.

1063. See Mazor, 'Jewish Court Physicians', pp. 43–5; Mazor, 'Ibn Ṣaghīr/Ibn Kūjik Family'.
1064. al-Sakhāwī, *al-Ḍawʾ al-Lāmiʿ*, vol. VI, p. 125.
1065. al-ʿUmarī, *Masālik al-Abṣār*, vol. IX, p. 363; Mazor, 'Jewish Court Physicians', p. 50.
1066. Ibn al-Nafīs was a personal physician of Sultan al-Ẓāhir Baybars (r. 1260–77); he moved from Damascus to Cairo, donated his home and library to the al-Manṣūrī hospital and even taught at the madrasa that was part of the hospital complex. On his social circle and professional network, which included Jewish students and physicians, see: Northrup, *Al-Bīmāristān al-Manṣūrī*, p. 26–7.
1067. For some examples of treatment see Mazor, 'Jewish Court Physicians', pp. 51–2.
1068. Mazor, 'Faraj Allāh Ibn Ṣaghīr'; Mazor, 'Jewish Court Physicians', p. 51.
1069. Mazor, 'Ibn Ṣaghīr/Ibn Kūjik Family'; Mazor, 'Jewish Court Physicians', pp. 50–2; Mazor, 'Faraj Allāh ibn Ṣaghīr'.
1070. Ashtor, *The History of the Jews in Egypt and Syria*, vol. II, p. 552.
1071. The loyal physician.
1072. Margoliouth, 'Ibn Al-Hītī's Arabic Chronicle', pp. 431–2; Mazor, 'Ibn Ṣaghīr/Ibn Kūjik Family'.
1073. Ashtor, *The History of the Jews in Egypt and Syria*, vol. II, p. 552.
1074. Meyerhof, 'Jewish Physicians Contemporaries of Maimonides', pp. 397–8. According to al-Ṣafadī, *Kitāb al-Wāfī bi-l-Wafayāt* (2000), vol. XV, p. 80, he died in 1342.
1075. Meyerhof, 'Medieval Jewish Physicians in the Near East', p. 456; al-Ṣafadī, *Kitāb al-Wāfī bi-l-Wafayāt* (2000), vol. XV, p. 80; Meyerhof, 'Jewish Physicians Contemporaries of Maimonides', pp. 397–8.
1076. Mazor, 'Ibn Ṣaghīr/Ibn Kūjik Family'.
1077. al-Ṣafadī, *Kitāb al-Wāfī bi-l-Wafayāt* (2000), vol. XV, p. 80; al-Ṣafadī, *Aʿyān al-ʿAṣr*, vol. II, p. 404; Meyerhof, 'Medieval Jewish Physicians in the Near East', p. 456.
1078. al-Ṣafadī, *Kitāb al-Wāfī bi-l-Wafayāt* (2000), vol. XV, p. 80; al-Ṣafadī, *Aʿyān al-ʿAṣr*, vol. II, p. 404.
1079. For more on the professional network of Ibn al-Nafīs see Northrup, *al-Bīmāristān al-Manṣūrī*, pp. 26–7.
1080. Mazor, 'Jewish Court Physicians', pp. 43–50; Mazor, 'Sadīd al-Dimyāṭī'; al-ʿUmarī, *Masālik al-Abṣār*, vol. IX, pp. 361–2.

1081. See Mazor, 'Jewish Court Physicians', pp. 43–5; Mazor, 'Ibn Ṣaghīr/Ibn Kūjik Family'.
1082. Mazor, 'Ibn Ṣaghīr/Ibn Kūjik Family'; Mazor, 'Jewish Court Physicians', p. 46.
1083. Ibid.
1084. Ashtor, *The History of the Jews in Egypt and Syria*, vol. II, p. 553–4.
1085. Ibid.
1086. Ashtor, *The History of the Jews in Egypt and Syria*, vol. III, pp. 89–90.
1087. Goitein, 'The Medical Profession', p. 181; Goitein, *A Mediterranean Society*, vol. II, p. 245.
1088. Ashtor, *The History of the Jews in Egypt and Syria*, vol. III, pp. 89–90; Goitein, 'The Medical Profession', p. 181; Goitein, *A Mediterranean Society*, vol. II, p. 245.
1089. Ibid.
1090. Ashtor, *The History of the Jews in Egypt and Syria*, vol. I, p. 275.
1091. See Mazor and Lev, 'Dynasties of Jewish Physicians'. For more about the Jews in Tabrīz see Netzer, 'The Fate of the Jewish Community of Tabriz'.
1092. al-Maqrīzī, *Durar al-'Uqūd*, vol. III, pp. 8–9; Ibn Ḥajar al-ʿAsqalānī, *al-Durar al-Kāmina*, vol. V, p. 169; Ibn Taghrī Birdī, *al-Manhal*, vol. VIII, pp. 376–7; Ashtor, *The History of the Jews in Egypt and Syria*, vol. I, pp. 323–4; Fischel, 'Azarbaijan in Jewish History', p. 19; Poliak, 'Nafīs b. David', pp. 84–5. According to some sources, it was Emir Sheikhū al-ʿUmarī, and not Qublāy, who was cured by Nafīs: see Ibn Taghrī Birdī, *al-Manhal*, vol. XIII, p. 377; al-Sakhāwī, *al-Ḍawʾ al-Lāmiʿ*, vol. VI, p. 166.
1093. For more on this family, and its medical activity, see dynasty 40.
1094. Ibn Taghrī Birdī, *al-Manhal*, vol. III, pp. 244–5; Ibn Ḥajar al-ʿAsqalānī, *Inbāʾ al-Ghumr*, vol. II, pp. 11–12, vol. III, pp. 258–9; Ashtor, *The History of the Jews in Egypt and Syria*, vol. I, pp. 323–4 (mistakenly mentioned as Badr al-Dīn Badīʿ).
1095. al-Maqrīzī, *Durar al-ʿUqūd*, vol. III, pp. 8 ff; Ibn Taghrī Birdī, *al-Manhal*, vol. VIII, pp. 375–7; al-Sakhāwī, *al-Ḍawʾ al-Lāmiʿ*, vol. VI, pp. 165–6; Ashtor, *The History of the Jews in Egypt and Syria*, vol. I, pp. 323–4; el-Leithy, 'Coptic Culture and Conversion', pp. 270–1, 333–4; Fischel, 'Azarbaijan in Jewish History', p. 19 n. 47.
1096. al-Maqrīzī, *Durar al-ʿUqūd*, vol. III, pp. 561–2; al-Sakhāwī, *al-Ḍawʾ al-Lāmiʿ*, vol. X, p. 292; Ashtor, *The History of the Jews in Egypt and Syria*, vol. I, p. 291.

1097. Ibid.
1098. Arad, 'The Community as an Economic Body', p. 61.
1099. Ashtor, *The History of the Jews in Egypt and Syria*, vol. II, pp. 27–8, 175.
1100. Jacoby, 'Jewish Doctors and Surgeons', pp. 438–43.
1101. Ibid., pp. 438–43.
1102. Ashtor, 'New Data for the History of Levantine Jewries', p. 87.
1103. Jacoby, 'Jewish Doctors and Surgeons', pp. 438–43.
1104. Ashtor, 'New Data for the History of Levantine Jewries', p. 87.
1105. Ashtor, *The History of the Jews in Egypt and Syria*, vol. II, pp. 448–9; Arad, 'The Community as an Economic Body', pp. 54–5 n. 165.
1106. For more about this family see 'Iscandari', *Encyclopaedia Judaica*, 2nd ed., vol. X, pp. 78–9; Arad, 'The Community as an Economic Body', pp. 54–6.
1107. Sambari, *Sefer Divrei Yosef*, p. 400; Ashtor, *The History of the Jews in Egypt and Syria*, vol. II, pp. 448–9.
1108. Arad, 'The Community as an Economic Body', p. 54 n. 165; Ashtor, *The History of the Jews in Egypt and Syria*, vol. II, pp. 488–9; Sambari, *Sefer Divrei Yosef*, pp. 400–1.
1109. Mosseri V 392.3.
1110. Arad, 'The Community as an Economic Body', pp. 54–5 n. 165; Sambari, *Sefer Divrei Yosef*, p. 400–1.
1111. When we discuss these dynasties, we should remember that we have used the information we have gathered so far, i.e., some of the dynasties may have lasted for more generations than we have presented, as one or more of their members may not have left any written trace in either Jewish or Muslim Arabic sources.
1112. Mazor and Lev, 'Dynasties of Jewish Physicians'.
1113. Ibid.
1114. These dynasties are discussed in depth in Mazor and Lev, 'The Phenomenon'. The main converted dynasties of the Mamluk period, whose members were all court physicians or otherwise distinguished, are Ibn Ṣaghīr (Karaite), Ibn Kūjik (Karaite), Ibn al-Maghribī, Nafīs b. Da'ūd b. ʿAnān al-Tabrīzī (Karaite), ʿAbdallah b. Da'ūd b. Abī al-Faḍl al-Da'ūdī (Karaite), ʿAbd al-Sayyid b. Isḥāq and Sukra al-Ḥalabī. There is a possibility that even a member of the Maimonidean dynasty had to convert for a period.
1115. This is not to say that the combination of the two positions, Head and court physician, was unknown, but that it was rarer than in former periods. See in detail Mazor and Lev, 'The Phenomenon'.

1116. Mazor and Lev, 'The Phenomenon'.
1117. See, for instance, the dynasties of Moses b. Elazar and Saʿadya b. Mevōrākh, discussed in Mazor and Lev, 'Dynasties of Jewish Physicians'.
1118. al-Dhahabī, *Taʾrīkh al-Islām*, vol. XLVIII, p. 299.
1119. We may add to these 'Heads' who were converts of Jewish origin also Sulaymān b. Junayba (d. 1410/11), who was 'Head of the Physicians' at the time of his death (al-Maqrīzī, *Kitāb al-Sulūk*, vol. IV, p. 598), and Zayn al-Dīn Khiḍr al-Isrāʾīlī in 1437–8 (al-Maqrīzī, *Kitāb al-Sulūk*, vol. IV, pp. 1041–2; Ashtor, *The History of the Jews in Egypt and Syria*, vol. II, pp. 89–90).
1120. Mazor and Lev, 'Dynasties of Jewish Physicians'.
1121. Marín, 'Biography and Prosopography', p. 8.
1122. See in detail Mazor and Lev, 'Dynasties of Jewish Physicians'.
1123. Pormann and Savage-Smith, *Medieval Islamic Medicine*, p. 81.
1124. Azar, 'Ibn Zuhr (Avenzoar)', pp. 64–102; Arnaldez, 'Ibn Zuhr'.
1125. Ibn Abī Uṣaybiʿa, *ʿUyūn al-Anbāʾ*, vol. II, pp. 119–20; ʿIsā, *Muʿjam al-Atibbāʾ*, pp. 230, 288, 304. For three-generation dynasties of distinguished physicians, see Ibn Abī Uṣaybiʿa, *ʿUyūn al-Anbāʾ*, vol. I, pp. 153–7 (9th-century Baghdad), 297–8 (12th-century Baghdad).
1126. See al-Jazarī, *Ḥawādith al-Zamān*, vol. II, pp. 167–8.
1127. Sourdel, 'Bukhtishūʿ'; Wilson, 'The Bakhitishuʿ'; Goitein, 'The Medical Profession', pp. 181–2.
1128. See for instance Ibn Abī Uṣaybiʿa, *ʿUyūn al-Anbāʾ*, vol. I, pp. 119–20, 184, 200, 202–3; for a Sabian dynasty of four generations (9th–10th centuries) see ibid., vol. I, pp. 215, 220, 224, 226.
1129. Mazor, 'Jewish Court Physicians', p. 61; Ibn Abī Uṣaybiʿa, *ʿUyūn al-Anbāʾ*, vol. II, pp. 121–3; Ashtor, 'Prolegomena', p. 152.

4

Professional, Social, Geographical, Religious and Economic Aspects of Jewish Medical Practitioners

The general history of the Jews in the Islamic world in the medieval period has been studied by scholars such as S. D. Goitein, Moshe Gil, Mark Cohen and Norman Stillman.[1] Another line of historical research has been conducted on a number of geographical regions such as Spain,[2] the Maghrib,[3] Sicily,[4] the Mediterranean,[5] Syria[6] and Egypt.[7] The life of Jews in the cities of Alexandria,[8] Aleppo,[9] Damascus,[10] Qayrawān[11] and Ashkelon has been studied as well.[12]

The exact number of Jews in the Muslim world in the relevant centuries is unknown, although some scholars have tried to estimate it. For instance, Goitein suggested that the Jews constituted something like 1 per cent of the population in the Muslim world of the Middle Ages, with a higher concentration in the big cities and small towns;[13] David J. Wasserstein argued that this estimate is 'a very rough approximation'.[14]

Stillman claimed that Islam was 'first and foremost an urban civilization', and since the majority of Jews living in the world during the medieval period came under Arab rule, they embarked on the transition from an agrarian to a cosmopolitan way of life. Jews took part in creating the new medieval Islamic civilisation. Moreover, they developed 'a flourishing Jewish culture along parallel lines'.[15]

The Jews in the Muslim world functioned as members of the *dhimmī* category, and according to Wasserstein, this affected the activities of the elite, to whom the Jewish medical practitioners belonged, perhaps more than other spheres of life. The medieval Jewish elite was a small group of intellectuals, merchants, religious leaders, community leaders, court officials and medical practitioners. Elites of minority groups are structured differently from those of the majority; they are actually dependent on the elite of the majority and its goodwill. Moreover, in the majority's eyes, in some cases, such an elite may actually not be considered an elite at all.[16]

Before I begin my discussion, I will repeat here the main questions that puzzled me while I conducted the research: Who were the Jewish practitioners in the medieval Muslim world? Where did they actually practise? Did they operate privately and individually, or were they somehow organised? What fees did they charge for their medical work? How many Jewish practitioners were active in each generation? Did Jewish practitioners treat Muslim and Christian patients in their private practices? If so, what was the essence of such a relationship? Were there any professional interactions with Muslim and Christian practitioners? If so, of what nature were these relations? What was their socio-economic status in the communities within which they operated? Were there any dynasties among the medical practitioners? What other kinds of duty did Jewish practitioners carry out in their communities? How often did Jewish physicians serve in the courts of the rulers, and what was their relationship with the authorities? Did each practitioner have his own library? If so, what works did it contain? How many Jewish practitioners actually worked in the city hospitals, and in what capacity? How did medieval Jewish practitioners acquire their medical skills and expertise? What was their professional standard? What was the theoretical background associated with the training of the Jewish practitioners? Did they specialise in various fields of medicine? What were the common medical problems which the practitioners had to deal with?

As mentioned above, Joseph Shatzmiller in his book raised several questions, some of which are relevant to my research,[17] I have tried to deal with them as well in my discussion.

In general, the Mediterranean medical milieu could be described as a 'disciple of the Greek, [heir] to a universal tradition, a spiritual brotherhood which transcended the barriers of religion, language, and countries'.[18] However, from a realistic point of view, and based on the Geniza documents as well as on Muslim Arabic writings, it should be stated that 'intercommunal tensions exist, and, despite the general climate of tolerance, frictions occurred'.[19]

Unlike the Muslim Arabic sources that were mentioned and used in the Introduction, the Cairo Geniza enables us to reach sporadic information on the personal as well as professional lives of Jewish practitioners in the Muslim world, mainly those of Egypt and the Middle East. Paulina Lewicka raised an issue regarding these 'missing' ordinary medieval Jewish physicians:

> But apart from those who achieved social prestige and rank there was also a crowd of Jewish physicians who lived their ordinary lives in ordinary neighbourhoods of Syria or Egypt and earned their income by attending to ordinary patients. This group constituted a majority of Jewish doctors living and working within the Muslim society; however, by virtue of its ordinariness this majority is generally missing from the Muslim Arabic historiography – as is usually the case with ordinary people. This implies that our picture of the past will always be somewhat distorted with respect to the present topic.[20]

In fact, these fragments of information that were 'mined' from the Geniza not only deal with the 'rich and famous' practitioners, but they describe the everyday life and actions of practitioners from various geographical locations in the Muslim world (big cities such as Cairo and Alexandria, as well as small villages such as Qūṣ or Bilbays). The records include gifts and donations for the poor, testimonies in court, recommendation letters, payments for treatments, involvement in trade and commerce, buying and selling houses, loaning money, activities for the community (such as charity), and private/personal information (marriage, divorce, personal letters within the family etc.).

Early Muslim Arabic sources such as al-Jāḥiẓ (9th century) described contemporary Jews as ignorant obscurantists: 'dyers, tanners, cuppers, butchers, cobblers'.[21] Al-Muqaddasī (a 10th-century Muslim Arab geographer) noticed that in his time most of the doctors in Jerusalem were Christians, while Jews were 'money changers, dyers and tanners'.[22] Max Meyerhof explained that this was simply because there were only a few qualified Jewish practitioners at that time.[23]

In general, the Muslim Arabic sources contributed much-needed information, mainly regarding professional issues of the Jewish practitioners, as well as their work in hospitals and courts of Muslim rulers, studying and teaching medicine, and establishing relationships with non-Jewish practitioners, administrators and rulers. These sources also imparted cultural and social perceptions of Muslims towards Jewish practitioners.

Shatzmiller pointed out that 'while Jews were among the first-known doctors in the early Islamic empire, and Ibn al-Qifṭī (d. 1248) gives the names of three of them, by contrast, almost half of the doctors – 52 out of 124 – were Christians'. Moreover, he added that no Jewish name is recorded for the hundred years between 950 and 1050, and only three out of seventeen doctors in the twelfth century are Jewish.[24] According to Françoise Micheau, who analysed the same source (*History of Learned Men* by Ibn al-Qifṭī), there were only 17 Jews among the 124 physicians who practised between 750 and 1230.[25] Conversely, decades before, Meyerhof traced forty-four medieval Middle Eastern Jewish doctors, of whom eighteen (40 per cent) were contemporaries of Maimonides.[26]

The findings of our research oppose Micheau's analysis, and further support Meyerhof's work by presenting names and information regarding dozens of Jewish physicians that were practising in the Muslim world during that period. The simple explanation for this is that Micheau studied only a single historical source, although it was an important one (Ibn al-Qifṭī), while Meyerhof made use of many other sources. The data we collected is based upon hundreds of Geniza documents written by many people from that period – officials, physicians and laymen. This exemplifies the importance of our research, and moreover, strengthens our choice of methodology.

In any case, it seems that the eleventh century marked a new era, and many more Jewish practitioners are recorded, as can also be learnt from our research, and this phenomenon gained even greater momentum towards the twelfth century. It is clear from our findings that the highest numbers of physicians and pharmacists are from the eleventh to the thirteenth centuries, that is, the Fatimid and the Ayyubid periods. Those periods represent a liberal regime that allowed minorities to flourish, and this points to the centrality of Cairo as the capital of the Muslim caliphate. Interestingly, this is the period that historians of medieval Jewish studies call the classical Geniza period. As mentioned above, the vast majority of the documents and fragments found in the Cairo Geniza are from this period. Therefore, we have more information regarding many matters, including Jewish practitioners.

Many medieval Egyptian Jews chose the medical profession for a wide range of reasons. The Geniza records constitute historical evidence supporting Maimonides' account of the great number of physicians in Cairo: 'In some cases a patient was healed of one ailment by ten physicians.'[27] The fact that a large number of Jews engaged in the medical profession in Egypt and other Muslim territories emerges from other historical sources as well, mainly the books written by medieval biographers and historians of medicine such as Ibn Abī Uṣaybiʿa. This writer mentioned more than fifteen Jewish practitioners he either met, knew or heard of in Cairo during his time and before.[28]

Goitein explains the phenomenon of Jewish predominance in medicine not as the continuation of a pre-Islamic tradition but as a contemporary development resulting from the revival of the Greek sciences under Islam, and from the flourishing trade with India and the Far East. In his opinion, medicine and pharmacy experienced then an unprecedented exuberance and became almost new professions.[29] Cohen stated that physicians were among the non-poor in the Jewish community.[30] In several cases, Jewish physicians were among the best-known and most prominent men in the community, such as Abraham Maimonides and Moses (Abū Saʿd) b. Nethanel ha-Levi.[31]

In this chapter I will discuss various issues dealing with Jewish medical practitioners in the Muslim world obtained from Muslim sources as well as the Jewish ones, that is, mainly the Cairo Geniza. I begin with a discussion about places of medical practice, the practitioners' education, female practitioners, physicians' libraries and the position of 'Head of the Physicians'; and I shall then resume the topics of personal issues, everyday life and activities of Jewish practitioners, physicians' possessions, their travels and means of transportation, and commercial activities. The next issues that will be dealt with are moral aspects, such as medical ethics, behaviour and artistic expression, fees and the 'Geniza' patients. Then I will proceed to religious and inter-religious aspects (practitioners and Jewish scholarship, Jewish practitioners serving in the Egyptian army and navy, Jewish practitioners in the Christian versus the Muslim world, inter-religious intellectual and professional relations, *wazīrs* and other high-ranking positions which Jewish practitioners held, and conversion of Jewish practitioners to Islam), and Jewish practitioners as famous scholars, authors, poets and diplomats, as well as community affairs such as the socio-economic position of Jewish practitioners, headship of the Jews, judges, *ḥazzānim*, charity and donations. I will finish Chapter 4 by discussing the geographical, sectoral and historical aspects (Karaite and Samaritan practitioners, and Jewish practitioners in Andalusia, north Africa, provincial Egyptian towns, Bilād al-Shām, Iraq, Iran, and Azerbaijan).

4.1 Professional Aspects

Medical care in the Islamic world was pluralistic, with various practices serving different needs and sometimes intermingling.[32] I will start my discussion here with the various titles of physicians found in the sources and continue with the main specialisations in the field of medicine.

Terminology

The titles or descriptors of physicians in Muslim Arabic sources as well as in Geniza documents varied: *al-mutaṭabbib*, *al-ṭabīb*, *ha-rōfē* and *al-ḥakīm* (all signifying medical 'doctor'). Based on the accumulated data, it can be said that most of the physicians mentioned in the Geniza worked privately in Cairo, Alexandria and other big cities around the Muslim world. Others pursued their careers in small villages, some practised in hospitals and a select few in rulers' courts. The Geniza records constitute historical evidence supporting Maimonides' account of the great number of physicians in Cairo.[33]

The vast majority of the Jewish physicians who have been identified as working in the Muslim world during the 8th–16th centuries were called al-Ṭabīb. Some of them were named al-Mutaṭabbib, for example Abū ʿAlī Ḥasan al-Mutaṭabbib al-Barqī; Ibrāhīm al-Mutaṭabbib b. Mukhtār; al-Asʿad al-Mutaṭabbib; Yaʿqūb (Abū Yūsuf) ʿImrān al-Mutaṭabbib; al-Muwaffaq ʿAbd al-Dāʾim b. ʿAbd al-ʿAzīz b. Muḥāsan, ʾIsrāʾīlī al-Mutaṭabbib; Sulaymān b. Mūsā al-Yahūdī al-Mutaṭabbib; and Abū Manṣūr al-Mutaṭabbib.[34]

The term *al-ḥakīm*, 'doctor', designated not only a physician but also a man of comprehensive secular education or physician/philosopher, for example Abū al-Bishr b. Aaron Ha-Levi al-Kirmānī al-Ḥakīm, Ibrāhīm b. Faraj b. Mārūth al-Sāmirī al-Ṭabīb (al-Ḥakīm), Yaḥyā b. Sulaymān al-ʾIsrāʾīlī al-Ṭabīb al-Ḥakīm, Japheth b. David b. Samuel Ibn Ṣaghīr (al-Ḥakīm al-Ṣafī), Abū Yaʿqūb al-Ḥakīm, Kamāl al-Dawla Abū ʿAlī b. Abī al-Faraj (Ibn al-Dāʿī al-ʾIsrāʾīlī al-Irbilī al-Ḥakīm), Masīḥ b. Ḥakam (Masīḥ b. Ḥakīm), al-Ḥakīm al-Iskandrī al-Murabbā al-Maghribī al-Nisba, ʿAbd al-Wāḥid ha-Kohen Ḥakīm, ʿImrān b. Ṣadaqa al-ʾIsrāʾīlī al-Ḥakīm Awḥad al-Dīn and R. Samuel b. Ḥakīm.[35] In one case, a pharmacist was called al-Ḥakīm (al-ʿAṭṭār al-Ḥakīm).[36] An interesting anecdote, from which we learn about the different uses of terms, is brought to us by Ibn al-Fuwaṭī, a Muslim historian (13th–14th centuries), who described Rashīd al-Dīn's father as *al-ḥakīm wa-l-ṭabīb* (a philosopher and a physician).[37]

Many of the Jewish physicians were called, on top of the Arabic descriptor, ha-Rōfē, which is the Hebrew name for a physician to the present day.

Moreover, doctors also bore honorific titles. According to Goitein, these titles were first confined to the more prominent members of the profession such as 'the physician to the exalted Majesty', referred to above, who bore the title 'The Sound'. Later on, certain titles became very common, three especially: al-Sadīd (the sound), al-Muwaffaq (the successful) and al-Muhadhdhab (the accomplished).[38] And indeed dozens out of the hundreds of physicians that are revealed and studied in this book were named al-Sadīd (for example Abū al-Bayān b. al-Mudawwar al-Sadīd, Abū Zikrī al-Sadīd b. Elijah and al-Sadīd al-Dimyāṭī al-Ṭabīb al-Yahūdī), al-Muhadhdhab (for example al-Sheikh al-Muhadhdhab al-Ṭabīb, al-Sheikh al-Jalīl al-Raʾīs al-Kāfī al-Muqarrab al-Ḥākim al-Muhadhdhab Tāj al-Ḥukamāʾ Thiqāt al-Mulūk wa al-Salāṭīn and Yūsuf b. Abī Saʿīd b. Khalaf al-Sāmirī al-Muhadhdhab al-Ṭabīb) or al-Muwaffaq (for example al-Muwaffaq al-Kohen al-Ṭabīb; al-Muwaffaq ʿAbd al-Dāʾim b. ʿAbd al-ʿAzīz b. Muḥāsan, ʾIsrāʾīlī al-Mutaṭabbib; and al-Muwaffaq al-Qaṣīr al-Ṭabīb al-Yahūdī).[39]

Besides the regular use of common titles there were others, more elaborate ones, such as Ibrāhīm b. Faraj b. Mārūth al-Sāmirī al-Ṭabīb (al-Ḥakīm), known as Shams al-Ḥukamāʾ 'The Sun of the Doctors'.[40] The person thus honoured was addressed with that title even in a short note of a few lines. One case is extraordinary, having an exceptional number of descriptors; ʿAbd al-Sayyid b. Isḥāq b. Yaḥyā al-Ḥakīm al-Faḍl Bahāʾ al-Dīn b. al-Muhadhdhab, al-Ṭabīb al-Kaḥḥāl.[41] All the information about this physician, who had converted to Islam, comes from Muslim Arabic sources.

Specialisation

In his work on ʿAlī Ibn Riḍwān (d. 1068) Michael Dols wrote: 'Medieval doctors were general practitioners but might also have a special skill in ophthalmology, bone-setting, pharmacology, or surgery.'[42] Similarly, the large hospitals were organised according to the fields of specialisation held by the medical staff, and the different diseases being treated (fevers, ophthalmology, surgery, dysentery, internal diseases, orthopaedics).[43] Indeed, we have information about some of the Jewish practitioners regarding their specialisations, for example:

a. **Ophthalmologists/oculists (*kaḥḥāl* in Arabic).** Eye diseases have been a major medical problem from early times, creating major health problems in hot climate environments around the world until the present day.[44] They were naturally prevalent in the less hygienic ancient world as well.[45] Many of the ophthalmological practices were similar in various cultures and places.[46] People in the medieval Muslim world suffered from eye diseases and the doctors had to treat them accordingly. Savage-Smith stated that 'ophthalmology was the only area, besides pharmacology, that could be called a specialty, and no wonder that an extensive specialist literature were developed'.[47] Arabic physicians displayed particular concern and skill in the diagnosis and treatment of eye diseases, perhaps because blindness was the major cause of disability throughout the Muslim world.

Moreover, ophthalmologists developed their own extensive specialist literature. Nearly every medical compendium had chapters on the subject. The most comprehensive coverage was to be found in the large number of monographs devoted solely to eye diseases. Ophthalmology was a topic in which medieval Islamic writers displayed considerable originality.[48]

Both ophthalmologists and oculists are specialists in the branch of medicine concerned with the study and treatment of disorders and diseases of the eye. Goitein stated that *kaḥḥāl* (who included women) were the specialists most frequently referred to in the Geniza records.[49] Interestingly enough, most of the parts of books that have been identified in the Geniza so far are either fragments of books on eye diseases or parts of general medical books which dealt with ophthalmology.[50] Moreover, many of the notebooks that have been identified in the Geniza deal with the treatment of eye diseases. Analysis of the prescriptions found in the notebooks, with the help of contemporary pharmacopoeias, shows that eye diseases were the most prevalent ailments,[51] and similarly, some of the Geniza's practical prescriptions that were studied include recipes for the treatment of eye diseases[52] as well as large numbers of medicinal substances.[53]

Several Jewish eye doctors were mentioned in the Geniza; according to Cohen, oculists were among the non-poor in the Jewish community, meaning that they were making a good living and donated generous sums of money compared to other community members of their time.[54] Some of them, and a few others, were mentioned by Muslim Arabic sources as well. Here are a few examples: Abū al-Faraj b. Abū al-Faḍā'il b. al-Nāqid (12th century), a respected ophthalmologist who was active in Cairo and converted to Islam;[55] Abū al-ʿIzz al-Kaḥḥāl and Makārim al-Kaḥḥāl, mentioned in a list of donors to aid payment of a head tax, dated to the thirteenth century,[56] and in a list of taxpayers or donors to a fund for the redemption of captives and so on;[57] and Yūsuf al-Kaḥḥāl, mentioned in a list of donors from c.1210.[58] More examples for other eye doctors are Abū al-Fakhr b. Abī al-Faḍl b. Abī Naṣr b. Abī al-Fakhr al-Yahūdī, known as Aaron ha-Levi Ibn al-Kirmānī al-Kaḥḥāl (1220), a Karaite physician;[59] Makārim b. Isḥāq b. Makārim, ophthalmologist (active in Cairo around 1245);[60] Asad al-Yahūdī,[61] a prominent physician in Egypt and Syria (Hama, Safed, Damascus and Aleppo as well as Cairo) under the Mamluks (13th–14th centuries), who worked as a general physician, surgeon and an ophthalmologist treating the military and political elite of the Mamluks;[62] Najīb al-Dawla (ophthalmologist in the court of Tabriz around 1305, convert);[63] and Khalaf al-Kaḥḥāl (around 1436).[64] From the Ottoman period there were Kamāl b. Mūsā, an ophthalmologist who worked in Jerusalem and was 'Head of the Physicians' of Jerusalem, around 1571; and Shaḥāda b. Abraham, physician (Jerusalem, around 1577), named al-Kaḥḥāl.[65]

A testimony to consultation with some ophthalmologists in Fusṭāṭ is learnt from a letter that was sent to a smaller town in which the writer reports that he

> went to the ophthalmologists [in the plural], informed them about his complaints, and they prescribed ointments and powders which I sent to him. However, the doctors said to me that the medicines would be of no avail, as long as he continued to work in sunlight, which his profession forces him to do.[66]

From an account about al-Muwaffaq al-Qaṣīr al-Ṭabīb al-Yahūdī, a physician from Damascus (13th–14th centuries) who fixed the sight problem of his Muslim friend (c.1300), we learn about the treatment and the use of the medical literature: fluid was seeping from the friend's eyes and he was blinded in one of them and his sight was weakening in the other. Al-Muwaffaq treated him with medicines mentioned by Ibn al-Bayṭār. He collected all the medicinal drugs he mentioned for stopping the discharge and prepared a remedy that improved the patient's condition and strengthened his vision.[67]

b. Surgeons. As mentioned above, the large hospitals were organised according to the fields of specialisation held by the medical staff, and surgery was among the important ones.[68] Only a few Jewish surgeons (*jarā'iḥī*) are known to us from both the Geniza and Muslim Arabic sources.[69] Al-Ṭabīb al-Ḥaqīr al-Nāfiʿ, also known as al-Jirāḥī al-Miṣrī (the Egyptian Surgeon), was a surgeon who dealt mainly with healing wounds without being well known. According to Ibn Abī Uṣaybiʿa,[70] he got his name from the caliph al-Ḥākim bi-Amr Allāh (r. 996–1020), after he successfully treated a wound in the caliph's leg in only three days when his private physicians had failed to do so. In return for his successful treatment, the caliph gave him a thousand dinars and honorary clothes, and nominated him among his personal physicians.[71]

Asad al-Yahūdī (d. 1330),[72] a prominent physician in Egypt and Syria (13th–14th centuries), worked as a general physician and ophthalmologist but was known specifically as a surgeon who treated fractures. He treated the military and political elite of the Mamluks, and was active in Hama, Safed, Damascus and Aleppo, as well as in Cairo.[73] Other surgeons from the Geniza that we know of are mainly from the fifteenth and sixteenth centuries: Judah from Damascus (15th century), who also worked in Candia, Crete;[74] Judah from Alexandria (who was employed by the Venetian colony in Alexandria in the fifteenth century);[75] and Isaac ha-Rōfē 2, born in Jerusalem, and working at the beginning of the sixteenth century.[76]

From sources we also learn about contemporary paramedical occupations. These are not the subject of this book, but I have decided to briefly present some of them here:

a. **Wound specialists.** The *kallām* (a wound specialist), as differentiated from the surgeon, appeared in several sources and publications. The word *kallām* is derived from *kalm*, meaning 'wound', 'cut' or 'slash', and Goitein claimed that it designated perhaps not a physician proper, but a male nurse bandaging wounds. Here are three examples: Abū al-Faraj b. al-Kallām, whose grandfather was a physician;[77] Abū al-Faḍl al-Kallām, mentioned in a letter to Nagid Samuel (12th century);[78] and Hiba b. al-Kallām, involved in commerce but the son of a wound specialist.[79]
b. **Stomach healers.** The *quḍāʿī*, healer of stomach problems, was mentioned in Geniza fragments; according to Goitein the term is also known as a Muslim family name.[80]
c. **Cuppers and phlebotomists.** *Ḥajjām* were somehow a subsection of the medical profession.[81] Prospective physicians tried to acquire surgical skills by means of the practice of bleeding. We find a cupper contributing to a public appeal and addressed as 'elder', another mentioned as an ancestor in a memorial list, and a third as recipient of a calligraphic letter dealing with a matter of inheritance, attended to by the *nagid*. Phlebotomists did not belong to the medical profession proper; however, they were required to have theoretical knowledge in addition to technical skills to perform bloodletting.[82] Abū al-Ḥasan b. Mūsā al-Fāṣid al-ʿAṭṭār might be an example of a pharmacist who was probably practising phlebotomy.[83]

4.1.1 Places of medical practice

During the medieval period, Jewish physicians and pharmacists practised the medical systems of the Christian and Muslim societies in which they lived. Pormann and Savage-Smith stated that there were four main places, in the medieval Arab world, where caring and curing took place: 'the markets [...] the home of the patient, the home of the physician, and the hospital'.[84] Our findings supply evidence for these locations as healing places for both Jewish practitioners and patients.

Private practice

As noted, most of the physicians worked privately. The healing process took place either in the home of the patient, or in the home of the physician, or in his clinic.

In the medieval period a doctor's clinic was called a *dukkān*, and according to several Geniza documents it was like any other open store in the market. In some cases, similar to present-day practice, two physicians shared a clinic. Reference is made in a letter to two joint clinics.[85] One example relating to the location of clinics that was found in the Geniza (11th century) concerns the store in Fusṭāṭ of Abū al-Faraj b. Maʿmar al-Sharābī (Nethanel ha-Levi b. Amram), a seller of medical potions, light beverages and wines. This store was probably spacious since it was used as a storeroom besides being a working place (clinic) for both a Jewish practitioner named R. Amram b. Saʿīd b. Mūsā and a Christian physician named Abū al-Ghālib; the latter wrote out prescriptions while people on the street could see a sign above the store publicising the physician's practice.[86]

An interesting anecdote was written by Ibn Abī Uṣaybiʿa about Ibn Jumayʿ,[87] who had a clinic in the Sūq al-Qanādīl (Market of Lamps) in Fusṭāṭ. Ibn Jumayʿ became famous after he managed to bring back to life a man believed to be dead who happened to pass by on a stretcher near the clinic. Ibn Jumayʿ noticed that the supposedly dead man's legs were stretched out and not dangling as would be expected.[88]

Clear evidence for clinics is also found in some late Geniza documents: Jacob ha-Rōfē 2, Moses ha-Rōfē 3 and Samuel ha-Rōfē are mentioned in a document from the Muslim court (1550), dealing with a rented shop in Jerusalem which was used as a clinic; Kamāl b. Mūsā (16th century), an ophthalmologist who also worked in Jerusalem, had a clinic located in a rented store in the Sūq al-ʿAṭṭārīn. He was also 'Head of the Physicians' of Jerusalem and received his salary from the public treasury.[89]

In some cases, the patient stayed at home – because there were no Jewish hospitals, and Jews did not use the Muslim ones – and the physician visited him or her on a daily basis. In a long letter from Tinnīs (Lower Egypt), a certain patient with a probably serious illness made reference to three other letters sent by him, mentioning that his physician came to see him every day. Sometimes, as we learn from a letter written by Menahem, a physician from Fusṭāṭ during the time of the *nagid* Abraham Maimonides, doctors travelled to visit patients in certain villages (in this case Ṭanān, in the Qalyūbiyya district near Cairo).[90]

In the case of serious medical treatment, the doctor's house served as a substitute for a hospital for patients who could afford it, or who were either his friends or members of his family. A father reported to his grandparents in Fusṭāṭ the death of his daughter in Alexandria, and described how she stayed with the physician, who sent her home only when he had established that her case was hopeless.[91]

According to a few Geniza fragments judge Nathan b. Samuel (a. 1122–53) maintained a private hospice for the sick and elderly people, but there is no hint that he was also a physician. Goitein suggested that this small 'institution' was run by his wife, a woman known otherwise as rich and charitable.[92]

There were also cases where diagnosis was made remotely. Our data, mainly based on physicians' letters, supports Goitein's suggestion that prescribing medicines without seeing the patient must have been a common practice for doctors. In such cases the illness would be described to them by a family member or in a letter, and they were expected to cure it by sending instructions and recipes for prescriptions. I will present here a few examples only:

a. In a set of letters sent from Alexandria to a prominent merchant in Fusṭāṭ, the merchant is asked to take a prescription from the *nagid* and court physician Abū al-Faḍl Mubārak (Mevōrākh b. Saʿadya). The son of the writer suffered 'from a dryness which appeared on his body, in particular boils and dry patches extending from his hips to his feet'. We have a reminder for this request in another letter and learn from a third letter that the young man for whom the medicine had been requested had died.[93]

b. Abū al-Riḍā al-Ṭabīb (Joseph ha-Levi) was a physician who was active in Cairo in the twelfth century; he was Maimonides' nephew and was mentioned by Ibn al-Qifṭī. In a letter addressed to him, a patient described the symptoms from which he was suffering and asked for a prescription.[94]

c. Another interesting case of distant diagnosis relates to Samuel ha-Nagid b. Hananiah, a court physician and the leader of the Jewish community in Fusṭāṭ (1140–59). We learn from a Geniza document that he apparently misdiagnosed Amram b. Isaac's wife's illness, and the drugs he prescribed for her only worsened her condition. Amram asked him to prescribe another drug after describing her illness in more detail.[95]

d. One of the most famous examples is the recipe for severe headaches which Maimonides prescribed in a letter for his former student Tuvia.[96]

e. Another example from the Geniza is a short letter containing thanks for forwarding a prescription from one physician and a request for a prescription from another, both for the writer's wife.[97]

f. Persons applying to a civic leader who happened to be a physician would also seize the opportunity to seek medical advice. In an autographed letter, Maimonides not only gave instructions relating to administrative matters to a community official, but also took care of his health by prescribing him a milk cure.[98]

g. A student of philosophy read one of Maimonides' books and asked the author questions relating to his new book, but at the same time consulted him about some dietetic problems. Maimonides, who (as he wrote) was himself in very poor health at that time, patiently gave the desired advice.[99]

Hospitals

The history of hospitals is long, diverse and interesting, ranging from the early classical period (ancient Greece), through the Roman and Byzantine periods, to the Kingdom of the Crusaders.[100] However, it is not within the scope of the current work.

The Muslim hospital, according to Savage-Smith, served several purposes: it was

> a center of medical treatment, a convalescent home for those recovering from illness or accidents, an insane asylum, and a retirement home giving basic maintenance needs for the aged and infirm who lacked a family to care for them. It is unlikely that any truly wealthy person would have gone to a hospital, unless they were taken ill while travelling far from home. Except under unusual circumstances, all the medical needs of the wealthy and powerful would have been administered in the home.[101]

The word 'hospital', *bīmāristān* ('place for the sick' in Persian), appeared in medieval Muslim Arabic sources and in documents found in the Geniza. Interestingly, when it is written in Hebrew characters in medieval historical sources it is always abbreviated to *māristān*, similar to less formal Arabic today.

The Muslim hospital was structured as a charitable institution for the welfare of the community. The rulers and holders of positions of influence, who initiated the establishment of hospitals, not only did so from within governmental considerations but also presented the philanthropic notion of 'the overall good'.[102]

The widespread distribution of hospitals in the Islamic world, whether in central cities or other areas from the eighth to the sixteenth centuries, attests to the equal importance placed on this form of institution by its various founders and those availing themselves of the services offered therein. In most cases, these hospitals were built according to a uniform and fixed model: close by a place of worship such as a mosque, domed tomb or school, which would allow for religious rites to be held. These were, according to Islamic faith, part of the healing process.[103]

Large, as well as small, hospitals were arranged according to a clear and accepted standard: division between men and women and segregation of the mentally ill from other patients. In most cases, a pharmacy would be found which provided medication to those who were hospitalised, as well as to day patients, free of charge. The large hospitals were organised into different wards according to the fields of specialisation held by the medical staff, and the different diseases being treated (fevers, ophthalmology, surgery, dysentery, internal diseases, orthopaedics). The large hospitals were also learning centres, within the walls of which generations of doctors studied both theoretical and practical aspects of medicine.[104] Various historical documents teach us about the way these hospitals operated, and how they financed and resourced their administrative and medical staff. Towards the end of the eighth century, the hospital became one of the characteristic institutions of almost every central Muslim city.[105] The Ayyubid rulers brought with them a tradition to endow or to maintain a hospital; this was acknowledged by Nūr al-Dīn Zengī, their former overlord.[106]

Uri Hazan presented information regarding many medical institutions in the East which were part of the Muslim Empire: one hospital in Samarkand; thirteen hospitals in Baghdad and six more in other locations in Iraq; six in Damascus, three in Aleppo and two more in other cities in Syria; eight medical institutions in the land of present-day Israel and Jordan; one hospital in Alexandria, four in Fusṭāṭ, four in Cairo; and three hospitals in Ḥijaz.[107]

Working in a hospital required practitioners to use more paperwork and writing than in their private practice. A detailed document (*dustūr*) was written for every patient, including the description of his or her diseases, medications and progress. These documents served as a means of communication with other practitioners and paramedical staff, and was important, together with other documents (requests for drugs and *materia medica*) to the administrator and especially the treasurer, who actually ran the hospital. Unfortunately, as far as we know, none of these documents (from all Islamic hospitals) have survived. Therefore, we have no evidence that they were also used for medical learning or education.

As mentioned above, professional medical life in hospital was not only about medical practice; education was an equally important aspect. A hospital medical education allowed more people through the 'gate' of the profession, thus distinguishing it from the medical education of the madrasa or European school of medicine; it actually served as 'a site for a pre-existing educational system that relied on the direct relation of master and student'.[108] For example, al-Bīmāristān al-Manṣūrī was important for ophthalmologists, surgeons, bone setters and phlebotomists, enabling them to participate in the lessons given by the chief physician.[109]

Based on medieval Muslim Arabic sources it appears that one of the main advantages of the hospital was the existence of stacks of ready-made drugs and medications that could be given on the spot to patients in critical conditions and in urgent cases. Ahmed Ragab suggested that 'although the medications themselves may not have been different from others produced in the market, their immediate availability gave the *bīmāristān* a significant edge'.[110]

In some cases, mainly when the patient was a child, a woman, poor or very sick, medication was taken to the home of the patient by a family member who would visit the hospital or the physician's clinic and explain the patient's condition to the physician. The family member would come away from the hospital with medication,[111] or from a private clinic with a prescription (as learnt from the Geniza), which would then be taken to a pharmacist to prepare the medication.[112] Moreover, from the study of dozens of Geniza fragments, mainly letters, we learn about another option; the writer would describe his own medical condition or that of a family member, or even that of his patient, and ask for a prescription from a doctor.[113]

Thanks to surviving documents from al-Bīmāristān al-Manṣūrī in Cairo, we learn that the main purpose of the institution was housing and feeding patients. It is clear that the *bīmāristān* paid relatively low salaries to the practitioners and therefore it was unable to recruit the most talented physicians. Similarly, al-Manṣūr Qalāwūn's medical patronage was also motivated by charity and care for the poor. Moreover, his interest in providing medical education at the hospital was motivated by concern from the Muslim elite and himself over the small number of Muslim medical practitioners on the one hand, and the dominance of Christian and Jewish practitioners on the other. This was mainly due to the high salaries of administrative positions in Muslim religious institutions, which attracted the Muslim physicians and intellectuals.[114]

Table 4 presents some examples of Jewish practitioners who according to contemporary sources worked in hospitals in the Muslim world, usually due to their prestige and high professional achievements. It is very clear that the last six physicians that appear at the end of the table, who were active in the Mamluk period, converted to Islam. Another point of interest is that nine out of the fourteen physicians presented in the table worked also in the courts of Muslim rulers. Interestingly, many of them came from dynasties of Jewish physicians. We have information on only one physician, Makārim b. Isḥāq b. Makārim (13th century), that received a lifetime appointment.

Neither Jewish hospitals nor Jewish patients being treated in Muslim hospitals were mentioned in the Geniza.[115] According to Goitein, 'this is somewhat surprising, for many Jewish doctors are mentioned both by the Geniza and in Muslim Arabic sources as working in what could be called government hospitals, namely those erected by Muslim rulers, whereas Jewish patients are never mentioned in Geniza documents as making use of them'.[116] Moreover, several Muslim Arabic sources specified that Islamic hospitals were exclusively designated for Muslim patients.[117]

Indeed, our research confirmed that although many Geniza documents refer to Jewish doctors working in hospitals, not even one document mentioned that Jewish patients were hospitalised there. This is probably due to Halakhic issues, mainly regarding dietary laws and the religious purity of the medicines in an institution that operated under Muslim auspices. Therefore, members of the Jewish community were treated by private Jewish practitioners as and when required.[118]

Table 4 Jewish physicians working in Muslim hospitals[119]

Name	*Dates*	*City*	*Hospital*	*Remarks*
Moses b. Maimon	1138–1204	Cairo		Court physician
Abraham b. Moses b. Maimon	1186–1237	Cairo		Court physician
Abū al-Faḍl Dāʾūd b. Sulaymān b. Abū al-Bayān al-ʾIsrāʾīlī al-Sadīd (David b. Solomon)	b. 1161	Cairo	al-Bīmāristān al-Nāṣirī	Court physician
Moses b. Nethanel ha-Levi (Abū Saʿd)	12th century	Cairo		Court physician
ʿImrān b. Ṣadaqa al-ʾIsrāʾīlī al-Ḥakīm Awḥad al-Dīn (Moses b. Ṣadaqa)	b. 1165	Damascus	al-Bīmāristān al-Kabīr, al-Bīmāristān al-Nūrī	Court physician
Ṣadaqa al-ʾIsrāʾīlī	12th–13th centuries	Mainly Damascus		Court physician
Makārim b. Isḥāq b. Makārim;	a. c.1245	Cairo		Ophthalmologist; lifetime appointment
Saʿd al-Dawla b. Ṣafī b. Hibat Allāh b. Muhadhdhib al-Dawla al-Abharī	d. 1291	Abhar, Iran; Baghdad; Tabriz	Financial supervisor of al-Bīmāristān al-ʿAḍudī	
Rashīd al-Dīn Ṭabīb Faḍl Allāh b. al-Dawla, Abū al-Khayr b. ʿAlī Abū al-Hamadānī (convert)	1247–1318	Hamadān, Tabriz	Famous for the establishment of hospitals	Court physician, *wazīr*
Jamāl al-Dīn Ibrāhīm (Ibn al-Maghribī dynasty) (convert)	d. 1355	Cairo		Court physician
Shihāb al-Dīn Aḥmad al-Maghribī (convert)	13th–14th centuries	Maghrib, Cairo, ?Damascus	'Head of the Physicians' in hospitals	Court physician, *wazīr*
Yūsuf (convert 1302)	d. 1356	Damascus	Physician, probably in the hospital	
ʿAbd al-Sayyid b. Isḥāq b. Yaḥyā al-Ḥakīm al-Faḍl Bahāʾ al-Dīn b. al-Muhadhdhab, al-Ṭabīb al-Kaḥḥāl (convert 1302)	d. 1315	Damascus	Physician (ophthalmologist) in al-Bīmāristān al-Nūrī	His son, Jamāl al-Dīn ʿAbd Allāh, also served as a physician in the Nūrī hospital
Zayn al-Dīn Khiḍr al-ʾIsrāʾīlī al-Zuwaylī (convert)	d. 1438	Cairo	Head physician of Qalāwūn hospital	

Working in a hospital was prestigious, as stated by Pormann and Savage-Smith: 'For physician to have a position in one of these hospitals was apparently quite desirable.'[120] This is well illustrated by a petition, found in the Geniza, which was written in 1240, for a salaried post at the Nāṣirī hospital.[121] The petition was to an Ayyubid sultan from the Jewish physician Makārim b. Isḥāq asking for a lifetime appointment in the hospital of (New) Cairo (presumably the one founded by Saladin) with the usual salary of three dinars per month. Accordingly, two of the sultan's personal physicians testified to the excellence of the applicant's qualifications.[122]

Physicians practising in hospitals, seeing dozens of patients, had little interaction with each one individually, and naturally could not have established that kind of monitoring; in most cases they did not have the patient's medical history despite its great importance. Therefore, they were expected to use their experience and their practical knowledge to make decisions and treatment recommendations (prescribe effective and rapidly working remedies), relying mainly on physical examination. Ragab therefore claimed that 'prescribing extreme remedies and trying new regiments may have been possible or even praiseworthy in hospital but were likely impossible and unwise with more affluent or more powerful clients'.[123] Geniza records, as well as Muslim Arabic sources, suggested that mainly prominent physicians worked in the hospitals; and, similar to the present day, physicians' duties at the medieval 'government' hospitals included night shifts.[124]

Courts

Jewish physicians were working in rulers' courts in Christian Europe,[125] and all over the medieval Muslim world.[126] In some cases, the ruler had several Jewish physicians, as in the case of Saladin: according to Eliyahu Ashtor (based on Ibn Abī Uṣaybiʿa), eight out of the twenty-one physicians that treated him were Jewish.[127] Daniel Nicolae claimed that the success of Jewish physicians at court was due, among other things, to the positive public perception of both Jewish and Christian physicians.[128]

In many cases, in the medieval Muslim world, people would not agree to transgress the injunctions of their religion, even if recommended for the sake of their health. For instance, Ashtor pointed out that Saladin refused to take wine, although one of his Jewish physicians had prescribed

Table 5 Jewish court physicians[129]

Name (dates) [century of activity in court]	*Place of medical activity (court)*
Masīḥ b. Ḥakam al-Dimashqī [8th]	Served in the court of Hārūn al-Rashīd (r. 786–809)
Israel b. Zechariah al-Ṭayfūrī [9th]	Served in the court of the Abbasid caliph al-Mutawakkil
Isḥāq b. Sulaymān al-ʾIsrāʾīlī (Isaac b. Solomon) [9th–10th]	Served as the court physician of the Aghlabī emir and of the Fatimid caliph of Qayrawān
Mūsā b. Elʿāzār al-ʾIsrāʾīlī (Moses b. Elazar) [10th]	Served the first Fatimid caliph, al-Muʿizz li-Dīn Allāh, *wazīr*
Isaac b. Moses (Isḥāq b. Mūsā) (son of Moses b. Elazar) [10th]	Chief leader of the Jews(?), d. 973; (court) physician, *wazīr*
Hārūn (Aaron) b. Isaac of Cordova [10th]	Served in Cordova under the Moorish rulers of Spain
Ḥasday b. Shaprūṭ (905–75) [10th]	Physician, and trusted adviser at the court of the Umayyad caliphs ʿAbd al-Raḥmān III and al-Ḥakam II in Cordova
Abū Ibrāhīm b. Qasṭār (Isaac b. Yashush) [10th–11th]	Physician in ordinary to Muwaffaq Mujāhid al-ʿĀmirī and of his son Iqbāl al-Dawla, kings of Dénia *taifa*, Andalusia
al-Ḥaqīr al-Nāfiʿ al-Ṭabīb (al-Jirāḥī al-Miṣrī) [10th–11th]	Served Caliph al-Ḥākim bi-Amr Allāh (r. 996–1020)
Ṣaqr al-Ṭabīb [10th–11th]	Served Caliph al-Ḥākim bi-Amr Allāh in 1007, replacing the Christian physician Ibn al-Nasṭās al-Naṣrānī (d. 1006)
Mūsā b. Yaʿqūb (grandson of Isaac b. Moses) [11th]	Served as court physician around 1039. Probably also served as the *Raʾīs al-Yahūd*
Abū Isḥāq Ibrāhīm b. ʿAṭā (Abraham b. Nathan) [11th]	Served as court physician to the rulers of Tunisia, Bādis and his son al-Muʿizz
Isaac ha-Kohen ha-Rofe b. Furāt [11th]	Served as court physician at Ramle
Abraham b. Isaac ha-Kohen b. Furāt [11th]	Physician of the Fatimid ruler in Ramle and court physician in Cairo
Ephraim b. al-Zaffān [11th]	Served as physician at the Fatimid court. Was also a merchant
Saʿadya b. Mevōrākh [11th]	Served as physician at the Fatimid court
Abū al-Faḍl (Ḥasday b. Joseph b. Ḥasday), [11th]	Served as court physician at Saragossa, for the Almoravid ruler
Aaron ha-Rōfē al-ʿAmmānī, [11th]	Served as court physician at Amman, Alexandria
Abū Zikrī al-Ṭabīb (Judah b. Saʿadya) (d. 1077) [11th]	Served as court physician and as *nagid* (1062–4)
Abū al-Faḍl Mubārak (Mevōrākh b. Saʿadya) (1040–1111) [11th–12th]	Served as court physician and was influential figure with the Fatimid caliph. *Nagid* 1078–82, 1099–1111

Name (dates) [century of activity in court]	*Place of medical activity (court)*
Moses b. Mevōrākh b. Saʿadya (b. 1080) [11th–12th]	Served as court physician and as *nagid* (1112–26)
Saʿadya b. Mevōrākh [11th–12th]	Probably served as court physician
Ḥasan Abū Kanū [12th]	Served as court physician of the Almoravid emir ʿAlī b. Yūsuf (r. 1106–42)
Meʾir (Abū al-Ḥasan) Ibn Qamniʾel [12th]	Served as court physician to Sultan Yūsuf b. Tāshufīn (r. 1061–1106) in Marrakesh (Almoravid)
Ibn Shūʿa (al-Muwaffaq) [12th]	Served as court physician to Saladin
Hibat Allāh Nethanel b. Moses ha-Levi [12th]	Served as court physician at Cairo
Abū al-Barakāt Hibat Allāh b. ʿAli b. Malkā al-Baladi al-Tabib al-Faḍl (convert) [12th]	Served as physician to Caliph al-Mustanjid biʾllāh (ruled Baghdad 1160–70)
Abū al-Maʿālī/Abū al-ʿAlā Tammām b. Hibat Allāh b. Tammām [12th]	Served as court physician to Saladin
Abū al-ʿAshāʾir Hibat-Allāh b. Zayn b. Ḥasan b. Ifrāʾīm b. Yaʿqūb b. Ismāʿīl Ibn Jumayʿ al-ʾIsrāʾīlī (Nethanel b. Samuel) [12th]	Served as court physician to Saladin
Moses b. Nethanel ha-Levi (Abū Saʿd) [12th]	Cairo, possibly court physician to Fatimid-Ayyubids, worked in hospital, was Head of the Jews
Elijah b. Zechariah, Abū al-Faraj b. al-Raʾīs [12th]	Served under the Ayyubid sultan al-Malik al-Kāmil
Abū Zikrī al-Sadīd b. Elijah b. Zechariah [12th]	Served as court physician to Sultan al-Malik al-ʿAzīz (r. 1193–8), the son of Saladin and his successor
Moses b. Maimon (Maimonides) [12th]	Served as court physician to the Ayyubids, as Head of the Jews, and worked in hospital
Abraham Maimonides (1186–1237) [13th]	Court physician to al-Malik al-Kāmil Muḥammad b. Abī Bakr b. Ayyūb, served as Head of the Jews, and worked in hospital
Ibrāhīm al-Sāmirī, known as 'Shams al-Ḥukamāʾ' [12th]	Served as court physician to Saladin
Abū al-Ḥajjāj Yūsuf b. Yaḥyā b. Isḥāq al-Sabti al-Maghribi [12th]	Served as court physician at Aleppo, Ayyubid
Abū Ayyūb al-Yahūdī (al-ʾIsrāʾīlī) (Solomon b. al-Muʿallim) (Seville) [12th]	Served in the court of the Almoravid emir ʿAlī b. Yūsuf b. Tāshufīn (1106–42) in Marrakesh
Abū Naṣr Samawʾal b. Judah b. ʿAbbās al-Maghribī (converted to Islam 1163, d. 1170) [12th]	Served as court physician to Bahlawān in Azerbaijan and settled in the capital, Marāgha

Table 5 continued

Name (dates) [century of activity in court]	*Place of medical activity (court)*
Samuel b. Hananiah (Abū Manṣūr) [12th]	Served as court physician, Head of the Jews, Cairo, Fatimid
Ibrāhīm b. Khalaf al-Sāmirī [12th–13th]	Served as court physician to Saladin
Abū al-Bayān b. al-Mudawwar al-Sadīd [12th–13th]	Karaite, served as court physician to Fatimid-Ayyubids at Cairo
Abū al-Faḍl Dā ʾūd b. Sulaymān b. Abū al-Bayān al-ʾIsrāʾīlī al-Sadīd (Karaite) (David b. Solomon) [13th]	Served as court physician at Cairo to Saladin and his heir al-ʿĀdil (r. 1200–18), worked in a hospital (al-Bīmāristān al-Nāṣirī)
Ṣadaqa al-ʾIsrāʾīlī [12th–13th]	Probably served as court physician, worked in a hospital
Zechariah the Alexandrian (12th–13th]	Probably served as court physician
Sukra al-Yahūdī al-Ḥalabī [12th]	Served as court physician to Nūr al-Dīn Zengī and Saladin
Abū al-Barakāt al-Quḍāʿī [12th]	Served as court physician to ʿUthmān, son of Saladin
ʿAfīf b. ʿAbd al-Qāhir Sukra [12th–13th]	
ʿImrān b. Ṣadaqa al-ʾIsrāʾīlī al-Ḥakīm Awḥad al-Dīn (Moses b. Ṣadaqa) (1165–1239) [12th–13th]	Served as court physician of the Ayyubid sultan al-Malik al-ʿĀdil, worked in hospitals (al-Bīmāristān al-Kabīr, al-Bīmāristān al-Nūrī)
Abū al-Ḥasan al-ʿAṭṭār 3 [12th–13th]	Served at the court at Alexandria, pharmacist
Yaḥyā b. al-Ṣāʾigh [13th]	Served as court physician to Abū al-Ḥajjāj (ruled Granada 1273–1302)
Yeshūʿā ha-Rōfē b. Aaron ha-Rōfē [13th]	Probably served as court physician in Cairo, around 1217
Elazar the King's physician [13th]	Served as court physician in Aleppo, to Saladin's son al-Malik al-Ẓāhir al-Ghāzī
Kamāl al-Dawla Abū ʿAlī b. Abī al-Faraj, Ibn al-Dāʿī al-ʾIsrāʾīlī al-Irbilī [13th]	Maybe physician in the Mongol court
Ṣadaqa b. Munajjā b. Ṣadaqa al-Sāmirī [13th]	Served as court physician to the Ayyubid sultan al-Ashraf Mūsā b. al-ʿĀdil b. Ayyūb, who ruled Ḥarrān, Baalbek and Damascus
Amīn al-Dawla Abū al-Ḥasan b. Ghazāl b. Abī Saʿīd al-Sāmirī (Samaritan) [13th]	Served as court physician to prince of Baalbek (al-Amjad Bahrām Shāh), *wazīr*
Yūsuf b. Abī Saʿīd b. Khalaf al-Sāmirī al-Muhadhdhab al-Ṭabīb (Samaritan) [13th]	Served as court physician to prince of Baalbek (al-Amjad Bahrām Shāh)
Moses b. Joseph ha-Levi (Abū ʿImrān b. al-Lawī al-Ishbīlī) [13th]	Served the last Moorish king of Seville, Andalusia
Rashīd al-Dīn Abū al-Khayr b. ʿAlī al-Hamadānī (1247–1318) [13th–14th]	Served as court physician at the Īl-Khānate in Tabriz, *wazīr*

Name (dates) [century of activity in court]	*Place of medical activity (court)*
Maghribī, Shihab al-Dīn Aḥmad (convert) [13th–14th]	Probably served as court physician
Jalāl al-Dīn b. al-Ḥazzān [13th–14th]	Served as court physician to Öljeitü Khān, from the Īl-Khānate dynasty in Azerbaijan
Najīb al-Dawla (probably a convert) [13th–14th]	Served as court physician (ophthalmologist) at Tabriz (Mongol Īl-Khāns)
al-Sadīd al-Dimyāṭī [14th]	Served in the court of the Mamluk sultan al-Nāṣir Muḥammad b. Qalāwūn (1285–1341)
Ibn Ṣaghīr, Karaite (convert) [13th–14th]	Probably served as court physician
Ibrāhīm b. al-Tharthār [14th]	Served as court physician to Muḥammad V al-Naṣrī in Granada
Ibn Kūjik, Karaite (convert) [14th]	Probably served as court physician
Jamāl al-Dīn Ibrāhīm b. al-Maghribī (convert) [14th]	'Head of the Physicians' in the court of al-Malik al-Nāṣir Muḥammad b. Qalāwūn, *wazīr*
Faraj Allāh (Yeshūʿā) Ibn Ṣaghīr [14th]	Served in Cairo in the court of al-Malik al-Nāṣir Muḥammad b. Qalāwūn (r. 1310–41) until his death
Asad al-Yahūdī [13th–14th]	Probably served as court physician at Hama
Nafīs ('ʿAbd al-Salām') b. Dāʾūd b. ʿAnān al-Dāʾūdī al-Tabrīzī (1354–1413), Karaite (convert) [14th–15th]	Probably served as court physician. Migration to Cairo 1354, conversion 1360
ʿAbd Allāh b. Daʾūd b. Abī al-Faḍl al-Daʾūdī (d. 1428), Karaite (convert) [14th–15th]	Probably served as court physician
Solomon b. R. Joseph (Samuel Rakkaḥ or Rakkakh) [15th]	Served as court physician to Mamluk sultan Qaitbāy, Cairo. *Nagid*
R. Joseph b. Khalīfa [15th]	Served as court physician to the sultan, Cairo. *Nagid*

it as a remedy for colic.[130] Similar advice was given by Maimonides to Saladin's successor, his son al-Malik al-Afḍal, when he recommended wine and music as a remedy for melancholy, although both were prohibited by the Muslim religion. Maimonides stressed that it is the doctor's duty to prescribe the right drug, leaving the patient to make his decision according to his conscience.[131]

Sometimes, Jewish court physicians used their influence for the benefit of their brothers in the community, as for example in the case of the Jewish leader who was also a court physician (probably Moses b. Mevōrākh

b. Saʿadya, b. 1080). From a letter he wrote to the ruler of Egypt, we learn about the procedure of redeeming a Jewish leader.[132]

Court physicians and those of rich people closely observed their patron, and therefore were able to monitor their health and change their diet or prescribe a drug upon noticing the first change of their steady state. As mentioned above, physicians practising in hospitals were seeing dozens of patients, had little interaction with any of them, and naturally could not have established this kind of monitoring.[133]

Table 5 presents some seventy-five Jewish practitioners that according to contemporary sources worked in courts of Muslim rulers. The number of Jewish physicians who worked in these courts was much higher than that of Jews practising medicine in hospitals. Only a few worked in both hospital and court (for example Moses b. Nethanel ha-Levi, Moses b. Maimon, Abraham Maimonides, Abū al-Faḍl Dāʾūd b. Sulaymān b. Abū al-Bayān al-ʾIsrāʾīlī al-Sadīd, Ṣadaqa al-ʾIsrāʾīlī and ʿImrān b. Ṣadaqa al-ʾIsrāʾīlī al-Ḥakīm Awḥad al-Dīn).[134]

Marina Rustow suggested that Jewish physicians and courtiers at times 'proved more capable of exercising power and more adept at negotiating the channels of government than the *Raʾīs al-Yahūd* himself'. She based her claim on a Mamluk decree found in the Geniza that contains the story of a physician whom the *Raʾīs* had prohibited from entering the synagogue of which he was a member. The physician got around the problem by seeking redress from the sultan; therefore, the *Raʾīs* was forced to rescind his ban.[135]

Jewish court physicians had a prestigious position in their society. Many of them served also as leaders of the Jews in their countries (for example Isḥāq b. Mūsā b. Elʿāzār, Mūsā b. Yaʿqūb, Judah b. Saʿadya, Abū al-Faḍl Mubārak, Moses b. Mevōrākh b. Saʿadya, Moses b. Nethanel Ha-Levi, Moses b. Maimon, Abraham Maimonides, Samuel b. Hananiah, Solomon b. R. Joseph and R. Joseph b. Khalīfa).[136]

There are quite a few Jewish court physicians who were fully trusted and appreciated by the Muslim rulers. Some of them were appointed as advisers (for example Ḥasday b. Shaprūṭ), and even as *wazīrs* (for example Mūsā b. Elʿāzār, Isḥāq b. Mūsā b. Elʿāzār, Yūsuf b. Abī Saʿīd b. Khalaf al-Sāmirī al-Muhadhdhab al-Ṭabīb, Amīn al-Dawla Abū al-Ḥasan b. Ghazāl b. Abī Saʿīd al-Sāmirī, Saʿd al-Dawla b. Ṣafī b. Hibat Allāh b. Muhadhdhib al-Dawla al-Abharī, Jamāl al-Dīn Ibrāhīm b. al-Maghribī, Rashīd al-Dīn Ṭabīb Faḍl Allāh b. al-Dawla and Abū al-Khayr b. ʿAlī Abū al-Hamadānī), thanks to their administrative abilities. In one case (Ḥasday b. Shaprūṭ), a Jewish court physician became a diplomat and special delegate of the ruler.[137]

Miri Shefer claimed that life as a court physician was far from easy. They had to demonstrate a 100 per cent success rate: 'A successful physician had to be cunning, crafty and quick with his thinking in order to save his patient in a situation where normal doctors would fail.'[138] Life as a non-Muslim court physician had advantages but also disadvantages, which probably prompted the conversions. For example, the Christian physician Ibn Muṭrān converted to Islam during the reign of Saladin, and one of his motives may have been the benefits which he was unlikely to have enjoyed as a Christian.[139]

Physicians in Muslim courts were not necessarily rich, but their fixed salaries were enough to prevent them from competing with other practitioners and healers for more clients. Shefer claimed that even though they were on a fixed wage they enjoyed many social and economic privileges. Indeed, being a court physician meant power; however, this could be a double-edged sword. Success at court depended on the caprices of a patron, and as a result it could be short-lived, ending tragically.[140] The biographies of Jewish court physicians presented in this book clearly support these claims.

Success of *dhimmī* physicians in general, and of the Jewish ones in particular, caused jealousy and polemics;[141] and in many cases Jewish physicians in the courts of the Muslim rulers were objects of jealousy from other courtiers. Pormann and Savage-Smith mentioned that 'inter-communal tensions existed, and, despite the general climate of tolerance, frictions occurred'.[142]

And indeed, similarly to their fellow courtiers, some of the Jewish court physicians met their death in court due to political intrigues, such as Isaac ha-Kohen ha-Rōfē b. Furāt (served in Cairo and Ramle, 11th century) and Abū al-Bayān Mūsā b. Abī al-Faḍl (Moses b. Mevōrākh b. Saʿadya) (served in Cairo, 11th–12th centuries). Interestingly, they were both members of medical dynasties.[143] Some lost their lives even after their conversion to Islam, for example Fatḥ Allāh b. Muʿtaṣim b. Nafīs (Fatḥ al-Dīn) (Karaite, served in Tabriz and Cairo, 14th–15th centuries).

Serving as a physician in court varied in length of time. In some cases, they gave only sporadic medical advice and in other cases only for a short period. Few Jewish physicians received a lifetime appointment or even a pension when they became old.

4.1.2 Practitioners' education

Being a physician was a prestigious occupation; according to Goitein, a physician's knowledge was 'esoteric, accessible to others only imperfectly'. Jewish physicians were students of the writings of the ancients[144] like other students of medicine in the medieval period. The medical knowledge that young Jewish students of medicine acquired was mainly based on the writings of Hippocrates and especially Galen, whose works 'had been profusely commented on and whose notions had been re-elaborated and adapted by Arab medical authors, who also made their own original contributions'.[145] Based on Geniza documents, we know that the names Hippocrates, Galen and Dioscorides were familiar even to laymen; the evidence is in general lists of books, a few of which mention medical ones.[146]

In both Muslim and Jewish medieval societies memorising information played a critical role in the process of mastering any knowledge, scientific as well as religious. Medical knowledge was studied and transmitted in various forms, all of which involved memorising.[147] The art of medicine was learnt from books and apprenticeship with a master; thus a relationship would develop between him and the medical student by transmitting both medical theory and practice. According to Carmen Caballero-Navas, prospective physicians were trained under such guidance and supervision, and the students attended to patients in the same manner, trying to implement what had been learnt both from books and from the experience of their masters. In most cases, Jews benefited from this system, which was equally applied by Muslims and Christians, without distinguishing between students and masters.[148]

The theoretical knowledge and practical skills needed for practising medicine in the medieval Arab world were acquired in various ways, but mainly from learning within the family (father, grandfather, friend of the family), self-learning, classes in hospitals and medical schools or study groups with a teacher. The students were learning from medical books and had to gain clinical experience. At the end of their studies, they had to pass examinations that tested their medical knowledge and training. The examination was oral and dealt with both theoretical and practical knowledge (but there was no practical examination as such).[149]

Another option of studying medicine in the Arabic tradition was reading public lectures to medical students.[150] In general where this was done, biographers made a special point of it. So far, we have not been able to find evidence for such practice in the Geniza, although according to Ibn Abī Uṣaybiʿa, Ibn Jumayʿ, the Jewish physician that served Saladin, 'held general meetings for all those who practised under him the art of medicine'.[151]

The medical educational system in the Muslim world during the medieval period was not monopolistic, and operated as an 'open system'. The various paths or tracks of learning medicine were all legitimate and open to members of all religious. In fact, every person could transfer medical knowledge and students could even study by themselves. There was a general consensus regarding the medical literature that the students had to read and learn; however, the way that these books were studied, and the knowledge that was acquired, were up to the students and the teachers. It is important to note that the Jews had an advantage over other medical students due to their knowledge of languages, something that made more medical literature available for them.[152]

In the Muslim world, there was a mechanism of control and ordination of physicians which enabled them to maintain their required standards. According to the Muslim perception of the governing bodies, the caliph, the religious and political leader of all Muslims, was responsible for the physical and psychological welfare of his subjects. Therefore, the rulers developed a mechanism to control the medical profession. This system included the office of the *muḥtasib*, and an ordination examination for physicians that intended to work independently. These examinations were mainly based on the vast medical literature written by the Arab physicians who discussed in depth ways to prevent medical quackery and charlatanism.[153]

Jews practised under that system, as was proved from the study of some Geniza fragments.[154] As far as we know, there was no anti-Jewish deviation in the work of the *muḥtasib*.[155] Towards the thirteenth century, the teaching of mathematical, philosophical and medical sciences progressively infiltrated into the religious teaching institutions; medicine and pharmacology were among the non-religious disciplines that were taught in a madrasa.

The process of teaching medicine by teachers who were legally appointed broadened access to medical knowledge beyond families of doctors, but it decreased the access of minority groups, including the Jews, to the study of these sciences. Sonja Brentjes claimed that these fields were learnt and taught among the Christian and Jewish communities; and not only in madrasas and mosques.[156]

The study of medicine included other sciences such as pharmaceutics, nutrition and climatology, as well as general sciences, such as logic and mathematics. The physician should have a mind trained in philosophy. As mentioned before, the term *ḥakīm*, 'doctor', designated not only a physician, but also a man of comprehensive secular education. In a bookish civilisation, acquaintance with ancient sources was highly respected. When a physician wished to assure his patient that he was receiving the best treatment available, he would tell him that it was recommended 'by the most ancient authorities' and name one of those mentioned above.[157]

The Geniza provides us with information regarding some of the various ways of studying medicine and becoming a physician, and of gaining practical medical experience in the medieval Muslim world.[158] These have been gleaned from documents and from letters found in the Geniza:

a. Apprenticeship to a physician of repute. Evidence of this course being chosen by Maimonides is discussed in detail by Joel Kraemer.[159]

b. From a letter addressed by Me'ir b. al-Hamadānī, father of a medical student, to the judge and physician Moses (according to Goitein most probably Maimonides), we learn that it was not easy to find the opportunity to study and practise under the guidance of a famous physician. In his letter Me'ir offered to pay the physician a higher fee than his former apprentice.[160] Friedman strongly (and gently) claimed this proves that the letter was not addressed to Maimonides.[161]

c. Working in a hospital improved the students' medical knowledge and enhanced their careers. However, this option was fairly difficult to acquire, as we learn from several letters. While hospital work was easily accessible to prominent doctors, the young candidate had to obtain a letter of recommendation from a person of authority and social standing, such as a governor or a judge, as well as a certificate of good character from the local chief of police.[162] Moreover, it enabled talented young physicians to complete their medical education and receive their licences.[163] In other cases it gave them the opportunity to belong to a network of physicians and scholars.[164]

In a letter sent to a young 'doctor' who was studying in Cairo and looking for an appointment in a hospital in Alexandria, his cousin wrote from there and advised him to obtain letters of recommendation from the chief of police, the *qadi* and 'the Successful' (probably the famous Ibn Jumayʿ).[165] It appears that a police certificate of good conduct was required in order to practise the medical profession in general and not only for working in hospitals. In a fragment addressed to a judge we read, 'No one is permitted to practise medicine either in Fusṭāṭ or [?in Cairo] without a certificate of good conduct.' Such a certificate was secured not so much by good conduct itself as by appropriate connections and presumably also gifts to the officials handling the matter.[166]

An interesting anecdote teaches us about residency. Residents were not allowed to practise independently, except under the supervision of a licensed physician, as we learn from an ophthalmologist's letter to his assistant: 'I heard that Menahem has already been licensed, while you are still only a *muʿallim* [unlicensed practitioner].'[167]

As mentioned above, biographical dictionaries were used as a unique source for the reconstruction of the world of Islamic knowledge, tracing networks of scholars, their connection with political power, and their professional careers.[168] Indeed, from Muslim Arabic sources we learn that Jewish physicians were learning from other Jewish ones, as in the case of Abū Sahl Dūnash b. Tamīm (d. 971), a court physician and author of medical books from Qayrawān. He was the student of Isḥāq b. Sulaymān al-ʾIsrāʾīlī.[169] Other examples include Abū al-Faḍl Dāʾūd b. Sulaymān b. Abū al-Bayān al-ʾIsrāʾīlī al-Sadīd (David b. Solomon) (1161–1236), who was the student of Ibn Jumayʿ and Ibn al-Nāqid (an ophthalmologist);[170] and Abū al-Khayr Salāma b. Mubārak b. Raḥmūn b. Mūsā al-Ṭabīb (11th–12th century), considered to be one of the best physicians in Egypt – he had studied medicine, for a long time, under the guidance of Ephraim b. al-Zaffān, and was his best student.[171] Some Jewish physicians studied medicine from Muslim ones, while others were teaching medicine. In most cases, their students were either Muslims or Christians.[172]

We also have evidence that Jewish practitioners consulted each other, as we can learn from the case of Asʿad al-Dīn (Ibn Ṣabra) al-Maḥallī al-Mutaṭabbib (Jacob b. Isaac), who according to Ibn Abī Uṣaybiʿa carried on a scientific correspondence with a Samaritan physician from Damascus, Ṣadaqa b. Munajjā b. Ṣadaqa al-Sāmirī.[173] Another case is a letter found in the Geniza in which one physician discusses with another certain eye conditions and their treatments.[174]

Sometimes the physicians pushed their sons to study and practise from an early age. Ibn Abī Uṣaybiʿa for example, described a doctor serving the caliph, who paid his son a few dirhams every day and had him bleed patients outside the door of his office, until he acquired great dexterity in this technique. When a courtier needed bleeding, the young man was invited to do the job; as suggested by the father, in the presence of the caliph. Thanks to his performance he was admitted to the court, where he remained throughout his life.[175] A similar case regarding a Jewish physician was studied from Geniza documents and presented by Goitein. Hibat Allah-Nethanel was head of the Jewish Rabbinical college in Fusṭāṭ and a court physician; as a son of a doctor, he was bribed in his youth with the very large sum of twenty-five dinars never to leave his house, not even for a visit to the public bathhouse, and to devote his time entirely to the study of medicine, languages, the Talmud and theology. We learn about this from letters he sent in which he complained bitterly about his separation from his boon companions.[176]

4.1.3 Female practitioners

Women played a hidden, though important, part in the health of the members of medieval societies. They took care of family health behind the curtain by cooking for and feeding their family members, and by solving and treating minor medical issues. Their role in medical history was astutely described by Pormann and Savage-Smith:

> It can be argued that health care, both in the medieval Islamic and in early modern Europe societies, was for the most part provided by women.

> Within the family they looked after the medical needs of the children, as well as after those of their husbands and other members of the extended family. As nurses and midwives, as careers and curers, they contributed fundamentally to the health of the wider society.[177]

Based on Arabic literary sources it seems that gynaecological care in the medieval Muslim world was mainly 'women consulting women' or midwives serving as adjuncts to male physicians, conducting examinations and manoeuvres to preserve the modesty of the patient.[178] According to Avner Giladi, childbirth was often the exclusive dominion of midwives and female attendants.[179]

The learned medical discourse was largely dominated by men. There is no historical record of the medical activity of women in medieval Islam. Female physicians are only identified when they are rarely mentioned in the bio-bibliographical and medical literature. It seems as though when orthodox medicine was perceived not to work, people turned to alternative practitioners, many of whom were probably female.

When we come to check this assumption in the Jewish societies of the Muslim world, the picture is very similar. For example, Pormann and Savage-Smith state that 'there are in fact a comparatively high number of instances where the female practitioners mentioned in our sources worked as ophthalmologists';[180] it is not surprising that a few female ophthalmologists (*kaḥḥālah*) were mentioned in the Geniza documents, for example in a list of people receiving alms, one of whom was a woman who was probably poor.[181] According to Goitein, women doctors appear quite frequently in the Geniza, including one female ophthalmologist. As those mentioned belonged to the lower strata of society, they certainly had not gone through the expensive apprenticeship of scientific medicine; but they were practitioners whose knowledge and skills had come to them by tradition. They were called *tabība*, and in one case al-Ṭubayba, 'the Little [or Beloved] Doctor'.[182] These women fulfilled an important role in the female society of the Geniza period, some also specialising in the removal of hair from women's bodies.[183] Some examples have been traced in the Geniza: Mubārak b. al-Ṭabība and Farij b. al-Ṭabība;[184] Awlād Ibn al-Ṭubyba;[185] (anonymous) al-Ṭabība, mentioned in a document dealing with a household receiving bread.[186] These might have been female physicians.[187] However, we do not learn anything of importance about the activities of these professionals – attending to a woman, for example, at childbirth.[188]

4.1.4 Physicians' libraries

Books were indispensable tools for the medieval scholar. Physicians were no exception, and the size of a physician's library can be an indication of his erudition, prominence and importance. If a physician had access to many books, he had access to the knowledge and experience of his predecessors. The more he knew through reading books, the more his contemporaries respected him and possibly relied on him.[189]

Thanks to the Geniza manuscripts we know quite a lot about the size and the content of the medical libraries of Jewish physicians in the Muslim world. Our knowledge is based on three main genres of manuscripts: the first is titles and categories of books that were found and identified in the Geniza,[190] the second is a doctor's book lists,[191] and the third is titles of medical books found in general lists of books.[192]

Medical libraries were composed of reference books, which the practitioners consulted in order to diagnose the medical problems of their patients and find the best way to cure them, and also of medical teaching literature. Brentjes claimed that the latter 'encompassed books that were studied in a number of Islamic societies over many centuries, and texts that were taught on a regional level'. The strong local character of medical teaching was due to various reasons: different languages, statistical connections between Muslim and non-Muslim inhabitants, and the presence or absence of other healing traditions.[193] Indeed, it seems as though the medical library of the medieval Jewish practitioners was unique. From preliminary research on the fragments of medical books that have been identified in the main Geniza collection (the Taylor-Schechter Collection at Cambridge University Library), it appears that most are written in Arabic (740), fewer in Judaeo-Arabic (470), and only 150 in Hebrew.[194] There is no doubt that books written in Judaeo-Arabic and Hebrew were used only by Jewish practitioners.

The strong interest in pharmacy is evidenced by the large number of pharmacopoeias and *materia medica* books that were identified as such. Some of these works were even written by members of the Jewish community.[195] In most cases, it is uncertain whether the owners of the books were physicians or pharmacists. Over and over again the Muslim Arabic sources give us information regarding the size of the libraries of the rich and famous; the Geniza informs us of their content. The relationship between the two professions was very close, with the pharmacists usually seen (from the physician's point of view) as carrying out the physicians' instructions. Although the physicians usually only wrote down prescriptions, they were considered as capable of making them up by themselves.[196]

Regarding the size of medical libraries, I present a few case studies from Muslim Arabic sources:

a. Saladin's famous secretary and counsellor al-Qāḍī al-Fāḍīl founded the Fāḍīliyyah madrasa in Cairo, which was allegedly endowed with a library containing more than 100,000 books.[197]

b. Ephraim b. al-Ḥasan al-Zaffān, a Cairene physician who was active during the eleventh century in Egypt (d. 1068), was the most prominent student of the famous Muslim physician ʿAlī Ibn Riḍwān.[198] He was the author of several medical books,[199] and his family was known as a family of traders and physicians.[200] According to Ibn Abī Uṣaybiʿa: 'He was in the service of the caliphs of his time, and received from them a very great amount of money and favours. He had an acute interest in acquiring and copying books, so that he accumulated many scores of them on medicine and other subjects.'[201] These efforts resulted in a unique library of 20,000 volumes desired by many people of his time.[202] This figure is probably after he sold 10,000 to the *wazīr* al-Afḍal. Some of the books that had a unique private ex-libris were seen two decades later.[203]

c. Ṣadaqa b. Munajjā b. Ṣadaqa al-Sāmirī al-Ṭabīb, a Samaritan physician (d. 1232) of the Ayyubid sultan, who ruled Ḥarrān, Baalbek and Damascus, had a big library with over 10,000 books and manuscripts. Ṣadaqa himself wrote many medical books (for example a commentary on Hippocrates and answers to questions asked by Asʿad al-Dīn (Ibn Ṣabra) al-Maḥallī al-Mutaṭabbib (Jacob b. Isaac).[204] According to Nicolae, the figure of 10,000 is not to be taken literally, but only as an indication that the book collection was comparatively large.[205]

Another method that was employed to estimate the size of libraries was practised by Nicolae. He described in detail what he called 'Ibn Jumayʿ's library',[206] claiming in his *Canon* commentary that Ibn Jumayʿ displayed an impressive array of sources. Ibn Jumayʿ cited about eighty authors and referred to probably no fewer than sixty different treatises. Nicolae added that 'it is difficult to imagine that the number of medical books available to him exceeded one or two hundred items'. Moreover, he added, 'Ibn Jumayʿ may have never had a personal library'. In any case, the existence of large libraries in Cairo indicates that the books Ibn Jumayʿ referred to may not necessarily have been in his personal collection, but rather part of a larger library to which he had access. Furthermore, we cannot be sure that Ibn Jumayʿ had direct access to a treatise just because he cited it.[207]

A few Geniza documents can teach us about the size and content of medical libraries that were owned by middle-class Jewish practitioners in medieval Egypt:

a. A document records a rich bride who had a staff of two maids and two personal attendants. Her dowry and nuptial gift (presented in the fragment from around 1140) included a library worth 250 dinars. Goitein suggested that she was probably the daughter of a rich physician who had recently died, and about to marry a physician who was after the books.[208] This bride's library might have contained about a thousand manuscripts.[209]

b. A library belonging to a physician and his wife was put up for sale in November 1190, after the physician's death. Some 102 volumes were sold, at an average price of approximately a quarter of a dinar. Interestingly, but not surprisingly, at least thirty-three of those volumes contained works by Galen. The most recent authors mentioned in the collection may have died around 120 years before the proprietor of that excellent library.[210]

c. A list was found in a Geniza fragment dated 1223, concerning two auctions, held on two successive Tuesdays. The library, which was auctioned in Fusṭāṭ, included works by the Spanish Muslim Ibn Rushd (Averroes), who died in 1198. Similar to the previous list, Galen and Hippocrates were the most important authors, followed by al-Rāzī (d. 925), one of the most original authors of Islamic medicine.[211]

Several more anecdotes give us further examples of the importance of books to Jewish intellectuals in general, and Jewish physicians in particular:

a. Aaron ha-Rōfē b. Yeshūʿā ha-Rōfē Ibn al-ʿAmmānī was a physician and Alexandrian judge who was also a book dealer. We know this from a letter he sent to a certain ʿAṭṭār, with other books among which were three volumes of Dioscorides.[212]

b. The Geniza has preserved the inventory of the estate of Ibn al-Sharābī, containing 200 bound volumes and an unspecified number of loose books.[213]

c. Another case is related to a public auction of a library of a deceased doctor (probably not left to any relative who would have had a claim on it and an interest in it), in which we further learn about the content of a library of a Jewish doctor.[214]

d. In a letter from Aden, southern Arabia, written in July 1202, to Cairo, Maḍmūn II b. David, the *nagid* of Aden, ordered all the medical writings of the master to be copied for him![215]

e. Abraham b. Hillel ha-Ḥasid (physician, poet and scholar, close to the Ben Maimon family, d. 1223) owned a large library of medical and religious Jewish writings.[216]

The foremost impression to be gathered from the lists of medical books so far found in the Geniza is the preponderance of works by classical authors as well as Arab medical authorities.[217] We also understand from several cases that medical books were lent from one physician to another, for example:

a. Ben ha-Sōfer ha-Dayyān (c. 1150) borrowed the famous book 'Ten Treatises on the Eye' by Ḥunain b. Isḥāq from a *warrāq* who was possibly also a physician.[218]

b. Abū al-Fakhr al-Ṭabīb's name is mentioned in the context of information regarding book purchases that was found in *Warrāq's Notebook*,[219] the diary of a book merchant, and it is written that he lent ten books, including four copies of a book called *The Craft of Healing*, in two parts: 'The Power of Medicines' and 'Spiritual Medicine'. He also had in his possession two booklets, one an abridgment of 'The Physician Is a Philosopher' and the other of 'The Craft of Healing', as well as another booklet entitled 'Being and Loss'. The prices of some of the books are noted.[220]

4.1.5 The 'Head of the Physicians'

The position of 'Head of the Physicians' in the Muslim world was responsible for the proper qualification of all practising physicians. The holder of this position had the authority to issue or to withdraw the medical licence of any physician.[221]

The high position of 'Head of the Physicians' could have been occupied by a Jewish physician in the Ayyubid period, as we learn from the case of Ibn Jumayʿ.[222] However, in the Mamluk period it was occupied only by Jews who had converted to Islam or belonged to converted Jewish dynasties.[223] Here are some examples:

a. Shihāb al-Dīn Aḥmad al-Maghribī (13th–14th centuries) and his son Jamāl al-Dīn Ibrāhīm (d. 1355).
b. The Karaite Nafīs b. Daʾūd b. ʿAnān al-Tabrīzī (1354–1413) and his son Ṣadr al-Dīn Badīʿ (d. 1394), who had probably converted with his father.
c. As previously mentioned above, the Karaite Ibn Ṣaghīr dynasty (14th–15th centuries) held this post as well.
d. The converted Sulaymān b. Junayba (1410–21) and Zayn al-Dīn Khiḍr al-Isrāʾilī (1437–8).[224]

4.2 Everyday Life

4.2.1 Personal issues and everyday life and activity

The sources, mainly the documents from the Geniza, enable us to acquire information relating to the personal matters of some of our practitioners, such as marriage, family, children, housing, other occupations and so on.

The biographies in this book contain a vast amount of chronological information. One issue of interest is the number of years a Jewish physician or pharmacist practised, and at what age they died. Some researchers, using quantitative history as a method and studying biographies of Muslim scholars, have examined a similar question. Richard Bulliet, for example, studied the age structure of medieval Islamic education in the eastern part of the Muslim world; using thousands of biographies of teachers and students of Muslim scholars, he learnt about the average age they started to study, the number of years they studied, how long the teachers were active, their average age and when they died.[225] María Luisa Ávila studied Islamic scholars' age at death in the Muslim West.[226] I tried to apply both methods and get some insight regarding the Jewish practitioners in the medieval Muslim world, but unfortunately our data on the Jewish practitioners does not allow us to make such research viable. We know the age of death of only a few known physicians, and interestingly enough, such information comes usually from Muslim Arabic sources! So far, I have managed to trace the age of just sixteen practitioners (out of 607). Their average age at death was surprisingly high, at seventy-two. We should take into consideration that usually we know this kind of detail (birth and death) only about prestigious practitioners who made such an impact during their lives that the sources (Muslim Arabic as well as the Cairo Geniza) mentioned these details. Clearly, the longer one lives, the greater the impact. Moreover, the practitioners who lived in the big cities, who were heads of communities and who worked in courts and hospitals were better known. In any case, here are some examples: Isḥāq (Abū Yaʿqūb) b. Sulaymān al-ʾIsrāʾīlī died at the age of 100,[227] Abū al-Barakāt Hibat Allāh b. ʿAli b. Malkā al-Tabib al-Faḍl died around the age of 80,[228] Rashīd al-Dīn was executed at the age of 71,[229] and Moses Ben Maimon (Maimonides) lived for 66 or 67 years.

Several studies have been published on the activities of physicians in the Muslim world during the Middle Ages,[230] a number of which deal with Jewish practitioners as well.[231] A Jewish doctor that served in either a court or a hospital usually began his day very early in the morning. From Geniza letters we learn that a private doctor did so as well, sometimes even 'when the stars were still visible'. In a letter written by a physician, the writer worries that he is unable to say his morning prayers at the prescribed time.[232]

According to S. D. Goitein, a physician would buy for himself a home worth 200 or 300 dinars or more. Residences in this range of prices apply not only to Egypt but also to Qayrawān, Tunisia, Palermo, Sicily, Seleucia and Asia Minor.[233] Since Jews were restricted in where they could ride on Saturdays due to Halakhic rules, noble families tried to live near the synagogue. When the city of Cairo was founded and a synagogue was erected there, three court physicians of the Fatimid caliphs (belonging to one family) had their houses round about it.[234]

4.2.2 Records of practical medical activity

Inventories of the physicians' possessions written after their death are our main source of knowledge. One particular document gives us some insight into the type of clothes worn by a twelfth-century physician (Abū al-Riḍā ha-Levi) and tells us about his carpets and some of his medical utensils. The document was ordered by Moses Maimonides on 13 April 1172. The physician and his brother Abū a1-Ḥasan are known from a document written in the provincial town of Minyat Ziftā. Abū al-Riḍā was probably a middle-class 'country doctor', settled in the capital. Some of the items that were used for medical purposes were recorded such as canisters, a mirror, a pestle (to grind medicinal substances), buckets, a bookcase made of bamboo canes containing black silk borders, an iron dipper, a bandage container, kohl containers (for the treatment of eye diseases), washbasins and tables, a pillow, a set of copper vessels, a lamp for wax candles, and a knife in a sheath.[235] Three carpets were described: a white centre carpet with blue borders (13.2 metres long); 'a middle piece', a red silk carpet (17.6 metres long); and another red carpet (10.6 metres long). Goitein suggested that a successful physician had to seat many visitors (as both Maimonides and Judah ha-Levi, who were physicians, emphasise in their letters), and silk was perhaps favoured because it could be cleaned more easily than other textiles. In general, most carpets were imported, including 'a physician's carpet', *namaṭ ṭabībī*.[236]

As we can learn from the above description and from other documents, some physicians prepared their own compounds, therefore they had to have the necessary tools, and when they visited patients they took with them certain remedies they had in stock. Another well-preserved fragment that seems to be an inventory gives us an idea of the objects they carried; the list contains instruments such as a mortar, a scale and glasses, indicating that the doctor or an assistant prepared the medicaments themselves.[237]

Records of practical medical activity such as prescriptions and medical recipes are rarely found in the early medieval period. Fortunately, thanks to the Cairo Geniza, some such documents have studied and identified in the last few decades. A selection of them are presented and briefly discussed below:

a. Maimonides' handwriting is unique and therefore recognisable; dozens of Geniza fragments have been identified as being written in his own hand. Most of them have been studied and published. One known case is of a recipe for the treatment of headaches which he prescribed in a letter[238] to his former student Tuvia.[239]

b. Lately, a practical prescription[240] written by Maimonides has been identified and will be published in the near future.[241]

c. A few prescriptions written in his handwriting and found in the Geniza have been identified as those of Berakhot b. Samuel, who was active in Egypt in the thirteenth century.[242]

d. Abraham b. Yijū, a Jewish merchant, scholar and poet with medical knowledge, was active in Egypt and India during the twelfth century.[243] There is rare evidence of his medical activity, however: two prescriptions were found[244] which were probably written in his handwriting.[245]

4.2.3 Travelling and means of transportation

In the Muslim world, people in general, and scholars in particular, travelled, as well as traders, pilgrims and geographers; the latter, mainly travelling for the sake of knowledge, in many cases stopped in the big cities and studied with others, including famous scholars and professionals.[246] In order to survive, some Jewish physicians moved and practised under both Muslim and Christian regimes, according to the historical developments.[247] Shefer noted that in Mamluk Egypt, physicians assembled in the scholarly centre of Cairo and rarely travelled outside Egypt.[248]

Brentjes claimed that the travels of Jewish (and Christian) students and teachers are more difficult to trace. Under the Ayyubid and Mongol dynasties, non-Muslim scholars and physicians eagerly travelled between Syria, Iraq and Iran, visiting famous scholars or looking for patrons. However, from the fourteenth century, information about them is scarce.[249]

Jewish physicians serving the rulers, or called to patients in smaller places, were to be found on the roads.[250] However, according to the 'Pact of 'Umar', *dhimmīs* were not allowed to ride on horses, although a lower-middle-class physician could have a modest riding donkey (price range around four dinars). If for any reason the practitioner did not keep one, he at least kept in the house saddles and harnesses for both mule and donkey to be used when he bought or hired a riding animal for travel. Such equipment was found in the estate of a Jewish druggist (1143), for example.[251] An interesting tale related to this concerns Ibn Shūʿa (al-Muwaffaq) (d. 1183), one of Saladin's physicians. He was hurt by a Muslim zealot who threw a stone at him which took out one of his eyes, and all because he was riding a horse in violation of the laws restricting the *dhimmīs*.[252]

From various documents we learn that physicians travelled a lot to Egyptian destinations such as Ashmūm, Salman and Dimyāṭ (Damietta). It should be mentioned here that travels, particularly over long distances and at sea, were dangerous, and since Jewish physicians were travelling frequently, some were captured by pirates. We learn for example about a Jewish physician and his wife who were on board a Christian ship captured by Muslim freebooters and brought to Alexandria.[253] In such cases, the Jewish communities collected money to pay the ransom and set them free.

Jews, including Jewish physicians, had over certain periods to pay taxes when travelling from one place to another. In one document, a young physician is advised not to travel from Egypt to Syria, 'for, as a Jew, you will have to pay 30 silver pieces as customs duties'.[254]

Jews hosted in their houses other Jews travelling from one place to another. In one case, a physician travelling from Cairo to Damascus was put up by the Jewish judge of Bilbays, on the eastern fringes of the Nile Delta.[255]

From a letter written by a physician from Qalyūb, we learn that he left his hometown and opened an office in Cairo. He wrote to his wife that due to the hostility of other physicians he could not risk coming over to examine her sore eyes and therefore asked her to join him.[256]

Abraham b. Yijū is only one example of a 'frequent traveller'; a man of many talents and initiatives who, as mentioned above, also had medical knowledge. He was born in al-Mahdiyya (Tunisia), travelled to India, where he was active between 1132 and 1149, and finally settled in Egypt in 1153. He was a Jewish scholar, wrote Halakhic responsa[257] and was also a merchant and a poet.[258]

4.2.4 Commercial activity of Jewish practitioners

It turns out that Jewish physicians, similarly to other Geniza people, were involved in commercial activities as a sideline (such as trade, industry, loans, property etc.). This was not unusual in medieval Muslim society. In her anthroponymic study on Muslim scholars connected with economic activities in Andalusian society (10th–12th centuries), Marín found 150 different occupational *laqabs*.[259] Some examples of Jewish practitioners' economic activities are presented below:

a. **Trade:** Among the many examples of practitioners involved in trade in general, and in India trade in particular, Maimonides advised one of his disciples to earn his livelihood through commerce and teaching medicine. Moreover, Maimonides promised to set up accounts for him with a merchant trading with India. A letter addressed to Maimonides from his brother David, when the latter was en route to India, shows that Maimonides himself was well versed in business affairs.[260] Other Geniza documents reveal that some physicians and their family members even acted as merchants' representatives (*wakil*).[261] According to the data collected so far, members of at least three dynasties of physicians were merchants beside being community leaders and in some cases even court physicians: Ephraim b. al-Zaffān (Cairo, 11th century) court physicians and merchants (dynasty 5); Moses b. Jekuthiel (Andalusia, Cairo, 11th–12th centuries), physicians, merchants and community leaders (dynasty 12);[262] and Zechariah the Alexandrian (Alexandria, Jerusalem, Cairo, 12th–13th centuries), court physicians, communal leaders, judges and merchants (dynasty 21). Worth mentioning, in particular, is Abū Yaʿqūb al-Ḥakīm (Jekuthiel b. Moses ha-Rōfē), a prominent 11th–12th-century representative of the merchants in Fusṭāṭ. It is reasonable to assume that he studied medicine and practised it a little.[263] He took part in both the Mediterranean and India trades and according to the documents was known as a tough merchant.[264] His son also acted as a representative of the merchants, whereas his grandson, Abū al-Faḍāʾil Jekuthiel II b. Moses II ha-Rōfē, went back to medicine, his great-grandfather Moses' profession.[265]
b. **Sugar factories:** From a few documents dealing with sugar production, we learn that physicians not only had a share in the factories, but also participated in their operation. In one document, two physicians, father and son, admitted a scholar as a partner in a 'sugar factory' belonging

to them; he brought in a total share of 100 dinars. Goitein claimed that since this was a comparatively small undertaking, it is not impossible that the two doctors actually looked after their sugar shop.[266] Elsewhere, the physician Japheth ([Abū] al-Maḥāsin) ha-Kohen b. Josiah was mentioned in a legal document dated 1220–1 in which he is said to be the partner of a sugar merchant named Abū al-ʿIzz b. Abū al-Maʿānī in operating a sugar factory. From this document we learn that they could no longer pay the high governmental taxes.[267] Another fragment described a broker who had received a loan from a physician, who sold sugar (around 1225). In the thirteenth century, sugar factories became a favourite and fashionable form of investment, repeatedly mentioned as owned by physicians.[268]

c. **Book trading:** Books played an important part in medieval Arab society. Stories about copying and trading books are mentioned by many medieval Muslim Arabic sources.[269] Book trading was an especially preferred business for physicians,[270] who were bibliophiles because of their profession.[271] For example, a letter to a prominent 12th-century physician who was in the army teaches us that like other physicians he was dealing with books,[272] while a medical notebook contains information regarding the trading and lending of books. Another letter enquires of the perfumer Abū Saʿīd of Fusṭāṭ about several books, including three volumes of an Arabic translation of Dioscorides. The wide diversity of the subjects of these books shows that they were destined for sale.[273] Aaron ha-Rōfē b. Yeshūʿā ha-Rōfē Ibn al-ʿAmmānī, a physician and a judge in Alexandria (12th century),[274] also dealt with books.[275]

d. **Teaching:** Education in general, and teaching young boys in particular, has always been highly important in Jewish tradition. *Melammēd* was the Hebrew term for this job in medieval society. A very few physicians bore this term as part of their name: Judah ha-Melammēd b. Aaron ha-Rōfē Ibn al-ʿAmmānī (Alexandria, 13th century) was a *melammēd* and a *ḥazzān* (cantor), a court clerk and in charge of the charity records (*ṣadāqā*).[276] Another physician bearing the name Melammēd was Elijah ha-R(ō)fē b. Samuel ha-Melammēd (14th century).[277]

Based on documents from the Geniza, Goitein claimed that teaching was a profitable job.[278] From a letter found in the Geniza we learn about a physician in Minyat Ziftā who undertook the teaching of schoolchildren in addition to his medical work, due to the absence of the local teacher; the physician became so enthusiastic about the additional income that he did not let the children go back to their former teacher when he returned.[279]

e. **Ship ownership:** From one document we learn that a Jewish physician owned a ship that sailed, among other destinations, to Tripoli (Libya), al-Mahdiyya and Egypt.[280]

f. **Real estate and mortgages:** Urban properties were an important form of investment, and many physicians were involved in buying and selling houses or parts of them, sometimes even mortgaging properties for loans.[281]

g. **Ammonia sellers:** Abū al-Faraj b. al-Nashādirī was an ammonia merchant, or belonged to a family that dealt with ammonia, appeared on a list of taxpayers or donors to a fund raised for the redemption of captives etc.[282]

h. **Bathing house owner:** Ibn Qarqa, a physician, was, according to al-Maqrīzī, the owner of a bathing house known as Hammām al-Ṭabīb Abū Saʿīd b. Qarqa, in the Jewish neighbourhood of Zuwayla, adjacent to the al-Masʿūdī market in Cairo, and his own house was near the bathing house.[283]

4.3 Moral Aspects, Fees and the 'Geniza Patient'

4.3.1 Medical ethics and behaviour

According to Lewicka, Ayyubid and Mamluk Muslim discourses are literary expressions of the thoughts, beliefs, disputes, stereotypes and values that created the cultural climate and social mood of these times, mainly in Egypt and Syria. Learning the sources – that is, bibliographical dictionaries, analytical works, chronicles and religious treatises – exposes two main strategies reflecting a process of radicalisation of Islam and its growing tendency to dominate.

First, authors promoted a 'strategy of selection', not recognising eminent Jewish and Christian physicians and their achievements. This absence could be influenced by a negative bias towards non-Muslim physicians or reflect a shift towards a conceptualisation of the superiority of Islamic religious education and skills. As a consequence, theoretical medical education became the domain of the *ʿulamāʾ*, while medical practice was left to professionals who were not of the *ʿulamāʾ*, in other words Christians and Jews. Therefore, Jewish and Christian physicians were excluded from the 'elite' who were famous for their books, knowledge or high positions; they were perceived as 'ordinary' medical practitioners who were not 'worthy' to be mentioned. In the second strategy, several authors followed a narrative of negative propaganda, such as spreading false, overgeneralised and negative stereotypes relating to *dhimmī* physicians in general, and Jewish practitioners in particular, as well as encouraging negative attitudes towards them.

These two strategies of religious bias were by no means used by the entire Muslim community, but primarily by radical religious scholars. The success of Jewish physicians (and Christian) and their generally good reputation and popularity among Muslim patients was perceived as weakening Islam. Lewicka differentiates between the individual level (physicians were linked to allegations of charlatan practices or insincerity) and the collective level (Jewish physicians characterised as having 'evil intentions'). They were blamed as a group of taking medicine away from Muslims, or of seriously threatening their Muslim patients' lives.[284]

A few examples of negative Muslim propaganda towards Jewish physicians can be found in various sources, for instance quoting the physician al-Kaskarī (Baghdad, 10th century): 'The physicians of the land are mostly Jews fond of using falsehood and deceit.'[285] According to Nicolae it is a clear indication that Jews had an important and well-established place in medicine.[286]

Another example, from Syria, is brought to us by Zayn al-Dīn al-Jawbarī, a thirteenth-century traveller who visited Iraq, India and Syria:

> Their physicians are the atheists of the atheists and they have hidden secrets that they reveal to no one. If they want to heal a person, they do everything they can and give him the right drug to be well shortly; but, if they wish him ill, they tell him to take harmful drugs. Moreover, they heal the patient from one illness in order to bring on him another one ... If the patient has an heir that gives hints to them, they contact him and weaken the patient slowly, slowly until his death. In case the patient's wife wishes his death and she hints this to the Jewish physician, he would allegedly refuse, saying he

> can't murder a person. If the wife continues to beg him, he asks for cash money, and if she is attractive the physician would also demand to have sex with her.[287]

Pormann and Savage-Smith stated that 'physicians needed to treat patients kindly and win their confidence. To this end, they were required to appear dignified, which they achieved by dressing and speaking in a specified or customary manner.' In one interesting example they elaborate on the Muslim physician Asad Ibn Jānī as 'not being able to attract enough patients because he neither spoke nor dressed like his Christian or Jewish competitors'.[288] Here we should mention a testimony from a Muslim source regarding a Jewish physician who was practising in the court of Sultan al-Nāṣir Muḥammad b. Qalāwūn in Cairo. The Muslim scholar Ibn Faḍl Allāh al-ʿUmarī (1301–49) praised Faraj Allāh Ibn Ṣaghīr in his encyclopedia[289] for his kind treatment and gentle approach towards his patients.[290]

Goitein claimed that it was taken for granted that Jewish practitioners believed in God, the prophets and the world to come, and they fulfilled the highest standards of morality and comportment including perfuming themselves when visiting a patient. All these ideas were already contained in the unique manuscript of Isḥāq al-Ruhāwī's *Adab al-Ṭabīb* ('The Education of a Physician'), written in the ninth century. It is interesting to note that on the title page of the manuscript, the name of the author was accompanied by the appellation *al-Yahūdī* (the Jew). This line was crossed out and the name was repeated without the words 'the Jew'. The book was written in the spirit of the Greek authors so copiously referred to by him.[291]

Another example for comparison can be learnt from a document describing a physician from Qalyūb (about 19 kilometres north of Fusṭāṭ), who had opened a clinic in the capital. He wrote to his wife that the response of the public had been excellent, but that the enmity of the other members of the profession was so strong that he did not dare interrupt his work even for one day.[292]

Some Jewish practitioners faced in their professional career complex dilemmas, for example Ibn Qarqa, a twelfth-century Jewish physician, engineer and head of the Jewish community who also worked for the caliph al-Ḥāfiẓ. He is noted to have prepared a poison, at the request of the caliph, in order to kill his son Ḥasan. Due to his consent to prepare the poison and Ḥasan's death, all his possessions were confiscated and transferred over to Samuel ben Hananiah (Abū Mansur), who had by contrast refused to make the poison for the caliph. In 1134 al-Ḥāfiẓ ordered Ibn Qarqa's execution.[293]

A stereotypical notion was that Jewish physicians took certain liberties that their Muslim colleagues might not have approved of (for example recommending wine to their patients), and that the scientific and medical practice of Jews was less restricted by religious strictures. Indeed, Ibn Jumayʿ wrote freely about alcoholic drinks, yet Nicolae claimed that we do not know what Ibn Jumayʿ would have suggested in a consultation with a Muslim. He mentioned alcoholic beverages in his treatise to Saladin, but merely to illustrate his argument: for instance, if somebody does not know what Hippocrates said about treating pains of the eye, namely that alcoholic beverages,[294] a bath, a bandage, bleeding and laxatives will ease the pain, how then can he perform the proper treatment if necessary?[295]

4.3.2 Fees

It is mentioned in the so-called ethical will of Judah b. Tibbon (Samuel's father), who was a physician and translator, that he had fled in the middle of the twelfth century from Muslim Spain to southern France. He praised medical charity, saying:

> Let thy countenance shine upon the sons of men; tend their sick and may thine advice cure them. Though thou take fees from the rich, *heal the poor gratuitously*; the Lord will require thee. Thereby wilt thou find favour in the sight of God and man.[296]

Fees for medical treatments and advice varied according to the physician's professional standing and the socio-economic status of the patient. According to Hans-Hinrich Biesterfeldt, who considered physicians' remuneration in medieval Islam, 'The problem of remuneration turns out to be critical whenever there is discrepancy between the demands of the medical art and the interests of those who practice'.[297] Pormann and Savage-Smith claimed that 'in real life some practitioners did need to charge a fee, and others were at least perceived as being motivated by avarice not only by their colleagues … but also by the non-medical public'.[298]

Muslim Arabic literature presents cases of physicians, usually highly trained and very skilful, who refused to accept payment when they treated laymen and the poor. Usually, those physicians were either very rich, had a patron, or were very religious; sometimes they earned their livelihood by doing other things such as copying books, or they engaged in commerce in general and in trade in books or drugs in particular. Several court physicians such as Ibn Tilmīdh (d. 1168), Ibn al-Muṭrān (d. 1191) and Maimonides (1138–1204) were known for their refusal to accept presents of payment except from the rulers.[299]

Similarly, Cohen suggested that some of the patients of the Jewish practitioners must have been indigent, in that they treated them without payment (a form of charity). To support this statement, he mentioned the famous letter from Maimonides (or his son Abraham) to Samuel b. Tibbon,[300] in which he described how he would return home after a long working day and find many patients waiting for his advice. According to Cohen, he probably treated them free of charge.[301] Indeed, the Geniza documents teach us that rich people and rulers gave much more than required to their doctors, while patients with chronic disabilities were exempt from paying any fees.[302] I tend to agree with Goitein that sick poor Jews were treated without charge by Jewish physicians. Cohen noted that although physicians and druggists were numerous in the Jewish community, there are only a few examples of charity (from the abundant records of both private and public charity) specifically designated for medical treatment.[303] A communal payroll registered the enormous sum of 60.75 dirhams designated for a doctor's visit, demonstrating another option: the community subsidising medical treatment for the poor (13th century).[304]

Information regarding doctors' fees is rare. A few Arabic contracts for medical treatment that were found in the Geniza deal with a doctor's payment according to his success or failure.[305] Such fragments teach us that fees ranged from three dirhams a week for the treatment of a sore eye to a thousand dinars, promised to a Jewish physician in Tripoli, Libya, for the successful healing of the sultan of Gabes, Tunisia. According to Goitein, in this case the physician received 100 dinars before he even left his own house. He was not eager to attempt to cure the sultan so he offered the Bedouin rulers of Tripoli a bribe of fifty dinars if they allowed him to ignore the sultan's summons. They insisted, however, that he treat the sultan, and, in their rough Bedouin manner, threw all the Jewish notables of the town into prison and held them there until the physician complied with the sultan's request. Finally, the doctor set out on his perilous expedition, but, fortunately for him, the sultan died before he arrived.[306]

A letter sent by a Jewish doctor teaches us that he had worked on a retainer of one dinar a month as a house physician for a noble Muslim family.[307] However, fees for private medical care could be excessively high: a blind woman was charged four dinars by a Muslim physician and had to ask the community for charity to pay the bill.[308] In some cases, fees depended on the degree of satisfaction from the patient: for example, a thirteenth-century contract (June 1245) found in the Geniza described the fee that was promised to be paid to the Jewish physician Makārim b. Ishāq b. Makārim as an honorarium for the successful treatment of a Nubian slave's left eye.[309] The same physician, Makārim b. Ishāq, is mentioned in a petition to an Ayyubid sultan in which he asks for a lifetime appointment in the hospital of (New) Cairo with the usual salary. The standard monthly salary of a physician in the hospitals of Cairo around 1240 was three dinars. At midday, the hospital physicians left for home and were free to attend to their private practice.[310] Similarly to the present day, a position in the hospital was perhaps sought for reasons of prestige, and physicians practised privately after fulfilling their duty in public institutions.

The issue of greed among medieval physicians was jokingly mentioned to a friend in a letter from a Jerusalemite doctor and head of a congregation: 'Although I am a doctor, a president, and from Jerusalem, so that all the reasons for being exacting are combined in me, I am not of this type, as far as you are concerned.'[311]

4.3.3 The 'Geniza patient'

A great deal has been written about 'Geniza society', but the patient remains obscure. Thanks to the study of Geniza medical documents, we can present here some insights into the patients as well. Like the physicians and the pharmacists who are the subject of this book, the patients who received a prescription in Judaeo-Arabic were probably Jewish; however, the patient that received prescriptions written in Arabic letters may have been a Muslim or a Christian. Moreover, from letters found in the Geniza we have learnt about the more common diseases (eye conditions for example) and people's attitude towards them. These also testify in most cases to a basic knowledge of drugs. According to Goitein, 'The fact that the Jewish community harbored a disproportionately high percentage of physicians, druggists, and traders in spices and pharmaceuticals might have contributed to the vivid interest and knowledgeability in medications found in the Geniza correspondence.'

Sufferers of medical conditions often knew which remedies worked best for them; especially for chronic or common ailments such as eye diseases (mainly ophthalmia).[312] And indeed, based on the Geniza we know that people often ordered for themselves medications not prescribed for them by a physician, but known to them otherwise.[313] In many cases one of the family members knew how to treat medical conditions. In general, during an acute illness the patient was asked to use a syrup or other medicine and eat various kinds of vegetables and in many cases also pullets.[314] And yet, obviously it helped to have a physician in the family.

Another issue is Jewish patients being treated at hospitals; as mentioned above, while Jewish physicians and pharmacists staffed the hospitals of medieval Cairo there is no evidence that a Jew was ever admitted as a patient.[315]

Only a few prescriptions with patients' names have been found in the Geniza, presumably because the patient's identity would be obvious as prescriptions were individual. Patients were expected to receive their prescription directly from the physician and then bring it to the pharmacist in order to have it made up. Even if a prescription was meant for someone too ill to leave the house, the bearer of the prescription would know whose it was. The rare examples of patients' names found in prescriptions, written in Judaeo-Arabic, include al-Karāmiyya (a woman, probably from the Karām family, a common name in the 12th–13th centuries); the elder Abū Yaḥyā (alternatively, the sheikh Abū al-Ḥayy), probably Naharay b. Nissīm;[316] and a dozen or so short prescriptions written on a single sheet of paper, all bearing names of males and females, some of whom were related to each other (probably 12th–13th century): al-Nafūs, al-Damīriyya, *zawjat* Ibrāhīm (wife of Abraham), *ibn* Siḥān (son of Siḥān), *zawjat* Ḥasan (wife of Ḥasan), Maḥāsin (male), *bintuhu* (his daughter), al-Najīb, *ibnuhu* (his son) Farīj, *umm* al-Zabbānī (mother of al-Zabbānī), *ibnuhā* (her son).[317]

Names of sick people and their medical conditions appear in many letters that were found in the Geniza, of which some have been studied and even published. However, in this book, I have chosen to focus particularly on practitioners and not on medical conditions, or patients.

4.4 Religious and Inter-religious Aspects of Jewish Practitioners

4.4.1 Practitioners and Jewish scholarship

The Jewish physicians and pharmacists known from the Geniza were observant, participated in the life of the community, and in most cases were well versed in Jewish scholarship. Goitein claimed that the combination of secular with religious scholarship, and accordingly, that of the profession of physician with the office of judge or Head of the Jews was

> not uncommon in the period under consideration and was even characteristic of it. Still, the physicians not known as religious scholars by far outnumber those who were. The secular vein in the culture of the period must therefore have been of considerable strength.[318]

Most researchers agree that among the Jewish practitioners of the medieval Muslim lands the most important Jewish scholar was Moses b. Maimon (Maimonides).[319] Besides being a court physician of the Fatimids and Ayyubids and Head of the Jews, he was one of the most influential Halakhic scholars ever. He wrote many books, including the fullest commentary ever written on the entire Mishna, *The Book of Commandments*, *Letter of Martyrdom*, *Mishne Tora: Sefer Yad ha-Chazaka* ('Repetition of the Torah: Book of the Strong Hand'), *The Guide for the Perplexed*, *Responsa* and *Commentary on the Jerusalem Talmud*. His offspring took over his position as the Head of the Jews, and some of them are known to have been physicians. Abraham Maimonides for example was a famous court physician, a Halakhic and the *nagid* of the Jewish community in Egypt.[320] In his capacity as the *nagid*, he was highly influential, heavily involved in community affairs and an arbiter in Halakhic matters, regulations and laws.[321] He was known for his piety and his liturgical and devotional reforms.[322] Abraham too wrote some books, including *Milchamot ha-Shem* ('The Book of the Wars for God', a compilation); *Kitāb Kifāyah al-ʿĀbidīn* ('A Comprehensive Guide for the Servants of God'); a commentary on the Torah; a book on Jewish law; Responsa (*Sefer Birkat Avraham*); and *Discourse on the Sayings of the Rabbis*.[323] David b. Abraham b. Moses b. Maimon, Maimonides' grandson, was also a *nagid* and probably a physician.[324] David held the title 'Head of the Yeshiva of the Torah' and was often in contact with Rabbinical scholars in Spain, Damascus and Italy, and spent much time defending Maimonides' doctrines.[325]

As an anecdote, it is interesting to note that the court physician Abraham b. Isaac ha-Kohen b. Furāt, the great benefactor and protector of the community, was flattered in a letter as an 'outstanding scholar of Jewish studies'. However, according to Goitein, he was not.[326] In another tale that sheds light on the issue, when a young physician announced his intention to marry a girl, he was told in reply that marrying a girl of a good family was certainly reasonable, but the study of the sacred law was even more meritorious. Both the young doctor and his brother, also a doctor, were bidden to participate in the courses given by the local 'judge'.[327]

Among the later practitioners we should mention R. Solomon Luria, a physician from Lublin, a Torah scholar and a Kabbalist who immigrated to Eretz-Israel at the beginning of the sixteenth century (when he was eighty) and settled in Jerusalem; and R. Ḥayyīm b. Joseph Vital (1543–1620), considered the most prominent and important student of Isaac Luria. He studied Kabbala and the Torah.[328]

4.4.2 Jewish practitioners serving in the Egyptian army and navy

Only a few Geniza documents mention Jewish physicians attached to the Egyptian armed forces. It appears that there was one army unit which must have been rather popular among the minority groups, which was that of the 'medical corps'. Some letters to and from Jewish physicians serving in the army were found in the Geniza, and are mentioned below:[329]

a. A letter (1100) to a physician who served in the army teaches us that like other physicians, he dealt with books.[330]

b. A letter dated 1137 from a Jewish Egyptian physician who had settled in Byzantium mentioned that he had previously written from the army camp in Jaffa.[331]

c. An army doctor complained that he had to cure a Mamluk and then to report back to his emir and supervise him taking medication.

d. Abū Zikrī, the elder son of the judge Elijah b. Zechariah, served around 1220 in the army of the Ayyubid prince al-Malik al-Muʿaẓẓam ʿIsā. Two issues of interest can be learnt from his letters. He must have been quite influential, since he promised to procure for his old father a pension from Sultan al-Malik al-Kāmil; but he could not get away from the army whenever he wished.

e. A letter to a physician serving in the army teaches us that while he was away, his son-in-law, the writer of the letter, collected his salary, which was obviously paid in the capital.

f. Abū al-Barakāt Hibat Allāh b. ʿAli b. Malkā al-Baladi al-Tabib al-Faḍl (12th century), known as 'Awḥad al-Zamān', served for some time as an army doctor.[332]

From a letter dealing with a loan, we learn about a Jewish physician serving on a battleship of the Muslim navy (*usṭūl*) in 1129. The physician also bought a saddled mount for four dinars upon arrival at the Mediterranean port of Damietta (probably on board ship).[333]

4.4.3 Jewish practitioners in the Christian vs the Muslim world

Thanks to the archives of European universities and cities, several researchers have dealt with Jewish practitioners in medieval Europe (mainly late medieval). Shatzmiller's book *Jews, Medicine, and Medieval Society* deals mainly with the role of the Jews in medicine in Mediterranean Europe during the High or Late Middle Ages (1250 onwards). His book is different from ours in many senses: those of the geographical area (Mediterranean Europe *vs* the Muslim Empire), the time span (13th–17th centuries *vs* 9th–16th), the cultural and religious atmosphere (Christian *vs* Muslim), and even the sources for both research projects (archives *vs* Jewish Geniza and Muslim Arabic literature). Nevertheless, it gives us a golden opportunity to compare various characteristics, to try analysing the similarities and differences, and to better understand 'global' processes.

There were some difficulties in identifying or distinguishing between Christian and Jewish physicians from the European Mediterranean sources, but in most cases the latter had the word *judeus* added to their name and professional description. Shatzmiller provides examples: *magister X phisicus judeus* for the superior doctor, 'well rounded in his education', and *magister X cirurgicus judeus*, 'the more inferior surgeon', of limited medical capacity who was expected to deal with wounds and to perform a variety of surgical operations. According to Shatzmiller, 'one can hardly find a Jewish community that did not count at least one medical doctor among its members' in Mediterranean Europe from 1250 onward; 'next to moneylending, medicine seems to have been the most preponderant profession among Jews'.[334]

I agree with Shatzmiller's suggestion that the process of the increasing numbers of Jewish practitioners in the Muslim world of the twelfth century had a similar pattern to that of the increasing numbers of Jewish physicians in the medieval West one or two centuries later (13th–14th centuries). Shatzmiller even tried to explain the connection between the two phenomena. According to him, in the thirteenth century, Jewish physicians of the Islamic world, who had already entered the field of medicine, brought with them their medical knowledge (including medical books that were translated into Hebrew) when they immigrated to western Europe and shared it with local Jewish doctors (he named Judah b. Tibbon from Granada as an example). Shatzmiller presented numerical data that attested to the extensive participation of Jews in the medical profession in Mediterranean Europe during the High or Late Middle Ages. He argued that this participation was 'out of proportion with contemporary demographics and the place of Jews in society'. According to his calculation the Jews accounted for about 1 per cent of the overall population and represented at the most 5–8 per cent of the population in great cities, but composed a significant share of about 50 per cent or more of the practitioners.[335]

Moreover, in his opinion, the medieval society of Mediterranean Europe went through a 'medicalisation' process between 1250 and 1450; this was phrased by Jacquart as 'a growing interest in and appreciation of scientific medicine'.[336] This process created a growing need for doctors, and since the Church opposed the clerical practice of medicine, Jews could enter into the medical profession.[337] At the same time, an opposing process happened in the East. The Mamluk period (1250–1517), and the zealous atmosphere of its regime, marked a deterioration in the position of *dhimmīs* in Egypt and in Syria, and that of Jewish physicians in particular. Muslim writers warned against hiring non-Muslim physicians as well as against buying medicines from them.[338] The decline of the Jewish physicians' status is also related to the general decline of the science of medicine in the Muslim world, and especially in the Mamluk sultanate. Mamluk sultans encouraged mainly Islamic religious studies, and Sufi sheikhs, who were believed by the people to create miracles, gained more and more honour and prestige among both people and rulers. The 'secular' physicians and their medical science seemed to be useless, especially in the light of the Black Death.[339]

More than half of the dynasties of Jewish practitioners from the Mamluk period converted to Islam. All of these converted dynasties included distinguished physicians who served rulers. During the fourteenth century, the dismissal of Jewish court physicians became frequent, and one may discern an increasing opposition from orthodox Muslims to the treatment of Muslim patients by Jewish or Christian physicians.[340]

4.4.4 Inter-religious intellectual and professional relations

Studying the well-documented lives of the two Jewish court physicians Ibn Jumayʿ and Maimonides can teach us many things about everyday medical practice in medieval Cairo, including their relationship with Muslim and Christian physicians. Learning their medical writings teaches us about the theory of their days. According to Nicolae, Ibn Jumayʿ showed that medical practice and theory in medieval Cairo 'were not written in stone, but were still open to change and debate and medieval Cairo in the late 12th century was probably one of the most vibrant inter-cultural and inter-religious sites of the era'. Moreover, he claimed that the work of Ibn Jumayʿ and Maimonides was a 'prime example of the fruitful and positive scientific exchanges of the Middle Ages that were not restricted by any religious divides'. Both of them worked in the court of Saladin, together with Muslim and Christian physicians, and it was there that they 'developed their practice of medicine, their notion of medicine, and their understanding of the human body'.[341]

Lewicka stated that the religious affiliation of a physician 'was often responsible for many aspects of his professional career, including the way he was treated by the authorities as well as the way he was perceived by the society'.[342] Goitein mentioned that the study of medicine during these periods was inter-religious. Jewish students studied with Muslim and Christian teachers, and famous Jewish physicians taught students of other religions.[343] Here I present some examples demonstrating the wide range and complexity of such a relationship in various ways.

Friendly relations among medical students and practitioners from different ethnic and religious backgrounds were created alongside their studies and practice, similarly to the way it happens today. There are a few examples, studied mainly in the Muslim Arabic sources, of professional, personal and friendly relationships between Muslim and Jewish practitioners. The following are taken from them:

- **a.** Abū al-Ḥajjāj Yūsuf b. Yaḥyā b. Isḥāq al-Sabatī al-Maghribī (Joseph b. Judah b. Simon) (12th century) was a friend of Ibn al-Qifṭī, who dedicated to him a chapter in his book *Taʾrīkh al-Ḥukamāʾ* ('History of Physicians'). Ibn al-Qifṭī noted that Yūsuf was clever and highly perceptive. Yūsuf and Ibn al-Qifṭī had a pact in which it was stated that the first one to die would return to tell the other one what occurs after death. Ibn al-Qifṭī reported that Yūsuf visited him in a dream, two years after his death, and they discussed the evolution of the body and soul.[344]
- **b.** Al-Sadīd al-Dimyāṭī al-Ṭabīb al-Yahūdī, the prominent Karaite physician (a. c.1339–42), was closely associated with his teacher al-Nafīs, the *qadi* and historian Ibn Wāṣil, and the historians Khalīl b. Aybak al-Ṣafadī (1297–1363) and Ibn Faḍl Allāh al-ʿUmarī (1301–49). Many of al-Dimyāṭī's patients were members of the political and military elite. Moreover, he was also praised by al-ʿUmarī for his medical knowledge and nice manners; his successes among the 'women of Cairo' was mentioned as well.[345]
- **c.** Amir Mazor published unique information regarding the Jewish physician Faraj Allāh Ibn Ṣaghīr (active in 14th-century Cairo), to whom al-ʿUmarī dedicated an extensive *tarjama* (biographical entry) from which it is clear that this physician was a very eminent one in his time. Faraj Allāh was highly praised by the Muslim Arabic sources for his marvellous medical knowledge and practical treatments, and he received 'a complete wage and rich salary'; Sultan al-Nāṣir Muḥammad b. Qalāwūn distinguished him as the only physician of the inhabitants of the palace, including the sultan's wives, concubines and children. Moreover, al-ʿUmarī proudly

testified about his strong friendship with Faraj Allāh that he was the only physician in the court who managed to diagnose his father's disease and prolonged his life.[346]

Some **professional and business partnerships** and cooperation between Jewish practitioners and Muslim or Christian ones were recorded as well:

a. An interesting account (based on the Geniza) can be studied in a deathbed declaration (1182) of Abū al-Faraj (known from other documents as Ibn al-Kallām), a rich Jewish merchant and a trustee of the court. Abū al-Faraj owed money to some of his associates; among them were al-Sheikh al-Muwaffaq (Ibn Jumayʿ), teacher Moses (Maimonides) and three Muslims: the notable Qāḍī Ibn Sanāʾ al-Mulk (1155–1211); a religious scholar, Ibn Ṣawla; and a certain Abū al-Khayr of Haifa. Goitein claimed that these two most prominent Jews and two illustrious Muslims belonged to 'a circle of closed acquaintances who certainly were united by common spiritual interests'. He added that 'such contacts, even under the most auspicious circumstances, were of very limited scope and ephemeral character'. His explanation was that Jewish and Muslim jurists (such as Maimonides and Qāḍī Ibn Sanāʾ al-Mulk) had practical contacts through legal matters and probably also discussed theological issues.[347]

b. Ibn Abī Uṣaybiʿa, who worked in a hospital for a while, wrote that ʿImrān b. Ṣadaqa al-ʾIsrāʾīlī al-Ḥakīm Awḥad al-Dīn al-ʾIsrāʾīlī (Moses b. Ṣadaqa) and his friend, the Muslim physician ʿAbd al-Raḥīm al-Dakhwār, had a very beneficial collaboration in treating patients.[348]

c. Another example is the store in Fusṭāṭ of Abū al-Faraj b. Maʿmar al-Sharābī (Nethanel ha-Levi b. Amram), which was mentioned in Geniza documents (11th century). This store hosted, among other things, the clinic of a Christian physician named Abū al-Ghālib and a Jewish practitioner named R. Amram b. Saʿīd b. Mūsā. It was a working place for both Christian and Jewish practitioners and potion makers.[349]

Friendly relationships with members of the Muslim elite existed as well; here are some examples:

a. Furāt b. Shaḥnāthā (Shaḥāthā) al-Yahūdī (8th century), a virtuous physician in his time, befriended ʿIsā b. Mūsā al-ʿAbbāsī, the heir to the throne in the days of al-Manṣūr, the Abbasid caliph (r. 754–75). ʿIsā b. Mūsā used to consult Furāt on everything, since he liked the nature of his opinions and thought. The two had a good and tight relation.[350]

b. Asad al-Yahūdī (13th–14th centuries), a prominent physician in Egypt and Syria under the Mamluks, was in contact with scholars of his time, including the Muslim theologian Ibn Taymiyya.[351]

c. Al-Muwaffaq al-Qaṣīr al-Ṭabīb al-Yahūdī, a physician from Damascus (13th–14th centuries), solved the problem of the sight of his Muslim friend al-Sheikh al-Ṣāliḥ Sharaf al-Dīn Maḥmūd, who was a Ḥadith scholar (c. 1300).[352]

d. Faraj Allāh (Yeshūʿa) Ibn Ṣaghīr (d. 1377) had a close association with the historian Ibn Faḍl Allāh al-ʿUmarī (1301–49). Al-ʿUmarī emphasised his strong friendship with Faraj Allāh and mentioned some of his own experiences as one of his patients. Most of his family members had converted to Islam by that time.[353]

In any case, most of the evidence of business, educational and friendly relationships between Jewish practitioners and Muslim or Christian scholars is from the tenth to the mid-fourteenth centuries. After that, there is hardly any similar evidence. This does not mean that there were no such relationships, but that we do not have reliable sources: the amount of Geniza documents from this period dropped dramatically, and the works that were written by Muslim scholars tend not to portray *dhimmīs* in a positive light nor describe their relationship with Muslims (compared to the biographical dictionaries of Ibn Abī Uṣaybiʿa and al-Qifṭī).

We have records of some **Jewish physicians teaching medicine to Muslim or Christian students** (in most cases).[354] Here are some examples:

a. Hārūn (Aaron) b. Isaac was a Jewish physician who practised in Cordova under the Moorish rulers of Spain in the tenth century. According to the sources he taught medical students and was the author of a medical treatise.[355]

b. Ibrāhīm b. Faraj b. Mārūth al-Sāmirī al-Ṭabīb (al-Ḥakīm), one of Saladin's physicians, 'gave lectures to physicians and students about medicine', including the Samaritan physician Yūsuf b. Abī Saʿīd b. Khalaf.[356]

c. Abū al-ʿAshāʾir Hibat-Allāh b. Zayn b. Ḥasan b. Ifrāʾīm b. Yaʿqūb b. Ismāʿīl Ibn Jumayʿ al-ʾIsrāʾīlī (Nethanel b. Samuel) (d. 1198) was a medical scholar who wrote several medical essays. According to Muslim Arabic writers, Ibn Jumayʿ was a *kātib* of the *wazīr*, served as 'Head of the Physicians' in Cairo under Saladin and later on also served his successor. He was a teacher for students of all religions and took part, as mentioned, in discussions about the standards of medicine.[357] Nicolae suggested that Ibn Jumayʿ was also the teacher of the Muslim physician Ibn al-ʿAyn Zarbī.[358]

d. ʿImrān b. Ṣadaqa al-ʾIsrāʾīlī al-Ḥakīm Awḥad al-Dīn (Moses b. Ṣedāqā)[359] (al-Ḥakīm Awḥad al-Dīn al-ʾIsrāʾīlī') (b. 1165, Damascus) was one of the teachers of Ibn Abī Uṣaybiʿa.[360]

e. Nuʿmān b. Abī al-Riḍā b. Sālim b. Isḥāq (13th–14th centuries), known for his famous medical book, was the teacher of the Muslim ophthalmologist Ṣalāḥ al-Dīn Ibn Yūsuf al-Ḥamawī.[361]

Nicolae suggested that Jewish physicians such as Maimonides and Ibn Jumayʿ may have sometimes favoured the teaching of their coreligionists, and maybe even tried to restrict their teaching to their Jewish successors. But it seems that religious preferences might have other reasons, such as personal relations, chance or even social conventions for instance. In this case, Muslim students may have preferred not to be taught by a Jew.[362]

Jewish physicians studied medicine with physicians of all religions, many of them Muslim. The Muslim Arabic literature is our main source of information for this phenomenon and, in many cases, for the names of both teachers and students. Here are some examples from different periods and various geographical regions:

a. Judah b. Joseph b. Abī al-Thanā (9th–10th centuries), a physician from al-Raqqah, Syria, mentioned by al-Masʿūdī (d. 957) as a student of the Muslim scholar Thābit b. Qurra (826–901).[363]

b. Ephraim b. al-Ḥasan al-Zaffān (d. 1068) was considered the most prominent medical student of the famous Muslim physician ʿAlī Ibn Riḍwān from Giza,[364] and the Jewish physician Salāma b. Raḥmūn was also his student.[365]

c. Yūsuf b. Abī Sa'īd b. Khalaf al-Sāmirī al-Muhadhdhab al-Ṭabīb (12th century), a Samaritan physician from Damascus, studied medicine at the al-Ṣalāḥiyya institute from the Muslim physicians al-Muhadhdhab b. al-Naqqāsh, Ismā'īl b. Abū al-Waqqār and 'Alī Abī al-Yamān al-Kindī.[366]

d. The physician Abū al-Khayr Salāma b. Mubārak b. Raḥmūn b. Mūsā al-Ṭabīb studied philosophy with the learned Fatimid prince al-Mubashshir b. Fātik. A distinguished physician from Spain, Abū al-Ṣalt Umayya b. 'Abd al-'Azīz al-Andalusī, witnessed the esteem in which Salāma was held when he arrived in Cairo (1096); he praised his medical and philosophical erudition. Moreover, Salāma was mentioned by Abū al-Ṣalt in a letter he wrote (1116), during a visit to Egypt, in which he referred to the physicians in the area and named Salāma as 'one of the smartest and wisest' among the Egyptian physicians.[367]

e. Faraj Allāh (Yeshū'a) Ibn Ṣaghīr, a prominent Karaite physician, studied the medical profession with his father, and with Ibn al-Nafīs (d. 1288).[368]

f. Al-Sadīd al-Dimyāṭī al-Ṭabīb al-Yahūdī (a. c.1339–42),[369] a Karaite, studied medicine under the Muslim physician 'Imād al-Dīn al-Nābulsī, and Ibn al-Nafīs.[370]

Data regarding inter-religious transfer of medical knowledge (teachers and students of medicine) was accumulated during the research, and Table 6 presents the outcome.

There were at the same time negative feelings towards Christian and Jewish physicians, mainly during the Mamluk period. Both Lewicka and Ragab discussed this by naming important Muslim physicians such as Raḍī al-Dīn al-Raḥbī (d. 1233), who in general did not teach medicine to non-Muslims, except to two Jews: Ibrāhīm b. Khalaf al-Sāmirī (late 12th century) and 'Imrān b. Ṣadaqa al-'Isrā'īlī al-Ḥakīm Awḥad al-Dīn (1165–1239).[371] A similar case, from an earlier period, is Abū al-Barakāt Hibat Allāh b. 'Alī b. Malkā al-Baladi al-Ṭabīb al-Faḍl (1087–1165), a Jewish physician from Iraq who studied medicine under the Muslim physician Abū al-Ḥasan Sa'īd b. Hibat Allāh (who usually abstained from teaching

Table 6 Inter-religious transfer of medical knowledge (bold = Muslim physician)

Student	*Teacher*	*Century*	*Place*
Isḥāq b. Sulaymān al-ʾIsrāʾīlī (Isaac b. Solomon)	Isaac b. ʿImrān	9th	Qayrawān
Mūsā b. Elʿāzār al-ʾIsrāʾīlī (Moses b. Elazar)	Isḥāq b. Sulaymān al-ʾIsrāʾīlī (Isaac b. Solomon)	9th–10th	Qayrawān
Judah b. Joseph b. Abī al-Thanā	**Thābit b. Qurra**	9th–10th	al-Raqqah, Syria
Various students	Hārūn (Aaron) b. Isaac	10th	Andalusia
Ephraim b. al-Ḥasan al-Zaffān	ʿAlī Ibn Riḍwān	11th	Cairo
Abū al-Khayr Salāma b. Mubārak b. Raḥmūn b. Mūsā al-Ṭabīb	Ephraim b. al-Zaffān	11th–12th	Cairo
Abū al-Barakāt Hibat Allāh b. ʿAlī b. Malkā al-Baladī al-Ṭabīb al-Faḍl	**Abū al-Ḥasan Saʿīd b. Hibat Allāh**	11th–12th	Baghdad
Abū al-Faḍl Dāʾūd b. Sulaymān b. Abū al-Bayān al-ʾIsrāʾīlī al-Sadīd (David b. Solomon)	Abū al-ʿAshāʾir Hibat-Allāh b. Zayn b. Ḥasan b. Ifrāʾīm b. Yaʿqūb b. Ismāʿīl Ibn Jumayʿ al-ʾIsrāʾīlī (Nethanel b. Samuel)	12th	Cairo
Ṣanīʿat al-Malik Abū al-Ṭāhir Ismāʿīl	Abū al-ʿAshāʾir Hibat-Allāh b. Zayn b. Ḥasan b. Ifrāʾīm b. Yaʿqūb b. Ismāʿīl Ibn Jumayʿ al-ʾIsrāʾīlī (Nethanel b. Samuel)	12th	Cairo
Abū al-Faḍl Dāʾūd b. Sulaymān b. Abū al-Bayān al-ʾIsrāʾīlī al-Sadīd (David b. Solomon)	Ibn al-Nāqid	12th	Cairo
Ibn al-ʿAyn Zarbī	Abū al-ʿAshāʾir Hibat-Allāh b. Zayn b. Ḥasan b. Ifrāʾīm b. Yaʿqūb b. Ismāʿīl Ibn Jumayʿ al-ʾIsrāʾīlī (Nethanel b. Samuel)	12th	Cairo
Students of all religious	Abū al-ʿAshāʾir Hibat-Allāh b. Zayn b. Ḥasan b. Ifrāʾīm b. Yaʿqūb b. Ismāʿīl Ibn Jumayʿ al-ʾIsrāʾīlī (Nethanel b. Samuel)	12th	Cairo
Yūsuf b. Abī Saʿīd b. Khalaf al-Sāmirī al-Muhadhdhab al-Ṭabīb	**al-Muhadhdhab b. al-Naqqāsh, Ismāʿīl b. Abū al-Waqqār ʿAlī Abī al-Yamān al-Kindī** Ibrāhīm b. Faraj b. Mārūth al-Sāmirī al-Ṭabīb (al-Ḥakīm) (Abū Isḥāq Ibrāhīm al-Muṣannif) (Shams al-Ḥukamāʾ)	12th	Damascus

Student	*Teacher*	*Century*	*Place*
Abū al-Maʿālī (Abū al-ʿAlā) Tammām b. Hibat Allāh b. Tammām	Maimonides	12th	Cairo
Abū al-Bayān b. al-Mudawwar al-Sadīd	?Zayn al-Ḥassāb	12th	Cairo
Ibn ʿAknīn	Maimonides	12th	Fez
Abū al-Ḥajjāj Yūsuf b. Yaḥyā b. Isḥāq al-Sabatī al-Maghribī (Joseph b. Judah b. Simon) (Ibn Samʿūn)	Maimonides	12th	Cairo
Ibrāhīm al-Sāmirī al-Ṭabīb	Yūsuf b. Abī Saʿīd b. Khalaf	12th	Syria
Ibrāhīm b. Khalaf al-Sāmirī	**Raḍī al-Dīn al-Raḥbī**	12th–13th	Syria
ʿImrān b. Ṣadaqa al-ʾIsrāʾīlī al-Ḥakīm Awḥad al-Dīn	**Raḍī al-Dīn al-Raḥbī**	12th–13th	Syria
Amīn al-Dawla Abū al-Ḥasan b. Ghazāl b. Abī Saʿīd al-Sāmirī (Wazīr al-Ṣāliḥ, and Sharaf al-Milla)	**Ibn Abī Uṣaybiʿa**	13th	Syria
Ṣalāḥ al-Dīn Ibn Yūsuf al-Ḥamawī	Nuʿmān b. Abī al-Riḍā b. Sālim b. Isḥāq	13th	Syria
Faraj Allāh (Yeshūʿa) Ibn Ṣaghīr	Ibn al-Nafīs	13th–14th	Cairo
al-Sadīd al-Dimyāṭī al-Ṭabīb al-Yahūdī	**ʿImād al-Dīn al-Nābulsī**	13th–14th	Cairo
al-Sadīd al-Dimyāṭī al-Ṭabīb al-Yahūdī	Ibn al-Nafīs	13th–14th	Cairo
Faraj Allāh (Yeshūʿa) Ibn Ṣaghīr	Father	14th	Cairo

Christians and Jews) and eventually remained one of his permanent students.[372]

The success of *dhimmī* physicians in general, and Jewish ones in particular, caused jealousy and polemics;[373] and, as mentioned above, the zealous atmosphere did not escape the non-Muslim physicians. During the Mamluk period a generally increasing opposition of orthodox Muslims to the treatment of Muslim patients by Jewish and Christian physicians is noticeable. Muslim scholars warned the public in their writing against hiring non-Muslim physicians, as well as buying medicines from them. It also appears that more Muslim physicians refused to teach non-Muslims.[374]

Moreover, complaints against Christian and Jewish practitioners, who dominated medical practice in the Muslim world, became a known notion, and complainants such as al-Raḥbī and Muhadhdhab al-Dīn ʿAbd al-Raḥīm b. ʿAlī (d. 1230), known as al-Dakhwār, were only a fraction of it. There were many explanations for these complaints; the one that was stated by Ibn al-Ukhūwa (13th–14th centuries) is of special interest. He claimed that non-Muslims dominated the field of medicine

> not due to any active action on their part against Muslims, rather, it was due to the unwillingness of Muslims to pursue a field that was far less profitable than the religious sciences and law, which could lead to a position in a madrasa or a role in the expanding Mamluk bureaucracy.[375]

This was a complex issue that had been altered over the years depending on the various Muslim rulers (on both the local and global scale). According to Lewicka, 'generally, religion was rarely used as an argument in the pre-Mamluk medical culture – medical errors or charlatan practices were not associated with religious denomination'.[376] Goitein suggested that the Geniza likewise contains no allusion to poisonous propaganda against the treatment of Muslim patients by Christian and Jewish physicians, rather, it frequently mentions Jewish physicians as serving Muslim rulers or working in Muslim hospitals.[377]

Nicolae, in his scholarly comparison between Muslim and Jewish physicians, claimed that the assumption that medieval Jewish and Muslim physicians differed in their attitudes towards the compatibility of religion and medicine is problematic and even wrong. Moreover, in his opinion, 'the reliance and acknowledgment of Galen is not only common to Muslim physicians, but also to Jewish court physicians'. When Ibn Jumayʿ criticised his Muslim predecessors (Ibn Sīnā and al-Rāzī) his criticism was not based on any religious assumptions; 'he rather follows his own observations, relating them both to what Galen had said, but also to the ideas of his Muslim predecessors'.[378]

Another interesting anecdote concerns the anti-*dhimmī* treatise written in the late thirteenth or early fourteenth century, described the following case:

> I have been informed by the most unimpeachable sources that the physician Moses (Maimonides) was ill, and the Qāḍī al-Fāḍil paid him a visit. The Jew was a scholar and a gentleman. So, he said to al-Fāḍil: 'Your sense of decency has made you come and visit me. Let me advise you not to receive any medical treatment from a Jew, because with us, whoever desecrates the Sabbath – his blood is licit for us.'

According to the sources, the *qāḍī* thereupon banned Jews from practising medicine or being employed in that capacity.[379]

One example, out of many, of a Jewish physician being the object of hatred is Ibrāhīm b. al-Tharthār, who practised medicine at the court of Muḥammad V al-Naṣrī in Granada in the fourteenth century. A Muslim physician named Muḥammad al-Lakhmī al-Shaqūrī wrote a book against the Jews in general and Ibrāhīm b. al-Tharthār in particular. In 1359, when Muḥammad V moved to Morocco, Ibrāhīm took off to Castile and from there to Morocco. He later returned to Granada with his patron.[380] Jews were banned from practising medicine in 1448 when Sultan Jaqmaq issued a decree that took the first concrete measures against Jewish and Christian physicians, prohibiting *dhimmī* physicians from treating Muslim patients;[381] however, in 1463, when the sultan reissued a previous ban on *dhimmī* employment in the state bureaucracy, he made the prudent exception of physicians and moneychangers.[382] It is important to add that this decree was not enforced for long, for the simple reason that the Muslims could not manage without *dhimmī* physicians.

There was a frequently repeated prohibition to employ Christians and Jews in government service. It was a law that in the Ayyubid periods was honoured in the breach rather than by implementation. The vast number of Jewish physicians that worked in Muslim hospitals and the number of Jewish court physicians prove this assumption.[383] Similarly, in some cases we learn about a Jewish physician treating Muslim patients and one who served as the family doctor in the house of a man called 'The Sword of Islam'.[384]

4.4.5 Wazīr *(Vizier) and other high-ranking positions held by Jewish practitioners*

A *wazīr* was a high-ranking official or chief administrator or minister in Muslim regimes starting with the Abbasid caliphate. From the limited examples available we elucidate that for a Jewish person it was hard to break the 'glass ceiling' and become a *wazīr*. However, it appears that it was not impossible. Here are the main examples of Jewish or converted physicians who became *wazīrs* or carried out other high-ranking official positions (presented in chronological order):

a. Ḥasday b. Shaprūṭ (905–75) was a scholar, physician and trusted adviser in the court of the Umayyad caliph al-Ḥakam II in Cordova. Ḥasday came from a well-established family and became the most distinguished Jew in Andalusia, enjoying great wealth and social status.[385] In about 940 he was appointed as a physician to the caliph ʿAbd al-Raḥmān III, due to his engaging manners, knowledge, character and extraordinary ability. He gained his master's confidence to such an extent that he became the caliph's confidant and faithful counsellor. Without bearing the title of *wazīr* he was in reality the minister of foreign affairs and also had control of customs and ship dues in the port of Cordova.[386]

b. Mūsā b. Elʿāzār and some of his siblings (10th–11th centuries) served for several generations as court physicians to the caliphs, chief leaders of the Jewish community, and *wazīrs* in charge of the state treasury in the Fatimid courts at Qayrawān and Cairo.[387]

c. Yūsuf b. Abī Saʿīd b. Khalaf al-Sāmirī al-Muhadhdhab al-Ṭabīb was a Samaritan from Damascus (12th century). He served the Ayyubid emir of Baalbek, Farrukh Shāh, and after he died (1179) he then served under his successor. The latter also appointed him as a consultant and later on as a *wazīr*. Yūsuf acquired wealth from his positions and was accused by the Samaritan community of nepotism. Eventually, they told the sultan about his doings, and he then arrested him and confiscated his property. He was the paternal uncle of Amīn al-Dawla.[388]

d. Amīn al-Dawla Abū al-Ḥasan b. Ghazāl b. Abī Saʿīd al-Sāmirī (Wazīr al-Ṣāliḥ) was a Samaritan physician (13th century) and served as the court physician of the prince of Baalbek. After converting to Islam, he became in 1237 the *wazīr* of the ruler of Damascus, al-Malik al-Ṣāliḥ (d. 1250). He performed very well, built many structures, renewed schools and scholarly institutions and amassed great power and wealth.[389] He was executed in Egypt by the Mamluks, who replaced the Ayyubid dynasty in 1250.[390]

e. Sa'd al-Dawla b. Ṣafī b. Hibat Allāh b. Muhadhdhib al-Dawla al-Abharī (13th century) served as the financial supervisor of the 'Aḍudī hospital in Baghdad and later on was appointed as deputy to the Mongolian military governor of the city. In 1287 he became his financial administrator followed by his appointment as the personal physician to Arghūn Khān (r. 1284–91) in Tabriz, Iran. Sa'd al-Dawla found favour in Arghūn's eyes, both as a physician and as a person. This eventually led to his promotion to *wazīr*, in charge of the whole Īl-Khānate empire. In this capacity he ruled over large areas, and made sure to appoint, as was customary, the ones closely associated with him to key positions in the administration. His appointment and those of his Jewish relatives to key positions ruling over the Muslim community, in addition to his success, created opposition towards him among the Mongolian population in general, and the elite in particular, and he was executed in 1291.[391]

f. Jamāl al-Dīn Ibrāhīm b. al-Maghribī served in Cairo as the 'Head of the Physicians' in the court of al-Malik al-Nāṣir Muḥammad b. Qalāwūn (14th century). According to al-Ṣafadī,[392] he was at the level of *wazīr*.[393]

g. Rashīd al-Dīn Ṭabīb Faḍl Allāh b. al-Dawla, Abū al-Khayr b. 'Alī Abū al-Hamadānī (d. 1318) was one of the greatest statesmen and historians of medieval Iran. He was born Jewish in Hamadān and was the son of a pharmacist from a family of pharmacists. He started his career as a physician in the court of the Īl-Khānate in Tabriz. Up until his conversion to Islam, he was a loyal member of the Jewish community, in which he was educated and learnt Hebrew and Jewish traditions and customs. In 1298 he was appointed by Ghāzān Khān (d. 1304) as a *wazīr*, or the deputy of the grand *wazīr*, and remained in office under several rulers until he was executed at the age of seventy-one following a plot by an adversary.[394]

4.4.6 Conversion of Jewish practitioners to Islam

Conversion to Islam in the medieval period has received considerable attention in contemporary academic scholarship, both in the form of focused thematic discussions and in the framework of broad historiographic accounts.[395] This subject has been approached from many angles, raising a variety of historical questions such as: what were the reasons for conversion to Islam, what was the scope of the phenomenon, what were its process and the responses to it. Its effects on society reflected the different ways in which scholars have understood the process. Some scholars have seen conversion to Islam as an act that was charged with spiritual meanings, while others have seen it mainly as the adoption of a confessional label, that is, purely for its social consequences.[396] Stephen Humphreys, for example, claimed that conversion is a matter of exchanging one set of beliefs and rituals for another.[397]

A useful way of comprehending the phenomenon of conversion is by paying attention to the breaking points in the life of the convert, whether these be spiritual, cultural, social or even political. They may take place on a spectrum of levels and in different combinations.[398] Many reasons for conversion were named in the literature, from the side of the Muslim: inducing, forcing, missionising, preaching and appealing.[399] However, from the side of the non-Muslim, conversion to Islam could be opportunistic, enchanting, dependent, inspired, culturally embedded or communally feeble.[400]

In general, the consensus is that individuals and groups chose to join the ranks of Islam for various reasons, while the prevailing circumstances in each historical moment rendered certain factors more prominent than others. In any case, it seems clear enough that their decision to become Muslims entailed a certain measure of change in their daily lives.[401] Bulliet, in his quantitative history, studied the phenomena of conversion to Islam, using the system of Arabic-Islamic names to establish the curve of conversion to Islam in its earliest days. He claimed that conversion was mainly a social act that in time gave the Muslim community its distinctive character.[402]

Often, converts were shrouded with ambiguity, and this has been seen as a sign of their intermediate position, allowing them to transfer ideas, norms and practices across religious boundaries.[403] In this process, various communal institutions, mainly social and political, in which non-Muslims participated took on an Islamic veneer and could be seen to have transferred the adoption of an Islamic confessional affiliation as the byproduct of socialisation.[404] Therefore, a variety of literary genres expressed suspicions towards converts to Islam, questioning their integrity as Muslims and the sincerity of their motives.[405]

Humphreys pointed out that 'the three scriptural religions shared a core vocabulary, and each was equally able to demonstrate the inanity of the other two'. At that time religion was socially determined, that is, not strictly a personal choice and more of the community in which one lived. Therefore, if the social situation changed, it was not difficult to exchange one religion for another. Religion in pre-modern societies was a way of life, therefore conversion was exchanging one life for another, affecting dress, rules of marriage and divorce, law and inheritance, and actually much of everyday life would alter. So, the decision was not in what one believed, but about how one wanted to lead one's life.[406]

The phenomenon of conversion to Islam did not pass Jewish medical practitioners by. They were usually intellectuals and in many cases leaders of their communities,[407] who in many cases had a close relationship with Muslims, as fellow professionals (working together in hospitals for example),[408] in a personal capacity, as patients, as dignitaries and even religious scholars,[409] and as rulers (since they served in courts).[410]

Table 7 presents some basic details of most of the Jewish practitioners for whom we have information that they converted to Islam. More information can be found in their detailed biographies.[411] In the discussion (at the end of this section after the table) an analysis of the phenomenon will be presented according to various criteria from the literature and others such as chronology, ethnicity and geography.

The conversion of Jewish practitioners to Islam in the medieval Muslim world was a known phenomenon. However, not much, if anything, has been written about it. In most cases it was just mentioned as part of a general trend, which was that of the conversion of Jewish leaders who were also physicians.[412] From the data I collected for this book, it is clear that this phenomenon was on a small scale during the Fatimid-Ayyubid period, and on a much larger one especially in the Mamluk period.

So far, we have information about only two Jewish physicians who converted to Islam in the tenth century: Ismāʿīl b. Mūsā b. Elʿāzār, the son of Mūsā b. Elʿāzār al-ʾIsrāʾīlī (Moses b. Elazar), and Abū Sahl Dūnash b. Tamīm; both were court physicians who practised in Egypt (Cairo) and Tunisia (Qayrawān) respectively. Among the few Jewish practitioners who converted to Islam in the Fatimid-Ayyubid period (nine) we can mention: Abū al-Munajjā (Solomon b. Shaʿyā) (Egypt); Abū al-Faḍl (Ḥasday b. Joseph b. Ḥasday) (Andalusia); Abū al-Barakāt Hibat Allāh b. ʿAlī b. Malkā al-Baladi al-Ṭabīb al-Faḍl (Baghdad); Abū Naṣr Samawʾal b. Judah b. ʿAbbās

Table 7 Practitioners who converted to Islam[413]

Name	*Occupation*	*Place*	*Dates or century*	*Date and place of conversion*	*Remarks*
Ismāʿīl b. Mūsā b. Elʿāzār	Physician		10th		It is likely that he was originally of a Jewish family of physicians and converted to Islam
Abū Sahl Dūnash b. Tamīm	Physician and linguist	Qayrawān	d. 971		Dūnash was Muslim when he died
Abū al-Munajjā (Solomon b. Shaʿyā), ?convert	Physician, perhaps in charge of agriculture under the deputy of the Fatimid ruler, al-Afḍal		10th–11th		According to the 14th century chronicler Ibn Duqmāq, al-Munajjā is the Ibn Ṣaghīr family, most of whom converted to Islam and became physicians to kings and sultans
Abū al-Faḍl (Ḥasday b. Joseph b. Ḥasday)	Physician	Saragossa	11th		According to the Muslim sources he converted to Islam after he fell in love with a Muslim girl
Abū al-Barakāt Hibat Allāh b. ʿAlī b. Malkā al-Baladī al-Ṭabīb al-Faḍl (Nethanel Baruch b. Melekh)	Physician, military physician	Baghdad	1087–1165		It became clear to him that if he wanted a good life, he would have to convert to Islam
Abū Naṣr Samawʾal b. Judah b. ʿAbbās al-Maghribī	Physician and mathematician	Lived and worked for a while in Baghdad and in Diyarbakır, and later moved to Iran. At the end of the 12th century he reached Azerbaijan	d. 1170/1175	1163	He was the author of a polemical attack on the Jews and Judaism as well as an autobiographical account of his conversion

Abū Jaʿfar Joseph b. Aḥmad b. Ḥasday, ?convert	Physician	Saragossa, Egypt	12th		Born to a father who converted to Islam
Abū al-Faraj b. Abū al-Faḍāʾil b. al-Nāqid	Ophthalmologist	Cairo	12th century		
Yaḥyā b. Isḥāq	Physician	Andalusia	12th		
Kamāl al-Dawla Abū ʿAlī b. Abī al-Faraj, Ibn al-Dāʿī al-ʾIsrāʾīlī al-Irbilī, ?convert	Physician/ philosopher (*ḥakīm*)	*Ḥakīm* – the intention here is probably a physician or even a physician in the Mongol court. Was sent to Möngke Khan (perhaps to serve as a physician in his court in Mongolia) in 1259	13th		It is unclear whether or not he converted to Islam
Abū al-Ḥajjāj Yūsuf b. Yaḥyā b. Isḥāq al-Sabatī al-Maghribī, ?convert	Physician and merchant	North Africa, Syria, India. Fez, Alexandria, Fusṭāṭ, Aleppo, Iraq, Baghdad	d. 1226 in Aleppo	Earlier than 1182–4 or around 1185–90, Fez/ Aleppo	It is not certain that he converted
Amīn al-Dawla Abū al-Ḥasan b. Ghazāl b. Abī Saʿīd al-Sāmirī	Physician, *wazīr*	Became in 1237 the *wazīr* of the ruler of Damascus	13th. Executed in Egypt in 1251	No later than 1237	
ʿAbd Allāh b. Dāʾūd b. Abī al-Faḍl al-Dāʾūdi, Taqī al-Dīn	Physician		Beginning of the Mamlūk period	Beginning of the Mamlūk period	

Table 7 continued

Name	*Occupation*	*Place*	*Dates or century*	*Date and place of conversion*	*Remarks*
Ibn Aḥmad b. al-Maghribī, ?convert	The son of Shihāb al-Dīn (Sulaymān) Aḥmad al-Maghribī	Was at the service of the sultan al-Naṣīr Muḥammad b. Qalāwūn probably as physician	13th	The father converted to Islam in 1291, his sons probably converted like him at a young age	
Saʿd b. Manṣūr b. Kammūna, ?convert	Physician, philosopher and scholar	Baghdad or Egypt, smuggled by the governor of Baghdad to Hilla	13th	1280	It is said that he converted to Islam in 1280
Jamāl al-Dīn Dāʾūd b. Abī al-Faraj b. Abī al-Ḥusayn b.ʿImrān al-Ṭabīb	Physician	Probably Damascus	1275/1276–1336/1337		Al-Jazarī mentioned his conversion to Islam but not that he was a Jew. According to the names of his ancestors it is evident that he was a Jew
Shihāb al-Dīn (Sulaymān) Aḥmad al-Maghribī	Physician, 'Head of the Physicians'	Egypt	d. 1318	1291	
Najīb al-Dawla, ?convert	Ophthalmologist	Court of Tabriz	c.1300	1305, with a number of Jewish physicians in Tabriz	Intended to become Muslim

ʿAbd al-Sayyid b. Isḥāq b. Yaḥyā	Physician	Physician in the Nūrī hospital (al-Bīmāristān al-Nūrī) in Damascus	d. 1315	July 1302	
Nafīs b. Dāʾūd b. ʿAnān al-Tabrīzī	Physician	Originally from Tabriz, in 1354 he moved to Cairo	1354	Cairo	
Fatḥ Allāh b. Muʿtaṣim b. Nafīs (Fatḥ al-Dīn), ?convert	Physician. 'Head of the Physicians', appointed by al-Ẓāhir Barqūq as secretary of the Chancery for around 14 years	Born in Tabriz, active in Egypt	1358–1413. Choked to death in prison		Probably born Muslim. His father and grandfather converted probably in the mid-1360s
ʿAbd al-Ḥaqq	Pharmacist	Damascus	15th century	1480/1481	
Zayn al-Dīn Khiḍr al-ʾIsrāʾīlī al-Zuwaylī	Physician	?Egypt	Executed in 1438		
Khiḍr, ?convert	Physician		Early 16th		It is unclear if he converted to Islam
Anonymous	Physician	Probably from Egypt	16th		Converted to Islam when he was arrested

al-Maghribī (Azerbaijan);Abū Jaʿfar Joseph b. Aḥmad b. Ḥasday (Andalusia and Egypt); Abū al-Faraj b. Abū al-Faḍāʾil b. al-Nāqid (Egypt); Yaḥyā b. Isḥāq (Andalusia); Kamāl al-Dawla Abū ʿAlī b. Abī al-Faraj, Ibn al-Dāʿī al-ʾIsrāʾīlī al-Irbilī (Mongol court); Abū al-Ḥajjāj Yūsuf b. Yaḥyā b. Isḥāq al-Sabatī al-Maghribī (north Africa, Syria, India. Fez, Alexandria, Fusṭāṭ, Iraq, Baghdad and Aleppo); and Amīn al-Dawla Abū al-Ḥasan b. Ghazāl b. Abī Saʿīd al-Sāmirī (Syria and Egypt). Only one of these physicians, Abū al-Faraj b. Abū al-Faḍāʾil b. al-Nāqid, was a member of a medical dynasty!

By contrast, fourteen Jewish practitioners converted to Islam during the Mamluk period. It should also be noted that we have fewer sources of information from this period, either Muslim Arabic or Jewish.[414] The basic data regarding these converted physicians is found in the table above and more details are found in the biographies.[415]

A quick look at Table 7 clearly shows that the converted practitioners were practising all over the Muslim world, from Andalusia through the Maghrib, Egypt and Syria, and up to Iraq and Iran/Azerbaijan. Thus, the phenomenon was not restricted to a geographical region or even to an ethnic group (among them were Rabbanites, Samaritans and Karaites).

Members of more than a dozen dynasties of Jewish physicians converted to Islam during the Mamluk period, including ʿAbd al-Sayyid b. Isḥāq (13th–14th centuries), Shihāb al-Dīn (Sulaymān) Aḥmad al-Maghribī (13th–14th centuries), the Karaite medical dynasty of Nafīs b. Daʾūd b. ʿAnān al-Tabrīzī (13th–14th centuries), the Karaite Ibn Ṣaghīr (13th–14th centuries) and the Karaite ʿAbd Allāh b. Daʾūd b. Abī al-Faḍl al-Daʾūdī (14th century).[416]

Life as a non-Muslim court physician had its advantages, but also its disadvantages, which probably prompted conversions. For example, the Christian physician Ibn Muṭrān converted to Islam during the reign of Saladin, and among his incentives may have been the various benefits which he was unlikely to have enjoyed as a Christian.[417] Moreover, being a court physician enabled practitioners to show their abilities and talents. In many cases they became trustworthy and consequently the rulers may have appointed them to the position of *wazīr*. Converting to Islam was an important or requested step in most cases. Such occurrences happened rarely, possibly once or twice in each geographical area. Therefore, no pattern can be detected. However, we learn from the sources that most of the Jewish (or former Jewish) *wazīrs* were executed at some point due to plots or after their patron died, for example the Samaritan physician Amīn al-Dawla Abū al-Ḥasan b. Ghazāl b. Abī Saʿīd al-Sāmirī, who was active in courts in Syria and Egypt. According to the sources he became a *wazīr* of the ruler of Damascus in 1237, but was then executed in Egypt in 1251.[418]

Special attention should be given to the Karaite and Samaritan practitioners. Being a minority within a minority group, few of the physicians from Karaite families converted to Islam; those who did so include Ibn Kūjik (13th century),[419] Ibn Ṣaghīr (13th–14th centuries),[420] Nafīs b. Daʾūd b. ʿAnān al-Tabrīzī (14th–15th centuries) and ʿAbd Allāh b. Daʾūd b. Abī al-Faḍl al-Daʾūdī (13th century).

In its Iberian context, conversion to Islam has been studied through legal sources, where it is portrayed as a mechanism for the creation or removal of social boundaries.[421] We will mention here two examples: Abū al-Faḍl (Ḥasday b. Joseph b. Ḥasday) and Yaḥyā b. Isḥāq.

Conversion to Islam resulted in a new communal membership, but not necessarily in the complete abandonment of one's former beliefs and practices.[422] For instance, Abū al-Barakāt Hibat Allāh b. ʿAlī b. Malkā al-Baladī al-Ṭabīb al-Faḍl (Nethanel Baruch b. Melekh), a physician from Baghdad (12th century), converted but the rest, or at least some, of his family members remained Jewish. His daughters did not convert with him, although they knew that they wouldn't be recipients of his inheritance.[423]

Interestingly enough, converts themselves are also presented as important agents of conversion, including prominent communal leaders, intellectuals, spouses, siblings, children, and slave owners whose conversion to Islam had an impact on their surroundings.[424] Abū Naṣr Samawʾal b. Judah b. ʿAbbās al-Maghribī (12th century) lived and worked for a while in Iraq (Baghdad and Diyarbakır), and later moved to Iran. Samawʾal refrained from converting for a long time out of respect for his father (a well-known poet, Judah b. Abūn, a friend of Judah ha-Levi). In his autobiography, he described his conversion (1163) as the product of a process of study and intellectual analysis which took place over a considerable period of time. He eventually became a Muslim shortly before his father's death. Samawʾal's conversion was one of several at the time, which included Abū al-Barakāt Hibat Allāh, a physician and philosopher who converted at the end of his life, and Isaac the son of Abraham

b. Ezra. As all three were acquaintances, there have been suggestions that Hibat Allāh may have influenced the other two to convert, or that all these converts were part of a circle of intellectuals with shared interests and paths to Islam.[425] Sarah Stroumsa argued persuasively that this supposition is unfounded and that the conversions were independent.[426]

An example of collective conversions is that of the physician Jamāl al-Dīn Dā᾽ūd b. Abī al-Faraj b. Abī al-Ḥusayn b.ʿImrān al-Ṭabīb (1296–1359), who lived under the reign of al-Malik Naṣīr Naṣr Allāh, probably in Damascus. According to the Muslim Arabic sources, he converted to Islam together with other Jews: ʿAbd al-Sayyid the *dayyān* and his son, and Nissim the tanner and his sons.[427]

While stressing his strong friendship with the prominent Karaite physician Faraj Allāh (Yeshūʿa) Ibn Ṣaghīr (Cairo, 14th century), al-ʿUmarī provided us with a unique insight into the process of conversion. He described his own experiences as one of Faraj Allāh's patients and ended his entry with the sentence: 'If only he had lived longer. My grief for a man like him, who died while still holding his Jewish faith ...' One may interpret this statement as an indication of Faraj Allāh's intention to convert, probably due to pressures from the Muslim environment and since, as it seems, most of his family members were converted by this time.[428]

4.4.7 Jewish practitioners as famous scholars, authors, poets and diplomats

Most of the Jewish practitioners of the medieval period were among the elite of their society. They were scholars and usually had been blessed with a set of qualifications that were highly useful in their communities and in many cases were also beneficial for the Muslim administration and rulers. Their intellectual abilities were expressed not only in their medical education and study, but also in writing medical books. In some cases, they also wrote religious essays and/or secular texts and even poetry.[429] Some of the practitioners were involved in commercial activities, others became administrators and worked in courts, and some dealt with local, national and even international political activities.

Authors of medical literature

Jewish practitioners made significant contributions to the theoretical medical knowledge by writing books that broadened the contemporary medical corpus. Many of them lived and practised in the world under Islamic rule, mainly in the east but also in the west. Thanks to the Geniza we have even gained insight into the copying, buying and selling of medical books in the medieval Muslim world. An example of how physicians wrote their medical works can be learnt for example from Maimonides' autograph drafts.[430]

Caballero-Navas claimed that the number of practitioners did not seem proportional to the relatively small number of known medical texts authored by Jews. She added: 'This picture is not surprising, given that the number of practicing physicians is generally larger than that of medical writers.'[431] Miri Shefer and Michael Chamberlain suggested that writing medical books and presenting them to patrons was one of the ways a physician drew the attention of influential rulers and later became a court physician.[432] Thanks to the current research, we can add figures to this issue. In any case, in my opinion, Caballero-Navas's suggestion should be studied in the future in relation to time (various periods), subjects and geographical origin of the writers. Dozens (more than fifty known until now) of the Jewish practitioners (mainly physicians) of the Muslim world wrote medical books.[433] I will present here only a few of the most well-known and important ones (set in chronological order):[434]

a. Māsarjawayh (Iraq, 683–750): when translating *Kunnāsh Ahron* from Syriac to Arabic, he added two articles, one on 'the power of food, its qualities and demerits' and one on 'the power of drugs, their qualities and demerits'.

b. Isḥāq b. Sulaymān al-ʾIsrāʾīlī (Egypt, Qayrawān, 832–932): among his main medical writings were a 'book of components', a 'book on dietetics', a 'book on fevers', a 'treatise on urine', a 'treatise on elements', a 'treatise on definitions and outlines' and 'The Garden of Knowledge', which deals with metaphysical matters.

c. Mūsā b. Elʿāzār al-ʾIsrāʾīlī (Moses b. Elazar) (Qayrawān, Cairo, 10th century): among his medical writings are a paper on coughs and two books dedicated to Caliph al-Muʿizz li-Din Allah: *al-Kitāb al Muʿizzī fi* *al-Ṭabīkh* and *Kitāb al-Qarābādhīn*, which according to Goitein was lost, but descriptions of medical conditions and recipes for medicines included in it are mentioned in other books.[435]

d. Abū al-Barakāt Hibat Allāh b. ʿAli b. Malkā al-Baladi al-Tabib al-Faḍl (1087–1165, Hamadān): *Kitāb al-Muʿtabar*, including logic, natural sciences and religion, and considered one of the best of its time on these topics; a summary of *Kitāb al-Tashrīḥ*; a summary of Galen, *Kitāb al-Aqrābādhin*; an article concerning a medicine he concocted named *Ṣifat Barshaʿthāʾ* (an Indian medicine); and *Risāla fī al-ʿAql wa-Māhiyatihi* (a letter about the brain and its essence).

e. Marwān (Abū al-Walīd) Ibn Janāḥ al-Qurṭubī (R. Jonah Marinus) (Cordova, Lucena, Saragossa, 10th–11th centuries): *Kitāb al-Talkhīṣ* ('The Book of Commentary'), a medical dictionary of simple drugs and weights and measurements that were used in medicine, containing about 830 columns and hundreds of synonyms in different languages.

f. Menahem b. al-Fawwāl (Saragossa, 11th century): *al-Adawiya al-Mufrada* (a book on simple drugs); innovation regarding the measurements and weights used in medicine, and drug dosages.

g. Yūsuf b. Isḥāq Ibn Biklārish (Saragossa, Almeria, 11th–12th centuries): *Kitāb al-Mustaʿīni*, one of the most important Arabic pharmacological treatises, containing information on hundreds of medicaments, and 'lists of substitute drugs with their properties and methods of use'.

h. Abū al-ʿAshāʾir Hibat-Allāh b. Zayn b. Ḥasan b. Ifrāʾīm b. Yaʿqūb b. Ismāʿīl Ibn Jumayʿ al-ʾIsrāʾīlī (Nethanel b. Samuel) (Cairo, d. 1198): *Kitāb al-Irshād li-Maṣāliḥ al-Nafs wa-l-Ajsād* (direction for the improvements of souls and bodies, 4 volumes), *Kitāb al-Taṣrīḥ bi-l-Maknūn fī Tankīḥ al-Qānūn* (criticism of Ibn Sīnā's Canon), *Maqāla fī al-Līmūn wa-Sharābihi wa-Manāfiʿihi* (on the benefits of lemons and their consumption), *al-Risāla al-Sayfiyya fī al-Adwiya al-Mulūkiyya*, a treatise on *qūlanj* (intestinal pain and spasms); *al-Maqāla al-Salāḥiyya fī Iḥyāʿ al-Ṣināʿa al-Ṭibbiya* (how to revive medicine), dealing with the reasons for the decline in the medical profession.

i. Ibn ʿAknīn (Joseph b. Judah b. Jacob) (Seville and Barcelona, 12th century): several essays including *Ṭibb al-Nufūs*, focused on psychology.

j. Moses b. Maimon, Maimonides (1138–1204): ten books/essays:

'Medical Aphorisms of Moses', 'The Art of Curing', 'Commentary on the Aphorisms of Hippocrates', 'Treatise on Haemorrhoids', 'Treatise on Cohabitation', 'Treatise on Asthma', 'Treatise on Poisons and Their Antidotes', 'Regimen of Health', 'Glossary of Drug Names'.

k. Abū al-Faḍl Dā'ūd b. Sulaymān b. Abū al-Bayān al-'Isrā'īlī al-Sadīd (David b. Solomon) (Cairo, 1161-1236): *al-Dustūr al-Bimāristānī fī 'l-Adwiya 'l-Murakkaba*, which included all of the medicines prevalent in hospitals, particularly Nāṣirī; a book of notes on Galen; a book of pains.

l. Abū al-Munā b. Abī Naṣr b. Ḥaffāẓ (al-Kohen al-'Aṭṭār al-'Isrā'īlī) (Karaite, Cairo, 13th century), pharmacist: *Minhāj al-Dukkān* a 25-chapter instruction manual for pharmacies, including explanations of medicine, preparation and advice concerning the preservation of materials. The manual was highly successful and widely used during the Middle Ages and continued to be used until the modern era.

m. Ḥayyīm Vital (Safed, lived also in Jerusalem, Damascus, 1543–1620): a book on medicines and mysticism.[436]

Practitioners and poets[437]

Poetry (and oratory) played an important role in pre-Islamic Arabia. According to Makdisi, poets and orators were the 'publicists of their tribes'; and they kept their prestige and positions of power in Islam. Arabic poetry was composed by all intellectuals in the Muslim medieval society.[438] It is no wonder that the Jews who lived in the Muslim world took part in and adopted this tradition, on top of the Jewish tradition of lyrical verse.

Another way of learning about various aspects of Jewish practitioners is through poetry, both secular (professional) and religious. Vast amounts of Hebrew and Arabic poems were found in the Geniza,[439] many of which were written by or about physicians; a leading example is that of the Alexandrian physician and judge Aaron Ibn al-'Ammānī.[440] It is interesting that another physician and poet, Judah ha-Levi, praised Aaron as a great physician who successfully fought the angel of death, bringing back to life patients who were considered incurable, and also as an encyclopaedic scholar, a powerful judge, an indefatigable teacher and a man of munificence.[441]

Medieval Jewish poetry has been extensively studied in the last century.[442] Poetry was a way of expressing personal feelings, political opinions and also communicating with society, friends, colleagues and even enemies. Here are some physicians who were also poets and scholars, some of whom are well known. Clearly, most of them are from Andalusia, and a few moved to Egypt, north Africa and even Iraq.[443]

a. Abū al-Faḍl (Ḥasday b. Joseph b. Ḥasday) (Saragossa, 11th century). A physician, poet and scholar; a member of one of the well-known Jewish families in Andalusia and a court physician to the Almoravid ruler. According to the Muslim sources he converted to Islam after he fell in love with a Muslim girl.

b. Abū al-Ḥasan (Judah b. Samuel ha-Levi) (Toledo, Cairo, 1080–1141). A physician, religious thinker and poet. In his youth he spent time in Granada where he joined the circle of Jewish public figures and intellectuals around Moses b. Ezra. His writings show his extensive knowledge of Hebrew grammar, literary tradition, the Bible, Rabbinic traditions, Arabic literature, Sufism, philosophy and medicine. He wrote *Kitāb al-Radd wa al-Dalīl fī al-Dīn al-Dhalīl* ('The Book of Rejoinder and Proof in Support of the Neglected Religion'), commonly known as the *Kuzari.*

c. Meʾir (Abū al-Ḥasan) Ibn Qamniʾel (Saragossa, Seville, Marrakesh, 11th–12th centuries). A Jewish physician and a poet. He moved to Morocco and served as the court physician of Sultan Yūsuf b. Tāshufīn. Known from the writings of Judah ha-Levi and Maimonides.

d. Abū Ayyūb al-Yahūdī (al-ʾIsrāʾīlī) (Solomon b. al-Muʿallim) (Seville, 1105–71). Court physician to an Almoravid emir in Marrakesh. He was a Jewish scholar and a poet. He was praised by Jewish dignitaries such as Moses b. Ezra, Judah ha-Levi and Judah al-Ḥarīzī.

e. Elias b. al-Mudawwar b. Ṣaddūd al-Yahūdī al-Ṭabīb al-Rundī (Andalusia, 12th century). A physician and a poet, especially mentioned by Arab historians as a poet.

f. Moses b. Abraham b. Saʿadya ha-Rōfē Darʿī (Alexandria, 12th century). A Karaite physician and a most gifted poet; in a collection of essays he wrote a *dīwān*, in which poems, prayers, praise, condemnations, complaints, lamentations, satires, riddles and more are included.

g. Aaron ha-Rōfē b. Yeshūʿā ha-Rōfē Ibn al-ʿAmmānī (active in Alexandria, 12th century). A physician and a judge,[444] he was a writer of *payṭan* (liturgical poetry), of which some has survived and can be found in the Cairo Geniza.[445]

h. Shem Tov b. Joseph b. Falaquera (Spain, 13th century). A physician, philosopher, poet and translator.[446]

An interesting anecdote is recalled about Ibn Shūʿa (al-Muwaffaq) (d. 1183), one of Saladin's physicians. Ibn Abī Uṣaybiʿa described him as easy-going and funny, and said that he used to play the guitar. Evidently, he liked to write poems: a scornful one written against his colleague Ibn Jumayʿ, and a humorous poem on a Muslim zealot who threw a stone that took out one of Ibn Shūʿa's eyes, because he was riding a horse in violation of the laws restricting *dhimmīs.*[447]

Intellectuals, thinkers and philosophers

For many Jewish intellectuals (both in the eastern and in the western parts of the Muslim World), practising medicine provided a means of earning their living and enjoying a respectable social position. This also enabled them to devote some of their time to other expertise and passions. I will present here four of the most important and well-known examples.

a. Isḥāq b. Sulaymān al-ʾIsrāʾīlī (Isaac b. Solomon) (Cairo, Qayrawān, 9th–10th centuries) was the best-known Jewish physician who preceded Maimonides. A philosopher, skilled in logic and several branches of science, Isaac wrote books in Arabic on medicine and philosophy. His philosophical writings were influenced by Neoplatonism and he was considered one of the earliest Jewish philosophers of the Middle Ages. His main contribution was introducing Neoplatonism to the world of Jewish thought. In spite of the critical attitude Maimonides had towards him and towards the greater publicity of his compatriot Saʿadya Gaon, Isaac influenced Solomon Ibn Gabirol and Joseph Ibn Ṣaddiq, as well as various mystic Jews.[448]

b. Mūsā b. ʿAbd Allāh al-ʾIsrāʾīlī al-Qurṭubī (Moses b. Maimon; Maimonides) (Cordova, Fez, Cairo, 12th–13th centuries) was a well-known and important physician, one of the most prominent Jewish philosophers of all time, an important scholar and Halakhic. Maimonides composed works of Jewish scholarship, Rabbinic law and philosophy. Among his most important books, which influenced not only the Jewish world, but also many Muslim philosophers and scholars, I will mention here only a few: *Mishne Torah* (14 volumes), a canonical authority as a codification of Talmudic law and the first full commentary on the entire Mishna; *Sefer ha-Mitzvot* ('The Book of Commandments'), 613 commandments traditionally contained in the Bible; *The Guide for the Perplexed*, a philosophical work harmonising and differentiating between Aristotle's philosophy and Jewish theology; *Responsa*, questions and answers of Jewish tradition (including a number of public letters); and *Sefer Ha-Shamad* ('Letter of Martyrdom').[449]

c. Marwān (Abū al-Walīd) Ibn Janāḥ al-Qurṭubī (Cordova, Lucena, 10th–11th centuries) was a well-known Jewish physician and intellectual, expert in logic and lexicography and a talented Arabic and Hebrew linguist and grammarian. Ibn Janāḥ was one of the most prominent Jewish authors of the time and contributed to the field of herbal medical research. His main works were *Kitāb al-Mustalḥaq* ('The Book of Criticism'), *Risālat al-Tanbīh* ('The Book of Admonition'), *Kitāb/Risālat al-Taqrīb wa al-Tashīl* ('The Epistle of Bringing Near and Making Easy'), *Kitāb al-Taswiya* ('The Book of Rebuke'), *Kitāb al-Tashwīr* ('The Book of Shaming') and *Kitāb al-Tanqīḥ* ('The Book of Minute Research'). He was also the author of *Kitāb al-Talkhīṣ* ('The Book of Commentary'), a medical dictionary that dealt with simple drugs and weights and measurements; it contained about 830 columns and hundreds of synonyms in different languages.[450]

d. An example of scientific and intellectual curiosity: ʿAbd al-Laṭīf b. Ibrāhīm b. Shams al-Baghdādī, a physician and a leader of the Jewish community in Cairo in the mid-fifteenth century.[451] He was described as a great scholar who lived for long periods in Syria and Egypt. ʿAbd al-Laṭīf wrote about his impressions of Cairene architecture and how he had the opportunity to review and explore skeletons and mummies in Cairo.[452] He expressed great knowledge of the wonders of nature.

A trusted courtier

Ḥasday b. Shaprūṭ (905–75) was a scholar, physician and trusted adviser to the court of the Umayyad caliphs in Cordova. Ḥasday became the most distinguished Jew in Andalusia, enjoying great wealth and social status. In about 940 he was appointed as a physician to the caliph ʿAbd al-Raḥmān III, who had declared an independent Iberian caliphate in 929. Due to his engaging manners, knowledge, character and extraordinary ability, Ḥasday gained his master's trust to such an extent that he became the caliph's confidant and faithful counsellor (minister of foreign affairs); he also had control of the customs and ship dues in the port of Cordova. In his capacity as a trusted courtier, he undertook a number of diplomatic missions and played a significant role in the negotiations between the caliph and the Byzantine emperor Constantine VII, which led to the exchange of delegations between Constantinople and Cordova. The Caliph appointed him *nāsī* (president or head) of the Jewish communities in Andalusia. As such, Ḥasday represented his coreligionists in court as their spokesman, defender and patron, promoting their welfare and appointing the spiritual leaders of the various communities.[453]

4.5 Community Affairs

4.5.1 The socio-economic position of Jewish practitioners

Muslim physicians' social positions varied greatly between both countries and communities. Even in the same locality conditions changed immensely over time.[454] The status of the medical profession and its practitioners was connected to several factors, mainly the characteristics of the various time frames. During the Fatimid and Ayyubid periods, due to the many wars, the importance of the medical profession peaked in comparison with the Mamluk period, which was characterised by periodic plagues, meaning massive numbers of deaths and helpless physicians.

A physician's rank was also influenced by his field of specialisation: those dealing with internal medicine were considered men of science, and therefore of a higher status than the other physicians. However, this was not true of the court physicians, who were held by their contemporaries in relatively high regard when compared to the others throughout all different periods – their eminence always remained. Hazan found out, based on the analysis of the bulk of primary sources, that during the time in which the medical profession was considered honourable, most doctors enjoyed the public's admiration and flourished financially; consequently, whether they worked in hospitals, practised medicine in private clinics or attended home visits, they were placed in the mid-to-high-level range. During times of crisis, when physicians could only stand aside helplessly as plague and devastation swept through the population, it appears that they lost some of their financial status and social prestige compared with the religious leaders.[455]

When Pormann and Savage-Smith dealt with the complexity of social life in the medieval world within which medical practitioners acted, they wrote: 'Yet, because of the lack of adequate documentation, we can only offer glimpses at what it might have been like to be a patient or practitioner in the period discussed here.'[456] Our findings, based on the information extracted from biographical data (including Geniza documents), can and will elaborate on the above mentioned issue and on many others.

Medicine was one of the few occupations in which Jews and Christians could acquire a rank and position of respect in medieval Muslim society. Therefore, they favoured it as a profession. Lewicka claimed that in general they were gifted doctors, 'both as scholars and practitioners'. Moreover, since the study and practice of medicine were a truly academic challenge, they were intellectually rewarding and brought personal satisfaction. Interestingly enough, according to some Muslim Arabic sources,[457] the patients clearly trusted them more than Muslim physicians, who were for some reason or other not considered successful in medicine.[458]

According to Goitein, a twelfth-century Jewish physician who worked in a government hospital either in Cairo or Aleppo was in most respects 'representative of the medical profession of his time in general, while a Jewish glassmaker, silk-weaver, or metal founder would use the same techniques and occupy approximately the same social position as his Christian or Muslim fellow workers'.[459] Due to the depth of Jewish integration in Islamic societies, especially during what is known as the classical period of Islam (700–1250), Jews in these professions enjoyed social prestige – often in stark contrast to their counterparts in the Christian world.[460]

From the socio-economic point of view, most of the physicians, pharmacists, druggists and perfumers were among the non-poor in the Jewish community, together with greengrocers, wax makers, vinegar makers, distributors of gallnuts, meat sellers, sellers of food delicacies, bakers, millers, honey sellers, clothiers, fullers, weavers, dealers in sal ammoniac, bead makers, net makers, merchants, heads of the money assayers, bankers in government service, brokers, government clerks, government workshop employees, suppliers of precious metals to the mint, phlebotomists and agents.[461] Important doctors (often acting as part-time or full-time court physicians) were part of the upper class in the Jewish community, together with high government officials and agents, chief judges and leading businessmen, especially if they were learned enough to act as community leaders also. Indeed, physicians, bankers and government officials were highly honoured in the Jewish community, and communal leaders were often chosen from their ranks.[462]

Many of the doctors appearing in the Geniza documents and in the Muslim Arabic sources were prosperous, influential and among the best-known and most prominent men in the community, such as Abraham Maimonides and Moses (Abū Saʿd) b. Nethanel ha-Levi.[463] For example, we learn from the deathbed declaration of Abū al-Faraj (1182), a rich Jewish merchant and a trustee of the court, that he owed money to some of his associates; these included two physicians, al-Sheikh al-Muwaffaq (Ibn Jumayʿ), and Maimonides, who were at the time probably among the richest in the community.[464]

Families of physicians who often treated rulers and governors were also likely to be close to the seats of power. A good example of how Jewish leaders made use of their good relations with the Muslim leadership, mainly due to their medical qualifications and positions, is a letter from a notable head of the Jewish community, who was also a court physician to the ruler of Egypt, regarding the redemption of a Jewish dignitary: 'I have written to the *nagid* – may he live forever – and asked him to request the commander of the fleet to rescue the *gaon* and his children in Tripoli when he happens to anchor there.'[465]

However, based on our findings, it appears that the social standing of Jewish practitioners did vary: some were poor, others took on additional jobs or had other businesses, and a few were rich, well known and very prestigious. Naturally, the greatest difference was between the urban and the rural practitioners. From legal documents, such as wills,[466] marriage contracts referring to doctors, or lists of contributions to public appeals, information on the poor financial status of some physicians was revealed. In other cases, it is stated expressly in letters. Moreover, it turns out that others possessed modest means only or were even poor.[467] One example comes from the will of the Jewish physician Abū al-Maḥāsin b. al-Kāmukhī b. Abū al-Faḍā'il (c.1241), in which he granted a modest sum to his widow. From this document we learn that not all medical practitioners enjoyed high income.[468]

It should also be mentioned that some physicians came from relatively humble backgrounds, and that becoming a physician offered the opportunity of social mobility. The Geniza documents enable us to read about a physician whose father was a tuna fishmonger, another whose father operated an oil press,[469] and a third who was the son of a fuller.[470]

*4.5.2 Headship of the Jews (*nagid*)*

Nagid (a Biblical word) is usually translated as 'prince' or 'leader'. The medieval meaning of this title, was according to Goitein, an 'abbreviation of such high-sounding phrases as "Prince of the Diaspora", "Prince of the People of the Lord (or: of Israel)", or "Prince of Princes".[471] In medieval Egypt, and in other locations of Jewish communities, it became the title for the territorial head of the Jewish community, who was also called *Ra'īs al-Yahūd*.[472]

I chose to start this discussion looking at it from a different angle, that is, how the Muslims saw the position of *nagid*. Qalqashandī noted the three sects of the Jews (Rabbanites, Karaites and Samaritans). The custom was that the Head of the Jews was exclusively drawn from the majority group (Rabbanites), who exercised jurisdiction over all members of these three sects.[473] The Geniza provided original and important material for the study of the public institution of the heads of the Jewish community in the Muslim world, mainly during the Fatimid and Ayyubid periods. The modern historical research of the territorial heads of the Jewish community in the last century was full of academic disputes between scholars which are beyond the scope of this book.[474] Since the issue has been dealt with in various publications by different scholars, I have chosen to present here some of the main points that were raised by Goitein:

a. The emergence of the title '*nagid*' is an internal Jewish issue, and the Muslim rulers had nothing to do with it.

b. This title evolved from the yeshiva's leadership (*geonim*) for their own needs, and it did not contradict the Rosh Gola.

c. The position of *nagid* came from the yeshiva's habit of appointing a 'clerk' in each country to collect questions and donations from the local Jewish communities, and meanwhile, to lead the people, judge them and stand up for them before the Muslim rulers.

d. Similar to other titles, the origin of the *nagid* was a yeshiva internal appointment. It was given usually to an enthusiastic supporter from a large family and 'exported' outside.

As far as we know today, the first to have borne the title '*nagid*' was Abū Isḥāq Ibrāhīm b. ʿAṭā, an eleventh-century physician of the rulers of Tunisia (Bādīs and his son al-Muʿizz). Abū Isḥāq Ibrāhīm b. ʿAṭā used his influential position to protect his Jewish fellows in a difficult period that saw an increase in fanaticism and disorders in that country. We know that he was a strong supporter of the Jewish scholars in Baghdad, in particular Hai Gaon (d. 1038). Therefore, and probably in recognition of his many merits, Hai Gaon conferred on him the title of '*nagid*' (1015). It is important to mention that Ibrāhīm's father, ʿAṭā (Nathan in Hebrew), had occupied a similar position of communal leader, but with the more widely used title 'head of the congregations'. The title '*nagid*' does not appear in Egypt until about 1065, almost a hundred years after the Fatimids' conquest, and it was not in continuous use even after its inception. Only from the beginning of the thirteenth century did the Hebrew title '*nagid*' become permanently attached to that of *Raʾīs al-Yahūd*, the Head of the Jews. According to Goitein, we have to distinguish between the title and the office, and, as far as the office is concerned, we have to keep in mind that the task was a combination of representing the Jewish community before the Muslim regime together with exercising its highest legal and religious authorities, which were developed in Egypt under very specific historical circumstances; and that was not easy. Disregard of these considerations led to the confusion still prevailing in Jewish historiography about this most important institution.[475]

As early as the tenth century, we learn that Ḥasday b. Shaprūṭ (Cordova) was assigned by the caliph to take on important functions and privileges, including oversight of the customs bureau. He also appointed him *nāsī* of

*Table 8 Jewish physicians as chief leaders of the Jewish communities (Head of the Jews/*nagid*)*[476]

Name and dates	*Title*	*Community*	*Remarks*
Mūsā b. El῾āzār al-᾿Isrā᾿īlī (Moses b. Elazar) (d. 974)	Chief leader of the Jews (*Ra᾿īs al-Yahūd*)	Cairo	Court physician to the first Fatimid caliph, al-Mu῾izz li-Dīn Allāh
Isḥāq b. Mūsā (Isaac b. Moses) (son of Moses b. Elazar) (d. 973)	?Chief leader of the Jews	Cairo	(court) physician, *wazīr*
Ḥasday b. Shaprūṭ (10th century)	*Nāsī*, 'Rish Cala'	Cordova	
Abū Isḥāq Ibrāhīm b. ῾Aṭā (Abraham b. Nathan) (11th century)	Goitein claimed that he was 'the first Nagid known to have borne this title in his capacity of "Head of a Jewish territorial community"'	Tunisia	Served two rulers of Tunisia, Bādis and his son al-Mu῾izz, as court physician
Judah b. Sa῾adya (Abū Zikrī) (d. 1077)	*Nagid* 1062–4	Cairo	Fatimid court physician
Mevōrākh Abū al-Faḍl b. Sa῾adya (Abū al-Faḍl Mubārak) (1040–1111)	*Nagid* 1078–82, 1099–1111	Cairo	Physician in the Fatimid caliph's court
Moses b. Mevōrākh b. Sa῾adya (b. 1080)	*Nagid* 1112–26	Cairo	
Samuel ha-Nagid b. Hananiah (Abū Manṣūr) (12th century)	Leader of the Jewish community in Fusṭāṭ 1140–59	Cairo	Served under the Fatimid caliph al-Ḥāfiz li-Dīn Allāh (r. 1130–49)
Hibat Allāh Nethanel b. Moses ha-Levi (d. 1185)	*Nagid*, active mainly in Cairo, 1159–69	Cairo	
Moses ben Maimon (Maimonides) (1138–1204)	*Nagid* 1171–3	Cairo	
Abraham Ben Maimon (Maimonides) (d. 1237)	Head of the Jews/ *Nagid*	Cairo	Court physician
Abū al-Ḥasan b. al-Muwaffaq b. al-Najm b. al-Muhadhdhab (13th century)	Head of the Jews 1285	Cairo	Associate of Sultan al-Manṣūr Qalāwūn
David b. Abraham b. Moses b. Maimon (Maimonides' grandson) (1212–1300)	*Nagid*	Cairo	
David II b. Joshua (d. 1415)	Head of the Jews	Cairo	
R. Joseph b. Khalīfa (15th century)	*Nagid*	Cairo	Physician to the sultan

Name and dates	*Title*	*Community*	*Remarks*
Solomon b. R. Joseph (Samuel Rakkaḥ or Rakkakh) (15th century)	*Nagid*	Cairo	Physician and associate of the Mamluk sultan Qaitbāy
ʿAbd al-Laṭīf al-Baghdādī (15th century)	Leader of the Jewish community in Cairo in the mid-15th century. It is possible that he was the head of the Jews, *Raʾīs al-Yahūd*	Cairo	

the Jewish communities in Andalusia. As such, Ḥasday represented his coreligionists as their spokesman in court as well as their defender and patron, promoting their welfare and appointing the spiritual leaders of the various communities.[477] As *nāsī* of Andalusian Jewry, Ḥasday was also named 'Rish Cala' or Abū Yūsuf.[478]

It was mainly in the Fatimid and Ayyubids period that eminent and court physicians were appointed to the Headship of the Jews, acting as the *nagid* in Egypt and Syria, that is, the supreme judicial authority of the Jews.[479] The Head of the Jews was responsible, *inter alia*, for the consolidation of the Jewish community, the administration of the community by observing its religious laws and the commandments according to the Jewish religion, ensuring compliance with the 'Pact of ʿUmar', supervision of religious and social services and maintenance of law and order by the community.[480] It was also during the latter part of this period that the Jewish leaders who resided in Fusṭāṭ gradually became more powerful in the wake of the decline of the Geonic academies in both Babylonia and Palestine. Gil wrote about physicians who served as Head of the Jews that they 'benefited from a preferred social status; a salient fact over the generations is the closeness to the rulers, of the Jewish physicians who treated them, and the opportunity openly given them to be spokesmen and intercessors for their people'.[481]

The timing and emergence of the formal position of Headship of the Jews in Egypt is a matter of controversy among scholars. Therefore, Jewish physicians who also assumed the leadership of Egyptian Jewry, though their precise position and official title are ambiguous, will be termed henceforth the chief leader of the Jewish community.[482] Information regarding the Headship of the Jews appears in Table 8.

Maimonides and his descendants continued to be the chief leaders of the Jewish community in Egypt for a long time. Their service as a dynasty of Heads was unique in several aspects, especially since the office was passed down from father to son for nearly 250 years, from 1171 until around 1415.[483] In addition to the position of Head of the Jews, several members of this family served as physicians, as discussed below.[484] This family embodies the golden age of dynasties of Jewish physicians (during the Fatimid and Ayyubid periods), in which dynasties of court physicians almost constantly occupied the office of Head of the Jews as well.[485] Four dynasties of Jewish physicians (besides Maimonides and his family members) in the Fatimid-Ayyubid period had members that were leaders of the Jewish community: Saʿadya b. Mevōrākh (11th–12th centuries), Moses b. Elazar (10th–11th centuries); Moses b. Nethanel ha-Levi (Abū Saʿd) (12th century) and Samuel b. Hananiah (Abū Manṣūr) (12th century). Members of one more probably held this post as well: Isaac ha-Kohen ha-Rōfē b. Furāt (11th century).[486]

Several dynasties in the Fatimid-Ayyubid period provided Jewish physicians as local community leaders: Zechariah the Alexandrian (12th–13th centuries), Moses b. Jekuthiel (11th–12th centuries), Aaron ha-Rōfē al-ʿAmmānī (11th–13th centuries) and Tiqva ha-Levi (13th century).[487] During the Mamluk period, members of other dynasties of Jewish physicians were local community leaders, for example Jacob ha-Rōfē (14th century) and Joseph b. Abraham Sakandarī (15th–16th centuries).[488]

There is evidence that distinguished non-converted Jewish physicians were community leaders, mainly in Syria, during the Mamluk period and were also associated with the ruling elite, including the sultans: Asad 'the Jew' (Asad al-Yahūdī), who was a court physician to the prince of Hama al-Malik al-Muʾayyad Abū al-Fidāʾ and to other emirs in Syria and Egypt (13th–14th centuries);[489] and a certain ʿAwḍ, who was a supreme judge (*dayyān al-Yahūd*) in Damascus and a physician of members of the Muslim elite (14th century). He was also a physician known among the Muslims for his successful castration surgeries.[490]

*4.5.3 Judges (*dayyānim*)*

The *dayyān*, a Jewish judge, was one of a few professional scholars who served the community. Since they devoted their time to the benefit of study and to the service of the community, *dayyānim* regarded it as a sacred duty to contribute to their upkeep. Indeed, the study of sacred law was a lifetime duty. It took place mainly in the yeshiva, and it was there that the *dayyān* conferred on the new scholar the licence to issue authoritative legal opinions, that is, to act as a judge. As a rule, only persons of mature age would qualify for such positions. Scholars and students attended court sessions as part of their course of study. Normally, the *dayyān* devoted most of his time to study (learning in company of other scholars) and teaching, regarding it as his main duty. Sermons connected to the usual synagogue service were normally given by the local judge. Similarly, public lectures were a regular feature of his routine work. The *dayyān* was also expected to speak at happy family events and at funerals.[491] Until the middle of the twelfth century, the Dayyān acted as supervisor and coordinator of social services in the community, taking care of orphans, widows, the poor, the sick, foreigners and captives. From the Geniza we learn that by the end of the twelfth century, the judge was managing community funds and administering these services in person.[492] As a community leader, the *dayyān* represented his community members before the local and central officials of the government and before the territorial and international authorities of the Jews. As such, he was involved in politics, dealing with legal cases and with administrative matters of all kinds.[493]

Over the years, some practitioners worked as *dayyānim* in the Jewish courts of their communities, and some of them even had the epithet Dayyān as part of their name. Here are a few examples:

a. Aaron ha-Rōfē b. Yeshūʿā ha-Rōfē Ibn al-ʿAmmānī (12th century), a physician and a judge.[494]

b. Ben ha-Sōfer ha-Dayyān is mentioned in the notebook of a Jewish physician, from around 1150 (Cairo). According to Goitein, it is most likely that Dayyān, who borrowed the book, practised medicine in order to earn his living.[495]

c. Elijah b. Zechariah (Abū al-Faraj) (Alexandria, 12th–13th centuries) was a physician and prominent judge in the court of Abraham Maimonides.[496]

d. Samuel b. Saʿadya ha-Levi was a *dayyān* and a scribe in the court of Maimonides (Alexandria, 12th century). When he was younger, apparently he worked as a pharmacist.[497]

e. Moses b. Peraḥya b. Yijū (13th century) was apparently a physician and a *dayyān* in Minyat Ziftā.[498]

f. ʿAbd al-Sayyid b. Isḥāq b. Yaḥyā al-Ḥakīm al-Faḍl Bahāʾ al-Dīn b. al-Muhadhdhab, al-Ṭabīb al-Kaḥḥāl, was formerly a *dayyān* among the Jews and then converted to Islam. His son Yūsuf ʿAbd al-Sayyid b. al-Muhadhdhab al-ʾIsrāʾīlī al-Mutaṭabib (Joseph b. al-Dayyān) was also a physician.[499]

g. ʿAwḍ was a Jewish physician (Damascus, 14th century) according to Muslim Arabic sources he was a *dayyān* (*qadi al-Yahūd*).[500]

h. Samuel b. Solomon al-Maghribī (Cairo, 14th–15th centuries), physician and *dayyān*. In 1434 he completed a book of religious laws in Arabic.[501]

i. Samuel Rakaḥ (Rakakh or Rabakh) (Cairo, 14th–15th centuries), physician. Mentioned as a *dayyān* by Meshullam of Volterra (1481).[502]

j. R. Joseph b. Abraham Sakandarī, left Spain for Egypt[503] and in Cairo served as a *dayyān* for many years. Towards the end of his life he emigrated to Eretz-Israel and settled in Safed.[504]

k. Ibrāhīm b. Faraj Allāh b. ʿAbd al-Kāfī, a Karaite physician in Cairo (d. 1441).[505] Muslim sources mentioned him as *qāḍī al-Yahūd* (Judge of the Jews).[506]

l. Kamāl b. Mūsā, a Jewish ophthalmologist and *dayyān*, worked in Jerusalem (16th century).[507]

m. Abraham Sakandarī was a physician and a *dayyān* in Cairo (16th–17th centuries). His father, Joseph, was a physician and *dayyān* and his son, Elazar, was also a physician.[508]

*4.5.4 Cantors (*ḥazzānim*)*

A *ḥazzān* in Hebrew is a cantor with a prestigious and powerful position in the community. We learn about a few physicians that held this title or actually bore this position:

a. Judah ha-Melammēd b. Aaron ha-Rōfē Ibn al-ʿAmmānī, (Alexandria, 13th century) was a *melammēd* (teacher) and a cantor, and was in charge of protocol in the community's court as well as keeping track of the amount of people who received *ṣadāqā* (charity).[509]

b. Jalāl al-Dīn b. al-Ḥazzān was a Jewish physician who served in the court of the ruler's dynasty in Azerbaijan.[510]

c. Judah ha-Rōfē b. Abraham Taurīzī (16th century), a Karaite physician who also served as a cantor in the Karaite synagogue in Cairo.[511]

d. ʿAbd al-ʿAzīz ha-Ḥazzān al-Ḥakīm (16th century), a physician and probably a cantor in Cairo.[512]

4.5.5 Charity and donations

Physicians were found in many lists of charities, donating different amounts. As mentioned before, in general, physicians were listed among the non-poor in Jewish society in the medieval Mediterranean. In some cases, they were at the top of the list, donating substantial sums of money (three to five, and even ten dinars). For example, only a wealthy person such as Mevōrākh b. Saʿadya (d. 1111), who served as chief leader of the Jewish community and a court physician, could afford to donate three dinars (enough to support a middle-class family for a month and a half), and according to Cohen 'we may be certain that it was not the first or only time he did'.[513] By contrast, practitioners would also experience economic hardships due to the strong competition,[514] in other words, they could be at the bottom of the list (in one case, a physician paid only one dinar, the same as various dyers).[515] This can teach us about the wide range of the socio-economic spectrum of physicians.

Charity could be dispensed in different ways, and one of them was free medical treatment for the poor. For example, a 'communal payroll' document registered the enormous sum of 60.75 dirhams that was designated for a doctor's visits, showing how the community subsidised medical treatment for the poor. Cohen stated that 'the very abundance of physicians and other medical practitioners (especially pharmacists) in the community suggests that some of their patients must have been indigent, and it stands to reason that they treated them without payment – a form of charity'. To support this statement, he mentioned Maimonides' (or his son Abraham's) famous letter to Samuel b. Tibbon, lamenting how, at the end of a long and hard day working as a physician in the sultan's palace in Cairo, he would return to find the waiting room of his home in Fusṭāṭ full of patients, both Jewish and Muslim. These 'must have included indigents whom he treated free of charge'.[516]

To sum up, Cohen's words regarding the medical charity of the Jewish communities of medieval Egypt are the best possible interpretation:

> In the mixture of private and public Jewish medical charity in the Geniza world we may see an aspect of community cohesion. The well and the sick lived in close proximity. Aid, in the nature of medical assistance from the community or individuals, or free health care by Jewish physicians, afforded opportunities to do good works – works of charity – on a personal level, fostering solidarity between people in the process. In this respect, as elsewhere, the charitable enterprise formed a unifying factor in medieval Jewish life.[517]

4.6 Geographical, Sectoral and Historical Aspects

In this section I present data on and analysis of the sectoral and geographical dispersion of medieval Jewish practitioners in the Muslim world. From the data that was collected it is quite clear that the vast majority of the known Jewish pharmacists were Rabbanites; in the case of Jewish physicians, we have more information regarding Karaites and even some Samaritans (see Chart 2).

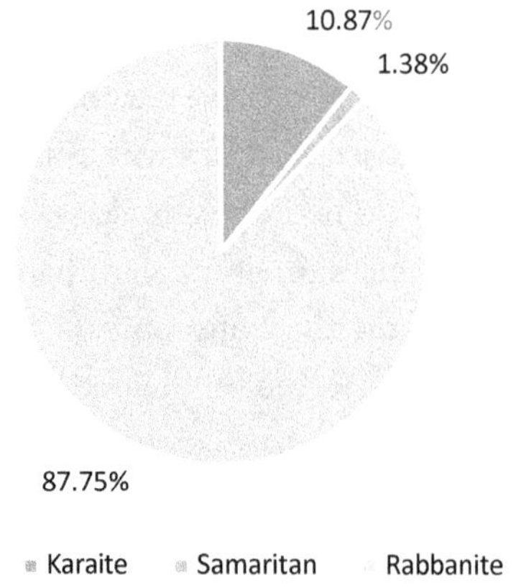

Chart 2 Religious affiliations of Jewish physicians in the Muslim world[518]

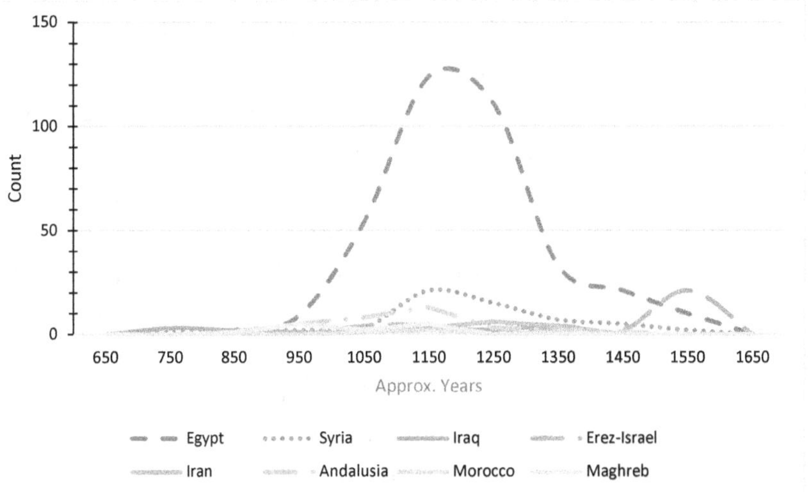

Chart 3 Dispersion of Jewish physicians in the Muslim world by year and location[519]

From the geographical point of view it is very clear that the vast majority of the pharmacists that we know of were active in Egypt in general and Cairo in particular between 950 and 1350 (see Chart 1 above, Section 3.2.1); this sounds logical, especially when taking into consideration that Cairo was the centre of the Muslim world during those historical periods and since the main source of information for this data is the Cairo Geniza.

The picture regarding the physicians is a bit different (see Chart 3); from the chart we learn that most of the Jewish physicians that we know of were active between 950 and 1650 in Egypt. But there were dozens who were active all over the Jewish diaspora in the Muslim world. The Cairo Geniza is the most important source of information; however, as mentioned above a few times, quite a few Arabic Muslim sources were studied, and contributed considerable information as well.

4.6.1 Karaite and Samaritan practitioners

The Karaites

Karaism is the longest-surviving form of sectarian Judaism.[520] Wasserstein suggested that the Karaites probably separated themselves from the bulk of Jewry in the ninth century, claiming that they followed only the sacred texts of scripture and rejected the writing of the sages (mainly the Mishna and the Talmud). This way they became a minority within a minority, remaining culturally alienated from the majority (the Rabbanites).[521]

The Karaites were the smallest group of Jews in the medieval world wherein the Rabbanites formed the majority. Rabbanites are followers of Rabbinic Judaism, considering themselves bound to the accumulated corpus of post-Biblical tradition contained in the Rabbinic literature and its commentaries. Karaites, on the other hand, dispensed with the post-Biblical corpus, contesting the Rabbinic claims of exclusive authority in determining Jewish practice, and focused their exegetical and legal energies on the Bible instead. Rabbanites and Karaites in the medieval Muslim world were in productive contact with each other in almost all aspects of their daily life, cooperating in business, maintaining formal and informal alliances and even marrying one another. Together, according to Rustow, they 'reshaped the medieval Jewish community under Islamic rule'.[522] Moreover, Wasserstein claimed that the conflict between the Karaites and the Rabbanites, was among the 'strongest fertilizing agents of medieval Jewish culture'.[523]

Table 9 presents the basic information from the biographies in this book regarding Karaite practitioners.[524] In general, medieval Karaites were not interested in science *per se*; however, similar to the Rabbanites they considered a few fields of science to be a tool for religious purposes and they were interested in medicine.[525] And indeed, Karaites were physicians in the medieval period both in the Christian West and particularly in the Muslim East.

It is important to note that members of seven dynasties of Karaite practitioners converted to Islam in the Mamluk period; almost all of them were court physicians or otherwise distinguished. The dynasties were Ibn Ṣaghīr, Ibn Kūjik, Ibn al-Maghribī, Nafīs b. Daʾūd b. ʿAnān al-Tabrīzī, ʿAbdallah b. Daʾūd b. Abī al-Faḍl al-Daʾūdī, ʿAbd al-Sayyid b. Isḥāq and Sukra al-Ḥalabī.

The non-converted dynasties of Karaite practitioners are R. Joseph b. Abraham Sakandarī, Ibn al-Kirmānī, another Karaite dynasty established by a certain Saʿadya, a Cairene dynasty established by Jacob the Physician, and two peripheral dynasties established by physicians named Obadia.[526]

Table 9 Karaite practitioners in the Muslim world[527]

Name and dates	*Occupation*	*Place of medical activity*	*Remarks*
Ibrāhīm b. Nūḥ al-Ṭabīb (10th century)	Physician	Egypt	Possibly Karaite
Abraham the Karaite (12th century)	Physician	Egypt	His son got married in Fusṭāṭ, 1117
Abū al-Bayān b. al-Mudawwar al-Sadīd (d. 1184)	Physician	Cairo	
Abū al-Barakāt Ibn Shaʿyā (12th–13th centuries)	Physician	Cairo	
Abū Manṣūr, the Karaite (12th century)	Physician	Cairo	
Aaron ha-Levi ha-Rōfē ha-Sōfer ha-Mahir (12th century)	Physician	Egypt	
Aaron ha-Rōfē al-Kāzrūnī (12th century)	Physician	Egypt, Syria	His family origin is the city of Kāzrūn, Iran
Elijah ha-Kohen (12th century)	Physician	Damascus	
Elisha ha-Rōfē (12th century)	Physician	Egypt	
David ha-Rōfē (12th century)	Physician	Egypt?	
Joseph ha-Rōfē (12th century)	Physician	Egypt	
Mevōrākh ha-Rōfē (12th century)	Physician	?	
Moses b. Abraham b. Saʿadya ha-Rōfē Darʿī (12th century)	Physician, poet	Born in Alexandria	
Faḍl b. Khalaf al-Raʾīs al-Sadīd (12th century)	Physician	Egypt	Lived in Alexandria
Abū al-Faḍl Dāʾūd b. Sulaymān b. Abū al-Bayān al-ʾIsrāʾīlī al-Sadīd (David b. Solomon) (1161–1236)	Physician	Cairo	Physician in the Nāṣirī hospital
Abū al-Munā b. Abī Naṣr b. Ḥaffāẓ (13th century)	Pharmacist	Egypt	
Ibn Kūjik (13th century)	Physician	Egypt	
Abraham ha-Levi ha-Rōfē (13th century)	Physician	Egypt	
Jekuthiel ha-Levi b. Petahya (13th century)	Physician	Damascus	Apparently Karaite
Abū Manṣūr Sulaymān b. Ḥaffāẓ (d. ?1295/1296)	Physician	Egypt	
Petahya ha-Levi ha-Rōfē (13th century)	Physician	Damascus	

Table 9 continued

Name and dates	*Occupation*	*Place of medical activity*	*Remarks*
Abū al-Fakhr b. Abī al-Faḍl b. Abī Naṣr b. Abī al-Fakhr al-Yahūdī (Aaron ha-Levi Ibn al-Kirmānī, al-Kaḥḥāl) (d. 1324)	Ophthalmologist (*kaḥḥāl*)	Cairo	Mentioned in documents of the Karaite community in Cairo. From a family of Karaite physicians
Abū al-Bishr b. Aaron Ha-Levi al-Kirmānī (a. 1324)	Physician	Cairo	
Ibn Ṣaghīr Abī Faraj Allāh (14th century)	Physician	Egypt	The father and tutor of a Karaite, Faraj Allāh (Yeshūʿā) Ibn Ṣaghīr, the sultan's private physician
Abraham ha-Levi (14th century)	Physician	Possibly Jerusalem	
Yūsuf b. Nūḥ (probably 14th century)	Physician	?	
Japheth b. David b. Samuel Ibn Ṣaghīr (14th century)	Physician	Egypt	
Nafīs b. Dāʾūd b. ʿAnān al-Tabrīzī (14th century)	Physician	Originally Tabriz, moved to Cairo in 1354	Converted to Islam
al-Sadīd al-Dimyāṭī (a. c.1339–42)	Physician	Cairo	
Faraj Allāh Ibn Ṣaghīr, (14th century, d. after 1337)	Physician	Cairo	
Samuel b. Solomon al-Maghribī (a. late 14th–early 15th centuries)]	Physician and *dayyān*	Cairo	Ashtor refers to this physician, but under the name Samuel b. Moses b. Yeshūʿā the Western (al-Maghribī)
Ibrāhīm b. Faraj Allāh b. ʿAbd al-Kāfī (d. 1441)	Physician	Cairo	
Isaac (a. mid-15th century)	Physician	Cairo	
Moses b. Abraham b. Saʿadya (15th century)	Physician	Born in Alexandria, moved to Cairo	
Ṣadaqa (15th century)	Physician	Cairo	
Samuel ha-Kohen (a. mid-15th century)	Physician	Cairo	Karaite according to Ashtor.

Samuel b. Jacob b. Japheth b. Moses (15th century)	Physician	Apparently Egypt	According to Steinschneider this is Samuel b. al-Mawlā al-Sheikh al-Muhadhdhab Abū al-Ḥasan al-Yahūdī al-Qarrāʾ al-Mutaṭabbib al-Shahīr bi-Alexandrī/bi-l-Iksandrī
Judah ha-Rōfē b. Abraham Taurīzī (16th century)	Physician, cantor	Cairo. Originally probably from Tabriz	
ʿAbd al-Karīm b. Mūsā (16th century)	Physician, 'Head of the Physicians'	Jerusalem 1532–52	
ʿAbd al-Karīm b. ʿAbd al-Laṭīf (16th century)	Physician	Jerusalem 1550–61	

The Samaritans

The Samaritans separated themselves from mainstream Judaism a few centuries before the Christians, and therefore in the medieval period they already constituted a separate and sizeable minority group from the Jews. Their holy books are the five books of Moses, together with the book of Joshua; they actually rejected all other Biblical books (which date after the supposed date of separation from the Israelites) and the sages' writings. In general, they tended not to move out of the Holy Land, though they had small sub-communities in Egypt and Damascus.[529]

Edmund Bosworth claimed that even though the Samaritans were not very numerous in the Medieval Muslim world in general, the sources occasionally mentioned a special 'Head of the Samaritans'. The Head of the Jews, the *nagid*, was authorised to appoint a subordinate head for the Karaites and the Samaritans; for example, in the Syrian province of the Mamluk Empire, the heads of the main sects of the Jews (Rabbanites and Karaites) were sitting in Damascus, while the head of the Samaritans was sitting in Nablus (Shechem) and his deputy was in Damascus.[530]

Table 10 presents the basic details about the Samaritan practitioners; it has been extracted from the biographies that are composed and presented in detail in other parts of the book.

4.6.2 Jewish practitioners in Andalusia

The Jewish presence in the Iberian peninsula, along the entire Mediterranean coast and in the Balearic archipelago dates back to the early Roman Empire (see Map 1). It is believed that already before the Visigoths arrived in the fifth and sixth centuries, large groups of non-Christians were living in urban areas. Jews seem to have been an important component of the societies in which they lived, side by side with other religious groups. In 711, Islamic troops began their incursions into the Iberian peninsula from Africa via the Strait of Gibraltar, and in 756 the Umayyad conquest of the peninsula was concluded. That same year, ʿAbd al-Raḥmān I 'the Immigrant' (731–88) proclaimed himself independent emir in Archidona, and established the capital of the new Umayyad emirate in Cordova. With the proclamation of the emirate, the Umayyad dynasty established itself in southern Spain and would go on to reign in Cordova for the following two and a half centuries.[531]

Table 10 Samaritan practitioners in the Muslim world[528]

Name and dates	*Occupation*	*Place of medical activity*	*Remarks*
Ibrāhīm b. Faraj b. Mārūth al-Sāmirī al-Ṭabīb (al-Ḥakīm) (Abū Isḥāq Ibrāhīm al-Muṣannif) (Shams al-Ḥukamāʾ) (12th century)	Physician		'al-Sāmirī'
Ibrāhīm b. Khalaf al-Sāmirī (12th–13th centuries)	Physician	Studied medicine in Damascus	
Yūsuf b. Abī Saʿīd b. Khalaf (12th–13th century, d. 1227)	Physician, appointed consultant and *wazīr* by al-Amjad Bahrām Shāh	Damascus. Treated Sitt al-Shām b. Ayyūb, the wife of the governor of Homs. Served the Ayyubid emir of Baalbek	
Amīn al-Dawla Abū al-Ḥasan b. Ghazāl b. Abī Saʿīd al-Sāmirī. (13th century)	Physician	Became in 1237 the *wazīr* of the ruler of Damascus, al-Malik al-Ṣāliḥ. Executed in Egypt by the Mamluks, who replaced the Ayyubid dynasty in 1251	Converted to Islam
Yūsuf b. Yaʿqūb b. Ghanāʾim – al-Muwaffaq al-Sāmirī [13th century	Physician	Damascus	Probably the son of Yaʿqūb b. Ghanāʾim. Converted to Islam
Yaʿqūb b. Ghanāʾim Abū Yūsuf al-Muwaffaq al-Sāmirī al-Ṭabīb (d. 1282)	Physician	Damascus	Converted to Islam
Ṣadaqa b. Munajjā b. Ṣadaqa al-Sāmirī, (12th–13th centuries, d. Ḥarrān 1223)	Physician	Physician to the Ayyubid sultan al-Ashraf Mūsā b. al-ʿĀdil b. Ayyūb, who ruled Ḥarrān, Baalbek and Damascus	

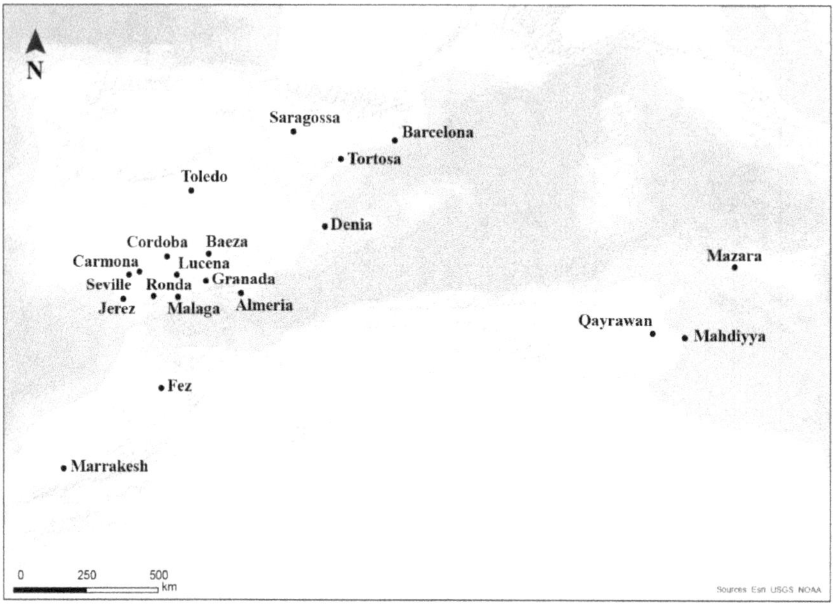

Map 1 Selected locations of Jewish medical activity in Andalusia, north Africa and Sicily

As mentioned above, Andalusia, the province of southern Spain (*al-Andalus* in Arabic), was well populated by Jews before 711. However, after the Muslim conquest, Jews from other Muslim territories, mainly Iraq, immigrated to the region and it became the cultural and social centre of Jewish life. Indeed, during the 500 years between the 10th and the 15th centuries, the Jews in the Iberian lands experienced alternating periods of inter-religious tolerance and zealotry.[532] In general, the Jewish communities flourished under the Muslim regime of the Umayyad (920–1009), the period of the *taifas* (independent Muslim kingdoms, 11th–13th centuries)[533] and the regime of the Almoravid dynasty (1090–1160). During those periods, the hundreds of Jewish communities of Iberia grew along with their intellectual and economic wealth. The atmosphere of inter-religious tolerance gave the Jews vast opportunities in many fields: commerce, administration, science, literature and even agriculture. In the twelfth century, the conquest of the Almohads ended this inter-cultural prosperity of the Jews (and Christians) in Andalusia, and they were persecuted.[534]

At the time of the first wave of the Christian *Reconquista*, in the second half of the twelfth century, well-established and large Jewish communities existed in major Iberian cities such as Cordova, Granada, Seville, Almeria, Lucena, Malaga, Carmona, Baeza and Jerez. Although much of the territory that was conquered by the Christians was taken back by the Muslims, in the mid-thirteenth century it was recaptured by the Christian forces.[535]

Bernard Reilly claimed that the population of Muslim Spain was six million, of which only 5 per cent resided in cities of more than 5,000 inhabitants. Some scholars estimate that the Jewish population in the Muslim world was 1 per cent, suggesting that the Jewish population of Muslim Spain was 60,000.[536] However, Wasserstein argued that this estimate is 'a very rough approximation'; he claimed that 'the largest Jewish community in Andalusia is unlikely to have counted more than eight or nine hundred individuals'.[537]

The history of the Jews in Andalusia is extensive, diverse, complex and decentralised, as a result of the twisted history of the region in the medieval period. Communities reached their peak (economic, cultural, independent ...) and then declined or were even destroyed. Some rebuilt themselves afterwards, and then, in an historical 'snakes and ladders', fell again.

Some of the Jewish practitioners who left Andalusia (or whose parents did) over the years are known to us because they became famous scholars and/or physicians and also due to their popularity. I will present four examples in chronological order:

a. Mūsā b. Abī al-Faḍā'il (Moses b. Jekuthiel ha-Rōfē) (11th–12th centuries), a physician, left Spain and moved to Egypt after his father was executed in 1039.[538] He was called 'the Spanish', and signed 'al-Andalusī' in a letter he wrote. His grandson was also a physician.[539]

b. Abū Naṣr Samaw'al b. Yaḥyā al-Maghribī (Samuel b. Judah b. ʿAbbās al-Maghribī), a physician and mathematician, converted to Islam (1163) and died in 1170 or 1175. He lived and worked for a while in Baghdad and later moved to Iran.[540] According to Ibn al-Qifṭī he originated from Andalusia, moved to the east with his father and became a well-known physician and scholar of the sciences, engineering and mathematics.[541] At the end of the twelfth century he reached Azerbaijan, settled in the capital, Marāgha, and served in court. He had several children, some of whom became physicians.[542] Samawʾal refrained from converting for a long time out of respect for his father (a well-known poet, Judah b. Abūn, a friend of Judah ha-Levi).[543]

c. Moses b. Maimon (Maimonides) (1138–1204), the most famous Jewish scholar of that period, physician, judge and Head of the Jews. He was born in Cordova,[544] immigrated with his family to Fez and later on settled in Egypt (1166). He lived in Fusṭāṭ.[545]

d. Joseph b. Abraham Sakandarī (15th–16th centuries), a physician and a judge, left Spain before the expulsion for Alexandria; later he moved to Cairo where he acted as the head of the *Mustaʿrib* congregation. His son, Abraham, and grandson, Elazar, were also physicians.[546] Towards the end of his life he immigrated to Eretz-Israel and settled in Safed, also living for a period in Jerusalem.[547]

Next I will present the most prominent physicians who practised medicine in Andalusia, and the information we have managed to gather about their lives, deeds and medical and intellectual activity. The practitioners are set as much as possible in chronological order. These will be followed by a short discussion.

a. Ibrāhīm b. Yaʿqūb al-ʾIsrāʾīlī al-Ṭurṭūshī (10th century), a Jewish traveller or merchant, born in Tortosa.[548] He is mainly known for making a long journey in Europe in 965, because he was either trading in horses or in slaves, or part of an official intelligence mission for the Umayyad caliphate of Spain. He crossed the Adriatic Sea, visited the countries of the West Slavs, Prague, eastern Germany and other Slavonic countries.[549] Al-Ṭurṭūshī was weightily cited by later writers such as al-Bakrī and al-Qazwīnī.[550] Some scholars expressed the view that Ibrahim was a physician or translator attached to a diplomatic mission at the court of the Holy Roman Emperor.[551]

b. Abū Ibrāhīm b. Qasṭār (Isaac b. Yashush) (982–1056), a physician, lived and practised in Spain. He was an astute person with genteel manners. He served as a physician at the command of the kings of the *taifa* of Dénia,[552] a maritime power on the eastern coast of al-Andalus.[553]

c. Ibn ʿAknīn (Joseph b. Judah b. Jacob) (12th century), a Jewish physician and scholar, born in Barcelona,[554] immigrated to Fez during the Almohad period.[555]

d. Elias b. al-Mudawwar b. Ṣaddūd al-Yahūdī al-Ṭabīb al-Rundī (12th century), a physician and poet, practised in Ronda.[556]

e. Abū al-Ḥasan (Judah b. Samuel ha-Levi) (1070/1080–1141), a poet, religious thinker and physician, was born in Toledo[557] and travelled as a youth to Granada[558] where he joined the circle of Jewish public figures and intellectuals. He practised as a physician in both Castile and Andalusia, and for most of his life he was a sought-after physician and a prominent, well-connected and well-adjusted member of the Andalusi Jewish aristocracy. His leadership, diligence and religious devotion were praised. In the summer of 1140, he left Spain and sailed for Egypt with the intention of dying in Eretz-Israel. He arrived in Alexandria on September 1140, spent over three months there and moved to Fusṭāṭ.[559]

f. Jacob b. Me'ir (12th–13th centuries), a physician, lived in Toledo. Al-Ḥarīzī described him as: 'the doctor and seer, Master Jacob b. Me'ir, light divine bright ore lifted from discernment's mine' and mentioned that he was the cousin of R. Joseph ha-Dayyān.[560]

g. Abū Ayyūb al-Yahūdī (al-'Isrā'īlī) (Solomon b. al-Mu'allim) (12th century), a physician, Jewish scholar and a poet, native of Seville,[561] lived and practised medicine in Spain between 1105 and 1171.[562] He was mentioned by Maimonides in his *Treatise on Asthma*, as one of the four physicians who served in the court of the Almoravid emir 'Alī b. Yūsuf b. Tāshufīn (r. 1106–42) in Marrakesh, and mistakenly killed him due to the use of wrong dosage of theriac.[563] Solomon carried the titles of *wazīr* and 'prince' and was praised by Jewish dignitaries such as Moses b. Ezra, Judah ha-Levi and Judah al-Ḥarīzī.[564]

h. Ḥasan Abū Kanū? (12th century), a physician, practised (probably at Seville), at the court of the Almoravid emir 'Alī b. Yūsuf.[565]

i. Abū al-Faḍl (Ḥasday b. Joseph b. Ḥasday) (11th century), a very knowledgeable physician, poet and scholar in various fields and a member of one of the most important and well-known Jewish families in Andalusia. He worked as a physician for the Almoravid ruler (probably in Seville), and according to the Muslim sources he converted to Islam after he fell in love with a Muslim girl.[566]

j. Ḥasday b. Shaprūṭ (10th century), a scholar, physician, trusted adviser in the court of the Umayyad caliphs in Cordova and the patron of the first Jewish intellectuals and poets in Andalusia.[567] Ḥasday was a scion of a well-established family. He gained his master's trust to such a degree that he became the caliph's confidant and faithful counsellor and was in actuality the minister of foreign affairs. He had also control of the customs and ship dues in the port of Cordova. In his capacity as a trusted courtier, Ḥasday undertook a number of diplomatic missions. When Ibn Shaprūṭ died around 975, Cordova had become the Jewish cultural centre that he had sought, and he had become the model of the Sephardi Jewish courtier and patron of scholarship and the arts.[568]

k. Hārūn (Aaron) b. Isaac of Cordova (10th century), a physician, practised in Cordova under the Moorish rulers of Spain. He was a teacher and the author of medical works (commentaries on Ibn Sīnā) and he is known for his contribution to a song that was written by Ibn Sīnā on fever.[569]

l. Marwān (Abū al-Walīd) Ibn Janāḥ al-Qurṭubī (R. Jonah Marinus) (985/990–1040), a Jewish intellectual, grammarian, Hebrew lexicographer and physician. He was educated in Lucena,[570] returned to Cordova, where he apparently studied medicine, and settled, after much wandering, in Saragossa,[571] where he practised medicine for the rest of his life. It is also documented in his book that in his search for information on drugs he consulted with tanners, pharmacists, physicians and even sorcerers and wandered in and around Saragossa to collect minerals and herbs.[572]

m. Munajjam (Menahem) b. al-Fawwāl (11th century) was one of the most important Jewish physicians and scholars in Andalusia. He lived and practised in Saragossa, and was mainly known thanks to his book *al-Adawiya al-Mufrada* ('On the Simple Drugs').[573]

n. Abū Jaʿfar Joseph b. Aḥmad b. Ḥasday (12th century), a physician, native of Saragossa. He practised in Moorish Spain and later moved to Egypt. Joseph wrote commentaries on Hippocrates and Galen.[574]

o. Yūsuf b. Isḥāq Ibn Biklārish (12th century), a physician and an authority on *materia medica*. He was born in Saragossa and practised in Almeria,[575] in the court of the Hūdid dynasty of Saragossa. In 1106 he completed what is probably the most important Arabic pharmacological treatise, *al-Kitāb al-Mustaʿīnī*. The existence of fragments of the book in the Cairo

Geniza can teach us about the route of the book's rapid distribution from Spain, where it was written, to Egypt, probably through the Maghrib. Dozens of Geniza documents have been identified as belonging to medical books, but no others were either written or tabulated by a Spanish Jewish author in Judaeo-Arabic.[576]

p. Ismaʿīl b. Yūnis (11th century), a physician from Almeria, who according to Ibn Ḥazm was trained in physiognomy, and was able to detect a person in love by looking at his or her face.[577]

q. Yūsuf b. al-Kazan (12th century), a physician, one of the notables in Almeria. He was the addressee of a letter from Ḥalfon b. Nethanel.[578]

r. Jacob ha-Rōfē (12th century), a physician, lived and practised in Andalusia. He was closely associated with Ḥalfon ha-Levi b. Nethanel (Alexandria and Fusṭāṭ), of the milieu of Judah ha-Levi. Two letters he wrote were preserved in the Geniza and have been found and studied lately.[579]

The main sources we have on the Jewish communities in general, and on Jewish practitioners in particular, are mostly from Muslims and written in Arabic. The information we gathered from the Jewish sources was mainly from the cultural and intellectual heritage of the members of the Jewish communities of medieval Andalusia, that is, books and poems. Indeed, the vast majority of the Jewish Andalusian practitioners who are described above were also scholars, intellectuals, poets and so on.

Some of the Jewish Andalusian physicians that are described above were deeply assimilated in Arabic culture. According to Stroumsa, it was a long and progressive process that stretched across several generations, but one in which even the converted members of the family kept some of their Jewish identity.[580]

Roth suggested that the Jews, who could not study medicine in the madrasas, studied medicine privately together with Muslims, and some of them were teaching Muslims privately.[581] It appears that the vast majority of the Jewish medical students studied within the family, from a family member physician. This was the way that medical dynasties were created.[582]

According to historical developments, in order to survive, some Jewish physicians moved and practised under both Muslim and Christian regimes.[583] Others, similar to their brothers who held different occupations and did not convert to Christianity or lived as *anusim* (*conversos* or *marranos*), left Spain (mainly during the fifteenth century) and moved, especially along the shores of the Mediterranean, to Europe, north Africa and the lands of the Ottoman Empire (including Egypt, Eretz-Israel etc.).

I have no doubt that more Jewish physicians practised medicine in the big cities of Andalusia as well as in the small towns. However, due to the harsh and violent way their communities were destroyed, no record has survived to tell us about their lives and activities. For example, so far, we have no records of Jewish physicians practising in Muslim Malaga, Carmona, Baeza or Jerez.

4.6.3 Jewish practitioners in north Africa (Maghrib) and Sicily[584]

Among the hundreds of known Jewish practitioners who worked in the medieval Muslim world, dozens were of north African origin. Some of them held the *nisba* 'al-Maghribī' for generations. For example:

a. Yaḥyā b. ʿAbbās al-Maghribī (Judah b. Abūn),[585] a physician and poet from Fez (d. 1138), moved to Baghdad and practised there. His son was the physician Abū Naṣr Samawʾal b. Judah b. ʿAbbās al-Maghribī. Samawʾal was a physician and mathematician who practised in Baghdad and Azerbaijan, and converted to Islam (1163).[586]

b. Abū al-Ḥajjāj Yūsuf b. Yaḥyā b. Isḥāq al-Sabatī al-Maghribī (Joseph b. Judah b. Simon) (Ibn Samʿūn), a physician and a merchant, born in Ceuta, Morocco. After he studied medicine, he moved to Egypt due to persecutions. He died in Aleppo in 1226.[587] Yūsuf was a friend of Ibn al-Qifṭī.[588]

c. Shihāb al-Dīn Aḥmad (Sulaymān) al-Maghribī al-Ishbīlī,[589] a physician to Sultan al-Nāṣir Muḥammad b. Qalāwūn (d. 1340). He converted to Islam in 1291 during the time of Sultan al-Ashraf Khalīl b. Qalāwūn, and his name was changed from Sulaymān to Aḥmad. He was appointed thereafter as 'Head of the Physicians'. His sons also served as the sultan's physicians, and one of them, Jamāl al-Dīn Ibrāhīm al-Maghribī (d. 1355), replaced him as 'Head of the Physicians'.[590] According to Muslim sources, descendants of this Jewish dynasty filled the office of 'Head of the Physicians' during the end of the thirteenth and the fourteenth centuries and continued to keep 'al-Maghribī' as part of their name.[591]

d. Samuel b. Solomon al-Maghribī, a Karaite physician and *dayyān* (15th century).[592]

In several cases, the *nisba* was more specific than 'al-Maghribī': some members of the Jewish community in Egypt and around the Mediterranean bore their Tunisian origin as part of their name, for example the physician Abū al-Ḥasan Yūsuf b. Josiah al-Tunisī (Joseph b. Isaiah).[593] The Muslim sources as well as the Geniza provide us with information about practitioners of Tunisian origin and others who were practising in the main cities. We have traced information regarding several Jewish physicians, in many cases distinguished members of their Jewish communities in the Maghrib, who actually practised there. I will present a few of them according to the main cites in which they lived and worked. In the case of Tunisia, Qayrawān and Mahdiyya will be dealt with together.[594] In both cities there were vibrant Jewish communities that had close and warm relationships with Jewish communities in Cairo, Alexandria, Sicily and other communities in the Maghrib. Many of the members of these communities were merchants that practised international trade.[595] Several Jewish physicians practised in the Tunisian cities, some of whom started important dynasties. I will mention some of them below:

a. The earliest known Jewish physician in Qayrawān is Mūsā b. El'āzār al-'Isrā'īlī (Moses b. Elazar),[596] who handed down the medical profession to several generations after him in the medical dynasty he started. They served as court physicians to the caliphs, as chief leaders of the Jewish community, and in some cases, as chief administrators (*wazīrs*), in charge of the state treasury.[597] Moses was originally from the city of Oria, southern Italy. In 925, a Fatimid corps invaded Oria and captured Moses, who was redeemed at Qayrawān.[598] In Tunisia, he served the Fatimid caliphs, and he arrived in Egypt after it was conquered by the Fatimids in 969. Having served in the Fatimid court for a long time, Moses became one of the most influential figures in Fatimid Cairo.[599] According to H. Z. Hirschberg, Moses b. Elazar, or Palṭiel, was also the leader of the Maghrib Jewry before he moved to Egypt.[600] His son Isḥāq b. Mūsā b. El'āzār (Abū Ya'qūb al-Ṭabīb) (al-Mutaṭabbib) was also a physician[601] and *wazīr*.[602]

It seems that he inherited this position also from his father, thus retaining even more power in his hands. According to some scholars, Isḥāq might also have succeeded his father's position as the Head of the Jews (*nagid*).[603] His brother Ismāʿīl b. Mūsā b. Elʿāzār was a known physician of the Fatimid caliph, he was appointed as the successor of his father and brother respectively as the chief administrator of the al-Muʿizz caliphate, and possibly also as a court physician after Isaac's death in 973.[604] As mentioned above, other members of the family, such as Yaʿqūb b. Isḥāq (grandson of Mūsā b. Elʿāzār al-ʾIsrāʾīlī) and Mūsā b. Yaʿqūb (great-grandson) held similar positions.[605]

b. Arguably, the most famous Jewish physician who preceded Maimonides was Isḥāq b. Sulaymān al-ʾIsrāʾīlī (Isaac b. Solomon), also a philosopher (9th–10th centuries).[606] He was born in Egypt (apparently in 832) and was a student of Isaac b. ʿImrān. In Qayrawān, he served as the court physician to the Aghlabī emir and the Fatimid caliph. He also served al-Mahdī ʿUbayd Allāh, the ruler of Ifrīqiyya.[607] Isaac wrote books on medicine and philosophy which were studied later in Europe for hundreds of years during the Middle Ages and Renaissance.[608]

c. Abū Sahl Dūnash b. Tamīm (Dūnash b. Tamīm) was a physician and linguist, born and raised in Qayrawān (10th century), and was educated in a family originating from Iraq. He served as a court physician to two Fatimid rulers, al-Manṣūr b. al-Qāʾim and his son al-Muʿizz li- Dīn Allāh. Dūnash was the student of Isḥāq b. Sulaymān al-ʾIsrāʾīlī. According to Saʿadya b. Danān, a Jewish linguist from Granada, Dūnash was a Muslim when he died in 971.[609]

d. Abū Isḥāq Ibrāhīm b. ʿAṭā (Abraham b. Nathan) was Qayrawān's *nagid* and physician (10th century). In 1015 he also received the title of 'Nagid ha-Gola' from Hai Gaon, of the Pumbedita Academy.[610] He was a physician to two emirs in al-Mahdiyya: Bādīs (r. 996–1016) and his son al-Muʿizz (r. 1016–62), and with the latter he joined their war campaigns.[611]

e. Yaḥyā Abū Zikrī al-Ṭabīb (Judah b. Moses) (11th century) was a merchant from Qayrawān (active mainly 1040–90). Since he was given the title 'al-Ṭabīb', he probably practised medicine to some extent.[612]

f. Solomon ha-Rōfē b. Rabīʿ (11th century) was a physician, active in

Qayrawān. He came from a prominent family of merchants and scholars who originated from M'Sila (Algeria today).[613]

g. Abraham b. Yijū, the famous trader (12th century), was born in al-Mahdiyya.[614] Abraham travelled to India where he was active between 1132 and 1149,[615] and finally settled in Egypt in 1153. He had some medical education as two Geniza prescriptions were found in his handwriting.[616] He served as the 'head of the community' in Dhū Jibla.[617]

Some of the present-day cities of Morocco had Jewish communities during the medieval period. I will mention only a few of the Jewish physicians who practised in Morocco. Interestingly, some of them were originally from Andalusia and in some cases, they moved to Morocco with or for the Muslim leaders they served under (mainly the Almohads and the Almoravids):

a. Saʿadya ha-Rōfē Darʿī (11th century),[618] a Karaite physician. His family arrived originally from Spain and settled in Morocco, in the *wadi* of the river Darʿa.[619] His son Abraham and grandson Moses were also physicians.[620]

b. Me'ir (Abū al-Ḥasan) Ibn Qamni'el (11th–12th centuries),[621] a Jewish poet and physician; born in Saragossa and a member of one of the most important Jewish families.[622] A poem by Judah ha-Levi indicates that he moved to Morocco and rose in the Almoravid court, facts confirmed by Maimonides in his *Book on Asthma*.[623] Thanks to Maimonides, it is known that Ibn Qamni'el was a court physician to Sultan Yūsuf b. Tāshufīn (r. 1061–1106) in Marrakesh.[624] He is named as one of the four court physicians, among whom was Solomon b. al-Muʿallim of Seville, who was also a friend of Judah ha-Levi; due to an error in preparing a dosage of theriac he brought about the sultan's death.[625]

c. Ibn ʿAknīn (Joseph b. Judah b. Jacob) (12th century), a Jewish physician and scholar from the time of Maimonides. He was born in Barcelona and immigrated to Fez[626] during the Almohad period. Ibn ʿAknīn wrote several unique essays, one of which, as far as we know, is the only one written by a Jewish physician in the Middle Ages that focuses on psychology.[627] Ibn ʿAknīn was a pupil of Maimonides in Fez during the period of forced conversion of Almohads. He described how he lived as a Muslim with feelings of guilt, and secretly observed the commandments and studied the Torah with Maimonides.[628]

d. Ibrāhīm b. al-Tharthār, a physician, practised in the court of Muḥammad V al-Naṣrī in Granada (r. 1354–9, 1362–91). In 1359, when Muḥammad V moved to Morocco, Ibrāhīm also moved to Morocco. He later returned to Granada with his patron.[629] He is apparently identical to Ibrāhīm b. Zarzar, who was mentioned by Ibn Khaldūn for refusing, as the court physician of the ruler of Granada, to travel to Fez in 1356 in order to take care of Abū ʿAnān, the sultan of Fez. The ruler, Muhammad V, asked for Abū ʿAnān's forgiveness.[630]

Sicily had a vibrant Jewish community mainly between the ninth and eleventh centuries;[631] the community was closely related to the ones in Egypt and north Africa. The Jews were living in Mazara (a port city located on the southern shore) and other cities.[632] We learn from the Geniza about Rabīb, a physician who was respected in Sicily and had a close relationship with the *nagid* of Egypt.[633]

4.6.4 Jewish practitioners in provincial Egyptian towns[634]

The life of the Jews in medieval Egypt in general, and in the provincial cities in particular, puzzled scholars, mainly historians from various fields of research. The number of Jews in Cairo and in the other cities was at the centre of another debate. Most of the researchers used, as a main source for that debate, the book of the Jewish traveller Benjamin of Tudela, who visited Egypt and Syria in the second half of the twelfth century.

Benjamin of Tudela reported that 2,000 Jews resided in the city of Cairo in the second half of the twelfth century.[635] However, according to Ashtor there were only 1,500.[636] Based on the descriptions of the Jewish communities which Benjamin visited in Egypt (fifteen in number), David Neustadt arrived at the conclusion that the total number of Egyptian Jews was no more than 20,000.[637] Ashtor, studying also other contemporary sources, mainly documents of the Cairo Geniza, added twenty-one more cities in which Jews lived. He concluded that at the end of the twelfth century, the number of Jews in Egypt did not exceed 10,000–12,000 souls.[638]

Most of the medieval Jewish practitioners traced and described in the current work lived and practised medicine in Fusṭāṭ[639] and in other large cities of the Muslim world.[640] Others pursued their career in small villages. However, similar to the present day, 'medical care available in remote and rural areas differed greatly from that in urban settings'.[641] In this case, the Cairo Geniza enables us to learn about physicians and pharmacists who worked in small towns in Egypt and in other cities in the Muslim world.

We discovered, for example, that physicians who practised in small cities moved to larger ones in order to get their medical education, to make a better living, and basically to improve their socio-economic status. We have records of physicians who worked in small cities where it was harder to make a living by practising medicine due to the small size of the Jewish communities. We can also learn about this phenomenon from several letters, one of which is from a physician who left his practice in a small village near Cairo and tried to establish a medical career in Cairo itself.[642] Another anecdote can teach us about centre–periphery relationships. In a letter from Alexandria, a prominent merchant from Fusṭāṭ was asked to take a prescription from the *nagid* prescribed by the court physician Abū al-Faḍl Mubārak (Mevōrākh b. Saʿadya) for his son who lived in Cairo.[643]

As previously mentioned, the vast majority of Jewish physicians and pharmacists presented in this book were practising in Fusṭāṭ. Given that all aspects of the life of this community are discussed in detail by Goitein, Gil, Cohen, Bareket and other scholars, and their biographies are presented in detail in this book, I have decided to focus on and bring to the reader's attention the medical activities in other cities and particularly in the small towns on the peripheries. The examples I present below are set in alphabetical order of the names of the places:

Abyār

Abyār or Ibyār was a town near the right bank of the Rosetta tributary of the Nile. It was a flourishing place, a centre for the textile industry[644] in which important merchants lived including a Jewish community. Judah ha-Levi, while travelling from Alexandria to Cairo, spent a Sabbath there. A local physician was mentioned as well.[645]

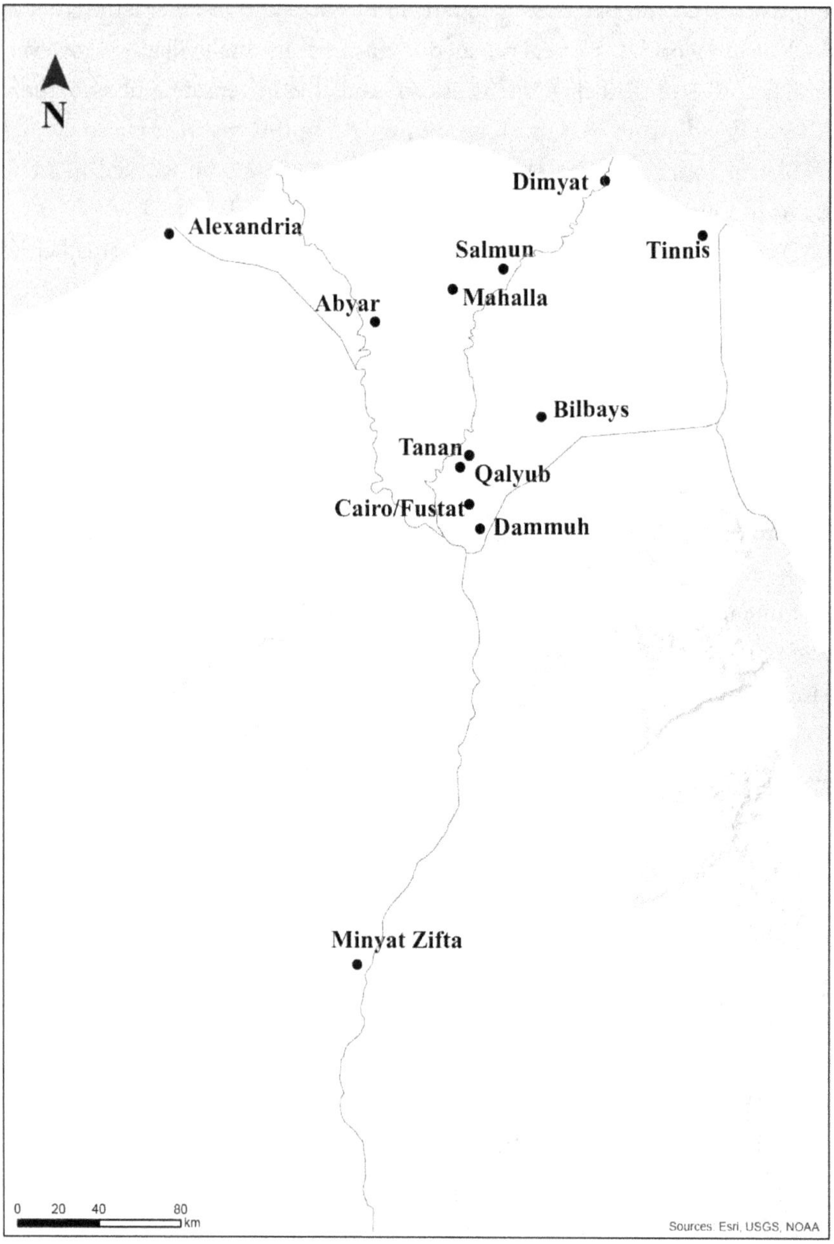

Map 2 Selected locations of Jewish medical activity in Egypt

Alexandria

Alexandria was, and still is, the second largest city and a major economic centre in Egypt, lying on the coast of the Mediterranean Sea in the north central part of Egypt. A vast number of documents relating to and originating in the city were found in the Geniza, thus enabling us to pursue and study the history of the Alexandrian Jewry.[646] Benjamin of Tudela counted 3,000 Jews in the city in the second half of the twelfth century.[647] However, according to Ashtor there were only 700.[648]

Thanks to Geniza documents, we have evidence of vibrant medical activities in the city by Jewish practitioners over hundreds of years. Some physicians who were born and even lived in Alexandria used to practise in other cities such as Cairo. For example: the Karaite physicians Moses b. Abraham b. Saʿadya ha-Rōfē Darʿī (12th century) and Moses b. Abraham b. Saʿadya (15th century), who were born in Alexandria, lived and practised in Cairo. Elijah b. Zechariah (12th–13th centuries) operated and lived in Jerusalem; Zechariah the Alexandrian (12th century) immigrated, settled and practised probably in Ashkelon. Samuel b. Elazar (13th century), who was born in Alexandria, was active at Qūṣ.[649]

It should be mentioned here that Alexandria was the landing port for Jewish immigrants from the Maghrib, Sicily and Andalusia. Among the new immigrants, who were mainly fleeing from persecution, were practitioners who took their first steps (personal as well as professional) in Egypt (and in some cases in the East) in this city. Some of them stayed, but the vast majority continued their journey to Cairo, as in the cases of the famous poet and physician Abū al-Ḥasan (Judah b. Samuel ha-Levi) (12th century), Abū al-Ḥajjāj Yūsuf b. Yaḥyā b. Isḥāq al-Sabatī al-Maghribī (12th–13th centuries) and R. Joseph b. Abraham Sakandarī (15th–16th centuries).[650]

We have information on some pharmacists who practised in the city, for example: Ephraim al-ʿAṭṭār (11th century)[651] and Abū al-Faraj al-ʿAṭṭār b. Abū al-Ḥasan al-ʿAṭṭār (13th century).[652] Some practitioners lived and worked most of their life in the city, for example Aaron ha-Rōfē b. Yeshūʿā ha-Rōfē Ibn al-ʿAmmānī (12th century), Samuel ha-Rōfē Ibn al-ʿAmmānī (12th–13th centuries)[653] and Japheth ha-Rōfē (13th century).[654]

Other practitioners had temporary activity in the city, such as Abū al-ʿAshāʾir Hibat-Allāh b. Zayn b. Ḥasan b. Ifrāʾīm b. Yaʿqūb b. Ismāʿīl Ibn

Jumayʿ al-ʾIsrāʾīlī (Nethanel b. Samuel), a well-known physician, known as 'al-Sheikh al-Muwaffaq Shams al-Riʾāsa', born and raised in Fusṭāṭ (d. 1198). He is mentioned in a letter sent to a young physician who was looking for a position in a hospital in Alexandria. In the letter, the physician's cousin, who wrote it, advises the young physician to show his recommendation letter to prominent figures in Alexandria, among them Ibn Jumayʿ.[655]

In one case, Alexandria was portrayed as a city of refuge. Mevōrākh Abū al-Faḍl b. Saʿadya (1040–1111), a physician and *nagid* (1078–82), was removed from his duty by David b. Daniel b. Azariah and was forced to escape to Alexandria.[656] Another interesting anecdote concerns Judah from Alexandria (15th century), who was a physician and a surgeon and was employed by the Venetian colony in Alexandria.[657]

Bilbays

Bilbays (Bilbais) is a fortress city on the eastern edge of the southern Nile Delta. It was the capital of the province of al-Sharqiyya, and there are many Geniza documents stemming from or referring to the Jews of Bilbays, mainly of the twelfth and the thirteenth centuries. It appears that the Jewish community experienced demographic development and economic prosperity during this period.[658] Benjamin of Tudela counted 3,000 Jews in the city in the second half of the twelfth century;[659] according to Ashtor's calculations there were 300.[660] The judge Elijah b. Zechariah (13th century) kept an orphan in his house, a relative, the son of a physician in Bilbays, who went to school in the capital.[661]

Dammūh

Dammūh (Damwah) is a small village a few kilometres south of Fusṭāṭ, with an ancient synagogue dedicated to Moses. The medieval Jews believed that this was the place where Moses prayed and slept after he spoke to Pharaoh. A small Jewish community existed in the village over certain periods.[662] The physician Ibrāhīm al-Mutaṭabbib b. Mukhtār left all his belongings, including money and medical books, to the synagogue of Dammūh.[663]

Dimyāṭ

Dimyāṭ (Damietta) is a port city located on the Damietta branch of the Nile, 15 kilometres from the Mediterranean Sea, about 200 kilometres north of

Cairo. The harbour was an emporium of Egyptian trade, and the city always had a Jewish community.[664] Benjamin of Tudela counted 200 Jews in the city in the second half of the twelfth century,[665] a figure that was accepted by Ashtor.[666] A few physicians who were mentioned in the Geniza bore the name of the city in their own name, as a sign of origin: Abū al-Ḥasan ha-Levi al-ʿAṭṭār, also known as Ibn al-Dimyāṭī, mentioned in a document from 1193;[667] and al-Sadīd al-Dimyāṭī al-Ṭabīb al-Yahūdī (13th–14th centuries, Karaite physician in Cairo).[668] The physician Abū al-Faraj al-Uṣṭūl (12th century) was mentioned arriving to Damietta.[669]

Maḥalla

Maḥalla is a town located in the middle of the Nile Delta on the western bank of the Damietta Branch. It was an important commercial centre in Lower Egypt from the tenth century and had a relatively large Jewish community. Benjamin of Tudela counted 500 Jews in the city in the second half of the twelfth century,[670] Ashtor agrees with this estimate.[671] Several physicians mentioned in the Geniza relate to this city. Asʿad al-Dīn (Ibn Ṣabra) al-Maḥallī al-Mutaṭabbib (Jacob b. Isaac) was a physician from the Ṣabra family of Maḥalla (13th century). He probably practised medicine there as his daughter married a physician who came to Maḥalla in order to study under Asʿad and be cured of a chronic illness. Asʿad himself died in Cairo.[672] Nethanel b. Abraham was a physician from Maḥalla,[673] as was Abū Isḥāq al-Maḥallī al-ʿAṭṭār (Abraham b. Sasson), who is mentioned in the Blessing of the Dead from the twelfth century.[674]

Minyat Ziftā

Minyat Ziftā was a flourishing town in Lower Egypt on the eastern tributary of the Nile opposite Minyat Ghamr. An important and vibrant Jewish community existed there in the Fatimid period. Benjamin of Tudela counted 200 Jews in the city in the second half of the twelfth century;[675] and according to Ashtor there were 500.[676]

Abū al-Riḍā al-Ṭabīb (Joseph ha-Levi) was a physician who was active in Cairo in the second half of the twelfth century.[677] He and his brother appeared in a document, originating in Minyat Ziftā, from which it can be learnt that the two brothers took care of an orphan.[678] Based on a document that contained a list of Abū al-Riḍā's possessions, which was written in 1172, probably shortly after his death; Goitein claimed that he served as a physician in one of Egypt's provincial towns and wasn't wealthy; however, Ora Molad-Vaza, in her research on clothing in Jewish society, came to the conclusion that Abū al-Riḍā was actually a well-off physician with a high social status.[679] Another person, apparently a physician, Moses b. Peraḥya b. Yijū, was active in the first half of the thirteenth century in the cities of Minyat Ziftā and Minyat Ghamr as a judge, and was also the author of many documents and letters written in the years between 1220 and 1234. Another physician (al-Muhadhdhab, 13th century) from Minyat Ziftā is mentioned in a letter to Abraham b. David.[680] The son of Shabbetay ha-Rōfē is mentioned in a colophon and was probably active around 1250, in the area of Minyat Ziftā.[681] A physician (al-Ṭabīb) from Minyat Ziftā is mentioned in a list of donors.[682]

Many documents in the Geniza describe Jewish life in the city.[683] An interesting anecdote is a complaint about a doctor's encroachment in which we learn about a physician in Minyat Ziftā who undertook the teaching of schoolchildren in addition to his medical work, due to the temporary absence of a local teacher. According to the document, the physician became so enthusiastic, mainly because of the additional income, that he did not let the children go back to their former teacher when he returned.[684]

We know of the number of practitioners in 1266 in Minyat Ziftā thanks to a Geniza document: two physicians, a veterinary surgeon and a druggist.[685]

Muṭaylib

Muṭaylib was a caravan station on the way from Eretz-Israel to Egypt. Thanks to a letter found in the Geniza it is known that the place was inhabited by Jews; the letter was from a doctor in Jerusalem writing that he was staying there.[686]

Qalyūb

Qalyūb is a small town located 19 kilometres north of Fusṭāṭ, at the mouth of the Nile Delta). It is mentioned in many Geniza documents, mainly of the twelfth and thirteenth centuries. However, according to Ashtor the Jewish community was of a medium size.[687] From a letter written by a physician from Qalyūb, we learn that he left his hometown and opened an office in the capital. He wrote to his wife that the response of the public had been excellent, but then the anger of the other members of the profession was so strong that he could not dare to interrupt his work even for one day to come out and examine her sore eyes; therefore, he asked his wife to join him there.[688]

Qūṣ

Qūṣ is a desert port on the Nile deep in the south of Upper Egypt. According to Ashtor, based on Geniza documents referring to or originating from Qūṣ, there was a large Jewish community in this city. It was the capital of Upper Egypt, had a mint (12th century) and was an emporium of Indian trade.[689] Benjamin of Tudela counted 30,000 Jews in the city in the second half of the twelfth century;[690] this figure was not accepted by Ashtor, who wrote 300.[691] Abū Mansur al-Mutaṭabbib (Elazar b. Yeshūʿā ha-Levi), a physician of Qūṣ, gave his two younger daughters the dowry of his late wife (1215–16), which he had inherited from her.[692] From a poem found in the Geniza that was written by Samuel b. Elazar ha-Rōfē, a physician from Alexandria, we learn that he practised in Qūṣ (c.1253).[693]

Salmūn

Salmūn is a town in Daqahlīyah governorate, northeast of Cairo. There is a letter written by an army doctor (in the service of the emir of Damietta) who had first to cure a Mamluk who resided on his fief in Salmūn, and then report back to his emir and supervise him to take his medicine.[694] According to Golb no evidence exists that Jews were permanently settled there.[695]

Tanān

Tanān is a town in the Qalyūbiyya district near Cairo, approximately 8 kilometres northeast of Qalyūb. Sometimes, as we learn from a letter written by Menahem, a physician from Fusṭāṭ during the time of the *nagid* Abraham Maimonides, doctors travelled to visit patients in the town.[696]

Tinnīs

Tinnīs is a small city on an island in Lake Manzala, southwest of Port Said. It was a populous place in the Fatimid period, and many Christians lived there.

Ashtor studied its description in the books of various Muslim travellers; they were impressed by the size of the city, the many boats anchored in the harbour and its linen industry.[697] Benjamin of Tudela counted forty Jews in the city in the second half of the twelfth century.[698] However, according to Ashtor, there were 150.[699] Abū Naṣr al-Ṭabīb b. al-Tinnīsī was a physician who is mentioned in two Geniza documents, one of them a contract signed in Fusṭāṭ 1146.[700] The other document, dated 1143, also mentioned his daughter.[701] In a long letter from Tinnīs, a certain patient with a probably serious illness made reference to three other letters sent by him, mentioning that his physician came to see him every day. This teaches us that there was a physician in the city, at least at this time.[702]

There are more villages and small cities in Egypt in which Jewish communities existed, according to documents found in the Geniza. However, no evidence has been found yet of medical activity of Jewish practitioners in those villages and small cities.

4.6.5 Jewish practitioners in Bilād al-Shām[703]

The Middle East region was ruled by many regimes during the Middle Ages: Umayyad, Abbasid, Fatimid, Ayyubid, Crusader, Mamluk and Ottoman, and therefore, borders in the Middle East have changed in rapid succession throughout history. Each of these regimes had its own perception of borders, so no single definition of the area or its borders can be found. One geographical area, including significant parts of present-day Syria, Lebanon, Israel and Jordan, used to be called Bilād al-Shām by the Arab rulers and scholars of the time.[704] During the rule of the Umayyads, Damascus was the capital of the Islamic caliphate; this region of Bilād al-Shām was divided into a number of districts.[705]

In medieval Syria, mainly in the big cities such as Damascus and Aleppo, many physicians were practising medicine. Based on Muslim Arabic sources Anne-Marie Eddé recorded fifty-six physicians, of whom four were Jews and three were Samaritans.[706]

The Jews lived in various towns and villages in Bilād al-Shām. They kept direct and intensive contact with their family members who moved to Egypt, mainly during the Fatimid, Ayyubid and Mamluk periods,[707] as we learn from the vast number of documents found in the Cairo Geniza. Actually, not

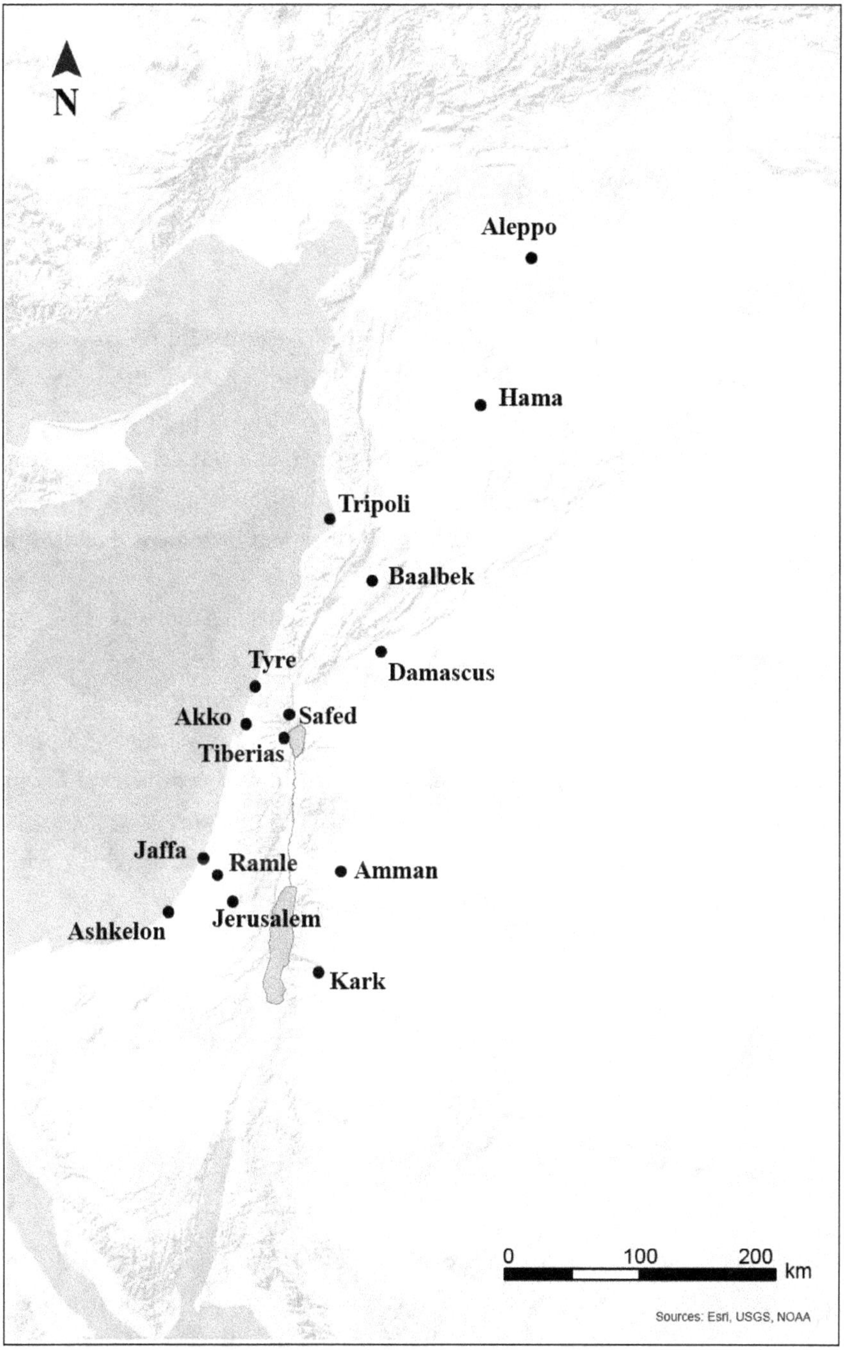

Map 3 Selected locations of Jewish medical activity in Bilād al-Shām

just letters and products were moving in between the various Jewish communities of Bilād al-Shām and Egypt; people were travelling to meet their family members, to conduct commerce and for other reasons.

Bilād al-Shām (general)[708]

I will start by mentioning some physicians who according to the sources spent time in Syria and practised there:

a. Amīn al-Dawla Abū al-Ḥasan b. Ghazāl b. Abī Saʿīd al-Sāmirī (Samaritan). He converted to Islam and became in 1237 the *wazīr* of the ruler of Damascus, al-Malik al-Ṣāliḥ. In 1252 he was executed in Egypt.

b. Ṣadaqa b. Munajjā b. Ṣadaqa al-Sāmirī (Samaritan physician, 13th century). He practised in the court of the Ayyubid sultan al-Ashraf Mūsā b. al-ʿĀdil b. Ayyūb, who ruled Ḥarrān, Baalbek and Damascus. He died in Ḥarrān.

c. Asad al-Yahūdī (13th–14th centuries), a physician who was active in Egypt (Cairo) and Syria (Hama, Safed, Damascus, Aleppo).

d. Nuʿmān b. Abī al-Riḍā Ibn Sālim Ibn Isḥāq (14th century).

e. David b. Joshua Maimon (14th–15th centuries), a physician who practised in Egypt (Cairo). During the 1370s, he was forced to leave Egypt and lived for a number of years in Aleppo and Damascus.

f. The physician to the sultan al-Muʾayyad Sheikh (15th century), a Jewish physician from Syria who was called to treat the sultan.

g. ʿAbd al-Laṭīf al-Baghdādī (15th century), a physician, and possibly *Raʾīs al-Yahūd*, according to some sources. He lived for a long period in Syria.

h. Shamlā al-ʿAṭṭār (15th century), a pharmacist.

Interestingly, a few of the above-mentioned practitioners were Samaritans (12th–13th centuries), some of whom converted to Islam.

Aleppo

Aleppo is a large ancient city in present-day Syria. It was the second city of importance in medieval Syria. In 637 the city was captured by the Muslims, and since then has been ruled by different Muslim dynasties (apart from short Byzantine and Mongol occupations). Aleppo has suffered a number of severe earthquakes through the ages.[709] The city had a Christian community during most of the medieval period, and a vibrant Jewish community as well. Benjamin of Tudela reported that 1,500 Jews resided in Aleppo in the second half of the twelfth century.[710]

The medieval Jewish community of Aleppo was described in detail by Frenkel,[711] including its leadership.[712] So far, we have information on sixteen Jewish physicians that practised in Aleppo during the period of our research. There is no doubt that there were more practitioners; however, they are not mentioned by any of our known sources. The names of the physicians are presented here in chronological order:

11th century: R. Zadok ha-Rōfē; Naḥman ha-Rōfē; Maḥfūẓ ha-Rōfē.
12th century: ʿAfif b. ʿAbd al-Qāhir Sukra; Yaḥyā b. ʿAbbās al-Maghribī (Judah b. Abūn), who lived in Aleppo when Benjamin of Tudela passed through, and had converted to Islam in Baghdad (1162); Sukra (ʿAbd al-Qāhir) al-Ḥalabī.
12th–13th centuries: Judah ha-Rōfē; Abū al-Barakāt b. Abū al-Kathīr (possibly Hananiah b. Bezalel); Elazar the king's physician; Pinḥas; Benjamin al-Sharīṭī ha-Rōfē, who lived in Aleppo when Benjamin of Tudela passed through; Abū al-Ḥajjāj Yūsuf b. Yaḥyā b. Isḥāq al-Sabatī al-Maghribī, merchant, physician and teacher, who moved from Egypt to Syria (sometime between 1185 and 1190), practised in Aleppo and may have converted to Islam.
13th century: Seth b. Japheth, physician and scribe, later moved to Iraq or Iran.
13th–14th centuries: Asad al-Yahūdī, who also practised in Cairo and other cities in Syria such as Hama, Safed and Damascus.
14th–15th centuries: David b. Joshua Maimon, forced to leave Egypt during the 1370s and lived for a number of years in Aleppo and Damascus.
16th century: a Jewish physician who treated Emir Khā'irbek al-Ashrafī in Aleppo.

We can clearly see that we have information on more Jewish practitioners in Aleppo in the twelfth and thirteenth centuries than in other periods. The reason for this is that the Fatimid and Ayyubid periods are the classical Geniza periods; that is, the community was at its peak, both at the centre of the Muslim world, and especially functioning as the heart of the Jews'. The vast majority of the documents from the Geniza are from this period, and therefore we have more information about practitioners and about every other segment or issue of Jewish society.

Damascus

Damascus is the capital of present-day Syria and has always been a major political and cultural centre of the Muslim world. It is located 80 kilometres inland from the Mediterranean on a high plateau (680 metres), on the banks of the river Barada. The city served as the capital in the Umayyad period (661–750), and after a long decline due to the rise of the Abbasid dynasty, Damascus regained its importance in the twelfth century and became a central city of the Ayyubids, Mamluks and Ottomans.[713] Throughout most of the medieval period, Damascus had vibrant Christian and Jewish communities.[714] Benjamin of Tudela reported that 3,000 Jews, 200 Karaites and 400 Samaritans resided in Damascus in the second half of the twelfth century.[715]

Being the capital of Syria, Damascus had a large Jewish community during the period of our research.[716] Therefore, it is not surprising that we should have found information on more than twenty-eight practitioners who lived and practised in the city for at least a period. Here we present the names of the main practitioners corresponding with the periods in which they were active in Damascus.

12th century: Ibrāhīm b. Khalaf al-Sāmirī, medical student (Samaritan); R. Zadok ha-Rōfē (mentioned by Benjamin of Tudela, in his description of the city).

12th–13th centuries: Abū al-Faḍl b. al-Ṣarīḥ; Baruch the physician; ʿImrān b. Ṣadaqa.

13th century: Yaʿqūb b. Ghanāʾim (Abū Yūsuf) al-Muwaffaq al-Sāmirī al-Ṭabīb (Samaritan); Jacob b. Isaac al-Maḥallī; Yūsuf b. Yaʿqūb b. Ghanāʾim – al-Muwaffaq al-Sāmirī (Samaritan); Jekuthiel ha-Levi b. Petahya and his father, Petahya ha-Levi ha-Rōfē (Karaites).

13th–14th centuries: al-Muwaffaq al-Qaṣīr; Asad al-Yahūdī; ʿAbd al-Sayyid b. Isḥāq b. Yaḥyā; Gregorios b. al-ʿIbrī, historian, physician, philosopher and theologian; Jamāl al-Dīn Dāʾūd b. Abī al-Faraj b. Abī al-Ḥusayn b. ʿImrān al-Ṭabīb (convert).
14th century: Yeshūʿā b. Menahem; ʿAwḍ, physician and *dayyān*.
15th century: ʿAbd al-Ḥaqq, pharmacist.

We have information on some physicians who were working in the Nūrī hospital (al-Bīmāristān al-Nūrī) in Damascus. These include ʿImrān b. Ṣadaqa (1165–1239), who was summoned by the rulers of other cities such as Homs, Karak (Jordan) and Hama, and who even travelled to Cairo for a while; and ʿAbd al-Sayyid b. Isḥāq b. Yaḥyā (d. 1315), who converted to Islam in 1302. Another interesting physician and unique figure was R. Joseph (possibly identical to Joseph ha-Nagid), a community leader around 1481. He was mentioned as the head of the community in Damascus during the visit of the traveller Meshullam of Volterra.

Some physicians left the city, such as Joseph from Damascus, a surgeon and moneylender from the beginning of the fifteenth century, who moved with his two sons (Judah and Nathan), also physicians, from Damascus to Candia, Crete.

Ḥarrān

Ḥarrān was a major city in ancient Mesopotamia (present-day Turkey). At the beginning of the Muslim period it was one of the main cities in the region. During the early Muslim period (8th–9th centuries) it was a centre for translating scientific works from Greek to Arabic, which later moved to Baghdad. Together with Raqqah the city served as a residence for the Ayyubid princes and was destroyed by the Mongols (1260).

Two Jewish physicians were recorded in the sources as practising in the city: Maṣlīaḥ (12th–13th centuries) and Ṣadaqa b. Munajjā b. Ṣadaqa al-Sāmirī, a Samaritan (13th century). Ṣadaqa practised in the court of an Ayyubid sultan, al-Ashraf Mūsā b. al-ʿĀdil b. Ayyūb, who ruled Ḥarrān, Baalbek and Damascus. He died in Ḥarrān.

Jerusalem

Jerusalem is an ancient city, located in the Judean Mountains between the Rift Valley and the Mediterranean. It is a holy city for the Jews, Christians and Muslims, and their many ancient and new temples, synagogues, churches and mosques are found in the city to the present day. The city has changed hands many times throughout its long history. Byzantine Jerusalem was conquered by the Muslims in 638 and was ruled by various Muslim dynasties and regimes until 1917, with a few decades of Christian rule during the Crusader period (1099–1187). The Jews returned to the city after the Muslim conquest and established a Jewish community throughout the medieval period; it included Rabbanites as well as Karaites. The Jewish community existed during the Ottoman period, absorbing immigrants from Spain and even Italy, some of whom were physicians.[717]

The Jewish physicians of Jerusalem were researched in the past as part of a general study on the history of medicine in the city,[718] and more intensively as well.[719] We have managed to trace more than twenty-five practitioners who were working and living throughout different periods in Jerusalem.

In the middle of the eleventh century, the physician Abū al-Ḥasan ʿAmmār ha-Rōfē practised in Eretz-Israel (apparently in Jerusalem). In the twelfth century, Elijah b. Zechariah (1160–1242), a physician and a judge, operated and lived in Jerusalem for a long time during the city's occupation by Saladin. In the fourteenth century we know that Abraham ha-Levi worked in the city, and in 1348 Meʾir b. Isaac Aldabi (b. probably 1310 in Toledo), a physician and religious philosopher, settled in the city.

However, the vast majority of Jewish physicians that we know of as practising in the city were from the Ottoman period, that is, the sixteenth century: ʿAbd al-Karīm b. ʿAbd al-Laṭīf, ʿAbd al-Karīm b. Mūsā (probably 'Head of the Physicians'), David b. Shushan, Ibrāhīm b. Shūmalī, Jacob ha-Rōfē 2, Joseph b. Isaac, Kamāl b. Mūsā,[720] Moses ha-Rōfē 3, R. Moses Vidalish ha-Rōfē, R. Samuel ha-Levi ha-Zāqēn (R. Samuel b. Ḥakīm), Samuel ha-Rōfē, Shaḥāda b. Abraham, Solomon b. Jacob, Sulaymān b. ʿAlī, Yaḥyā b. Joseph b. Solomon and Yūsuf b. Ibrāhīm. Others are known historical figures such as Ḥayyīm Vital (1543–1620), who was probably born in Safed and lived on and off in Jerusalem (however, we do not have information as to whether or not he practised medicine).[721]

Some of these physicians even came from Europe. For example, Solomon Luria, a physician from Lublin, immigrated to Eretz-Israel and settled in Jerusalem around 1520, when he was about eighty years old. Another example is Barbosa the physician, a Christian who converted to Judaism. He sailed to Ancona, from there moved to Turkey, and finally settled in Jerusalem.[722]

Karak

Karak is a city in Jordan, 140 kilometres south of Amman, on a hilltop of about 1,000 metres and surrounded on three sides by a valley. It is known for its large and impressive castle that was built by the Crusaders and was considered as one of the strongest and most celebrated fortresses of Syria. The city was captured by Saladin, and since then has been ruled by the Muslims.

Two Jewish physicians were recorded in the sources as practising in the city. The first was ʿImrān b. Ṣadaqa (1165–1239), a physician from Damascus. He stayed in Karak in order to cure its ruler. He also practised in Cairo, Hama, Homs and the Nūrī hospital in Damascus. The second physician was Isaac ha-Rōfē 2 (16th century), a surgeon from Jerusalem. In 1507 he practised as a physician in Karak.

Ramle

Ramle is a city in central Israel that lies at the intersection of the main road connecting Egypt (Cairo) and Syria (Damascus) with another road connecting Jerusalem and the port of Jaffa. It was founded in 705–15 by the Umayyads and was conquered by all the rulers of the land. Ramle was a principal city and district capital for the Muslims until the Crusader period. It had a small Jewish community (according to Benjamin of Tudela 300 people in 1163).[723]

Three Jewish physicians were recorded as practising in Ramle, all from the eleventh century: Amram ha-Kohen ha-Rōfē b. Aaron, mentioned and signed in a letter from Abraham b. Samuel III in Ramle to Solomon b. Judah in Jerusalem; Isaac ha-Kohen ha-Rōfē b. Furāt, a physician born in Fusṭāṭ who was active around 1029 in Ramle; and Abraham b. Isaac ha-Kohen b. Furāt, a physician who resided in Ramle for about twenty years, and was probably later the *Raʾīs al-Yahūd.*

Safed

Safed is a small town located on a mountain (900 m) in northern Israel. It was a fortified city in the Crusaders' kingdom that changed hands and was finally captured by the Mamluks in 1266. Then, the town also became an administrative centre. Safed functioned as the capital of Galilee, and had a small Jewish community during the early Muslim and through the Mamluk and Ottoman periods. Since the sixteenth century, Safed has been considered one of the four Jewish Holy Cities and it has become a centre of Jewish spirituality and mysticism (Kabbalah).

A few Jewish physicians were recorded as practising medicine in Safed. Asad al-Yahūdī (13th–14th centuries) practised in Egypt (Cairo) and Syria (Hama, Safed, Damascus, Aleppo). Solomon Qāmīs (16th century), a physician, originally from Portugal, at some point arrived in Safed, and from there he continued to Cyprus. R. Joseph b. Ezra (1543–1620), known in Arabic as ʿAfif. Ḥayyīm Vital, was probably born in Safed and lived there, and in Jerusalem on and off (where he did not practise medicine).[724]

Other cities

In other cities in Bilād al-Shām, only one physician was recorded as practising medicine. These cities are outlined in alphabetical order:

Acre:[725] David b. Abraham b. Moses b. Maimon, *nagid*, and probably a physician (13th century). At the end of his life he was forced to leave Cairo and move to Acre.

Amman:[726] Aaron ha-Rōfē al-ʿAmmānī (11th century), founder of the al-ʿAmmānī dynasty of physicians; his descendants immigrated to Alexandria and practised there for a long period (eight generations, 11th–13th centuries).[727]

Ashkelon:[728] Zechariah the Alexandrian,[729] probably a physician (12th century). Possibly originating from Alexandria, and immigrated and settled in Eretz-Israel, perhaps in Ashkelon.

Baalbek:[730] Yūsuf b. Abī Saʿīd b. Khalaf (Samaritan, d. 1227).

Hama:[731] Asad al-Yahūdī (13th–14th centuries), practised in Egypt (Cairo) and Syria (Hama, Safed, Damascus, Aleppo).

Jaffa:[732] An anonymous physician from Seleucia (12th century) was recorded. It is possible that he accompanied the Fatimid army, which was defeated by the Venetians on a coast near Jaffa in 1124.

Raqqah:[733] Judah b. Joseph b. Abī al-Thanā, philosopher and physician (10th–11th centuries).

Tiberias:[734] R. Nehorai, physician and medical herb seller (12th century). Thanks to the Geniza we know about a community of lepers who lived in the city, mainly because of the hot springs that were nearby.[735]

Tripoli:[736] – Obadia ha-Rōfē (14th century)[737] possibly lived and practised here.

Tyre[738] – Samuel ha-Rōfē 2, a physician (13th century), mentioned as living in Tyre in 1283.

4.6.6 Jewish practitioners in Iraq, Iran and Azerbaijan[739]

A large number of scholars agree that for most of the medieval period. Jewish physicians seem to have been better received in Egypt, Syria and north Africa than in Iran and Iraq.[740] Below I present the information we have about medical activity by Jewish practitioners in this part of the Muslim world.

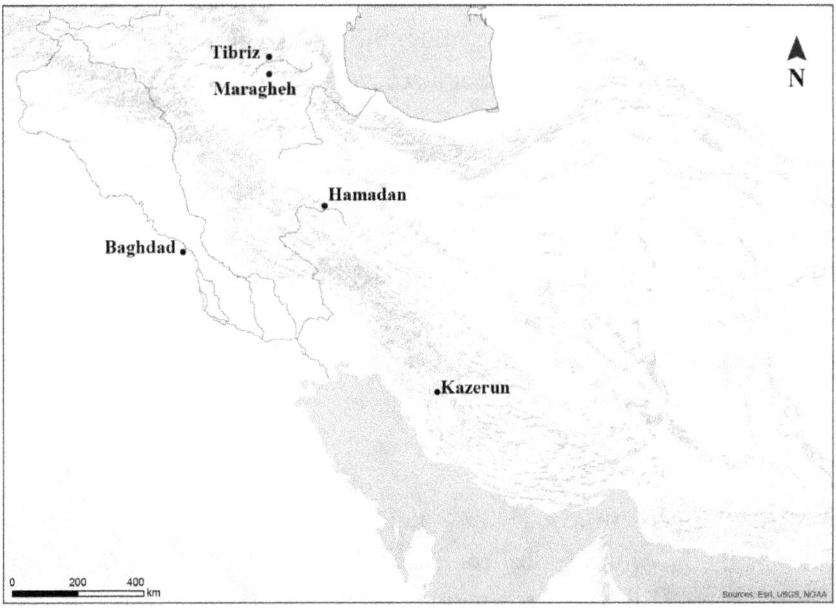

Map 4 Selected locations of Jewish medical activity in Iraq, Iran and Azerbaijan

Iraq

The Jewish community of Iraq became smaller after the fall of the Abbasid caliphate, and many of its members moved elsewhere, mainly to the new capital, Cairo.[741] Therefore, the low number of Jewish practitioners in Iraq on whom we could gather information in comparison to the number in Egypt is not surprising. Here are some of the Jewish physicians, mainly those who practised in Baghdad:[742]

a. Yaḥyā b. ʿAbbās al-Maghribī (Judah b. Abūn), a physician and poet from Fez who immigrated to Baghdad (11th–12th centuries).[743]

b. Abū al-Barakāt Hibat Allāh b. ʿAli b. Malkā al-Baladi al-Tabib al-Faḍl, who appeared in Ibn Abī Uṣaybiʿa as Awḥad al-Zamān al-Baladī,[744] was a Jewish physician and resident of Baghdad (1087–1165). He served in the medical corps and then became the physician to the caliph al-Mustanjid biʾllāh (r. 1160–70). He died aged 77 or 78, in the city of Hamadān, from where his coffin was carried to Baghdad.[745]

c. Abū Naṣr Samawʾal b. Judah b. ʿAbbās al-Maghribī (d. 1170), who converted to Islam (1163), worked for a while in Baghdad.[746]

d. ʿIzz al-Dawla Saʿd b. Manṣūr b. Kammūna, a Jewish physician, philosopher and scholar (13th century), lived in Baghdad. He wrote many scientific treatises. It is said that he converted to Islam in 1280.[747]

Bīra (Birecik)[748]

Jekuthiel b. Uziel ha-Dayyān (al-Muwaffaq ʿAbd al-Dāʾim b. ʿAbd al-ʿAzīz b. Muḥāsan, ʾIsrāʾīlī al-Mutaṭabbib) was a physician from Bīra who lived in the beginning of the fourteenth century. It appears that his father and grandfather were physicians, as he adds the epithet 'Ḥakīm' to their names. He finished writing a book on physics and metaphysics in 1315.[749]

Iran and Azerbaijan[750]

After the massive destruction of the states in central Asia, Iran, Iraq, Syria and Anatolia by the Mongol tribal confederation during the thirteenth century, the new Mongol Īl-Khānate dynasty (r. 1256–1335) created conditions for the recovery of intellectual activities, including medicine and pharmacology.

They brought together scholars and administrators from all ethnic groups and origins, including Jewish physicians.[751]

Based on Muslim Arabic sources we know about a few Jewish physicians (most of whom had converted) who practised in Azerbaijan and Iran:

a. Abū Naṣr Samaw'al b. Judah b. ʿAbbās al-Maghribī (d. 1170) converted to Islam (1163). He was the author of works on science and at the end of the twelfth century he reached Azerbaijan and settled in the capital, Marāgha.[752]

b. Saʿd al-Dawla b. Ṣafī b. Hibat Allāh b. Muhadhdhib al-Dawla al-Abharī (d. 1291) was born in Abhar, western Iran. Among other jobs he was the personal physician to Arghūn Khān in Tabriz,[753] the capital of the Īl-Khānate dynasty, in Azerbaijan.[754]

c. Abū Manṣūr Muhadhdhab al-Dawla (13th century) practised in Azerbaijan, as did Jalāl al-Dīn b. al-Ḥazzān (14th century), who served in the court of Öljeitü Khān, from the Īl-Khānate dynasty in Azerbaijan.[755]

d. The most famous of all was Rashīd al-Dīn Ṭabīb Faḍl Allāh b. al-Dawla, Abū al-Khayr b. ʿAlī Abū al-Hamadānī (1247–1318), who was the greatest recorded historian of medieval Iran. Born Jewish in Hamadān[756] as the son of a pharmacist into a family of pharmacists, he was a physician in the court of the Īl-Khānate in Tabriz. In 1298 he was appointed by Ghāzān Khān (d. 1304) as *wazīr*, or deputy of the grand *wazīr* Ṣadr al-Dīn al-Zinjānī. He remained in office under the rulers Öljeitü and Abū Saʿīd Khan.[757]

e. Aaron ha-Rōfē al-Kāzrūnī was a Karaite physician. According to his name, he or his family originated from the city of Kāzrūn, Iran.[758]

Yemen[759]

We have information regarding three Jewish physicians who were practising in Yemen:

a. A Yemenite physician, who in 1240–1 was riding a mule in fancy clothes and accompanied by servants; this angered a Yemenite *faqīh* who then knocked him off the mule.[760]

b. 'A skilled physician from the Jews of Egypt', sent by Sultan al-Ẓāhir

Barqūq to the sultan of Yemen (1397), using him as part of a gift. The Jewish physician died less than a month after his arrival there.[761]

c. Yaḥyā b. Sulaymān al-ʾIsrāʾīlī al-Ṭabīb al-Ḥakīm (Zechariah b. Solomon) (15th century) was a physician who was active in Dhamār. Since he was the only one among the Yemenite Jewish learned men who was called 'al-Ṭabīb' Yosef Tobi deduced that he was also known as a physician outside the Jewish community.[762]

Notes

1. Goitein, *Jews and Arabs*; Gil, *In the Kingdom of Ishmael*; Gil, *Jews in Islamic Countries*. Cohen, *Under Crescent and Cross*; Stillman, *The Jews of Arab Lands*.
2. Ashtor, *The Jews of Moslem Spain*.
3. Ben-Sasson, *The Emergence of the Local Jewish Community*.
4. Ben-Sasson, *The Jews of Sicily*.
5. Goitein, *Jews and Arabs*.
6. Gil, *Palestine during the First Muslim Period*.
7. See for example: Ashtor, *The History of the Jews in Egypt and Syria*; Cohen, *Jewish Self-Government*.
8. Frenkel, *The Compassionate and Benevolent*.
9. Frenkel, 'The Medieval Jewish Community of Aleppo'.
10. Cohen, 'The Jewish Community in Damascus'.
11. Ben-Sasson, *The Emergence of the Local Jewish Community*.
12. Yagur, 'Between Egypt and Jerusalem'.
13. Goitein, 'Jewish Society and Institutions under Islam', p. 173.
14. Wasserstein, 'Jewish Élites in al-Andalus', p. 107.
15. Stillman, 'The Jew in the Medieval Islamic City', p. 3.
16. Wasserstein, 'Jewish Élites in al-Andalus', pp. 103–4.
17. Shatzmiller, *Jews, Medicine, and Medieval Society*, pp. x–xi.
18. Goitein, 'The Medical Profession', p. 177.
19. Pormann and Savage-Smith, *Medieval Islamic Medicine*, p. 102.
20. Lewicka, 'Healer, Scholar, Conspirator', p. 122.
21. See Finkel, 'A Risāla of al-Jāḥiẓ', p. 328; Perlmann, 'Notes on the Position of Jewish Physicians', pp. 315–16.
22. al-Muqaddasī, *ʾAḥsan al-Taqāsīm*, p. 106; Prawer, *The History of the Jews*, p. 121.
23. Meyerhof, 'Von Alexandrien nach Bagdad', pp. 424–5.

24. Shatzmiller, *Jews, Medicine, and Medieval Society*, p. 12.
25. Micheau, 'Hommes de sciences'.
26. Meyerhof, 'Medieval Jewish Physicians in the Near East'.
27. Maimonides, *Treatise on Asthma*, p. 117.
28. Ibn Abī Uṣaybiʿa, *ʿUyūn al-Anbāʾ*, vol. II, pp. 117–18.
29. Goitein, *A Mediterranean Society*, vol. II, p. 266.
30. Cohen, *Poverty and Charity*, pp. 64–6.
31. Goitein, *A Mediterranean Society*, vol. II, pp. 250, 528.
32. Savage-Smith, 'Ṭibb'.
33. Maimonides, *Treatise on Asthma*, p. 117.
34. See biographies in Chapter 3.
35. Ibid.
36. ENA 2967.3.
37. Netzer, 'Rashīd al-Dīn', p. 122.
38. Goitein, *A Mediterranean Society*, vol. II, pp. 246–7.
39. See biographies in Chapter 3.
40. Ramaḍān, *al-Yahūd fī Miṣr*, p. 44; Luṭf, *Yahūd Miṣr al-Ayyūbiya*, p. 93.
41. Ibn Kathīr, *al-Bidāya wa-l-Nihāya*, vol. XIV, p. 86; see biography in Chapter 3.
42. Dols and Gamal, *Medieval Islamic Medicine*, p. 36.
43. Hazan, 'Medical, Administrative and Financial Aspects', pp. ii, 22, 62–3; Goitein, *A Mediterranean Society*, vol. II, p. 251.
44. Sandford-Smith, *Eye Diseases in Hot Climates.*
45. Hirschberg, *The History of Ophthalmology.*
46. Albert and Edwards, *The History of Ophthalmology*, p. 1.
47. Savage-Smith, 'Medicine', pp. 948–50.
48. Savage-Smith, 'Ṭibb'.
49. Goitein, *A Mediterranean Society*, vol. II, p. 255.
50. Personal observation, work in progress; for fragmentary information see Isaacs, *Medical and Para-medical Manuscripts*, index; Lev, 'Work in Progress'.
51. Lev, 'Mediators between Theoretical and Practical', p. 496 n. 48.
52. See Lev and Chipman, *Medical Prescriptions*, index; for a detailed study of some of these prescriptions see: Hoki, 'Logic in Compound Drugs'.
53. See Lev and Amar, *Practical Materia Medica*, index.
54. Cohen, *Poverty and Charity*, pp. 64–6.
55. Ibn Abī Uṣaybiʿa, *ʿUyūn al-Anbāʾ*, vol. II, pp. 115–16; Meyerhof, 'Medieval Jewish Physicians in the Near East', p. 445.

56. ENA 2591.6.
57. Strauss, 'Documents for the Economic and Social History of the Jews', pp. 142–5; Bodl. MS heb. c. 28, fol. 47 (2876-47).
58. TS AS 151.5.
59. Richards, 'Arabic Documents', pp.108–11; Mann, *Texts and Studies*, p. 261; Goitein, *A Mediterranean Society*, vol. IV, pp. 100 nn. 101, 102, 103.
60. Richards, 'A Doctor's Petition', p. 301; Goitein, *A Mediterranean Society*, vol. II, pp. 256–7.
61. Lewicka, 'Healer, Scholar, Conspirator', pp. 129–30.
62. Mazor, 'Asad al-Yahūdi'; Mazor, 'Jewish Court Physicians', pp. 54–60.
63. Fischel, 'Azarbaijan in Jewish History', p.17 n. 36; al-Yūnīnī, *Early Mamluk Syrian Historiography*, vol. II, p. 119.
64. Ashtor, *The History of the Jews in Egypt and Syria*, vol. I, p. 174.
65. Amar and Lev, *Physicians, Drugs and Remedies*, p. 110.
66. Goitein, *A Mediterranean Society*, vol. II, p. 255.
67. al-Yūnīnī, *Early Mamluk Syrian Historiography*, vol. II, p. 237.
68. Ragab, *The Medieval Islamic Hospital*; Hazan, 'Medical, Administrative and Financial Aspects', pp. ii, 22, 62–3; Goitein, *A Mediterranean Society*, vol. II, p. 251.
69. Meyerhof, 'Medieval Jewish Physicians in the Near East', p. 442; Goitein, *A Mediterranean Society*, vol. II, p. 255.
70. al-Ḥaqīr al-Nāfiʿ translates as 'the Wretched and Helpful' – wretched because he was unknown and helpful because he was able to cure the caliph.
71. Ibn Abī Uṣaybiʿa, *ʿUyūn al-Anbāʾ*, vol. II, p. 89; Ibn al-Qifṭī, *Taʾrīkh al-Ḥukamāʾ*, p. 178; Meyerhof, *Medieval Jewish Physicians*, p. 442; Ramaḍān, *al-Yahūd fī Miṣr*, p. 436.
72. Lewicka, 'Healer, Scholar, Conspirator', pp. 129–30.
73. Mazor, 'Asad al-Yahūdī'; Mazor, 'Jewish Court Physicians', pp. 54–60.
74. Jacoby, 'Jewish Doctors and Surgeons', pp. 438–43; Ashtor, 'New Data for the History of Levantine Jewries', p. 87.
75. Ashtor, 'New Data for the History of Levantine Jewries', p. 76.
76. Amar and Lev, *Physicians, Drugs and Remedies*, p. 108.
77. Goitein, *A Mediterranean Society*, vol. V, p. 447, vol. II, p. 255 n. 73.
78. TS 10J17.22.
79. TS NS 321.40.
80. Goitein, *A Mediterranean Society*, vol. II, p. 255.

81. Marín, 'Anthroponymy and Society', p. 273.
82. Goitein, *A Mediterranean Society*, vol. I, p. 91 nn. 48, 49.
83. Ibid., vol. II, pp. 485, 508, App. C 139.
84. Pormann and Savage-Smith, *Medieval Islamic Medicine*, p. 95.
85. Frenkel, *The Compassionate and Benevolent*, pp. 557–61. The writer regrets that the addressee, the physician Yedūthūn, had separated from his partner.
86. Goitein, *A Mediterranean Society*, vol. II, p. 253, vol. V, pp. 314–19, 592 nn. 23–4; see biography in Section 3.1.1.
87. Nethanel (Hibat Allāh) b. Zayn b. Ḥasan b. Ephraim Ibn Jumayʿ al-Isrāʾīlī, see full biography in Chapter 3.
88. Ibn Abī Uṣaybiʿa, *ʿUyūn al-Anbāʾ*, vol. II, pp. 112–15; al-Dhahabī, *Taʾrīkh al-Islām*, vol. XLVIII, p. 299; Ramaḍān, *al-Yahūd fī Miṣr*, pp. 442–4; Jadon, 'A Comparison of the Wealth', pp. 6, 70–1, 74–5; Miller, 'Doctors without Borders', pp. 112–13, 117–18; Ashtor-Strauss, 'Saladin and the Jews', p. 310; Luṭf, *Yahūd Miṣr al-Ayyūbiya*, p. 80; Goitein, *A Mediterranean Society*, vol. I, pp. 121–2 n. 44, vol. II, pp. 249–51 with n. 42; al-Maqrīzī, *al-Mawāʿiẓ*, vol. II, p. 368; Steinschneider, *Die Arabische Literatur der Juden*, no. 145; Meyerhof, 'Medieval Jewish Physicians in the Near East', pp. 444–5.
89. Amar and Lev, *Physicians, Drugs and Remedies*, pp. 109–10.
90. Goitein, *A Mediterranean Society*, vol. II, pp. 254, 579 n. 67.
91. Ibid., vol. II, p. 21.
92. Ibid., vol. II, p. 252.
93. Gil, *In the Kingdom of Ishmael*, vol. III, pp. 560–4; Goitein, *A Mediterranean Society*, vol. II, p. 255.
94. TS AS 152.4.
95. Goitein and Friedman, *India Book IV/B*, no. 79, pp. 431–41; Goitein and Friedman, *India Book IV/A*, pp. 227 ff.
96. In this case Maimonides repeated the symptoms: Stern, 'Maimonidis Commentarius'; Stern, *Corpus Codicum Hebraicorum.*
97. Goitein, *A Mediterranean Society*, vol. II, pp. 254–5. For more about the Geniza's prescriptions see Lev, 'Medieval Egyptian Judaeo-Arabic Prescriptions'; Chipman and Lev, 'Arabic Prescriptions'.
98. Shilat (ed.), *Letters and Essays of Moses Maimonides*, vol. I, pp. 242–5.
99. Ibid.
100. Risse, *Mending Bodies, Saving Souls.*
101. Savage-Smith, 'Ṭibb'.
102. Hazan, 'Medical, Administrative and Financial Aspects', p. 1; on the various

kind of hospitals in the Muslim lands see Ragab, *The Medieval Islamic Hospital*, pp. 185–201; Hamarneh, 'Development of Hospitals in Islam'.

103. Hazan, 'Medical, Administrative and Financial Aspects', pp. i–ii.
104. Ragab, *The Medieval Islamic Hospital*; Hazan, 'Medical, Administrative and Financial Aspects', pp. ii, 22, 62–3.
105. For other aspects of the medieval Islamic hospital, see Tabbaa, 'The Functional Aspects'.
106. This hospital, erected in Damascus shortly after 1154, continued to operate until 1899.
107. Hazan, 'Medical, Administrative and Financial Aspects', pp. 10–70.
108. Ragab, *The Medieval Islamic Hospital*, pp. 220–2.
109. Ibid.
110. Ibid., pp. 187–9.
111. Ibid., p. 87.
112. More than 145 practical prescriptions were found in the Geniza and studied: Lev and Chipman, *Medical Prescriptions*; Lev, 'Medieval Egyptian Judaeo-Arabic Prescriptions'; Chipman and Lev, 'Arabic Prescriptions'; Lev, Chipman and Niessen, 'Chicken and Chicory Are Good for You'.
113. See for example Ashur and Lev, 'Medical Recipes'; Stern, 'Maimonidis Commentarius'; Stern ,*Corpus Codicum Hebraicorum.*
114. Ragab, *The Medieval Islamic Hospital*, pp. 228–9.
115. Cohen, *Poverty and Charity*, p. 240. Cohen added that many more Jewish physicians served in hospitals than the famous ones inscribed in Arabic biographical dictionaries. See Cohen, 'The Burdensome Life', for the example of al-Tabīb al-Maristān (the Physician of the Hospital), who donated to public charity; Goitein, *A Mediterranean Society*, vol. II, pp. 508–9.
116. Goitein, *A Mediterranean Society*, vol. II, p. 133 n. 36.
117. Lev, *Charity, Endowments, and Charitable Institutions*, pp. 122–3.
118. Goitein, *A Mediterranean Society*, vol. II, p. 251.
119. The idea of the table is to assemble all the data regarding physicians and pharmacists who practised in hospitals and present it to the reader. The practitioners are arranged in chronological order (as far as possible). The information in this table is based on the various biographies in Chapter 3; therefore, and for the sake of simplicity, I have omitted the references.
120. Pormann and Savage-Smith, *Medieval Islamic Medicine*, p. 95.
121. Richards, 'Arabic Documents'.
122. Goitein, *A Mediterranean Society*, vol. II, pp. 256–7.

123. Ragab, *The Medieval Islamic Hospital*, pp. 201–9.
124. Cohen, 'The Burdensome Life'; Goitein, *A Mediterranean Society*, vol. II, p. 250.
125. See Shatzmiller, *Jews, Medicine, and Medieval Society*.
126. For more about the history of physicians in Muslim courts see Shefer, 'Physicians in the Mamluk and Ottoman Courts', pp. 115–18.
127. Ashtor-Strauss, 'Saladin and the Jews'.
128. Nicolae, 'A Medieval Court Physician at Work', p. 56.
129. In this table I have tried to assemble all the available data regarding the main Jewish physicians and pharmacists that practised at the courts of Muslim rulers and present it all together. The practitioners are arranged in chronological order (wherever possible). The information in this table might be partial, but it is based on the various biographies in Chapter 3 (physicians in Section 3.1.1, pharmacists in Section 3.1.2, members of dynasties in Section 3.3.2); therefore, and for the sake of simplicity, I have omitted the references.
130. Ashtor-Strauss, *Saladin and the Jews*, p. 311.
131. Meyerhof, 'The Medical Work of Maimonides', p. 288.
132. Goitein, *A Mediterranean Society*, vol. I, pp. 329–30 n. 15.
133. Ragab, *The Medieval Islamic Hospital*, pp. 201–9.
134. See biographies in Chapter 3 (physicians Section 3.1.1, members of dynasties Section 3.3.2).
135. T-S Ar. 38.131; Rustow, 'At the Limits of Communal Autonomy', p. 150. See also Goitein, *A Mediterranean Society*, vol. II, pp. 168, 327.
136. Ibid.; regarding the position of headship of the Jews see in detail Section 4.5.2.
137. Ibid.; regarding the position of *wazīr* see in detail Section 4.4.5.
138. Shefer, 'Physicians in the Mamluk and Ottoman Courts', p. 120.
139. Nicolae, 'A Medieval Court Physician at Work', p. 59; Jadon, 'A Comparison of the Wealth', p. 68.
140. Shefer, 'Physicians in the Mamluk and Ottoman Courts', p. 120.
141. Nicolae, 'A Medieval Court Physician at Work', p. 56; Pormann and Savage-Smith, *Medieval Islamic Medicine*, p. 102.
142. Pormann and Savage-Smith, *Medieval Islamic Medicine*, p. 102.
143. See biographies in Section 3.3.2.
144. Goitein, *A Mediterranean Society*, vol. II, p. 241.
145. Caballero-Navas, 'Medicine among Medieval Jews', p. 328.
146. See for example Allony, *The Jewish Library in the Middle Ages*, pp. 18, 30, 40, 130, 143, 157, 169, 181–2, 211, 259–61, 346–52, 379–82, 405–19.

147. Berkey, *The Transmission of Knowledge*, pp. 28–9.
148. Caballero-Navas, 'Medicine among Medieval Jews', p. 328.
149. Leiser, 'Medical Education in Islamic Lands'.
150. Ibid.
151. Ibn Abī Uṣaybiʿa, *ʿUyūn al-Anbāʾ*, vol. II, p. 113.
152. Weisz, 'The Jewish Physicians', pp. 18–21.
153. See in detail Karmi, 'State Control of the Physicians in the Middle Ages', pp. 66–7.
154. Goitein, 'The Medical Profession'.
155. See Leiser, 'Medical Education in Islamic Lands'; Karmi, 'State Control of the Physicians in the Middle Ages'; Goitein, 'The Medical Profession'.
156. Brentjes, *Teaching and Learning*, pp. 71, 91, 94; for more about teaching medicine in madrasas see pp. 92–7.
157. Ibn Abī Uṣaybiʿa, *ʿUyūn al-Anbāʾ*, vol. V, pp. 419–20.
158. Leiser, 'Medical Education in Islamic Lands'; Goitein wrote about this issue that 'normally one or several students would get what we would call private tutoring from a physician of established fame and would also practice under his or another's supervision, the two aspects of study not always being combined'. Goitein, *A Mediterranean Society*, vol. II, p. 248.
159. Kraemer, 'Six Unpublished Maimonides Letters'.
160. Goitein, *A Mediterranean Society*, vol. II, p. 248.
161. Friedman, 'Did Maimonides Teach Medicine?'.
162. Goitein, *A Mediterranean Society*, vol. II, p. 250. Muslim students could also be trained as physicians in a mosque or madrasa; see Amar and Lev, *Physicians, Drugs and Remedies*, p. 63.
163. Goitein, *A Mediterranean Society*, vol. II, pp. 249–50.
164. Linda Northrup dealt with network analysis of physicians; see Northrup, *al-Bīmāristān al-Manṣūrī,* pp. 25–8.
165. Frenkel, *The Compassionate and Benevolent*, pp. 410–17.
166. Goitein, *A Mediterranean Society*, vol. II, p. 250.
167. Ibid., vol. II, p. 246.
168. Marín, 'Biography and Prosopography', p. 8.
169. Ibn Murād, *Buḥūth*, pp. 93–5.
170. Ibn Abī Uṣaybiʿa, *ʿUyūn al-Anbāʾ*, vol. II, p. 118–19; Meyerhof, 'Jewish Physicians Contemporaries of Maimonides', pp. 393–4; Ramaḍān, *al-Yahūd fī Miṣr*, p. 449–50; Steinschneider, *Die Arabische Literatur der Juden*, no. 154; Meyerhof, 'Medieval Jewish Physicians in the Near East',

p. 452. Regarding findings of Abū al-Faḍl's book in the Geniza see: Lev, Chipman and Niessen, 'A Hospital Handbook for the Community', pp. 103–18.

171. Abū al-Ṣalt, 'al-Risāla al-Miṣriyya', vol. I, pp. 35–7; Ibn al-Qifṭī, *Ta'rīkh al-Ḥukamā*, pp. 209–10; Ibn Abī Uṣaybi'a, *'Uyūn al-Anbā'*, vol. II, p. 107; Ramaḍān, *al-Yahūd fī Miṣr*, pp. 437–8.
172. See in detail Section 4.4.4.
173. Ibn Abī Uṣaybi'a, *'Uyūn al-Anbā'*, vol. II, p. 218; Goitein, *A Mediterranean Society*, vol. V, p. 271 nn. 80–1.
174. Ashur and Lev, 'Medical Recipes'.
175. Ibn Abī Uṣaybi'a, *'Uyūn al-Anbā'*, vol. II, p. 109; Goitein, *A Mediterranean Society*, vol. II, p. 247.
176. Goitein, *Jewish Education in Muslim Countries*, pp. 201–2.
177. Pormann and Savage-Smith, *Medieval Islamic Medicine*, pp. 103–4.
178. Giladi, *Muslim Midwives*, pp. 74–5; Pormann and Savage-Smith, *Medieval Islamic Medicine*, p. 107.
179. Giladi, *Muslim Midwives*.
180. Pormann and Savage-Smith, *Medieval Islamic Medicine*, p. 104.
181. Goitein, *A Mediterranean Society*, vol. I, pp. 127–8.
182. Ibid., vol. III, pp. 63–4 n. 68.
183. Ibid., vol. I, pp. 127–8 n. 8.
184. TS K15.96; Goitein, *A Mediterranean Society*, vol. II, p. 441.
185. TS K15.66; Goitein, *A Mediterranean Society*, vol. II, p. 440.
186. TS 24.76; Goitein, *A Mediterranean Society*, vol. II, pp. 438–9.
187. For more regarding woman physicians, see Goitein, *A Mediterranean Society*, vol. III, pp. 63–4.
188. Ibid., vol. III, p. 232 n. 55.
189. Nicolae, 'A Medieval Court Physician at Work', p. 74; see also: Jadon, 'The Physicians of Syria', p. 325.
190. For titles that were already identified in the Geniza see for example Isaacs, *Medical and Para-medical Manuscripts*, indexes; Lev, 'Work in Progress'; Lev, 'A Catalogue of the Medical and Para-medical Manuscripts'; Lev and Niessen, 'Addenda to Isaacs's "Catalogue"'; Lev and Smithuis, 'A Preliminary Catalogue'. For publications regarding specific medical books that were identified in the Geniza see for example Lev, 'An Early Fragment'; Lev, Chipman and Niessen, 'A Hospital Handbook for the Community'; Lev and Chipman, 'Texts/Documents/Translations', Chipman and Lev, 'Take a Lame and Decrepit

Female Hyena'; Serry and Lev, 'A Judaeo-Arabic Fragment'; Chipman and Lev, 'Syrups from the Apothecary's Shop'.

191. Baneth, 'A Doctor's Library'; see also Nicolae, 'Jewish Physicians at the Court of Saladin', pp. 25–6.
192. Frenkel, 'Book Lists from the Geniza'; Allony, *The Jewish Library in the Middle Ages*.
193. Brentjes, *Teaching and Learning*, p. 247.
194. I intend to reconstruct the medical library of the Jewish practitioners in the medieval period in the near future.
195. See in detail Section 4.4.7.
196. Chipman, *The World of Pharmacy and Pharmacists*, p. 71. For the Geniza's prescriptions see Lev and Chipman, *Medical Prescriptions*.
197. Makdisi, *The Rise of Humanism*, p. 59; Nicolae, 'A Medieval Court Physician at Work', p. 75.
198. Miller, 'Doctors without Borders', pp. 113–17.
199. Ibid.; Meyerhof, 'Von Alexandrien nach Bagdad'; Meyerhof, 'Medieval Jewish Physicians in the Near East', pp. 442–3; Ramaḍān, *al-Yahūd fī Miṣr*, p. 436.
200. See biography in Section 3.1.1 for more details.
201. Ibn Abī Uṣaybiʿa, *ʿUyūn al-Anbāʾ*, vol. II, p. 105.
202. Pormann and Savage-Smith, *Medieval Islamic Medicine*, p. 94.
203. Ibn Abī Uṣaybiʿa, *ʿUyūn al-Anbāʾ*, vol. II, p. 105.
204. al-Ghazūlī, *Maṭāliʿ al-Budūr*, p. 421; al-Ṣafadī, *Kitāb al-Wāfī bi-l-Wafayāt* (2000), vol. XVI, pp. 173–5; Meyerhof, 'Jewish Physicians Contemporaries of Maimonides', p. 395; Wedel, 'Transfer of Knowledge', pp. 3.78–3.79.
205. Nicolae, 'A Medieval Court Physician at Work', p. 74.
206. Ibid., pp. 74–86.
207. Ibid., pp. 74–5.
208. Goitein, *A Mediterranean Society*, vol. IV, p. 311.
209. Ibid.; see Ashtor, *Histoire des prix et des salaires*, p. 567.
210. Allony, *The Jewish Library in the Middle Ages*, pp. 241–51; see also Baneth, 'A Doctor's Library'; Nicolae, 'Jewish Physicians at the Court of Saladin', pp. 25–6.
211. Allony, *The Jewish Library in the Middle Ages*, pp. 256–63.
212. Frenkel, *The Compassionate and Benevolent*, pp. 95–6; Goitein, *A Mediterranean Society*, vol. II, pp. 258, 264, 580 nn. 96, 99.
213. Goitein, *A Mediterranean Society*, vol. II, p. 264. This was a very large private library for those days, when all books were written by hand.

214. Bacher, 'La Bibliothèque d'un médecin juif'. According to Goitein such a library usually consisted of two parts, one Hebrew and the other Arabic, and the auctions were held at two different meetings, Gentiles taking a prominent part in the Arabic sale; see Goitein, *A Mediterranean Society*, vol. II, p. 248.
215. Goitein, *Letters of Medieval Jewish Traders*, p. 219, sec. G.
216. Bareket, 'Abraham Ben Hillel'.
217. Allony, *The Jewish Library in the Middle Ages*, pp. 241–51; see also Baneth, 'A Doctor's Library'.
218. Goitein, 'The Oldest Documentary Evidence', pp. 301–2; see biographies in Chapter 3.
219. The notebook, dated 1157, includes medical prescriptions, commercial bills and records of book loans.
220. Allony, *The Jewish Library in the Middle Ages*, pp. 161, 164–5, 174, 211.
221. Behrens-Abouseif, *Fatḥ Allā and Abū Zakariyya*, pp. 5–6.
222. al-Dhahabī, *Taʿrīkh al-Islām*, vol. XLVIII, p. 299.
223. Ashtor, *The History of the Jews in Egypt and Syria*, vol. II, pp. 89–90.
224. al-Maqrīzī, *Kitāb al-Sulūk*, vol. IV, p. 598.
225. Bulliet, 'The Age Structure of Medieval Islamic Education'.
226. Ávila, *La sociedad hispanomusulmana*.
227. Finkel, 'An Eleventh Century Source', pp. 50–1; Roth, 'Medicine', p. 434; al-Andalusī, *Science in the Medieval World*, p. 80; Ibn Juljul, *Ṭabaqāt al-Aṭibbāʾ*, pp. 87–8.
228. al-Ṣafadī, *Kitāb al-Wāfī bi-l-Wafayāt* (2008–10), vol. XXVII, p. 300–2; al-ʿUmarī, *Masālik al-Abṣār*, vol. IX, pp. 247–50; Ibn al-Qifṭī, *Taʾrīkh al-Ḥukamāʾ*, p. 343; Steinschneider, *An Introduction to the Arabic Literature of the Jews II*, 13(1), p. 94; Gil, *Jews in Islamic Countries*, p. 470; Stillman and Pines, 'Abū al-Barakāt al-Baghdadī'.
229. Moreen, 'Rashīd al-Dīn Ṭabīb'; Fischel, 'Azarbaijan in Jewish History', pp. 16–18.
230. For example Rosenthal, 'The Physician in Medieval Muslim Society'; Biesterfeldt, 'Some Opinions'; Behrens-Abouseif, 'The Image of the Physician'; Hazan, 'Medical, Administrative and Financial Aspects', pp. 111–15.
231. For example, the classic articles by Meyerhof, 'Medieval Jewish Physicians in the Near East', and Goitein, 'The Medical Profession'.
232. Cohen, 'The Burdensome Life'.
233. Goitein, *A Mediterranean Society*, vol. IV, pp. 86–7.
234. Ibid., vol. II, p. 243, vol. III, p. 37 n. 9, vol. IV, p. 265 n. 23.

235. The full list can be found ibid., vol. IV, p. 335 nn. 196–9.
236. Ibid., vol. IV, p. 125 nn. 115–16.
237. Isaacs, *Medical and Para-medical Manuscripts*, p. xiv.
238. TS Ar.30.286.
239. Stern, 'Maimonidis Commentarius'; Stern, *Corpus Codicum Hebraicorum.*
240. Mosseri I.115.1. Dr Amir Ashur identified and edited the fragment. For a physical description and content see Lev, 'A Catalogue of Medical and Para-medical Manuscripts'.
241. Ashur and Lev, 'Practical Prescriptions by Maimonides'.
242. TS 8J15.20; see image, transcription and discussion in Lev and Chipman, *Medical Prescriptions*, pp. 48–50. More fragments are at Bodl. MS heb. a. 3, fol. 18; TS 10J17.27 – I plan to publish these fragments with Dr Amir Ashur in the near future.
243. Goitein and Friedman, *India Book III*; Goitein and Friedman, *India Traders of the Middle Ages*, vol. I, pp. 52–89 (Abraham's medical knowledge, p. 68). For his journey back from India, especially from a material cultural point of view, see Lambourn, *Abraham's Luggage.*
244. TS Ar. 41.81.
245. Lev and Chipman, *Medical Prescriptions*, pp. 108–10.
246. Marín, 'Biography and Prosopography', p. 8; on Muslim scholars travelling for the sake of knowledge see Brentjes, *Teaching and Learning*, pp. 135–9.
247. See in detail Weisz, 'The Jewish Physicians'.
248. Shefer, 'Physicians in the Mamluk and Ottoman Courts', p. 117.
249. Brentjes, *Teaching and Learning*, p. 144.
250. Goitein, *A Mediterranean Society*, vol. I, p. 273.
251. Ibid., vol. II, p. 257 n. 87, vol. IV, pp. 263–4 nn. 13, 16.
252. Ibn Abī Uṣaybiʿa, *ʿUyūn al-Anbāʾ*, vol. II, pp. 116–17; Jadon, 'A Comparison of the Wealth', p. 65; Kraemer, *Maimonides*, pp. 214–15; Meyerhof, 'Medieval Jewish Physicians in the Near East', p. 446; Ramaḍān, *al-Yahūd fī Miṣr*, p. 444; Ashtor-Strauss, 'Saladin and the Jews', p. 310.
253. Goitein, *A Mediterranean Society*, vol. III, p. 340.
254. Ibid., vol. I, p. 345, vol. II, p. 289 n. 58.
255. Ibid., vol. II, p. 162, vol. IV, pp. 227–8 n. 6.
256. Ibid., vol. II, p. 257.
257. He dealt, among other things, in laws of inheritance, bills and marriages; see for example Goitein and Friedman, *India Book III.*
258. Goitein and Friedman, *India Traders of the Middle Ages*, vol. I, p. 84.

259. Marín, 'Anthroponymy and Society'.
260. Shilat, *Letters and Essays of Moses Maimonides*, vol. I, pp. 72–6.
261. Stillman, 'The Eleventh Century Merchant House'; for more examples see Goitein, *A Mediterranean Society*, vol. I, pp. 79 n. 16, 191 n. 23, vol. II, p. 258.
262. See in detail Section 3.3.2.
263. Goitein and Friedman, *India Book I*, p. 39, and n. 46 on the possibility of him being a physician; Cohen, *Poverty and Charity*, p. 66 n. 167.
264. Goitein and Friedman, *India Book I*, pp. 39–42, 45–116.
265. Ibid., p. 41.
266. Goitein, *A Mediterranean Society*, vol. I, p. 89.
267. Ibid., vol. II, p. 258, vol. I, pp. 252, 463 n. 134.
268. Ibid., vol. I, pp. 252 n. 134, 233 n. 74.
269. See in detail Makdisi, *The Rise of Humanism*, pp. 71–6.
270. Goitein, 'Ministrants and Physicians as Booksellers'.
271. Goitein, *A Mediterranean Society*, vol. II, pp. 258–9, 264, 580 n. 96; Frenkel, *The Compassionate and Benevolent*, pp. 95–6.
272. Goitein, *A Mediterranean Society*, vol. I, p. 379 n. 47.
273. Ibid., vol. II, p. 258.
274. Frenkel, *The Compassionate and Benevolent*, p. 97; Goitein, *A Mediterranean Society*, vol. II, p. 576 n. 21.
275. Frenkel, *The Compassionate and Benevolent*, pp. 95–6; Goitein, *A Mediterranean Society*, vol. II, pp. 258, 264, 580 nn. 96, 99.
276. Frenkel, *The Compassionate and Benevolent*, p. 27; Zeldes and Frenkel, 'The Sicilian Trade', p. 136.
277. Mosseri VIII.80.1.
278. Goitein, *Jewish Education in Muslim Countries*, p. 195.
279. Ibid.; Goitein, *A Mediterranean Society*, vol. II, pp. 189 n. 24, 258.
280. Goitein, *A Mediterranean Society*, vol. I, p. 322 n. 65.
281. Ibid., vol. IV, pp. 67, 83, 277, 283–4, 287.
282. Strauss, 'Documents for the Economic and Social History of the Jews', pp. 142–5; Bodl. MS heb. c. 28, fol. 47 (2876-47).
283. It is unlikely that a non-Jew would have a bathhouse for Jews in a Jewish neighbourhood.
284. Lewicka, 'Healer, Scholar, Conspirator'; Conermann, *Muslim–Jewish Relations*, pp. 15–17.
285. See in detail Pormann, 'The Physician and the Other', p. 213.

286. Nicolae, 'A Medieval Court Physician at Work', p. 56; Pormann and Savage-Smith, *Medieval Islamic Medicine*, p. 102.
287. Höglmeier, *al-Ǧawbarī und seine Kašf al-asrār*, pp. 137–8; Ashtor, *The History of the Jews in Egypt and Syria*, vol. I, pp. 341–2.
288. Pormann and Savage-Smith, *Medieval Islamic Medicine*, p. 89; Mazor, 'Jewish Court Physicians'.
289. al-ʿUmarī, *Masālik al-Abṣār*, vol. IX, p. 365 (in the section that deals with 'the physicians of Egypt').
290. Mazor, 'Jewish Court Physicians', p. 51.
291. Levey, *Medical Ethics of Medieval Islam*; Goitein, *A Mediterranean Society*, vol. V, pp. 419–20, 625 n. 26.
292. Goitein, *A Mediterranean Society*, vol. II, p. 257.
293. Ramaḍān, *al-Yahūd fī Miṣr*, pp. 438–9.
294. For the use of *sharāb* as a euphemism for wine, see Chipman, *The World of Pharmacy and Pharmacists*, p. 24.
295. Nicolae, 'A Medieval Court Physician at Work', p. 68.
296. Cohen, *Poverty and Charity*, p. 241; Abrahams, *Hebrew Ethical Wills*, p. 67.
297. Biesterfeldt, 'Some Opinions', p. 17; see detailed bibliography there in note 9.
298. Pormann and Savage-Smith, *Medieval Islamic Medicine*, p. 95.
299. Biesterfeldt, 'Some Opinions', pp. 18–19.
300. The Hebrew translator of Maimonides' Arabic 'Guide for the Perplexed'.
301. Cohen, *Poverty and Charity*, p. 241; Cohen, 'The Burdensome Life'.
302. Goitein, *A Mediterranean Society*, vol. II, p. 256.
303. Cohen, *Poverty and Charity*, pp. 239–342
304. Ibid., p. 241.
305. TS Ar. 34.94; see Khan, *Arabic Legal and Administrative Documents*, pp. 275–6; Goitein, *A Mediterranean Society*, vol. II, p. 257 n. 86.
306. Cohen, *Poverty and Charity*, p. 241.
307. Goitein, *A Mediterranean Society*, vol. I, p. 259, vol. II, pp. 256, 580 n. 88. Regarding income of physicians in Muslim lands see Rosenthal, 'The Physician in Medieval Muslim Society'.
308. Cohen, *Poverty and Charity*, p. 241.
309. The idea that payment should be made to a physician only after successful treatment was even then thousands of years old (see the Hammurabi Codex, paragraphs 215 ff. for example).
310. Goitein, *A Mediterranean Society*, vol. II, pp. 256–7.
311. Ibid., vol. II, p. 257.

312. For more on eye disease and its treatment see Lev and Chipman, *Medical Prescriptions*, pp. 151–3.
313. Goitein, *A Mediterranean Society*, vol. V, p. 112.
314. Lev and Chipman, *Medical Prescriptions*, pp. 153–4. Regarding the medicinal substances see Lev and Amar, *Practical Materia Medica.*
315. Sabra, *Poverty and Charity*, p. 73; Cohen, *Poverty and Charity*, p. 240.
316. Goitein, *A Mediterranean Society*, vol. II, pp. 266–7 nn. 29, 44.
317. Lev, Chipman and Niessen, 'Chicken and Chicory Are Good for You'.
318. Goitein, *A Mediterranean Society*, vol. II, pp. 260–1.
319. Among many publications dealing with life and scholarship: Ben-Sasson, 'The Maimonidean Dynasty'; Kraemer, *Maimonides*; Stroumsa, *Maimonides in his World*; Isaacs, 'An Encounter with Maimonides'; Goitein, 'Maimonides' Life'.
320. Ibn Abī Uṣaybiʿa, *ʿUyūn al-Anbāʾ*, vol. II, p. 118; Steinschneider, *Die Arabische Literatur der Juden,* no. 159; Meyerhof, 'Medieval Jewish Physicians in the Near East', p. 451; Ramaḍān, *al-Yahūd fī Miṣr*, p. 450; Sarton, *Introduction*, II, p. 376.
321. Frenkel, *The Compassionate and Benevolent.*
322. There is extensive research on Abraham's pietist lifestyle and leadership, recently discussed in Russ-Fishbane, *Judaism, Sufism, and the Pietists of Medieval Egypt.*
323. For detailed references, see the biographies in Chapter 3.
324. Fenton, 'Maimonides, David ben Abraham', Goitein, *A Mediterranean Society*, vol. VI, pp. 28–9.
325. Fenton, 'Maimonides, David ben Abraham'; Katsh, 'From the Moscow Manuscript', pp. 140–1.
326. Goitein, *Palestinian Jewry*, pp. 185–6; Goitein, *A Mediterranean Society*, vol. V, pp. 419–20 n. 27.
327. Goitein, *A Mediterranean Society*, vol. II, p. 193 n. 7.
328. Amar and Lev, *Physicians, Drugs and Remedies*, pp. 108–11.
329. Goitein, *A Mediterranean Society*, vol. II, p. 380.
330. Ibid., vol. I, p. 379 D note 47.
331. Ibid., vol. I, p. 73 n. 29.
332. Ibid., vol. II, p. 380 nn. 31–4; Steinschneider, *Die Arabische Literatur der Juden*, p. 183.
333. Goitein, *A Mediterranean Society*, vol. I, p. 73 n. 30, p. 252 n. 131, vol. III, p. 475 n. 6, vol. IV, pp. 263–4 n. 12.
334. Shatzmiller, *Jews, Medicine, and Medieval Society*, pp. ix–x, 1.
335. Ibid., pp. 1, 13.

336. Jacquart, *Le Milieu medical en France*, p. 231; Shatzmiller, *Jews, Medicine, and Medieval Society*, pp. 2–8.
337. Shatzmiller, *Jews, Medicine, and Medieval Society*, pp. 8–12.
338. Perlmann, 'Notes on the Position of Jewish Physicians', pp. 316–19; Ashtor, 'Prolegomena', pp. 154–5; Baron, *A Social and Religious History*, vol. XVII, p. 175; Behrens-Abouseif, *Fatḥ Allāh and Abū Zakariyya*, pp. 13–14; Stillman, *The Jews of Arab Lands*, p. 72; Mazor and Lev, 'The Phenomenon'.
339. Behrens-Abouseif, 'The Image of the Physician', pp. 335–6, 342–3; Behrens-Abouseif, *Fatḥ Allāh and Abū Zakariyya*, pp. 14–19.
340. Mazor and Lev, 'The Phenomenon'.
341. Nicolae, 'Jewish Physicians at the Court of Saladin', p. 45; see in detail pp. 8–41.
342. Lewicka, 'The Non-Muslim Physician', p. 501.
343. Goitein, *Jewish Education in Muslim Countries*, p. 195; Stillman, 'The Non-Muslim Communities', p. 209; Goitein, *A Mediterranean Society*, vol. II, p. 241.
344. Miller, 'Doctors without Borders', p. 113; Yahalom and Blau, *The Wanderings of Judah Alharizi*, pp. 33–4; Meyerhof, 'Jewish Physicians Contemporaries of Maimonides', p. 393; Kraemer, *Maimonides*, pp. 363–4.
345. Mazor, 'Jewish Court Physicians', pp. 43–50; Mazor, 'Sadīd al-Dimyāṭī'; al-ʿUmarī, *Masālik al-Abṣār*, vol. IX, pp. 361–2; Meyerhof, 'Medieval Jewish Physicians in the Near East', p. 456; al-Ṣafadī, *Kitāb al-Wāfī bi-l-Wafayāt* (2000), vol. XV, p. 80; Meyerhof, 'Jewish Physicians Contemporaries of Maimonides', pp. 397–8.
346. Mazor, 'Jewish Court Physicians'.
347. Goitein, 'The Moses Maimonides–Ibn Sanāʾ al-Mulk Circle', pp. 403–4.
348. Ibn Abī Uṣaybiʿa, *ʿUyūn al-Anbāʾ*, vol. II, p. 214.
349. Goitein, *A Mediterranean Society*, vol. V, pp. 314–19, 592 nn. 23–4.
350. Ibn al-Qifṭī, *Taʾrīkh al-Ḥukamāʾ*, pp. 225, 317.
351. Mazor, 'Asad al-Yahūdī'; Mazor, 'Jewish Court Physicians', pp. 54–60; Lewicka, 'Healer, Scholar, Conspirator', pp. 129–30.
352. al-Yūnīnī, *Early Mamluk Syrian Historiography*, vol. II, p. 237.
353. Mazor, 'Faraj Allāh Ibn Ṣaghīr'; Mazor, 'Jewish Court Physicians', p. 51.
354. Northrup dealt with the issue of teacher–student chain and named it *Silsila*; Northrup, *al-Bīmāristān al-Manṣūrī*, p. 26.
355. Friedenwald, *The Jews and Medicine*, p. 633.
356. Ramaḍān, *al-Yahūd fī Miṣr*, p. 44; Luṭf, *Yahūd Miṣr al-Ayyūbiya*, p. 93; Ashtor-

Strauss, 'Saladin and the Jews', p. 311; Kedar, 'The Frankish Period'; Wedel, *Kitāb aṭ-Ṭabbāḫ*, p. 147; Ben-Hayyim, *The Literary and Oral Tradition*, vol. I, p. 30; Meyerhof, 'Jewish Physicians Contemporaries of Maimonides', p. 395; Crown, Pummer and Tal, *A Companion to Samaritan Studies*, pp. 6–7.

357. Ibn Abī Uṣaybiʿa, *ʿUyūn al-Anbāʾ*, vol. II, pp. 112–15; Kaḥāla, *Muʿjam al-Muʾallifīn*, vol. IV, p. 56; al-Dhahabī, *Taʾrīkh al-Islām*, vol. XLVIII, p. 299; Steinschneider, *Die Arabische Literatur der Juden*, no. 145; Meyerhof, 'Medieval Jewish Physicians in the Near East', pp. 444–5; Jadon, 'A Comparison of the Wealth', pp. 65, 70–1, 74–5; Miller, 'Doctors without Borders', pp. 112–18; Ashtor-Strauss, 'Saladin and the Jews', p. 310.
358. Nicolae, 'A Medieval Court Physician at Work', p. 62.
359. Steinschneider, 'An Introduction to the Arabic Literature of the Jews II', 13(1), p. 93 n. 1; Meyerhoff, 'Medieval Jewish Physicians in the Near East', p. 453.
360. Ibn Abī Uṣaybiʿa, *ʿUyūn al-Anbāʾ*, vol. II, p. 193; Steinschneider, 'An Introduction to the Arabic Literature of the Jews II', 13(1), p. 93.
361. Meyerhof, 'Jewish Physicians Contemporaries of Maimonides', p. 398; Steinschneider, 'An Introduction to the Arabic Literature of the Jews I', 11(2), p. 308.
362. Nicolae, 'A Medieval Court Physician at Work', p. 64.
363. Steinschneider, 'An Introduction to the Arabic Literature of the Jews II', 13(2), p. 298.
364. In the words of Ibn Abī Uṣaybiʿa: 'He had studied the art of medicine with ʿAlī Ibn Riḍwān and was his most illustrious pupil.' Ibn Riḍwān (d. 1061) was a renowned physician, medical author and polemicist, who was appointed chief physician of Egypt by the Fatimid caliph.
365. Ibn Abī Uṣaybiʿa, *ʿUyūn al-Anbāʾ*, vol. II, pp. 105–6; Roth, 'Medicine', p. 435; Roth, *Jews, Visigoths and Muslims*, p. 180; Miller, 'Doctors without Borders', pp. 113–17; Ramaḍān, *al-Yahūd fī Miṣr*, pp. 436–7; Meyerhof, 'Von Alexandrien nach Bagdad'; Meyerhof, 'Medieval Jewish Physicians in the Near East', pp. 442–3; Pormann and Savage-Smith, *Medieval Islamic Medicine*, p. 94.
366. Meyerhof, 'Jewish Physicians Contemporaries of Maimonides', p. 395; Ibn Abī Uṣaybiʿa, *ʿUyūn al-Anbāʾ*, vol. II, pp. 233–34; al-Ṣafadī, *Kitāb al-Wāfī bi-l-Wafayāt* (2000), vol. XXIX, p. 89.
367. Abū al-Ṣalt, 'al-Risāla al-Miṣriyya', vol. I, pp. 35–7; Ibn al-Qifṭī, *Taʾrīkh al-Ḥukamā*, pp. 209–10; Ibn Abī Uṣaybiʿa, *ʿUyūn al-Anbāʾ*, vol. II, p. 107; Ramaḍān, *al-Yahūd fī Miṣr*, pp. 437–8; Steinschneider, *Die Arabische Literatur*

der Juden, n. 143; Meyerhof, 'Medieval Jewish Physicians in the Near East', p. 443; Roth, *Jews, Visigoths and Muslims*, p. 180.

368. On the professional network of Ibn al-Nafīs, see: Northrup, *al-Bīmāristān al-Manṣūrī*, p. 26–7.
369. Meyerhof, 'Jewish Physicians Contemporaries of Maimonides', pp. 397–8. According to al-Ṣafadī, *Kitāb al-Wāfī bi-l-Wafayāt* (2000), vol. XV, p. 80, he died in 1342.
370. Mazor, 'Ibn Ṣaghīr/Ibn Kūjik Family'.
371. Ragab, *The Medieval Islamic Hospital*, pp. 164–70; Lewicka, *Medicine for Muslims?* p. 16; Jadon, 'A Comparison of the Wealth', p. 66. See in detail their biographies in Sections 3.1.1 and 3.3.2.
372. Stillman and Pines, 'Abū al-Barakāt al-Baghdadī'; Steinschneider, 'An Introduction to the Arabic Literature of the Jews II' 13(1), p. 93. See in detail his biography in Section 3.1.1.
373. Nicolae, 'A Medieval Court Physician at Work', p. 56; Pormann and Savage-Smith, *Medieval Islamic Medicine*, p. 102.
374. Mazor, 'Jewish Court Physicians', pp. 40–1; Ashtor, *Toledot ha-Yehudim*, vol. I, pp. 107–8, 341–3; Lewicka, 'Healer, Scholar, Conspirator', pp. 124, 134–8; Stillman, *The Jews of Arab Lands*, pp. 71–2.
375. Ragab, *The Medieval Islamic Hospital*, pp. 164–70; Lewicka, *Medicine for Muslims?* p. 16; Lewicka, 'The Non-Muslim Physician', p. 501.
376. Lewicka, 'Healer, Scholar, Conspirator', p. 122.
377. Goitein, *A Mediterranean Society*, vol. II, p. 288.
378. Nicolae, 'Jewish Physicians at the Court of Saladin', pp. 44–5.
379. Nicolae, 'A Medieval Court Physician at Work', p. 57; Stillman, *The Jews of Arab Lands*, p. 276; Gottheil, 'Dhimmis and Moslems in Egypt', pp. 396–7.
380. al-Khālidī, *al-Yahūd Taḥta Ḥukm al-Muslimīn*, p. 357.
381. Nicolae, 'A Medieval Court Physician at Work', p. 57; Stillman, *The Jews of Arab Lands*, p. 71.
382. Rustow, 'At the Limits of Communal Autonomy', p. 133.
383. See Sections 3.1.1 and 3.3 and Tables 2 and 3.
384. Goitein, *A Mediterranean Society*, vol. I, p. 259, vol. II, p. 288 n. 57.
385. Cano, 'Ḥasday Ibn Shaprūṭ'.
386. Ibn Abī Uṣaybiʿa, *ʿUyūn al-Anbāʾ*, vol. II, p. 50; al-Andalusī, *Ṭabaqāt al-ʾUmam*, pp. 203–4.
387. See in detail Section 3.3.2, dynasty 1.
388. Meyerhof, 'Jewish Physicians Contemporaries of Maimonides', pp. 395, 396;

Ibn Abī Uṣaybiʿa, *ʿUyūn al-Anbāʾ*, p. II, p. 233–4; al-Ṣafadī, *Kitāb al-Wāfī bi-l-Wafayāt* (2008–10), vol. XXIX, p. 205; al-ʿUmarī, *Masālik al-Abṣār*, vol. XIX, pp. 290–1; Ashtor, *The Jews and the Mediterranean Economy*, pp. 152–3.

389. He appeared in Ibn Abī Uṣaybiʿa as Al-Ṣāḥib Amīn al-Dawla: Ibn Abī Uṣaybiʿa, *ʿUyūn al-Anbāʾ*, vol. II, pp. 234–5; al-Ṣafadī, *Kitāb al-Wāfī bi-l-Wafayāt* (2008–10), vol. XII, pp. 104–5; al-ʿUmarī, *Masālik al-Abṣār*, vol. IX, p. 292; Meyerhof, 'Jewish Physicians Contemporaries of Maimonides', p. 396; Wedel, 'Transfer of Knowledge', 3.80–3.81.
390. al-Ṣafadī, *Kitāb al-Wāfī bi-l-Wafayāt* (2008–10), vol. XII, p. 105; al-ʿUmarī, *Masālik al-Abṣār*, vol. IX, pp. 291–2; Meyerhof, 'Jewish Physicians Contemporaries of Maimonides', p. 396.
391. Fischel, 'Azarbaijan in Jewish History', pp. 6–10; Amitai, 'Saʿd al-Dawla'; Meyerhof, 'Jewish Physicians Contemporaries of Maimonides', pp. 398–9.
392. al-Ṣafadī, *Aʿyān al-ʿAṣr*, vol. II, p. 404.
393. al-ʿUmarī, *Masālik al-Abṣār*, vol. IX, pp. 360–1; al-Dhākirī, *al-Ṭibb wa-l-Aṭibbāʾ fī l-Quds*, 56.
394. Moreen, 'Rashīd al-Dīn Ṭabīb'; Fischel, 'Azarbaijan in Jewish History', pp. 13–18.
395. For a detailed review see Bulliet, *Conversion to Islam*, p. 3; Morony, 'The Age of Conversions', p. 137; Carlson, 'Contours of Conversion'; Bulliet, 'Process and Status'.
396. Peacock, 'Introduction', p. 4.
397. Humphreys, *Islamic History*, p. 274.
398. Tannous, *The Making of the Medieval Middle East*, p. 361.
399. Arnold, *The Preaching of Islam*; Hodgson, *The Venture of Islam*; Little, 'Coptic Conversion to Islam'; Lev, 'Persecutions and Conversion to Islam'; Levy-Rubin, 'New Evidence'.
400. Levtzion, *Conversion to Islam*, pp. 7–12; Levtzion, 'Conversion to Islam in Syria and Palestine'; Gervers and Bikhazi, *Conversion and Continuity*, pp. 4–5; el-Leithy, 'Coptic Culture and Conversion', pp. 35, 65, 362–3; Wasserstein, 'Conversion and the *Ahl al-Dhimma*', pp. 185–7; Carlson, 'Contours of Conversion'.
401. Wasserstein, 'Conversion and the *Ahl al-Dhimma*', pp. 199–200.
402. Bulliet, *Conversion to Islam*.
403. Tannous, *The Making of the Medieval Middle East*, pp. 387, 398.
404. Carlson, 'Contours of Conversion'; Peacock, 'Introduction'; Tannous, *The Making of the Medieval Middle East*, p. 363.

405. El-Leithy, 'Coptic Culture and Conversion', pp. 29–33, 140–1; Safran, 'Identity and Differentiation', p. 579; Simonsohn, 'Conversion to Islam'.
406. See in detail Humphreys, *Islamic History*, pp. 274–83.
407. See Sections 4.4.1, 4.4.5 and 4.4.7.
408. See in detail Section 4.1.1.
409. See for example Section 4.4.4.
410. See in detail Sections 4.4.1 and 4.4.5.
411. Physicians in Section 3.1.1, pharmacists in Section 3.1.2 and members of dynasties in Section 3.3.2.
412. See in detail Mazor, 'Jewish Court Physicians', pp. 43–6.
413. The purpose of the table is to assemble all the data regarding Jewish practitioners that converted to Islam and present it to the reader. The information in this table is fragmentary and based on the various biographies in Chapter 3 (physicians in Section 3.1.1, pharmacists in Section 3.1.2, members of dynasties in Section 3.3.2); therefore, and for the sake of simplicity, I have omitted references. For detailed references, see the biographies.
414. The biographical dictionaries of physicians (by Ibn Abī Uṣaybiʿa and Ibn al-Qifṭī) are from the thirteenth century, and the vast majority of the Geniza is from the 11th–13th centuries.
415. For physicians see Section 3.1.1, for pharmacists see Section 3.1.2 and for members of medical dynasties see Section 3.3.2.
416. Mazor and Lev, 'The Phenomenon'.
417. Nicolae, 'A Medieval Court Physician at Work', p. 59; Jadon, 'A Comparison of the Wealth', p. 68.
418. See detailed biography in Section 3.3.2, dynasty 27.
419. Ashtor, *The History of the Jews in Egypt and Syria*, vol. I, p. 280–2; Goitein, *A Mediterranean Society*, vol. III, p. 12 n. 69.
420. See Mazor, 'Ibn Ṣaghīr/Ibn Kūjik Family'; Goitein, *A Mediterranean Society*, vol. III, pp. 10–11 n. 62.
421. Zorgati, *Pluralism in the Middle Ages*.
422. DeWeese, *Islamization and Native Religion*, p. 27; Crone, The Nativist Prophets of Early Islamic Iran, p. 14; Peacock, Introduction, p. 5.
423. Stillman and Pines, 'Abū al-Barakāt al-Baghdadī'; Steinschneider, 'An Introduction to the Arabic Literature of the Jews II', 13(1), p. 93.
424. Zorgati, *Pluralism in the Middle Ages*, chh. 4, 5; Simonsohn, 'Conversion to Islam'; Simonsohn, 'Conversion, Exemption, and Manipulation', pp. 203–6; Sahner, *Christian Martyrs under Islam*.

425. Wasserstein, 'Samau'al ben Judah'.
426. Stroumsa, 'On Jewish Intellectuals Who Converted'.
427. al-Dhahabī, *Dhuyūl al-ʿIbar*, vol. IV, p. 3.
428. Mazor, 'Faraj Allāh Ibn Ṣaghīr'; Mazor, 'Jewish Court Physicians', p. 51.
429. For more on the literary culture and products of the Andalusian Jews see Brann, 'The Arabized Jews'.
430. CUL Or.1080 2.70; T-S Ar. 44.51.
431. Caballero-Navas, 'Medicine among Medieval Jews', p. 327.
432. Shefer, 'Physicians in the Mamluk and Ottoman Courts', p. 116; Chamberlain, *Knowledge and Social Practice*, pp. 136–7.
433. So far, we have been able to trace records of more than 607 Jewish practitioners.
434. My intention here is to shed light on another aspect of the Jewish practitioners, therefore the information in this section is fragmentary. Neither all the Jewish practitioners of the Muslim territories nor all the authors of medical books are represented here. I have no doubt that this issue deserves a separate research project and publication. When the Arabic book titles are presented, the English translation appears in brackets; when they are not, the English name or description of the book appears in inverted commas. Every translation was either taken from earlier publications or undertaken by members of my research group. Titles have been capitalised only in the case of known and accredited names (Maimonides' books for example).
435. Ibn al-Qifṭī, *Taʾrīkh al-Ḥukamā*, p. 320; Ibn Abī Uṣaybiʿa, *ʿUyūn al-Anbāʾ*, vol. II, p. 86; Meyerhof, 'Medieval Jewish Physicians in the Near East', p. 442; Goitein, 'The Medical Profession', p. 179; Ramaḍān, *al-Yahūd fī Miṣr*, pp. 433.
436. For detailed references, see the biographies in Chapter 3.
437. In this section I present some examples that evidence the poetry writing of Jewish practitioners which has been found, studied and published; it is only a fragmentary list to show the reader another aspect of the rich intellectual life of the practitioners. Naturally this issue is not the main topic of the book and deserves a more intensive study.
438. See in detail Makdisi, *The Rise of Humanism*, p. 333.
439. For a good and up-to-date introduction and many examples, see Ahmed, 'An Initial Survey of Arabic Poetry'.
440. See for example, Schirmann, 'Studies of the Research Institute'; Scheiber, 'Unbekannte Gedichte'.
441. Goitein, 'The Biography of Rabbi Judah ha-Levi'.

442. See for example Brann, *The Compunctious Poet*; Guetta and Itzhaki, *Studies in Medieval Jewish Poetry*; Tobi, *Between Hebrew and Arabic Poetry*; Yeshaya, *Medieval Hebrew Poetry*.
443. The poets are presented in chronological order.
444. Frenkel, *The Compassionate and Benevolent*, p. 97; Goitein, *A Mediterranean Society*, vol. II, p. 576 n. 21.
445. Frenkel, *The Compassionate and Benevolent*, pp. 95–6; Goitein, *A Mediterranean Society*, vol. II, pp. 258, 264, 580 nn. 96, 99.
446. For detailed references, see the biographies in Chapter 3.
447. Ibn Abī Uṣaybiʿa, *ʿUyūn al-Anbāʾ*, vol. II, pp. 116–17, 113–14; Jadon, 'A Comparison of the Wealth', p. 65; Meyerhof, 'Medieval Jewish Physicians in the Near East', p. 446; Ramaḍān, *al-Yahūd fī Miṣr*, p. 444; Ashtor-Strauss, 'Saladin and the Jews', p. 310; Kraemer, *Maimonides*, pp. 214–15; Goitein, *A Mediterranean Society*, vol. II, pp. 257–8.
448. Lasker, 'Israeli, Isaac ben Solomon'.
449. Kraemer, *Maimonides*.
450. See selected bibliography: Ibn Abī Uṣaybiʿa, *ʿUyūn al-Anbāʾ*, vol. II, p. 50; al-Andalusī, *Ṭabaqāt al-ʾUmam*, p. 204; Kaḥāla, *Muʿjam al-Muʾallifīn*, vol. III, p. 844; Delgado, 'Ibn Janāḥ'; Fenton, 'Jonah Ibn Ğanāḥ's Medical Dictionary', pp. 108, 116; Tenne, 'Ibn Janāḥ, Jonah'; Roth, *Jews, Visigoths and Muslims*, p. 78; Finkel, 'An Eleventh Century Source', p. 52; al-Andalusi, *Science in the Medieval World*, p. 8; Assis, 'Jewish Physicians and Medicine', p. 35; Amar and Serri, 'Compilation'; Kozodoy, 'The Jewish Physician in Medieval Iberia', p. 104; Caballero-Navas, 'Medicine among Medieval Jews', p. 328.
451. Cohen, 'Jews in the Mamlūk Environment'; Gottheil, 'Dhimmis and Moslems in Egypt', p. 384.
452. Wiet, *Cairo*, pp. 45–6, 55–6.
453. For detailed references, see the biography in Chapter 3.
454. Pormann and Savage-Smith, *Medieval Islamic Medicine*, p. 80.
455. Hazan, 'Medical, Administrative and Financial Aspects', pp. vi–vii.
456. Pormann and Savage-Smith, *Medieval Islamic Medicine*, p. 81.
457. See in detail Pormann, 'The Physician and the Other', p. 214.
458. Lewicka, 'The Non-Muslim Physician', p. 502.
459. Goitein, *A Mediterranean Society*, vol. I, p. 71 n. 2.
460. On the prominent position of Jews as bankers in the Muslim world, see for instance Fischel, *The Origin of Banking*. For Jews as long-distance merchants, see for instance Goitein's studies; Goldberg, *Trade and Institutions*, pp. 50–5,

116–17, 210–11, 350, 354–8. For Jewish careers in medieval Muslim territories and Europe, see Cohen, *Under Crescent and Cross*, pp. 77–103 (trade and banking), 134–5, 196 (medicine).

461. Cohen, *Poverty and Charity*, pp. 64–6; Cohen, *The Voice of the Poor*, pp. 165, 172–4, 176; based on dozens of lists of contributors (some lists had several doctors).
462. Goitein, *A Mediterranean Society*, vol. I, p. 76 n. 4, p. 248 nn. 109, 110.
463. Ibid., vol. II, pp. 250, 528.
464. Goitein, 'The Moses Maimonides–Ibn Sanā' al-Mulk Circle'.
465. Goitein, *A Mediterranean Society*, vol. I, pp. 329–30 n. 15.
466. Ibid., vol. I, p. 78, vol. II, p. 257.
467. Ibid., vol. II, p. 257.
468. Ibid., vol. I, p. 424 n. 100, vol. III, p. 251 n. 8.
469. Ibid., vol. I, p. 80 n. 17.
470. Ibid., vol. III, p. 503 n. 143.
471. Ibid., vol. II, pp. 23–4.
472. On the Jewish elite in medieval Egypt see Bareket, *Fustat on the Nile*.
473. Bosworth, 'Christian and Jewish Religious Dignitaries', p. 212.
474. See in detail Friedman, 'Maimonides *Rayyis al-Yahūd*'.
475. Goitein, *A Mediterranean Society*, vol. II, pp. 23–4; Goitein, *The Yemenites*, pp. 75–7.
476. The idea of the table is to assemble all the possible data regarding physicians that were chief leaders of the Jewish communities and present it together to the reader. The information in this table is based on the various biographies in Chapter 3 (physicians in Section 3.1.1, pharmacists in Section 3.1.2 and members of dynasties in Section 3.3.2); therefore, and for the sake of simplicity, I have omitted the references. For detailed references, see the biographies.
477. Cano, 'Ḥasday Ibn Shaprūṭ'.
478. Ashtor, *The Jews of Moslem Spain*, vol. I, pp. 162–3; Cano, 'Ḥasday Ibn Shaprūṭ'.
479. Goitein, *A Mediterranean Society*, vol. II, p. 247; Mann, *The Jews in Egypt and in Palestine*, vol. II, p. 282.
480. Bareket, 'Nagid' (I); Bareket, 'Nagid' (II); Ben-Sasson, 'The Maimonidean Dynasty', pp. 11–12; Goitein, *A Mediterranean Society*, vol. II, pp. 33–40, 243–5; Russ-Fishbane, *Judaism, Sufism, and the Pietists of Medieval Egypt*, p. 21.
481. Gil, *Jews in Islamic Countries*, p. 605.

482. The main debate is around the question of whether the formal position of the Headship of the Jews was established by the Fatimids on their conquest of Egypt around 969, or only about a century later. In addition, the Hebrew title *nagid* – a Biblical word having royal connotations – started to be used as an equivalent to *Raʾīs al-Yahūd* only in the first half of the thirteenth century. For the different views, see for instance Bareket, 'Nagid' (I); Bareket, 'Nagid' (II); Rustow, *Heresy and the Politics of Community*, pp. 102–7; Cohen, *Jewish Self-Government*; Stillman, 'The Non-Muslim Communities', pp. 204–5.
483. Ben-Sasson, 'The Maimonidean Dynasty', pp. 1–2.
484. Most of the data we have, though, concerns the first two members of this dynasty, i.e. Moses Maimonides and his son Abraham.
485. Mazor and Lev, 'Dynasties of Jewish Physicians'; Goitein, *A Mediterranean Society*, vol. II, p. 244.
486. See in detail Mazor and Lev, 'Dynasties of Jewish Physicians'.
487. Ibid.
488. Mazor and Lev, 'The Phenomenon'.
489. Mazor, 'Jewish Court Physicians'; Mazor, 'Asad al-Yahūdī'.
490. Ashtor, *The History of the Jews in Egypt and Syria*, vol. I, p. 346, vol. II, p. 174.
491. Goitein, *A Mediterranean Society*, vol. II, pp. 211–18.
492. Goitein claimed that 'this change was certainly attributable to the influence of the model of the Muslim Qadi, and also to the intrinsically institutional character of the later period'.
493. Goitein, *A Mediterranean Society*, vol. II, pp. 211–18.
494. TS 13J14.25; TS 10J26.2.
495. Goitein, 'The Oldest Documentary Evidence', p. 301.
496. Goitein, 'Meeting in Jerusalem', pp. 46–7; Goitein, *A Mediterranean Society*, vol. III, p. 245 nn. 158, 159; Motzkin, 'A Thirteenth-Century Jewish Physician', p. 344; Amar and Lev, *Physicians, Drugs and Remedies*, p. 105.
497. Goitein, *A Mediterranean Society*, vol. II, pp. 268–9.
498. Goitein and Friedman, *India Traders of the Middle Ages*, vol. I, 86. According to Goitein, the addressed Moses is Maimonides and not Moses b. Peraḥya.
499. al-Yūnīnī, *Early Mamluk Syrian Historiography*, vol. II, p. 255 (English translation vol. I, pp. 206–7): Ibn Ḥajar al-ʿAsqalānī, a*l-Durar al-Kāmina*, II, p. 476; al-Ṣafadī, *Aʿyān al-ʿAṣr*, vol. III, p. 65; Ibn Kathīr, *al-Bidāya wa-l-Nihāya*, vol. XIV, p. 86; el-Leithy, 'Coptic Culture and Conversion', pp. 173–4.
500. Ashtor, *The History of the Jews in Egypt and Syria*, vol. I, p. 346.

501. Steinschneider, *Die Arabische Literatur der Juden,* n. 199; Meyerhof, 'Medieval Jewish Physicians in the Near East', p. 45; Poznański, 'Recent Karaite Publications', p. 445; Margoliouth, 'Ibn Al-Hītī's Arabic Chronicle', 430; Meyerhof, 'Jewish Physicians Contemporaries of Maimonides', p. 399.
502. Adler, *Jewish Travelers*, p. 173; Ashtor, *The History of the Jews in Egypt and Syria,* vol. II, p. 44; Eisenstein, *Ozar Massaoth*, p. 94.
503. Ashtor, *The History of the Jews in Egypt and Syria*, vol. II, pp. 448–9; Arad, 'The Community as an Economic Body', pp. 54–5 n. 165.
504. Sambari, *Sefer Divrei Yosef,* p. 400; Ashtor, *The History of the Jews in Egypt and Syria,* vol. II, pp. 448–9.
505. al-Sakhāwī, *al-Ḍaw' al-Lāmi'*, vol. I, pp. 116–17.
506. al-Maqrīzī, *al-Mawā'iẓ*, vol. II, p. 409.
507. Amar and Lev, Physicians, Drugs and Remedies, p. 110.
508. Arad, 'The Community as an Economic Body', p. 54 n. 165; Ashtor, *The History of the Jews in Egypt and Syria,* vol. II, pp. 488–9; Sambari, *Sefer Divrei Yosef,* p. 400.
509. Frenkel, *The Compassionate and Beloved,* p. 27; Zeldes and Frenkel, 'The Sicilian Trade', p. 136.
510. Fischel, 'Azarbaijan in Jewish History', p. 18.
511. RNL Yevr. Ar. II 1378; Arad, 'A Pleasant Voice', p. 26.
512. Arad, 'The Community as an Economic Body', p. 61 n. 213.
513. Cohen, *Poverty and Charity*, p. 230.
514. Cohen, *The Voice of the Poor*, for example pp. 167–8, 172, 175; Cohen. *Poverty and Charity*, p. 60; Goitein, *A Mediterranean Society*, vol. I, p. 79, vol. II, p. 588.
515. Goitein, *A Mediterranean Society*, vol. I, p. 79 n. 10, vol. II, p. 588.
516. Cohen, 'The Burdensome Life'; Cohen, *Poverty and Charity*, p. 241.
517. Cohen, *Poverty and Charity*, p. 241.
518. The chart is based on the available data collected in this research.
519. The graph is based on the available data collected in this research.
520. Regarding the history of the Karaites, see in detail Lasker, 'Medieval Karaism and Science', p. 427; Astren, *Karaite Judaism*; Polliack, *Karaite Judaism*; Polliack, 'Rethinking Karaism'. Regarding their origin, see Gil, 'The Origin of the Karaites'; Gil, *Jews in Islamic Countries*, pp. 260–9. For an interesting point of view on how Muslim sources portrayed the Karaites, see Adang, 'The Karaites as Portrayed'.
521. Wasserstein and Wasserstein, *The Legend of the Septuagint*, p. 217.

522. Rustow, *Heresy and the Politics of Community*, pp. xv–xvii; see in depth Rustow, 'Karaites Real and Imagined'. On the Karaite communities in the Middle East during the medieval period, see Bareket, 'Karaite Communities in the Middle East'. Regarding their share in the Headship of the Jews, mainly during the Fatimid period, see Sela, 'The Headship of the Jews'.
523. Wasserstein and Wasserstein, *The Legend of the Septuagint*, p. 217.
524. Three more Karaites were mentioned as physicians by the translator of Ibn Al-Hītī's chronicle: Daniel al-Qūmisī, Sayyid ʿAnān and Yūsuf al-Baṣīr (10th–11th centuries); see Margoliouth, 'Ibn Al-Hītī's Arabic Chronicle', pp. 431–6. According to modern scholars (Dr David Sklare and Dr Avi Tal, personal communication), their identification as physicians was a translator's error. Yūsuf al-Baṣīr (Joseph b. Abraham ha-Roʾeh), a theologian and authority on Karaite law (960/970–1037/1039), studied medicine and philosophy; see Schwarb, 'Yūsuf al-Baṣīr'.
525. Lasker deals in detail with the accusation that Karaites did not believe in the use of medical care; see 'Medieval Karaism and Science', pp. 427–9; 'Karaism and Jewish Studies', pp. 21–5.
526. See in depth Mazor and Lev, 'The Phenomenon'.
527. The idea of the table is to assemble all the data regarding physicians and pharmacists of Karaite origin and present it to the reader. The information in this table is based on the various biographies in Chapter 3 (physicians in Section 3.1.1, pharmacists in Section 3.1.2 and members of dynasties in Section 3.3.2); therefore, and for the sake of simplicity, I have omitted references. For detailed references, see the biographies.
528. In this table I have assembled all available data regarding physicians and pharmacists of Samaritan origin and presented it together to the reader. The information in this table is based on the various biographies in Chapter 3 (physicians in Section 3.1.1, pharmacists in Section 3.1.2 and members of dynasties in Section 3.3.2); therefore, and for the sake of simplicity, I have omitted references. For detailed references, see the biographies.
529. On the Samaritans see in detail Pummer, *The Samaritans*; various chapters in Crown, *The Samaritans*; Montgomery, *The Samaritans*; Wasserstein and Wasserstein, *The Legend of the Septuagint*, p. 217.
530. Bosworth, 'Christian and Jewish Religious Dignitaries', p. 210.
531. Ashtor, *The Jews of Moslem Spain*.
532. A vast literature has been written on Muslim Spain; for example see Kennedy, *Muslim Spain and Portugal*. Regarding the Jews in Muslim Spain see for exam-

ple Roth, 'Andalucia'; Ashtor, *The Jews of Moslem Spain*; Scheindlin, *The Jews in Muslim Spain.*

533. See in detail Roth, *Jews, Visigoths and Muslims*, pp. 73–112; Wasserstein, *The Rise and Fall of the Party-Kings*, pp. 190–223; Brann, *Power in the Portrayal.*
534. Roth, *Jews, Visigoths and Muslims*, pp. 113–29; Weisz, 'The Jewish Physicians', p. 11.
535. See in detail: Roth, 'Andalucia'.
536. Reilly, *The Contest of Christian and Muslim Spain*, pp. 9, 15; Wasserstein, *The Rise and Fall of the Party-Kings*, pp. 191–2.
537. Wasserstein, 'Jewish Élites in al-Andalus', pp. 107–9.
538. See in detail dynasty 12.
539. Gil, *Palestine during the First Muslim Period*, vol. II, pp. 491–2; Goitein, *A Mediterranean Society*, vol. III, p. 207; Goitein and Friedman, *India Book I*, pp. 39–42, 45–6.
540. Ibn Abī Uṣaybiʿa, *ʿUyūn al-Anbāʾ*, vol. II, pp. 30–1; al-ʿUmarī, *Masālik al-Abṣār*, p. 264.
541. Ibn al-Qifṭī, *Taʾrīkh al-Ḥukamāʾ*, p. 209.
542. Fischel, 'Azarbaijan in Jewish History', p. 3; Ibn al-Qifṭī, *Taʾrīkh al-Ḥukamāʾ*, p. 209.
543. Wasserstein, 'Samauʾal ben Judah'; Stroumsa, 'On Jewish Intellectuals Who Converted'.
544. Cordova was conquered in 711 by the Muslims (Umayyads). It became the capital of the Muslims (716), and later of the caliphate of Cordova (766). The city became a centre of learning and scholarship; and by the tenth century had grown to be the largest in Europe (with hundreds of thousands of inhabitants); and one of the most advanced cities of the world from political, cultural and financial aspects, and an important industrial, agricultural and economic centre. Reilly claimed that the population of Cordova at that time was estimated at 90,000; see Reilly, *The Contest of Christian and Muslim Spain*, p. 9. The decline of the city started in 1002, its rulers died one after the other, and in 1031 the caliphate collapsed and the city became part of the *taifa* of Cordova. It returned to Christian hands in 1236. According to Ashtor, the number of the Jews of the city in the eleventh century was about 974; see Ashtor, 'The Number of Jews in Moslem Spain', pp. 50–1.
545. See in detail dynasty 3.
546. Ashtor, *The History of the Jews in Egypt and Syria*, vol. II, pp. 448–9; Arad, 'The Community as an Economic Body', pp. 54–5 n. 165.

547. Sambari, *Sefer Divrei Yosef*, p. 400; Ashtor, *The History of the Jews in Egypt and Syria*, vol. II, pp. 448–9.
548. Tortosa is a small city in present-day Catalonia, by the river Ebro on the slope of the mountains of the Cardó Massif. It was under Muslim rule for more than 400 years until conquered by the Crusaders, who were on their way to the Holy Land (1148).
549. 'Ibrahim Ibn Yaʿḳub, The Israelite', http://www.jewishencyclopedia.com/articles/8045-ibrahim-ibn-ya-kub-the-israeliteJewishEncyclopedia.com (accessed 29 September 2020).
550. al-Qazwīnī, *ʿAjāʾib al-Makhlūqāt.*
551. Miquel, 'Ibrāhīm b. Yaʿḳūb'; al-Khālidī, al-Yahūd Taḥta Ḥukm al-Muslimīn, p. 107; Ashtor, 'Ibrahim Ibn Yaʿqūb'.
552. Denia is an historical small coastal town between Alicante and Valencia. After the Muslim conquest it became the capital of a *taifa* kingdom that ruled over part of the Valencian coast and Ibiza. The city changed hands between Saqaliba, lord of Saragossa, and the Almoravids. The latter built the castle fortress after 1091. The town was reconquered by the Christians in 1244. On the Jews of Deniza see in depth Bruce, 'The Taifa of Denia'.
553. Roth, *Jews, Visigoths and Muslims*, p. 94; Friedenwald, *The Jews and Medicine*, p. 633; Finkel, 'An Eleventh Century Source', p. 52; al-Andalusī, *Ṭabaqāt al-ʾUmam*, pp. 204–5; Delgado, 'Ibn Yashūsh, Isaac'; Roth, 'Medicine', p. 436; Steinschneider, *Die Arabische Literatur der Juden*, p. 135; Neubauer, 'Sur la lexicographie hébraïque'. p. 249; Ashtor, *The Jews of Moslem Spain*, vol. II, p. 293; Ashtor, *Ibn Yashush*, vol. IX, p. 699.
554. Barcelona is a big city with a long and diverse history; it is the capital of Catalonia and located on the Mediterranean coast. After being conquered by the Muslims at the beginning of the eighth century it was then conquered in 801 by the Christians. In 985, Barcelona was conquered again by the Muslims. In 1137 it fell once more into Christian hands.
555. Prats, 'Ibn ʿAknīn'; Roth, 'Medicine', p. 436; Kraemer, *Maimonides*, pp. 116–17, 92.
556. Ronda is a small town located about 100 kilometres west of the city of Malaga. It was conquered by the Muslims and became the capital of a *taifa* (a small kingdom ruled by the Berbers) after they broke away from the caliphate of Cordova. In 1065, Ronda was conquered by the *taifa* of Seville. The Islamic domination of Ronda ended in 1485. Al-Maqqarī, *Nafḥ al-Ṭīb*, vol. III, pp. 528–9; Friedenwald, *The Jews and Medicine*, p. 634; Roth, *Jews, Visigoths and Muslims*,

p. 174; Ibn Saʿīd al-Andalusī, *al-Mughrib*, vol. I, p. 336; Hammer-Purgstall, *Literaturgeschichte der Araber*, vol. VI. p. 482; Steinschneider, *Jewish Literature from the Eighth to the Eighteenth Century*, p. 170. al-Khālidī, *al-Yahūd Taḥta Ḥukm al-Muslimīn*, p. 356.

557. Toledo is a city located in central Spain; the capital of the Visigoth kingdom (542–725). After the Muslim conquest (8th century), Toledo was ruled from Cordova under the command of the Umayyad caliph in Damascus. The city was controlled and fought over by various forces, Muslim as well as Christian. After the fall of the Umayyad caliphate in the early eleventh century, Toledo became the capital city of one of the richest *taifas* of Andalusia, and due to its central location, the city had a substantial role to play in the struggles between the Muslim and Christian rulers of northern Spain. The conquest of Toledo in 1085 marked the first time that a major city in Andalusia was captured by Christian forces. According to Ashtor, the number of inhabitants of the city in the eleventh century was about 37,000, of which 10 per cent (3,700) were Jews; see Ashtor, 'The Number of Jews in Moslem Spain', pp. 39–40. It is important to mention here that Wasserstein argued that 'there are too many uncertainties and variables and excessively large margins of error in Ashtor's methods to make his results either acceptable or useable'; see Wasserstein, 'Jewish Élites in al-Andalus', p. 107. However, Reilly claimed that the population of Toledo at this time was estimated as 28,000, including a Jewish population of about 4,000' see Reilly, *The Contest of Christian and Muslim Spain*, pp. 9, 15.

558. Granada is located at the foot of the Sierra Nevada mountains, at an average elevation of 738 metres. The city was conquered by the Muslims (Umayyads) at the beginning of the eighth century and became one of the most important cities of Andalusia in the early eleventh century. After the collapse of the Umayyad caliphate (early 11th century) the Berbers established an independent kingdom, the *taifa* of Granada. The Zirid *taifa* of Granada became a centre of Jewish culture and scholarship. From 1027 to 1066 Granada had a powerful and fruitful Jewish community, partly headed by Samuel b. Nagrila (who was also a *wazīr* 1037–56), and included several known scholars such as Moses Ibn Ezra, Judah ha-Levi and Ibn Gabirol. The massacre of the Jews took place in 1066, at the end of the Golden Age of Jewish culture in Spain. The Almoravids ruled the city from 1090 until 1166, then were replaced by the Almohads. The Nasrids took over in 1228, and they officially became the emirate of Granada in 1238. During Moorish rule, various religions and ethnic groups such as Muslims, Arabs, Berbers, Christians and Jews lived there in separate quarters.

The emirate of Granada surrendered to the Christians in 1492, the event which marked the completion of the Reconquista of al-Andalus. According to Ashtor, the number of the inhabitants of the city in the eleventh century was about 26,000, of which 20 per cent (about 5,392) were Jews; see Ashtor, 'The Number of Jews in Moslem Spain', pp. 51–2. Reilly claimed that the population of Granada at this time was estimated at 20,000; see Reilly, *The Contest of Christian and Muslim Spain*, pp. 9, 15.

559. Scheindlin, 'Judah (Abū al-Ḥasan) ben Samuel ha-Levi'; Gil and Fleischer, *Yehuda ha-Levi and His Circle*; Silman, *Philosopher and Prophet*; Goitein, *A Mediterranean Society*, vol. V, pp. 448–51; Goitein, 'The Biography of Rabbi Judah ha-Levi'.
560. Yahalom and Blau, *The Wanderings of Judah Alharizi*, p. 51, ll. 43–4; Segal, *The Book of Taḥkemonī*, p. 335, gate 46.
561. Seville was conquered by the Muslims in 712. During Muslim rule, Seville was under the jurisdiction of the caliphate of Cordova before becoming independent. Later it was ruled by the Almoravids and the Almohads until the Christian conquest in 1248. According to Ashtor, the number of the Jews in the city in the eleventh century was 5,222; see Ashtor, 'The Number of Jews in Moslem Spain', pp. 53–4. Reilly claimed that the population of Seville at that time was estimated at 52,000, including a Jewish population of about 5,000; see Reilly, *The Contest of Christian and Muslim Spain*, pp. 9, 15.
562. Friedenwald, *The Jews and Medicine*, p. 634; Alfonso, 'Ibn al-Muʿallim, Solomon'; Roth, *Jews, Visigoths and Muslims*, p. 175.
563. Bos, *Maimonides on Asthma*, pp. 102–5; Alfonso, 'Ibn al-Muʿallim, Solomon'; Friedenwald, *The Jews and Medicine*, p. 634; Roth, 'Medicine', p. 436; al-Khālidī, *al-Yahūd Taḥta Ḥukm al-Muslimīn*, pp. 190–1; Weisz, 'The Jewish Physicians', p. 27.
564. Alfonso, 'Ibn al-Muʿallim, Solomon'; al-Ḥarīzī, *Taḥkemoni*, no. 45.
565. al-Zarhūnī, *al-Ṭibb*, p. 58.
566. Friedenwald, *The Jews and Medicine*, p. 633; Ibn Abī Uṣaybiʿa, *ʿUyūn al-Anbāʾ*, vol. II, pp. 50–1; al-Shantarīnī, *al-Dhakhīra*, pp. 458–9; al-Andalusī, *Ṭabaqāt al-ʾUmam*, pp. 204–5; Steinschneider, *Die Arabische Literatur der Juden*, p. 100, n. 3.
567. See in detail dynasty 2.
568. Cano, 'Ḥasday Ibn Shaprūṭ'; Roth, 'Medicine', p. 434; Ashtor, *The Jews of Moslem Spain*, vol. I, pp. 162–3, 167; Finkel, 'An Eleventh Century Source', p. 51; Ibn Abī Uṣaybiʿa, *ʿUyūn al-Anbāʾ*, vol. II, p. 50; al-Andalusī, *Ṭabaqāt*

al-ʾUmam, pp. 203–4; al-Zarhūnī, *al-Ṭibb*, p. 35; Ibn Juljul, *Ṭabaqāt al-Aṭibbāʾ*, p. 22.

569. Friedenwald, *The Jews and Medicine*, p. 633.
570. Lucena is a town in southern Spain, 140 kilometres east of Seville, 60 kilometres southeast of Cordova and 105 kilometres west of Granada. It is situated on the river Lucena, at an important crossroads in the centre of Andalusia. It was inhabited almost exclusively by Jews, similar to Granada and Tarragona. The Jews were involved in industry and commerce, and many of them were scholars and considered wealthy. The Jews lived peacefully until the Almoravid conquest. Lucena was conquered by the Christians in 1240.
571. The city of Saragossa (Zaragoza) lies at an elevation of 199 metres. Following the destruction of the caliphate of Cordova, for 100 years (1018–1118) Saragossa was a *taifa* kingdom. In 1118, the Christians conquered the city and made it the capital of the kingdom of Aragon. See in detail Beech, *The Brief Eminence*. According to Ashtor, the number of the inhabitants of the city in the eleventh century was about 20,000, of which 6.3 per cent (2,760) were Jews; see: Ashtor, 'The Number of Jews in Moslem Spain', pp. 42–3. Reilly claimed that the population of Saragossa at this time was estimated at 17,000, including a Jewish population of about 1,200; see Reilly, *The Contest of Christian and Muslim Spain*, pp. 9, 15.
572. Tenne, 'Ibn Janāḥ, Jonah'; Roth, *Jews, Visigoths and Muslims*, p. 78; Delgado, 'Ibn Janāḥ'; Fenton, 'Jonah Ibn Ǧanāḥ's Medical Dictionary', pp. 108–18; Ibn Abī Uṣaybiʿa, *ʿUyūn al-Anbāʾ*, vol. II, p. 50; al-Andalusī, *Ṭabaqāt al-ʾUmam*, p. 204; Finkel, 'An Eleventh Century Source', p. 52; al-Andalusi, *Science in the Medieval World*, p. 81; Assis, 'Jewish Physicians and Medicine', p. 35; Roth, 'Medicine', p. 436; Amar and Serri, 'Compilation'; Kozodoy, 'The Jewish Physician in Medieval Iberia', p. 104; Kaḥāla, *Muʿjam al-Muʾallifin*, vol. III, p. 844.
573. Ibn Abī Uṣaybiʿa, *ʿUyūn al-Anbāʾ*, vol. II, p. 50; al-Andalusī, *Ṭabaqāt al-ʾUmam*, p. 204; Finkel, 'An Eleventh Century Source', p. 52; Kozodoy, 'The Jewish Physician in Medieval Iberia', p. 104; Roth, *Jews, Visigoths and Muslims*, p. 176; Roth, 'Medicine', p. 436; Friedenwald, *The Jews and Medicine*, p. 633.
574. Steinschneider, *Die Arabische Literatur der Juden*, pp. 148–9; Friedenwald, *The Jews and Medicine*, pp. 174, 633; Alfonso, 'Ibn Ḥasday, Joseph'; Sarton, *Introduction to the History of Science*, vol. II, pp. 229–30; Roth, 'Medicine', p. 435.
575. Almeria is a small town located on the Mediterranean Sea. It was conquered by

the Muslims at the beginning of the tenth century and the citadel (*mariyyah*) that gave the town its name was built (955). During the tenth and the eleventh centuries the town was part of the caliphate of Cordova and became wealthy thanks to the textile and silk industries and trade. After the fall of the caliphate of Cordova (1031), Almeria was ruled by local Muslim *taifa* emirs. Almeria fell within a decade into the hands of the Almoravids and became again a Christian town in 1489. According to Ashtor, the number of the inhabitants of the city in the eleventh century was about 27,000, of which 7.4 per cent (2,000) were Jews; see Ashtor, 'The Number of Jews in Moslem Spain', p. 50.

576. Serry and Lev, 'A Judaeo-Arabic Fragment'; Dietrich, 'Ibn Biklārish', Levey, 'The Pharmacology of Ibn Biklārish'; Burnett, *Ibn Baklarish's Book of Simples*; Kozodoy, 'The Jewish Physician in Medieval Iberia', p. 103; Ullmann, *Islamic Medicine*, pp. 201, 275; Ibn Abī Uṣaybiʿa, *ʿUyūn al-Anbāʾ*, vol. II, p. 52; Steinschneider, *Die Arabische Literatur der Juden*, p. 147.
577. Ibn Ḥazm al-Andalusī, *Rasāʾil Ibn Ḥazm*, vol. I, p. 114; Kozodoy, 'The Jewish Physician in Medieval Iberia', p. 104; Roth, *Jews, Visigoths and Muslims*, p. 180; al-Khālidī, *al-Yahūd Taḥta Ḥukm al-Muslimīn*, 356.
578. TS 8J18.9.
579. Goitein and Friedman, *India Book IV/B*, pp. 226–34 nn. 44, 45.
580. Stroumsa, 'Between Acculturation and Conversion', pp. 28–9.
581. Roth, 'Medicine', p. 439–40.
582. On this phenomenon see in detail Section 3.3.
583. On this phenomenon see in general Weisz, 'The Jewish Physicians'; Shatzmiller, *Jews, Medicine, and Medieval Society*.
584. See Map 1.
585. See in detail dynasty 10.
586. Ibn Abī Uṣaybiʿa, *ʿUyūn al-Anbāʾ*, vol. II, pp. 30–1; al-ʿUmarī, *Masālik al-Abṣār*, p. 264; Ibn al-Qifṭī, *Taʾrīkh al-Ḥukamāʾ*, p. 209.
587. Ibn al-Qifṭī, *Taʾrīkh al-Ḥukamāʾ*, pp. 392–4; Lasker, 'Ibn Simeon, Judah b. Joseph'; Yahalom and Blau, *The Wanderings of Judah Alharizi*, pp. 33–4; Meyerhof, 'Jewish Physicians Contemporaries of Maimonides', p. 393.
588. Miller, 'Doctors without Borders', p. 113; Yahalom and Blau, *The Wanderings of Judah Alharizi*, pp. 33–4; Meyerhof, 'Jewish Physicians Contemporaries of Maimonides', p. 393; Kraemer, *Maimonides*, pp. 363–4.
589. See in detail dynasty 39.
590. Mazor, 'Jewish Court Physicians', p. 61.
591. See Mazor and Lev, 'Dynasties of Jewish Physicians'.

592. Steinschneider, *Die Arabische Literatur der Juden*, n. 199; Meyerhof, 'Medieval Jewish Physicians in the Near East', p. 445; Poznański, 'Recent Karaite Publications', p. 445; Margoliouth, 'Ibn Al-Hītī's Arabic Chronicle', p. 430; Meyerhof, 'Jewish Physicians Contemporaries of Maimonides', p. 399; Ashtor, *The History of the Jews in Egypt and Syria*, vol. II, p. 557–9.
593. TS AS 146.24.
594. Qayrawān, also known as Kairouan, is a city in present-day Tunisia that was founded by the Umayyads (around 670) and became an important Islamic centre. Mahdiyya is the former capital city of the Fatimid caliphate, situated not far from Qayrawān.
595. Ben-Sasson, *The Emergence of the Local Jewish Community.*
596. See in detail dynasty 1.
597. See in detail Mazor and Lev, 'Dynasties of Jewish Physicians'.
598. Ben-Sasson, *The Emergence of the Local Jewish Community*, pp. 182, 381.
599. Ibn al-Qifṭī, *Taʾrīkh al-Ḥukamāʾ*, p. 320; Mann, *The Jews in Egypt and in Palestine*, p. 18; Miller, 'Doctors without Borders', pp. 111–12.
600. Hirschberg, *The History of Ophthalmology*, p. 205.
601. Meyerhof, 'Medieval Jewish Physicians in the Near East', p. 442.
602. al-Maqrīzī, *al-Muqaffā*, vol. II, p. 57.
603. Sela, 'The Head of the Rabbanite, Karaite and Samaritan Jews', p. 264.
604. al-Maqrīzī, al-*Muqaffā*, vol. II, p. 57; Ibn Abī Uṣaybiʿa, *ʿUyūn al-Anbāʾ*, vol. II, p. 86; al-Maqrīzī, *Ittiʿāẓ al-Ḥunafāʾ*, vol. I, p. 146.
605. Bareket, 'Ibn Furāt Abraham', p. 3 n. 9; Lewis, 'Palṭiel'; Sela, 'The Head of the Rabbanite, Karaite and Samaritan Jews', pp. 262–4; Gottheil, 'An Eleventh-Century Document', p. 467.
606. Miller, 'Doctors without Borders', pp. 117–18.
607. Ben-Sasson, *The Emergence of the Local Jewish Community*, p. 381.
608. Lasker, 'Israeli, Isaac ben Solomon'.
609. Ibn Murād, *Buḥūth*, pp. 93–5.
610. Ben-Sasson, *The Emergence of the Local Jewish Community*, pp. 348–62; Goitein, *Three Letters from Qayrawan*, pp. 166–9, 174–5; Goitein, 'The Qayrawan United Appeal', pp. 160–2; Stillman, 'Ibn ʿAṭāʾ, Abū Isḥāq Ibrāhīm'.
611. Stillman, 'Ibn ʿAṭāʾ, Abū Isḥāq Ibrāhīm'; Ben-Sasson, *The Emergence of the Local Jewish Community*, pp. 23, 353.
612. Wechsler, 'Ibn Sughmar Family'.
613. Goitein, *A Mediterranean Society*, vol. III, pp. 202 n. 195, 469 n. 95; Bareket, *The Jewish Leadership in Fusṭāṭ*, pp. 166–8.

614. On Abraham see Goitein and Friedman, *India Traders of the Middle Ages*, p. 52–89; on his medical knowledge see ibid., 68.
615. Lambourn, *Abraham's Luggage.*
616. TS Ar. 41.81.
617. Goitein and Friedman, *India Traders of the Middle Ages*, p. 84.
618. See in detail dynasty 8.
619. A long (about 190 kilometres) cultivated and populated valley which stretches along the two banks of the river Darʿa. The river rises on the southern slope of the High Atlas and flows west into the Atlantic on the edge of the Sahara. Jews lived in the area until the twentieth century.
620. Yeshaya, 'Darʿī, Moses ben Abraham'; Weinberger, 'Moses Darʿī', pp. 445, 450, 452, 454.
621. See in detail dynasty 9.
622. Roth, *Jews, Visigoths and Muslims*, p. 115.
623. Bos, *Maimonides on Asthma*, pp. 102–5; Alfonso, 'Ibn al-Muʿallim, Solomon'.
624. A major city of Morocco (until the present day), located on the northern foothills of the Atlas Mountains. Founded in 1062, it was much improved in the twelfth century by the Almoravids. After a period of decline, in the sixteenth century Marrakesh became again the capital of Morocco.
625. Roth, *Jews, Visigoths and Muslims*, p. 88; Salvatierra, 'Ibn Qamni'el, Me'ir'.
626. A major city in northern inland Morocco, located northeast of the Atlas Mountains, where roads to the main cities of Morocco meet. Fez was founded in the 8th–9th centuries, and under Almoravid rule, the city expanded and was considered one of the largest in the world (12th century).
627. Prats, 'Ibn ʿAknīn, Joseph b. Judah Jacob'; Roth, 'Medicine', p. 436.
628. Kraemer, *Maimonides*, pp. 116–17, 92.
629. al-Khālidī, *al-Yahūd Taḥta Ḥukm al-Muslimīn*, p. 357.
630. Ibn Khaldūn, *Taʾrīkh al-ʿAlāma*, pt. 1, vol. VII, p. 632.
631. The Jews lived in many Sicilian cities such as Messina, Catania and Palermo from early periods. Sicily was attacked a few times by the Muslims, who finally conquered it in 965, enabling the Jewish communities to prosper. From 1072 to 1194 the Normans ruled parts of the island, and later the Crusaders and other Christian regimes.
632. On the Jews in Sicily see in depth Roth, 'Sicily'; Gil, *Jews in Islamic Countries*, pp. 563–93; Ben-Sasson, *The Jews of Sicily*; Simonsohn, *The Jews in Sicily*, pp. xi–xxxv.

633. Goitein and Friedman, *India Book III*, p. 362.
634. See Map 2.
635. Asher, *The Itinerary of Rabbi Benjamin*, p. 147; Ashtor, 'The Number of Jews in Mediaeval Egypt', 18(1–4), pp. 13, 20.
636. Ashtor, 'The Number of Jews in Mediaeval Egypt', 19(1–4), p. 12.
637. Neustadt, 'Contribution to the Economic History'.
638. Ashtor, The Number of the Jews in Mediaeval Egypt', 19(1–4), p. 13.
639. On Old Cairo see Section 2.3 and more, for example Vorderstrasse and Treptow, *A Cosmopolitan City*.
640. On the life of the Jews in the medieval Islamic city see Stillman, 'The Jew in the Medieval Islamic City'.
641. Pormann and Savage-Smith, *Medieval Islamic Medicine*, p. 108.
642. Goitein, *A Mediterranean Society*, vol. II, p. 288. It might be interesting for the reader to look at a study made by Carl Petry of geographical origins of the Muslim learned elite of fifteenth-century Cairo; see in detail Petry, *The Civilian Elite of Cairo*.
643. Gottheil and Worrell, *Fragments from the Cairo Genizah*, vol. III, p. 22, ll. 7–10; Goitein, *A Mediterranean Society*, vol. II, p. 255.
644. Ashtor, 'The Number of Jews in Mediaeval Egypt', 19(1–4), p. 6.
645. Goitein, *A Mediterranean Society*, vol. IV, p. 401 n. 123.
646. See in depth Frenkel, *The Compassionate and Benevolent*; Ashtor, 'The Number of Jews in Mediaeval Egypt', 19(1–4), pp. 8–12.
647. Asher, *The Itinerary of Rabbi Benjamin*, p. 158; Ashtor, 'The Number of Jews in Mediaeval Egypt', 18(1–4), p. 13.
648. Ashtor, 'The Number of Jews in Mediaeval Egypt', 19(1–4), p. 12.
649. Ibid.
650. For more details and references, see biographies at Chapter 3.
651. Ashtor, 'The Number of Jews in Mediaeval Egypt', 19(1–4), p. 9 n. 328.
652. Wien, N: H 85 (PER H 85); Goitein, *A Mediterranean Society*, vol. III, pp. 160–1, 461.
653. See in detail dynasty 14.
654. Frenkel, *The Compassionate and Benevolent*, pp. 338–9.
655. See Goitein, *A Mediterranean Society*, vol. II, pp. 249–51 with n. 42.
656. Rustow, 'Mevorakh ben Saʿadya'; Sela, 'The Head of the Rabbanite, Karaite and Samaritan Jews', p. 260.
657. .Ashtor, 'New Data for the History of Levantine Jewries', p. 76.
658. Ashtor, 'The Number of Jews in Mediaeval Egypt', 18(1–4), pp. 23–7.

659. Asher, *The Itinerary of Rabbi Benjamin of Tudela*, p. 154; Ashtor, 'The Number of Jews in Mediaeval Egypt', 18(1–4), p. 13.
660. Ashtor, 'The Number of Jews in Mediaeval Egypt', 19(1–4), p. 12.
661. Goitein, *A Mediterranean Society*, vol. II, p. 446 sec. 31, vol. III, p. 303 n. 124, 125.
662. Asher, *The Itinerary of Rabbi Benjamin of Tudela*, p. 154; Ashtor, 'The Number of Jews in Mediaeval Egypt', 18(1–4), pp. 18–19.
663. Golb, 'The Topography of the Jews VI', pp. 124–5; Golb, 'The Topography of the Jews', pp. 249–51; Goitein, *A Mediterranean Society*, vol. II, pp. 111, 485 n. 37.
664. Asher, *The Itinerary of Rabbi Benjamin of Tudela*, p. 158; Ashtor, 'The Number of the Jews in Mediaeval Egypt', 19(1–4), pp. 2–3.
665. Ashtor, 'The Number of Jews in Mediaeval Egypt', 18(1–4), p. 13.
666. Ibid., 19(1–4), p. 12.
667. Goitein and Friedman, *India Book IV/B*, p. 39.
668. Meyerhof, 'Jewish Physicians Contemporaries of Maimonides', pp. 397–8; Mazor, 'Ibn Ṣaghīr/Ibn Kūjik Family'; Mazor, 'Jewish Court Physicians', p. 46; Mazor, 'Sadīd al-Dimyāṭī'; al-Ṣafadī, *Kitāb al-Wāfī bi-l-Wafayāt* (2008–10), vol. XV, pp. 127–8.
669. Goitein, *A Mediterranean Society*, vol. I, p. 252 n. 131, vol. II, p. 130 n. 30.
670. Asher, *The Itinerary of Rabbi Benjamin of Tudela*, p. 154; Ashtor, 'The Number of Jews in Mediaeval Egypt', 18(1–4), p. 13.
671. Ashtor, 'The Number of Jews in Mediaeval Egypt', 19(1–4), p. 12.
672. Richards, 'A Doctor's Petition', p. 303.
673. TS 10J17.19.
674. TS NS 226.30; Goitein, *A Mediterranean Society*, vol. II, pp. 485, 508, App. C 139.
675. Asher, *The Itinerary of Rabbi Benjamin of Tudela*, p. 154; Ashtor, 'The Number of Jews in Mediaeval Egypt', 18(1–4), p. 13.
676. Ashtor, 'The Number of Jews in Mediaeval Egypt' 19(1–4), p. 12.
677. Steinschneider, 'An Introduction to the Arabic Literature of the Jews I', 11(1), p. 118.
678. Goitein, *A Mediterranean Society*, vol. II, pp. 48–9, vol. IV, p. 335 n. 196.
679. Molad-Vaza, 'Clothing in the Mediterranean Jewish Society', pp. 331–5.
680. Ashtor, 'Some Features of the Jewish Communities', p. 65.
681. TS Misc. 20.183.
682. Ashtor, 'Some Features of the Jewish Communities', p. 69.

683. See for example the letters at https://cudl.lib.cam.ac.uk/search?keyword =Minyat%20Zifta&page=1 (accessed 8 September 2020).
684. Goitein, *A Mediterranean Society*, vol. II, p. 189 n. 24; a letter from Minyat Ziftā addressed to Abraham II Maimonides.
685. Goitein, *A Mediterranean Society*, vol. II, p. 46 n. 81.
686. Bodl. MS heb. d. 66, fol. 57 (2878); Golb, 'The Topography of the Jews VI', p. 134.
687. Ashtor, 'The Number of Jews in Mediaeval Egypt', 18(1–4), pp. 21–2.
688. Goitein, *A Mediterranean Society*, vol. II, p. 257.
689. Ashtor, 'The Number of Jews in Mediaeval Egypt', 18(1–4), pp. 14–16.
690. Asher, *The Itinerary of Rabbi Benjamin of Tudela*, p. 147.
691. Ashtor, 'The Number of Jews in Mediaeval Egypt', 18(1–4), p. 13; ibid., 19(1–4), p. 12.
692. Goitein, *A Mediterranean Society*, vol. III, p. 390; Ashtor, 'The Number of Jews in Mediaeval Egypt', 18(1–4), p. 15, Appendix B, no. 1.
693. Golb, 'The Topography of the Jews VI', pp. 136–7; Goitein, *A Mediterranean Society*, vol. II, pp. 258–9.
694. Goitein, *A Mediterranean Society*, vol. II, p. 380 n. 32.
695. Golb, 'The Topography of the Jews VI', p. 145.
696. Ibid., p. 142; Goitein, *A Mediterranean Society*, vol. II, p. 254.
697. Ashtor, 'The Number of Jews in Mediaeval Egypt', 19(1–4), pp. 4–6.
698. Asher, *The Itinerary of Rabbi Benjamin of Tudela*, p. 159; Ashtor, 'The Number of Jews in Mediaeval Egypt', 18(1–4), p. 13.
699. Ashtor, 'The Number of Jews in Mediaeval Egypt', 19(1–4), p. 12.
700. Goitein and Friedman, *India Book I*, p. 262; Goitein, *A Mediterranean Society*, vol. IV, pp. 317–18.
701. Ashtor, 'The Number of Jews in Mediaeval Egypt', 19(1–4), p. 5 n. 288; Goitein and Friedman, *India Book I*, p. 254.
702. Goitein, *A Mediterranean Society*, vol. II, p. 254.
703. See Map 3.
704. Bacher, 'Scham als Name Palästina's'.
705. For a detailed description of Bilād al-Shām and its various districts, see Le Strange, *Palestine under the Muslims*, pp. 14–43.
706. See in depth Eddé, 'Les Médecins dans la société syrienne'.
707. See for example Hofer, 'The Ideology of Decline'.
708. The information on the practitioners in this section has been extracted from the biographies in Chapter 3. In many cases the names also appear in some of

the tables and other sections of the book; therefore, and for the sake of better reading, references have been omitted.

709. For more about the history of the city, mainly in the late medieval–early modern periods, see Boogert, *Aleppo Observed.*

710. Asher, *The Itinerary of Rabbi Benjamin of Tudela*, p. 88.

711. Frenkel, 'The Medieval Jewish Community of Aleppo'.

712. Frenkel, 'The Leadership of the Community in Aleppo'.

713. On intellectual life in the city see Chamberlain, *Knowledge and Social Practice.*

714. On the Jewish community in Damascus during the classical Geniza period see Cohen, 'The Jewish Community in Damascus'.

715. Asher, *The Itinerary of Rabbi Benjamin of Tudela*, pp. 85–6.

716. Ibid.

717. For the Jewish communities in Eretz-Israel in general and in Jerusalem in particular, see Goitein, *Palestinian Jewry.*

718. Amar and Lev, *Physicians, Drugs and Remedies.*

719. Amar, *The History of Medicine in Jerusalem.*

720. Ophthalmologist and *dayyān*, his clinic was located in a rented store in Sūq al-ʿAṭṭārīn.

721. See detailed biographies in Section 3.1.1.

722. For more about the Jewish physicians in medieval Muslim Jerusalem see Amar and Lev, *Physicians, Drugs and Remedies*, pp. 105–11; Amar, *The History of Medicine in Jerusalem*, pp. 135–8.

723. For more about medieval Ramle and its Jewish community see in depth Gil, *Palestine during the First Muslim Period*; Asher, *The Itinerary of Rabbi Benjamin of Tudela*, p. 79.

724. For more about the town and Jewish life and activity in medieval Safed see in depth Gil, *Palestine during the First Muslim Period.*

725. Acre (Akko) is an ancient city on the coastal plain of northern Israel, sitting in a natural harbour on the Mediterranean Sea. It has always been an important trade centre; after the city was captured by the Muslims (638) it served as the main port of Palestine during the rule of the Umayyads, Abbasids, Mamluks and Crusaders (during that period, for a good dozen years it was even the capital of the Jerusalem kingdom). The city had a Jewish community throughout most of those periods. For a description of the city and its Jewish community in the second half of the twelfth century, see Asher, *The Itinerary of Rabbi Benjamin of Tudela*, p. 64.

726. Amman is the capital of present-day Jordan. It lies on the fringe of the Syrian

Desert and was even called 'Harbour of the Desert'. The Roman/Byzantine city was captured by the Muslims in 630; it was part of the Umayyad caliphate, which rebuilt it, but it was repeatedly destroyed by earthquakes. The city was functioning during the Abbasid, Fatimid, Crusader, Ayyubid and Mamluk regimes and had a small Jewish community.

727. See Section 3.3.2, dynasty 14.
728. Ashkelon (Ashqelon, Ascalon) is a coastal fortified ancient city in southern Israel, 50 kilometres south of Jaffa. Its seaport served all the rulers of the land including the various Muslim regimes and the Crusaders until it was destroyed (1270). Ashkelon changed hands many times and suffered from heavy battles. The medieval Jewish community numbered a few hundred Rabbanite and Karaite Jews; upon the destruction of the city they moved to Jerusalem. For more on the community see Yagur, 'Between Egypt and Jerusalem'.
729. See in detail dynasty 21.
730. Baalbek is an ancient (Greek, Roman, Byzantine) city in northern Lebanon, 85 kilometres northeast of Beirut, in the Beqaa Valley. It was conquered by the Muslims in 634 and fortified, and since then has changed hands between the various Muslim and Christian powers. The city also suffered during the medieval period from various earthquakes and other natural disasters.
731. Hama is a city in central western Syria, 213 kilometres north of Damascus, on the banks of the river Orontes. Hama was conquered by the Muslims (638/639) and became a market town surrounded by a wall. Between the tenth and the twelfth centuries it was under the rule of Aleppo. The city changed hands throughout its history and was ruled by various Muslim and Crusader regimes.
732. Jaffa (Yaffa) is an ancient commercial port city in present-day Israel; it was conquered by the Muslims (636) and served as a port of their provincial capital Ramle. The city was captured by the Crusaders in 1099 and served as the main port of Jerusalem and the Crusaders' kingdom. In 1187 the city was conquered again by the Muslims (Saladin) and later changed hands a few times. In 1268 it was captured by the Mamluks. For a description of the city and its Jewish community in the second half of the twelfth century, see Asher, *The Itinerary of Rabbi Benjamin of Tudela*, p. 79.
733. Raqqah is an ancient fortified city on the road between Iraq and Syria, located on the banks of the river Euphrates, about 160 kilometres east of Aleppo. It was conquered by the Muslims (639/640) and afterwards became an important city to the various Muslim regimes. An active Christian community was

reported in the Middle Ages as well as a Jewish one that survived until about the twelfth century.

734. Tiberias is a city on the western shore of the Sea of Galilee known for its hot springs. It was always an important centre of Judaism and from the sixteenth century on was considered one of the Four Holy Cities. It was conquered by the Muslims in 634 and served as the regional capital; during most of the Muslim rule it had a Jewish community. Jewish scholarship flourished in the city mainly between the eighth and the tenth centuries. The city was destroyed by a series of earthquakes and was ruled for about a dozen years by the Crusaders. Maimonides is believed to be buried in this city. For a description of the city and its Jewish community in the second half of the twelfth century, see Asher, *The Itinerary of Rabbi Benjamin of Tudela*, p. 81.
735. See for example: Gil, *Palestine during the First Muslim Period*, vol. II, pp. 458–75.
736. Tripoli is an ancient port city in northern Lebanon, 85 kilometres north of Beirut. It became a commercial and shipbuilding centre under the various Muslim regimes and was occupied by the Crusaders for about 180 years. Tripoli is also the name of a port city in present-day Libya, on the edge of the desert. The city was founded by the Phoenicians; it was conquered by the Muslims (642/643) and since then has been ruled by various dynasties.
737. Mazor and Lev, 'The Phenomenon'.
738. Tyre (Ṣūr) is an ancient port city on the southern Mediterranean shore of Lebanon, about 80 kilometres south of Beirut. The city was ruled by the Muslims until it was captured by the Crusaders (1124) and became one of the most important cities of the kingdom of Jerusalem. In 1291, Tyre was retaken by the Mamluks. For a description of the city and its Jewish community in the second half of the twelfth century, see Asher, *The Itinerary of Rabbi Benjamin of Tudela*, p. 127.
739. See Map 4; on the Jewish communities in these regions see in depth Gil, *Jews in Islamic Countries*, pp. 49–240, 273–534.
740. See for example Chipman, 'The Jewish Presence in Arabic Writings', p. 398.
741. On the history of the Jews in Iraq see for example Rejwan, *The Jews of Iraq,* mainly 85-93.
742. The city was built by the Abbasids in 762 on the western shore of the river Euphrates and served as their capital. The number of its inhabitants at its peak was estimated at 2,000,000. A big Jewish community existed in the city. It was the most important Jewish centre since the Jewish academies and courts of jus-

tice (*yeshivot*) Sura and Pumbedita moved and operated in the city. Regarding the Jewish population of Baghdad see Rejwan, *The Jews of Iraq*, pp. 94–103; for a description of the city, its Jewish communities and its medical services in the second half of the twelfth century, see: Asher, *The Itinerary of Rabbi Benjamin of Tudela*, pp. 93–105.

743. Ibn Abī Uṣaybiʿa, *ʿUyūn al-Anbāʾ*, vol. II, pp. 30–1; al-ʿUmarī, *Masālik al-Abṣār*, p. 264; Ibn al-Qifṭī, *Taʾrīkh al-Ḥukamāʾ*, p. 209.
744. From the city of al-Balad on the river Tigris, near Mosul.
745. al-Ṣafadī, *Kitāb al-Wāfī bi-l-Wafayāt* (2008–10), vol. XXVII, pp. 300–2; al-ʿUmarī, *Masālik al-Abṣār*, vol. IX, pp. 247–50; Ibn al-Qifṭī, *Taʾrīkh al-Ḥukamāʾ*, p. 343; Steinschneider, 'An Introduction to the Arabic Literature of the Jews II', 13(1), p. 94; Gil, *Jews in Islamic Countries*, p. 470; Stillman and Pines, 'Abū al-Barakāt al-Baghdadī'.
746. Ibn Abī Uṣaybiʿa, *ʿUyūn al-Anbāʾ*, vol. II, pp. 30–1; al-ʿUmarī, *Masālik al-Abṣār*, p. 264.
747. Steinschneider, *Die Arabische Literatur der Juden*, no. 178; Meyerhof, 'Medieval Jewish Physicians in the Near East', p. 456; Meyerhof, 'Jewish Physicians Contemporaries of Maimonides', p. 397.
748. Known also as Bir, and during the Crusades as Bile, Birecik is a town and district in present-day Turkey on the Euphrates.
749. Ashtor, *The History of the Jews in Egypt and Syria*, vol. I, p. 277; Mazor and Lev, 'The Phenomenon'; Meyerhof, 'Jewish Physicians Contemporaries of Maimonides', p. 399.
750. On the Jews of medieval Iran see in depth Yeroushalmi, *The Jews of Iran,* mainly pp. 3–36. On the Jews of Azerbaijan in the history of this region see in depth Fischel, 'Azarbaijan in Jewish History'.
751. Brentjes, *Teaching and Learning*, p. 24.
752. Wasserstein, 'Samauʾal ben Judah'. Marāgha is an ancient city in the province of East Azerbaijan (present-day Iran). The city is built on the bank of a river, 130 kilometres from Tabriz.
753. One of the capitals of Iran, Tabriz is located in the Quru valley (elevation 1,350–1,600 metres) in Iran's historic region of Azerbaijan. The development of the city began after the Muslim conquest and it was rebuilt in 791 after a devastating earthquake. After the Mongol invasion, Tabriz became the capital of the Īl-Khānate. During the Middle Ages, a Jewish community existed in the town. On the Jewish community in the city see Netzer, 'The Fate of the Jewish Community of Tabriz'.

754. Fischel, 'Azarbaijan in Jewish History', p. 6; Amitai, 'Saʿd al-Dawla'.
755. Fischel, 'Azarbaijan in Jewish History', pp. 8, 18.
756. Hamadān is an ancient city, 1,850 metres in altitude, in a green area in the foothills of Alvand Mountain (3,574 m) in the mid-West part of Iran, 360 kilometres southwest of Tehran. The city stands on the Silk Road and has always had strong trade and commercial activity. It fell in the hands of the Muslims in 633, and in the eleventh century, the Seljuks moved their capital to the city. For a description of the city and its Jewish community in the second half of the twelfth century, see Asher, *The Itinerary of Rabbi Benjamin of Tudela*, p. 127.
757. Fischel, 'Azarbaijan in Jewish History', pp. 13–18; Moreen, 'Rashīd al-Dīn Ṭabīb'.
758. Mann, *Texts and Studies*, p. 281.
759. Regarding the Jews in Yemen during their history, see in detail Tobi, *The Jews of Yemen*. See also Goitein, *The Yemenites*, for the history of their communal organization and spiritual life.
760. Lewicka, 'Healer, Scholar, Conspirator', p. 133.
761. al-Khazrajī, *al-ʿUqūd al-Luʾluʾiyya*, vol. II, p. 242; Ashtor, *The History of the Jews in Egypt and Syria*, vol. II, pp. 173–4, 243.
762. For additional information about Zechariah, see Tobi, 'Ben Solomon, Zechariah ha-Rofeh'.

5

Epilogue

The information I gathered for the current research has made it possible to discuss various issues regarding the lives of Jewish practitioners in the medieval Muslim world. It has yielded several conclusions, some of which support (with historical evidence) previous scholars' observations, while others are new and shed more light on the social issues and professional activities of this segment of medieval Jewish society living under Muslim regimes.

I took into consideration Patricia Crone's statement that 'early Islamic history has to be almost exclusively prosopographical',[1] and Michael Ebstein's remark, based on his own experience, that this method is a 'sophisticated tool for organizing the numerous details scattered throughout the vast corpus of classical Arabic literature'.[2] And therefore, from a methodological point of view, the use of the prosopographical approach in my work was the right thing to do. This tool enabled me to collect and organise not only the data scattered throughout the hundreds of thousands of Geniza documents, but also the details found in Muslim Arabic sources of the period. This combination turns out to be highly fruitful.

About 63 per cent of the biographies are based only on the information from the treasure trove of the Geniza; in other words, Muslim historians did not mention in their treatises (not even in biographical dictionaries dedicated to physicians) every single distinguished Jewish practitioner. On the other hand, in some cases (about 14 per cent of the biographies) we found in the Muslim Arabic sources data on important physicians which had no echo in the Jewish ones. This is because the main Jewish source material for our discussion came from the Geniza, which is not a systematic archive. The documents which made their way into this repository did so at the random hand of fate.[3]

The combined information from both sources (about 5 per cent of the biographies) supplies us with a better and clearer picture. The Muslim Arabic sources enabled me to learn more about the professional medical activity of the Jewish practitioners, mainly since the sources were either physicians themselves, or scholars; in any case, they were intellectuals. In some cases, they were driven out of hatred towards the Jews. However, in other cases they personally knew the practitioners about whom they wrote, and occasionally they were even friends. In most cases the professional and personal appreciation towards the Jewish practitioners was clearly reflected in their writing. To our knowledge another important contribution from the Muslim Arabic sources is the case of conversion. Usually, and clearly out of interest, they supply us with unique details related to the conversion of Jewish practitioners; an issue which the Jewish sources hardly dealt with.[4]

On the other hand, the Jewish sources, mainly the Cairo Geniza, provide us with vast amounts of detail regarding the daily lives of the Jewish practitioners, and their personal and communal contacts. These small pieces of information are scattered among the many thousands of documents and have been collected and published by many scholars over the last 120 years. In general, these publications had no particular intention of studying the medical milieu.

There are many examples of biographies in the book which were composed of information from both kinds of sources. The most interesting one, in my opinion, is the case of the twelfth-century Abū al-ʿAshāʾir Hibat-Allāh b. Zayn b. Ḥasan b. Ifrāʾīm b. Yaʿqūb b. Ismāʿīl Ibn Jumayʿ al-ʾIsrāʾīlī (Nethanel b. Samuel), who practised medicine in Cairo. This fascinating paradigm of taking advantage of the rare opportunity of using two sets of sources will be dealt with in a future publication.

The research yielded 607 biographies: 111 of Jewish pharmacists and 496 of Jewish physicians. These biographies reveal how varied the life stories of Jewish practitioners were.

Here I present only some of the knowledge that the research has yielded. I will start with a chronological review in which old and new insights will be presented and proceed with some topics which are not period related.

The Fatimid caliphate in Egypt and Syria is considered a golden age for the *dhimmīs*. Subsequently, this period was also a golden age for Jewish practitioners in general and for Jewish court physicians in particular. Despite a general decline in the position of the *dhimmīs* in the Ayyubid period, the position of Jewish physicians does not seem to have been critically affected. The Fatimid-Ayyubid period (900–1250) is considered the classical period of Islam, in which Muslim, Christian or Jewish practitioners enjoyed a very high status.[5] The data that is collected and presented in this book proves and supports this assumption.[6]

It is clear, mainly from Cairo Geniza material, that between the eleventh and the thirteenth centuries, physicians and pharmacists in Egypt and Syria were considered an important part of the elite of the community. In general, they were notables who were, in many cases, community leaders and were also well connected to the courts of the rulers. This elite class also included other groups, such as high governmental officials and agents, chief judges and leading businessmen.[7] Jewish physicians also played a prominent role in the medieval Islamic world of this period. They made significant contributions to the development of medical science in the Muslim world, both as successful physicians in the courts of the different Muslim rulers, and as authors or translators of dozens of important medical treatises.[8]

The medical profession was a highly attractive option for an ambitious Jew who wanted to achieve an honourable and scholarly career. Being a physician was highly esteemed by members of both his own community and the Muslim one, especially since most of the other options for eminent careers were blocked for either Jews or Christians.[9] The biographical writings of al-Qifṭī, Ibn Abī Uṣaybiʿa and other sources teach us that the early Ayyubid period saw an intellectual revival which also opened the way for contacts between the members of different religions.[10] According to Max Meyerhof's count of Jewish, Christian and Muslim physicians mentioned by Ibn Abī Uṣaybiʿa, Christian physicians dominated in the ninth and tenth centuries, while Jews were less frequent and Muslims the exception.[11] Thus, it is also in the Ayyubid period that we find greater numbers of Jewish court physicians.[12] The picture then changed from the end of the eleventh century onwards when Muslims entered the profession in larger numbers and eventually dominated the field.[13] Saladin's court physicians at the end of the twelfth century are somewhat representative of this trend, since most of them were Muslims.[14]

It was mainly in this classical age, and to a certain extent also in the late Middle Ages (14th century), that distinguished physicians were appointed also as the *Raʾīs al-Yahūd* or *nagid* (head of the Jews in Egypt and Syria).[15] Interestingly enough, in times of tension, the privileges of these *dhimmī* physicians tended to be interpreted as a manifestation of their superiority, going against the Islamic order that non-believers should be humbled. Thus the physicians fell victim to specific rules and regulations against them, in addition to the ongoing oppression and distress imposed on their community members.[16]

However, the zealous atmosphere of the Mamluk regime did not pass over the non-Muslim practitioners. (This trend can be easily seen in Chart 4.) During the fourteenth century, the dismissal of Jewish court physicians became frequent, and one discerns an increasing opposition by orthodox Muslims to the treatment of Muslim patients by Jewish and Christian physicians. The Mamluks questioned the rights of Jewish (and Christian) physicians to treat Muslim patients. I will present two examples: first, the Muslim

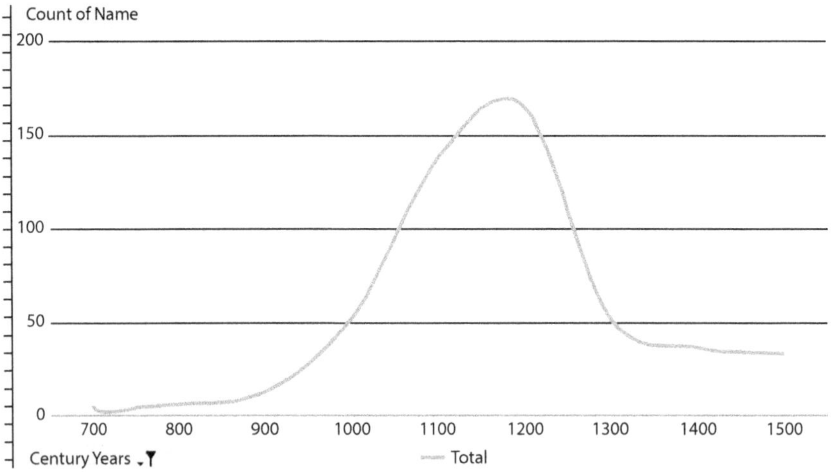

Chart 4 Number of Jewish physicians in the Muslim world over time[17]

theologian Ibn Taymiyya (13th–14th centuries) wrote that a Muslim was allowed to seek medical advice from an unbeliever, provided this unbeliever could be trusted and provided there was no probability of some dirty tricks being involved, such as sovereignty or superiority over Muslims.[18] Second, presenting Jewish and Christian physicians as a 'threat to Muslim patients' had been developed by Ibn al-Ḥājj (1258–1337), an extreme Muslim judge from Cairo who claimed that in principle non-Muslim physicians could not treat Muslim patients. His explanation was that 'simply because they were programmed to hate Muslims and to conspire against them, rather than help them'. Moreover, he denounced the *dhimmīs* as 'those who deliberately took over the control of medicine, ophthalmology and accounts in order to harm Muslims'. Ibn al-Ḥājj added that the strategic objective of the *dhimmī* physicians was to destroy the intellectual and religious elite of Islam, and therefore, he proclaimed against buying medicines from them.[19] Yael Weisz showed that there was a gap between the negative perceptions, attitudes and rhetoric of some Muslim scholars towards the Jewish physicians and their actual position.[20] The findings of my research, especially the large number of medical dynasties, court physicians, and other famous and successful Jewish practitioners, fully support this assumption.[21]

The decline of the Jewish physicians' status is also related to the decline of the science of medicine in the Muslim world, and especially in the Mamluk sultanate. The increasing power of orthodox Islam and mystical Sufism contributed to the deterioration of secular Greek studies, which constituted the basis for medical science. On the one hand, Mamluk sultans encouraged mainly Islamic religious studies in the numerous institutions they established. On the other hand, Sufi sheikhs and saints, who propagated popular Sufism and were believed by the people to create miracles, gained more and more honour and prestige among people and rulers. The 'secular' physicians and their medical science seemed to be useless, especially in light of the Black Death.[22] However, despite the clear decline in the position of distinguished Jewish physicians in the Mamluk period, this situation should not be overstated, especially regarding the whole quarter-millennium during which this period lasted.[23]

These historical developments raise several questions regarding the phenomenon of Jewish physicians in the Mamluk period. The first concerns the position of distinguished Jewish physicians versus Muslim society and the Muslim elite. According to Doris Behrens-Abouseif, Jewish physicians in general could not act as prominent or court physicians during the Mamluk period; 'great doctors, especially those attached to the court, had to convert to Islam'.[24] From the data presented in this volume, we clearly see this trend in hospitals.[25] And it is indeed the case that many Jewish practitioners, mainly physicians and especially court physicians, converted to Islam during the Mamluk period.[26] For example, we traced nine Jewish physicians practising in Muslim courts in the fourteenth and fifteenth centuries; seven of them had converted to Islam.[27] The rest of the practitioners remained Jewish but they continued to work in the courts of the Mamluk rulers.

It should be mentioned that despite certain calls to prevent Jewish physicians from treating Muslims, the Muslim authorities continued to give them work permits, the rulers continue to hire them, and the general Muslim public did not stop from calling on them for medical advice. Moreover, in line with Weisz's conclusions, it appears that in general, the ordination procedures of physicians in the Muslim world did not discriminate specifically against *dhimmī* physicians.[28] From a socio-economic point of view, it seems that the public's need for medical services defeated the theoretical social hierarchy between Muslim and Jews (and Christians) that was based on religious considerations.[29]

There are a few historical, social, economic and inter-religious issues that are worth mentioning here. In general, many of the life stories found in the hundreds of biographies of Jewish practitioners reveal friendly relationships which were built between Jewish physicians and Muslim or Christian ones and other intellectuals.[30] Regarding medical education, studying the hundreds of biographies clearly highlights the general notion that there was no formal monopoly on medical education in the medieval Muslim world. We see that this reality gave freedom of action to all members of the Muslim society, as well as to the *dhimmīs*.[31] The biographies clearly show that this atmosphere allowed the Jewish physicians to study medicine in various ways: with their family members, with and under the supervision of Muslim, Christian or Jewish physicians, in their home or even in the public hospitals.[32]

Christian and Jewish practitioners, mainly physicians, were often rich and respected, and in some cases influential.[33] I agree with Paulina Lewicka's claim that they 'were masters of life and death of Muslims, of whose weak side and the most intimate problems they were aware'.[34] Indeed, intimate relationships were built between Muslim rulers and their Jewish practitioners, mainly due to the personal closeness of a therapist to his patient. In this way, new opportunities for gaining wealth and political power were opened for those physicians. Weisz added that, possibly, in some cases, mystical perceptions regarding Jewish physicians (knowing foreign languages, having secretive medical knowledge, being different) were the reasons that Muslim rulers, as well as ordinary members of Muslim society, were inclined to approach Jewish physicians.[35]

Moreover, based on the historical evidence and the biographies which have been created, it is clear that S. D. Goitein was correct in stating that the combination of the two positions of court physician and Head of the Jews was, in a way, 'natural and understandable'. As a personal physician to the sultan, the Jewish leader could develop direct and informal relations with the Muslim ruler, for the benefit of his community. This way, the rulers also enjoyed better and more effective control over their Jewish subjects. It is not surprising, therefore, that physicians were the heads of congregations in local communities also.[36]

Weisz claimed that there were neither real nor genuine restrictions, rather goodwill and sympathy from the rulers to their Jewish physicians. In many cases this sympathy was based on their linguistic abilities, administrative qualifications and strong loyalty towards their Muslim patrons.[37] However, this was a highly sensitive issue which received considerable criticism from other courtiers and some Muslim dignitaries and scholars.[38]

Another aspect of the successful social integration of the Jewish practitioners (mainly the physicians) in Muslim society is the fact that the rulers saw the benefits of employing a non-Muslim neutral professional, for the Jews tended to stay out of the political coalitions in the courts.[39] Our biographies show that a number of Jewish court physicians were killed due to court intrigues; in some cases this happened while the rulers they served were still in power – for example Rashīd al-Dīn (14th century), Fatḥ Allāh b. Muʿtaṣim b. Nafīs (15th century) and Elazar Sakandarī (16th century) – but mainly when their patron died or lost his power, for example Amīn al-Dawla Abū al-Ḥasan b. Ghazāl b. Abī Saʿīd al-Sāmirī (Cairo, 13th century), when the Mamluks replaced the Ayyubids. Interestingly enough, some of these unfortunate physicians had converted to Islam long before they were executed.

As mentioned above, the fact that many Jewish intellectuals, both in the eastern and western parts of the Muslim world, earned their living as physicians gave them the opportunity to practise and express their other skills and expertise.[40] Examples include, to name a few, Marwān (Abū al-Walīd) Ibn Janāḥ al-Qurṭubī (R. Jonah Marinus), Moses b. Maimon (Maimonides) and Abū al-Faḍl Dāʾūd b. Sulaymān b. Abū al-Bayān al-ʾIsrāʾīlī al-Sadīd (David b. Solomon), and there are many more.[41] Moreover, it is clear from our findings that the high position that some of the Jewish practitioners (mainly physicians) had, serving sultans and high-ranking officials, helped them to earn prestige and recognition, and enabled social mobility. Caballero-Navas named some eminent medical Jewish practitioners who improved their social and political situation due to their success as physicians. In most cases, this was also reflected in their home communities: Ḥasday b. Shaprūṭ, Meʾir (Abū al-Ḥasan) Ibn Qamniʾel and Ibn Biklārish in the west,[42] and in the east Moses b. Maimon (Maimonides) and many others.[43]

People were travelling in the Muslim world for various reasons including trade and pilgrimage. Scholars were travelling mainly out of curiosity (for example geographers), and similarly physicians, for the sake of acquiring knowledge. They usually stopped in the big cities and studied with other scholars, especially the famous and professional ones.[44] There is reliable information regarding the travels of Jewish practitioners, some due to the abovementioned reasons, and others due to family visits and expulsions.[45]

Centre–periphery relationships, which included travelling, can also be learnt, for example, from a phenomenon in which a young man who wanted to study medicine moved to a big city in order to benefit from its medical education. Similarly, physicians who practised in the small cities of the Egyptian periphery, where it was harder to make a living by practising medicine due to the small size of these Jewish communities, moved to Cairo or Alexandria in order to make a better living and improve their socio-economic status.[46] And indeed, most of the medieval Jewish practitioners traced and described in the current work lived and practised medicine in Egypt in general and in Old Cairo (Fusṭāṭ) in particular.[47]

In this book, I have tried to present as complete a picture as possible of the socio-economic profile, number, professionalism and other aspects of Jewish physicians and pharmacists in the medieval Muslim world. When Peter Murray Jones tried to assess from a medieval English context 'what use [...] a 15th century medical practitioner [would] have for written information', he immediately posed the methodological problem that 'historians must rely on written documents alone for evidence'. His solution was that 'a little imagination is required; let us imagine our practitioner for a moment as a man'.[48] Thanks to the multitude of the Geniza documents, we can follow Jones's path and build up a general profile of the 'Geniza' practitioners, but using mainly historical records with hardly any imagination. The average Geniza physician was a man who was able to read and write both Arabic and Hebrew. He studied medicine with older, often well-known, physicians in their homes or in hospitals. In many cases he had his own medical library and had access to additional books in the hospital where he worked, or he borrowed them from other physicians who were fellow members of the Jewish community, where he was actively involved in its leadership. He regularly donated money to the poor and to redeem Jewish captives. In many cases he would travel to visit a family, to treat dignitaries and rulers, and from time to time even as part of his military service. Sometimes he was involved in economic activities such as local trade (books, sugar etc.), international trade (such as spices, perfumes and drugs), and intermittently in growing agricultural products and their industrial production (sugar for example).

It is probable that alongside the continuation of the Geniza research and the study of Muslim Arabic sources, more names and data about Jewish practitioners will be revealed and more information regarding known ones will appear. Readers are very welcome to send such new material to the author (elev@univ.haifa.ac.il). I will be happy to receive additional information regarding the practitioners who are discussed in this book, or concerning others who are not included, in order to add it to a future database. I hope that this contribution will be the beginning of a more ambitious, though much-needed, project – a Prosopography of Jewish Professionals in Medieval Egypt and the Mediterranean, as well as an online database with this information.

Notes

1. Crone, *Slaves on Horses*, pp. 16–17.
2. Ebstein, 'Shurṭa Chiefs in Baṣra', p. 130.
3. See in detail Mazor and Lev, 'Dynasties of Jewish Physicians'.
4. It should be noted that social issues such as conversions, socio-economic status etc. changed throughout the researched period due to, or thanks to, different regimes and various rulers, local as well as regional.
5. Goitein, 'The Medical Profession', p. 177; Goitein, *A Mediterranean Society*, vol. II, p. 241.
6. Mazor and Lev, 'Dynasties of Jewish Physicians'.
7. Goitein, *A Mediterranean Society*, vol. I, p.76.
8. See in detail Section 4.4.7.
9. Ashtor, 'Prolegomena', p. 153.
10. Goitein, *A Mediterranean Society*, vol. V, pp. 447–78; Goitein, 'The Moses Maimonides–Ibn Sanā' al-Mulk Circle', p. 404.
11. Meyerhof, 'Notes sur quelques médecins juifs egyptiens', pp. 116–17; Nicolae, 'A Medieval Court Physician at Work', pp. 57–8; Pormann, 'The Physician and the Other', p. 213.
12. Meyerhof, 'Sultan Saladin's Physician', p. 169; Kraemer, *Maimonides*, pp. 212–13. See also Section 4.1.1, Table 5.
13. Nicolae, 'A Medieval Court Physician at Work', pp. 57–8; Meyerhof, 'Notes sur quelques médecins juifs egyptiens', pp. 116–17; Pormann, 'The Physician and the Other', p. 213.
14. Nicolae, 'A Medieval Court Physician at Work', pp. 57–8; Jadon, 'A Comparison of the Wealth', p. 66; Jadon, 'The Physicians of Syria', p. 326.
15. Mazor and Lev, 'The Phenomenon'; Goitein, *A Mediterranean Society*, vol. II, pp. 243–5. See in detail Section 4.5.2.
16. Lewicka, 'The Non-Muslim Physician', p. 504.
17. The graph is based on the available data collected in this research.
18. Lewicka, 'The Non-Muslim Physician', pp. 511–12.
19. Translation by Paulina Lewicka; See in detail Lewicka, 'The Non-Muslim Physician', p. 511; Ibn al-Ḥājj, *al-Madkhal ilā Tammiyat*, vol. IV, pp. 108–9, 113–14; Perlmann, 'Notes on the Position of Jewish Physicians', pp. 316–19; Ashtor, 'Prolegomena', pp. 154–5; Baron, *A Social and Religious History*, vol. XVII, p. 175; Behrens-Abouseif, *Fatḥ Allāh and Abū Zakariyya*, pp. 13–14;

Stillman, *The Jews of Arab Lands*, p. 72; Mazor and Lev, 'The Phenomenon'. See in detail Section 4.4.4.

20. Weisz, 'The Jewish Physicians', p. 31.
21. See in detail Section 4.4.4.
22. Behrens-Abouseif, 'The Image of the Physician', pp. 335–6, 342–3; Behrens-Abouseif, *Fatḥ Allāh and Abū Zakariyya*, pp. 14–19.
23. Mazor and Lev, 'The Phenomenon'.
24. Behrens-Abouseif, *Fatḥ Allāh and Abū Zakariyya*, p. 12.
25. The information appears in Table 3, Section 3.3.1, and Table 4, Section 4.1.1.
26. See in detail Section 4.4.6, and Table 7 in that section.
27. See Table 5, Section 4.1.1.
28. See in detail Weisz, 'The Jewish Physicians', pp. 31–2.
29. Ibid., p. 32.
30. See in detail Section 4.4.4; various examples can be found in the biographies in Sections 3.3.2 and 3.1.1.
31. Ibid., p. 31.
32. See in detail Section 4.1.2.
33. See examples in Section 4.4.4.
34. Lewicka, 'The Non-Muslim Physician', p. 504.
35. See in detail: Weisz, 'The Jewish Physicians', p. 33.
36. Goitein, *A Mediterranean Society*, vol. II, pp. 243–5; on the role of medical practitioners in the Jewish leadership see in detail Section 4.5.2.
37. See in detail Sections 4.4.5 and 4.4.7.
38. Weisz, 'The Jewish Physicians', p. 32.
39. Ibid.
40. See for example Section 4.4.7; Caballero-Navas, 'Medicine among Medieval Jews', pp. 327–8; Perlmann; 'Notes on the Position of Jewish Physicians'.
41. See in detail Section 4.4.7.
42. Caballero-Navas, 'Medicine among Medieval Jews', pp. 327–8.
43. See in detail Sections 3.3.2, 4.4.5 and 4.4.7.
44. Marín, 'Biography and Prosopography', p. 8; on the travels of Muslim scholars for the sake of knowledge see Brentjes, *Teaching and Learning*, pp. 135–9.
45. See in detail sec. 4.2.3.
46. Goitein, *A Mediterranean Society*, vol. II, p. 288. It might be interesting for the reader to look at a study made by Carl Petry of the geographical origins of the

Muslim learned elite in fifteenth-century Cairo: see in detail Petry, *The Civilian Elite of Cairo*.

47. See Chart 3, Section 4.6.
48. Jones, 'Harley MS 2558', p. 35.

Bibliography

Abrahams, Israel (trans. & ed.), *Hebrew Ethical Wills*. Philadelphia: Jewish Publication Society, 1926.

Abū al-Munā al-Kūhīn al-ʿAṭṭār, *Minhāj al-Dukkān wa-Dustūr al-Aʿyān*, ed. Ḥ. Al-ʿĀṣī. Beirut: Dār Manāhil, 1992.

Abū al-Ṣalt, Umayya ibn ʿAbd al-ʿAzīz, 'Al-Risāla al-Miṣriyya', in ʿAbd al-Salām Muḥammad Hārūn (ed.), *Nawādir al-Makhṭūṭāt*. Cairo: Maṭbaʿat Lajnat al-Taʾlīf wa-l-Tarjama wa-l-Nashr, 1951, pp. 5–56.

Adang, Camilla, 'The Karaites as Portrayed in Medieval Islamic Sources', in Meira Polliack (ed.), *Karaite Judaism: A Guide to its History and Literary Sources*. Leiden: Brill, 2003, pp. 179–97.

Adler, E. Nathan. (ed.), *Jewish Travelers: A Treasury of Travelogues from 9 Centuries*, 2nd edn. New York: Hermon Press, 1966.

Ahmed, Asad Q., *The Religious Elite of the Early Islamic Hijaz: Five Prosopographical Case Studies*. Oxford: Unit for Prosopographical Research, 2011.

Ahmed, Mohamed A. H., 'An Initial Survey of Arabic Poetry in the Cairo Genizah', *Al-Masāq*, 30, 2018, pp. 212–33.

Albert, Daniel M. and Diane D. Edwards, *The History of Ophthalmology*. Cambridge, MA: Blackwell Science. 1996.

Alfonso, Esperanza, 'Ibn Ḥasday, Joseph (Abū ʿAmr)', in Norman A. Stillman (ed.), *Encyclopedia of Jews in the Islamic World Online*. Leiden: Brill, 2013.

Alfonso, Esperanza, 'Ibn al-Muʿallim, Solomon', in Norman A. Stillman (ed.), *Encyclopedia of Jews in the Islamic World Online*. Leiden: Brill, 2013.

Allony, Nehemia, 'Hebrew Manuscript in New York Libraries', *Israel Journal for Libraries and Archives*, 20(1–2), 1981, pp 29–35 [Hebrew].

Allony, Nehemia, *The Jewish Library in the Middle Ages: Book Lists from the Cairo*

Geniza, ed. Miriam Frenkel, Haggai Ben-Shammai and Moshe Sokolow. Jerusalem: Yad Ben-Zvi / Hebrew University of Jerusalem, 2006 [Hebrew].

Alpin, Prosper, *La Médecine des Égyptiens, 1581–1584*. Cairo: Institut Français d'Archéologie Orientale, 1980.

Altmann, Alexander and Hanoch Avenary, "Moses ben Joseph Ha-Levi", *Encyclopedia Judaica*, available at https://www.encyclopedia.com/religion/encyclopedias-almanacs-transcripts-and-maps/moses-ben-joseph-ha-levi (accessed 11 September 2020).

Amar, Zohar, *The History of Medicine in Jerusalem*, BAR International Series 1032. Oxford: Archeopress, 2002.

Amar, Zohar and Efraim Lev, *Arabian Drugs in Early Medieval Mediterranean Medicine*. Edinburgh: Edinburgh University Press, 2017.

Amar, Zohar and Efraim Lev, *Physicians, Drugs and Remedies in Jerusalem from the 10th to the 18th Centuries*. Tel Aviv: Eretz, 2000 [Hebrew].

Amar, Zohar and Efraim Lev, 'The Significance of the Genizah's Medical Documents for the Study of Medieval Mediterranean Trade', *Journal of the Economic and Social History of the Orient*, 50(4), 2007, pp. 524–41.

Amar, Zohar and Efraim Lev, 'Trends in the Use of Perfumes and Incense in the Near East after the Muslim Conquests', *Journal of the Royal Asiatic Society*, 23(1), 2013, pp. 11–30.

Amar, Zohar and Efraim Lev, 'Watermelon, Chate Melon and Cucumber: New Light on Traditional and Innovative Field Crops in the Middle Ages', *Journal asiatique*, 299(1), 2011, pp. 193–204.

Amar, Zohar and Yaron Serri, 'Compilation from Jonah Ibn Ǧanāḥ's *Dictionary of Medical Terms*', Lĕšonénu, 63(3–4), 2000–1, pp. 279–91 [Hebrew].

Amar, Zohar and Yaron Serri, *The Land of Israel and Syria According to al-Tamīmī's Description*. Ramat Gan: Bar-Ilan University Press, 2004 [Hebrew].

Amitai, Reuven, 'Saʿd al-Dawla', in Norman A. Stillman (ed.), *Encyclopedia of Jews in the Islamic World Online*. Leiden: Brill, 2013.

al-Andalusī, Said, *Science in the Medieval World: Book of the Categories of Nations*. Austin: University of Texas Press, 1996.

al-Andalusī, Ṣāʿid ibn Aḥmad ibn Ṣāʿid, *Ṭabaqāt al-ʾUmam*, ed. Ḥayāt Būʿalwān. Beirut: Dār al-Ṭalīʿa li-l-Ṭibāʿat wa-l-Nashr, 1985.

Arad, Dotan, 'The Community as an Economic Body: The Property of the Cairo Mustaʿrib Community in Light of Geniza Documents', *Ginzei Qedem*, 7, 2011, pp. 25–69 [Hebrew].

Arad, Dotan, '"A Pleasant Voice and an Expert on Every Matter" on Karaite and

Rabbanite Cantors in 16th Century Egypt', *Ginzei Qedem*, 12, 2016, pp. 9–32 [Hebrew].

Arnaldez, Roger, 'Ibn Zuhr', in *The Encyclopedia of Islam*, new edn. Leiden: Brill, 1960–2007, vol. III, pp. 976–9.

Arnold, Sir Thomas Walker, *The Preaching of Islam: A History of the Propagation of the Muslim Faith*. London: Constable, 1913.

Asher, Adolf (trans. & ed.), *The Itinerary of Rabbi Benjamin of Tudela*. New York: Hakesheth, 1840.

Ashtor, Eliyahu, 'The Diet of Salaried Classes in the Medieval Near East', *Journal of Asian History*, 4(1), 1970, pp. 1–24.

Ashtor, Eliyahu, *Histoire des prix et des salaires dans l'Orient médiéval*. Paris: S.E.V.P.E.N, 1969.

Ashtor, Eliyahu, *The History of the Jews in Egypt and Syria under the Mamluk Regime*. Jerusalem: Mosad Harv Kook, 1951. [Hebrew].

Ashtor, Eliyahu, 'Ibrāhīm Ibn Yaʿqūb of Tortosa', in Michael Berenbaum and Fred Skolnik (eds), *Encyclopedia Judaica*, 2nd ed. Farmington Hills, MI: Macmillan Reference USA, 2007, vol. IX, pp. 701–2.

Ashtor, Eliyahu. *The Jews and the Mediterranean Economy, 10th–15th Centuries*. London: Variorum Reprints, 1983.

Ashtor, Eliyahu. *The Jews of Moslem Spain*. Philadelphia: Jewish Publication Society of America, 1973–84.

Ashtor, Eliyahu, 'New Data for the History of Levantine Jewries in the Fifteenth Century', *Bulletin of the Institute of Jewish Studies*, 3, 1975, pp. 67–102.

Ashtor, Eliyahu, 'The Number of Jews in Mediaeval Egypt', *Journal of Jewish Studies*, 18(1–4), 1967, pp. 9–42.

Ashtor, Eliyahu, 'The Number of Jews in Mediaeval Egypt', *Journal of Jewish Studies*, 19(1–4), 1968, pp. 1–22.

Ashtor, Eliyahu, 'The Number of Jews in Moslem Spain', *Zion*, 28(1–2), 1963, pp. 34–56 [Hebrew].

Ashtor, Eliyahu, 'Prolegomena to the Medieval History of Oriental Jewry', *Jewish Quarterly Review*, n.s., 50(2), 1959, pp. 147–66.

Ashtor, Eliyahu, 'Some Features of the Jewish Communities in Medieval Egypt', *Zion*, 30, 1965, pp. 61–78 [Hebrew].

Ashtor-Strauss, E., 'Saladin and the Jews', *Hebrew Union College Annual*, 27, 1956, pp. 305–26.

Ashur, Amir, 'Engagement and Betrothal Documents from the Cairo Geniza'. PhD dissertation, Tel Aviv University, 2006 [Hebrew].

Ashur, Amir and Efraim Lev, 'Medical Recipes from the Cairo Geniza', *Ginzei Qedem*, 9, 2013, pp. 9*–35*.

Ashur, Amir and Efraim Lev, 'Practical Prescriptions by Maimonides', forthcoming.

Assaf, Simha, 'Old Geniza Documents from Palestine, Egypt, and North Africa (from the Jewish Sources)', *Tarbiz*, 9, 1937–8, pp. 11–34, 196–218.

Assaf, Simha, 'Slavery and the Slave-Trade among the Jews during the Middle Ages', *Zion*, 4(2), 1939, pp. 91–125 [Hebrew].

Assis, Yom Tov, 'Jewish Physicians and Medicine in Medieval Spain', in Samuel S. Kottek and Luís García-Ballester (eds). *Medicine and Medical Ethics in Medieval and Early Modern Spain: An Intercultural Approach.* Jerusalem: Magnes Press, 1996, pp. 33–49.

Astren, Fred, *Karaite Judaism and Historical Understanding*. Columbia: University of South Carolina Press, 2004.

Ávila, María Luisa, *La sociedad hispanomusulmana al final del califato: aproximación a un estudio demográfico*. Madrid: Consejo Superior de Investigaciones Cientificas, 1995.

Azar, Henry A., 'Ibn Zuhr (Avenzoar), Supreme in the Science of Medicine since Galen', PhD dissertation, University of North Carolina at Chapel Hill, 1998.

Bacher, Wilhelm, 'La Bibliothèque d'un médecin juif', *Revue des études juives*, 40, 1900, pp. 55–61.

Bacher, Wilhelm, 'Scham als Name Palästina's', *Jewish Quarterly Review*, 18(3), 1906, pp. 564–5.

Bachrach, Bernard S., 'Introduction: What Directions Will the Prosopography of the Middle Ages Take?', *Medieval Prosopography*, 8(2), 1987, pp. 41–8.

Baker, Colin F., ''Abū al-Ḥasan Saʿīd's *Maqāla fī Khalq al-ʾInsān*', PhD dissertation, University of Cambridge, 1990.

Baker, Colin F., 'Islamic and Jewish Medicine in the Medieval Mediterranean World: The Geniza Evidence', *Journal of the Royal Society of Medicine*, 89(10), 1996, pp. 577–80.

Baker, Colin F. and Meira Polliack, *Arabic and Judaeo-Arabic Manuscripts in the Cambridge Genizah Collections*. Cambridge: Cambridge University Press, 2001.

al-Bakrī, Abū ʿUbayd ʿAbd Allāh b. ʿAbd al-ʿAzīz, *Kitāb al-Masālik wa-l-Mamālik*. Beirut: Dār al-Kutub al-ʿIlmiyya, 2003.

Baneth, D. Z. H., 'A Doctor's Library in Egypt at the Time of Maimonides', *Tarbiz*, 30(2), 1960, pp. 171–85.

Banner, Lois W., 'Biography as History', *American Historical Review*, 114(3), 2009, pp. 579–86.

Bareket, Elinoar, 'Abraham ben Hillel', in Norman A. Stillman (ed.), *Encyclopedia of Jews in the Islamic World Online*. Leiden: Brill, 2013.

Bareket, Elinoar, 'Abraham ha-Kohen b. Isaac ibn Furat', *Hebrew Union College Annual,* 70/71, 1999–2000, pp. 1–19 [Hebrew].

Bareket, Elinoar, 'Abu 'l-Munajja Solomon ibn Sha'ya', in Norman A. Stillman (ed.), *Encyclopedia of Jews in the Islamic World Online*. Leiden: Brill, 2013.

Bareket, Elinoar, 'Alexandria', in Norman Roth (ed.), *Medieval Jewish Civilization: An Encyclopedia,* New York: Routledge, 2003.

Bareket, Elinoar, 'David ben Joshua Maimonides', in Norman A. Stillman (ed.), *Encyclopedia of Jews in the Islamic World Online*. Leiden: Brill, 2013.

Bareket, Elinoar, *Fustat on the Nile, the Jewish Elite in Medieval Egypt*. Leiden, Brill, 1999.

Bareket, Elinoar, 'Ibn Furāt Abraham ben Isaac ha-Kohen', in Norman A. Stillman (ed.), *Encyclopedia of Jews in the Islamic World Online*. Leiden: Brill, 2013.

Bareket, Elinoar, 'Jewish First Names as a Source of the Social and Cultural Status of the Jews in the Islamic Society during the Early Middle Ages', *Te'uda*, 24, 2011, pp. 101–36 [Hebrew].

Bareket, Elinoar, *The Jewish Leadership in Fusṭāṭ in the First Half of the Eleventh Century*. Tel Aviv: Diaspora Research Institute, Tel Aviv University, 1995 [Hebrew].

Bareket, Elinoar, *The Jews of Egypt, 1007–1055, Based on Documents from the 'Archive' of Efrain Ben Shemarya*. Jerusalem: Ben-Zvi Institute, 1995 [Hebrew].

Bareket, Elinoar, 'Karaite Communities in the Middle East during the Tenth to Fifteenth Centuries', in Meira Polliack (ed.), *Karaite Judaism: A Guide to Its History and Literary Sources*. Leiden: Brill, 2003, pp. 237–52.

Bareket, Elinoar, 'Nagid' (I), in Michael Berenbaum and Fred Skolnik (eds), *Encyclopedia Judaica*, 2nd ed. Farmington Hills, MI: Macmillan Reference USA, 2007, vol. XIV, p. 731.

Bareket, Elinoar, 'Nagid' (II), in Norman A. Stillman (ed.), *Encyclopedia of Jews in the Islamic World Online*. Leiden: Brill, 2013.

Bareket, Elinoar, 'Nethanel ben Moses ha-Levi', in Norman A. Stillman (ed.), *Encyclopedia of Jews in the Islamic World Online*. Leiden: Brill, 2013.

Bareket, Elinoar, 'Note on Jewish Naming Patterns in the Cairo Geniza during the Fatimid Reign (Tenth–Eleventh Centuries)', *European Journal of Jewish Studies,* 5(1), 2011, pp. 81–92.

Bareket, Elinoar, 'Samuel (Abu Mansur) ben Hananiah', in Norman A. Stillman (ed.), *Encyclopedia of Jews in the Islamic World Online*. Leiden: Brill, 2013.

Bareket, Elinoar, 'Struggles over Jewish Leadership in Fusṭāṭ in the Mid-Eleventh Century', *Zion*, 54, 1989, pp. 161–8 [Hebrew].

Baron, Salo W., *A Social and Religious History of the Jews*, 2nd edn. New York: Columbia University Press, 1952–83.

al-Bayhaqī, Ẓahīr al-Dīn, *Tārīkh Ḥukmāʾ al-Islām*. Cairo: Maktabat al-Thaqāfa al-Dīniyya, 1996.

Beech, George, *The Brief Eminence and Doomed Fall of Islamic Saragossa*. Saragossa: Instituto de Estudios Islámicos y del Oriente Próximo, 2008.

Beech, George, 'Prosopography', in James M. Powell (ed.), *Medieval Studies: An Introduction*. Syracuse, NY: Syracuse University Press, 1976.

Beeston, A. F., *Arabic Nomenclature: A Summary for Beginners*. Oxford: Oriental Institute, 1971.

Behrens-Abouseif, Doris, *The Book in Mamluk Egypt and Syria (1250–1517) – Scribes, Libraries and Market*. Leiden: Brill, 2018.

Behrens-Abouseif, Doris, *Fatḥ Allāh and Abū Zakariyya: Physicians under the Mamluks*. Cairo: Institut Français d'Archéologie Orientale, 1987.

Behrens-Abouseif, Doris, 'The Image of the Physician in Arab Biographies of the Post-Classical Age', *Der Islam*, 66(2), 1989, pp. 331–43.

Ben-Hayyim, Zeʾev, *The Literary and Oral Tradition of Hebrew and Aramaic amongst the Samaritans*. Jerusalem: Bialik Institute, 1957–79 [Hebrew].

Ben-Sasson, Menahem, *The Emergence of the Local Jewish Community in the Muslim World: Qayrawan, 800–1057*. Jerusalem: Magnes Press, 1996. [Hebrew].

Ben-Sasson, Menahem, *The Jews of Sicily, 825–1068*. Jerusalem: Magnes Press, 1991 [Hebrew].

Ben-Sasson, Menahem, 'The Maimonidean Dynasty, between Conservatism and Revolution', in Jay M. Harris (ed.), *Maimonides after 800 Years: Essays on Maimonides and His Influence*. Cambridge, MA: Harvard University Press, 2007.

Ben-Shammai, Meir Hillel, 'Aldabi, Meir ben Isaac', in Michael Berenbaum and Fred Skolnik (eds), *Encyclopedia Judaica*, 2nd ed. Farmington Hills, MI: Macmillan Reference USA, 2007, vol. I, p. 605.

Berger, Natalie (ed.), *Jews and Medicine: Religion, Culture, Science*. Philadelphia: Jewish Publication Society, 1995.

Berkey, Jonathan, 'al-Subkī and His Women', *Mamluk Studies Review*, 14, 2010, pp. 1–17.

Berkey, Jonathan, *The Transmission of Knowledge in Medieval Cairo: A Social History of Islamic Education*. Princeton, NJ: Princeton University Press, 1992.

Berto, Luigi Andrea, *In Search of the First Venetians: Prosopography of Early Medieval Venice.* Turnhout, Belgium: Brepols, 2014.

Biesterfeldt, H. H., 'Some Opinions on the Physician's Remuneration in Medieval Islam', *Bulletin of the History of Medicine*, 58(1), 1984, pp. 16–27.

Boogert, Maurits H. van den, *Aleppo Observed: Ottoman Syria through the Eyes of Two Scottish Doctors, Alexander and Patrick Russell.* London: Arcadian Library / Oxford: Oxford University Press, 2010.

Bos, Gerrit (trans. & ed.), *Maimonides on Asthma: A Parallel Arabic-English Text.* Provo, UT: Brigham Young University Press, 2002.

Bosworth, C. Edmund, 'Christian and Jewish Religious Dignitaries in Mamlûk Egypt and Syria: Qalqashandî's Information on Their Hierarchy, Titulature, and Appointment (II)', *International Journal of Middle East Studies*, 3(2), 1972, pp. 199–216.

Brann, Ross, 'The Arabized Jews', in Maria Rosa Menocal, Raymond P. Scheindlin and Michael Sells (eds), *The Literature of al-Andalus*, Cambridge: Cambridge University Press, 2000, pp. 435–54.

Brann, Ross, *The Compunctious Poet: Cultural Ambiguity and Hebrew Poetry in Muslim Spain.* Baltimore: Johns Hopkins University Press, 1991.

Brann, Ross, *Power in the Portrayal: Representations of Jews and Muslims in Eleventh- and Twelfth-Century Islamic Spain.* Princeton, NJ: Princeton University Press, 2002.

Brentjes, Sonja, *Teaching and Learning the Sciences in Islamicate Societies (800–1700).* Turnhout, Belgium: Brepols, 2018.

Brezzi, Paolo and Egmont Lee (eds), *Sources of Social History: Private Acts of the Late Middle Ages.* Toronto: Pontifical Institute of Mediaeval Studies, 1984.

Broady, Donald, 'French Prosopography: Definition and Suggested Reading', *Poetics*, 30(5–6), 2002, pp. 381–5.

Brody, H., 'Ahron Al'amani und seine Söhne', *Zeitschrift für Hebraeische Bibliographie*, 6, 1902, pp. 18–24.

Brody, Robert, *The Geonim of Babylonia and the Shaping of Medieval Jewish Culture.* New Haven, CT: Yale University Press, 1998.

Bruce, Travis, 'The Taifa of Denia and the Jewish Networks of the Medieval Mediterranean: A Study of the Cairo Geniza and Other Documents', *Journal of Medieval Iberian Studies*, 10(2), 2018, pp. 147–66.

Buchman, Yael, and Zohar Amar, *Practical Medicine of Rabbi Hayyim Vital (1543–1620).* Ramat Gan: Division of the History of Medicine, Bar-Ilan University, 2006 [Hebrew].

Buckley, R. P., 'The Muḥtasib', *Arabica*, 39(1), 1992, pp. 59–117.

Bulliet, Richard W., 'The Age Structure of Medieval Islamic Education', *Studia Islamica* 57 (1983), pp. 105–17.

Bulliet, Richard W., 'The Conversion Curve Revisited', in A. C. S. Peacock (ed.), *Islamisation: Comparative Perspectives from History*. Edinburgh: Edinburgh University Press, 2017, pp. 69–79.

Bulliet, Richard W., *Conversion to Islam in the Medieval Period: An Essay in Quantitative History*. Cambridge, MA: Harvard University Press, 1979.

Bulliet, Richard W., 'Process and Status in Conversion and Continuity', in Michael Gervers and Ramzi Jibran Bikhazi (eds), *Conversion and Continuity: Indigenous Christian Communities in Islamic Lands Eighth to Eighteenth Centuries*. Toronto: Pontifical Institute of Mediaeval Studies, 1990, pp. 1–12.

Bulliet, Richard W., 'A Quantitative Approach to Medieval Muslim Biographical Dictionaries', *Journal of Economic and Social History of the Orient*, 13(1), 1970, pp. 195–211.

Bulst, Neithard and Jean-Philippe Genet (eds), *Medieval Lives and the Historian: Studies in Medieval Prosopography*. Kalamazoo, MI: Medieval Institute, 1986.

Burnett, Charles (ed.), *Ibn Baklarish's Book of Simples: Medical Remedies between Three Faiths in Twelfth-Century Spain*. London: Arcadian Library / Oxford: Oxford University Press, 2008.

Caballero-Navas, Carmen, 'Medicine among Medieval Jews: the Science, the Art, and the Practice', in Gad Freudenthal (ed.), *Science in Medieval Jewish Cultures*. New York: Cambridge University Press, 2011, pp. 320–42.

Cameron, Averil (ed.), *Fifty Years of Prosopography: The Later Roman Empire, Byzantium and Beyond*. Oxford: Oxford University Press, 2003.

Campbell, Donald, *Arabian Medicine and Its Influence on the Middle Ages*. London: Kegan Paul, Trench, Trubner, 1926.

Cano, J. M., 'Ḥasday ibn Shaprūṭ', in Norman A. Stillman (ed.), *Encyclopedia of Jews in the Islamic World Online*. Leiden: Brill, 2013.

Carlson, Thomas A., 'Contours of Conversion: The Geography of Islamization in Syria, 600–1500', *Journal of American Oriental Society*, 135(4), 2015, pp. 791–816.

Chamberlain, Michael, *Knowledge and Social Practice in Medieval Damascus, 1190–1350*. Cambridge: Cambridge University Press, 1994.

Chipman, Leigh, 'The ʿAllāma and the Ṭabīb: A Note on Biographies of Two Doctors, Rashīd al-Dīn and Quṭb al-Dīn' al-Shīrazī', in Anna Akasoy, Charles Burnett and Ronit Yoeli-Tlalim (eds), *Rashīd al-Dīn: Agent and Mediator of Cultural Exchanges in Ilkhanid Iran*. London: Warburg Institute, 2013, pp. 115–26.

Chipman, Leigh, 'Islamic Pharmacy in the Mamlūk and Mongol Realms: Theory and Practice', *Asian Medicine*, 3, 2008, pp. 264–77.

Chipman, Leigh, 'The Jewish Presence in Arabic Writings on Medicine and Pharmacology during the Medieval Period', *Religion Compass*, 7(9), 2013, pp. 394–401.

Chipman, Leigh, *The World of Pharmacy and Pharmacists in Mamlūk Cairo*. Leiden: Brill, 2010.

Chipman, Leigh and Efraim Lev, 'Arabic Prescriptions from the Cairo Genizah', *Asian Medicine*, 6, 2011, pp. 75–94.

Chipman, Leigh and Efraim Lev, 'Syrups from the Apothecary's Shop: A Geniza Fragment Containing One of the Earliest Manuscripts of *Minhāj al-Dukkān*', *Journal of Semitic Studies*, 51(1), 2006, pp. 137–67.

Chipman, Leigh and Efraim Lev, '"Take a Lame and Decrepit Female Hyena …": A Geniza Study of Two Additional Fragments of Manuscripts of Sābūr Ibn Sahl's "*al-Aqrābādhīn al-Ṣaghīr*"', *Early Science and Medicine*, 13(4), 2008, pp. 361–83.

Cohen, Hayyim J., 'The Economic Background and the Secular Occupations of Muslim Jurisprudents and Traditionists in the Classical Period of Islam (until the Middle of the Eleventh Century)', *Journal of Economic and Social History of the Orient*, 13(1), 1970, pp. 16–61.

Cohen, Ilan, 'The Jewish Community in Damascus during the Classic Geniza Period', MA thesis, University of Haifa, 2015.

Cohen, Mark R., 'The Burdensome Life of a Jewish Physician and Communal Leader: A Geniza Fragment from the Alliance Israelite Universelle Collection', *Jerusalem Studies in Arabic and Islam*, 16, 1993, pp. 125–36.

Cohen, Mark R., *Jewish Self-Government in Medieval Egypt: The Origins of the Office of Head of the Jews, ca. 1065–1126*. Princeton, NJ: Princeton University Press, 1980.

Cohen, Mark R., 'Jews in the Mamlūk Environment: The Crisis of 1442 (a Geniza Study),' *Bulletin of the School of Oriental and African Studies*, 47(3), 1984, pp. 425–48.

Cohen, Mark R., *Poverty and Charity in the Jewish Community of Medieval Egypt*. Princeton, NJ: Princeton University Press, 2005.

Cohen, Mark R., *Under Crescent and Cross: The Jews in the Middle Ages*. Princeton, NJ: Princeton University Press, 1994.

Cohen, Mark R., *The Voice of the Poor in the Middle Ages: An Anthology of Documents from the Cairo Geniza*. Princeton, NJ: Princeton University Press, 2005.

Cohen, Mark R. and Sasson Somekh, 'In the Court of Yaʿqūb Ibn Killis: A Fragment from the Cairo Geniza', *Jewish Quarterly Review*, n.s., 80(3–4), 1990, pp. 283–314.

Conermann, Stephan (ed.), *Muslim–Jewish Relations in the Middle Islamic Period: Jews in the Ayyubid and Mamluk Sultanates (1171–1517)*. Göttingen: V&R unipress, 2017.

Conrad, Lawrence I., 'Arab-Islamic Medicine', in: W. F. Bynum and Roy Porter (eds), *Companion Encyclopedia of the History of Medicine*. London: Routledge, 1993, vol. I, pp. 676–727.

Crone, Patricia, *The Nativist Prophets of Early Islamic Iran: Rural Revolt and Local Zoroastrianism*. Cambridge: Cambridge University Press, 2012.

Crone, Patricia, *Slaves on Horses: The Evolution of the Islamic Polity*. Cambridge, Cambridge University Press, 1980.

Crown, Alan D. (ed.), *The Samaritans*. Tübingen: J. C. B. Mohr (Siebeck), 1989.

Crown, Alan D., Reinhard Pummer and Abraham Tal, *A Companion to Samaritan Studies*. Tübingen: Mohr (Siebeck), 1993.

David, Abraham and Lea Bornstein-Makovetsky, 'Paltiel', in Fred Skolnik (ed.), *Encyclopedia Judaica*, 2nd ed. Detroit: Macmillan Reference USA, 2007, vol. XV, p. 607.

De Lange, Nicholas, 'Byzantium in the Cairo Genizah', *Byzantine and Modern Greek Studies*, 16, 1992, pp. 34–47.

DeWeese, Devin, *Islamization and Native Religion in the Golden Horde: Baba Tükles and Conversion to Islam in Historical and Epic Tradition*. University Park, PA: Penn State University Press, 2010.

al-Dhahabī, Muḥammad b. Aḥmad, *Dhuyūl al-ʿIbar fī Khabar man Ghabar*. Beirut: Dar al-Kutub al-ʿIlmiyya, 1985.

al-Dhahabī, Muḥammad b. Aḥmad, *Taʾrīkh al-Islām wa-Wafayāt al-Mashāhīr wa-l-Aʿlam*, ed. ʿAbd al-Salām Tadmurī. Beirut: Dār al-Kitāb al-ʿArabī, 1987–2004.

al-Dhākirī, Muḥammad Fuʾād, *al-Ṭibb wa-l-Aṭibbāʾ fī l-Quds, nihāyat al-Qarn al-ḥādī ʿashar al-hijrī*, ed. Manshūrāt al-Hayʾa al-ʿĀmma al-Suriyya li-l-Kitāb. Damascus: Wuzārat al-Thiqāfa, 2009.

Dietrich, Albert, 'Ibn Biklārish', *The Encyclopedia of Islam*, new edn. Leiden: Brill, 1960–2007.

Dietrich, Albert, *Zum Drogenhandel im islamischen Ägypten*. Heidelberg: Carl Winter, 1954.

Dols, Michael W., *The Black Death in the Middle East.* Princeton, NJ, Princeton University Press, 1979.

Dols, Michael W. (trans.) and Adil S. Gamal (ed.), *Medieval Islamic Medicine: Ibn Riḍwān's Treatise 'On the Prevention of Bodily Ills in Egypt'.* Berkeley: University of California Press, 1984.

Ebstein, Michael, 'Shurṭa Chiefs in Baṣra in the Umayyad Period: A Prosopographical Study', *Al-Qantara*, 31(1), 2010, pp. 103–47.

Eddé, Anne-Marie, 'Les Médecins dans la société syrienne du VIIe/XIIIe siècle', *Annales islamologiques*, 29, 1995, pp. 91–109.

Eddé, Anne-Marie, *Saladin*, trans. Jane M. Todd. Cambridge, MA, and London: Belknap Press, 2011.

Eisenstein, David J. (ed.), *Ozar Massaoth: A Collection of Itineraries by Jewish Travellers to Palestine, Syria, Egypt and other Countries.* Newark, NJ: David J. Eisenstein, 1927 [Hebrew].

Ellenblum, Ronnie, *The Collapse of the Eastern Mediterranean: Climate Change and the Decline of the East, 950–1072.* Cambridge: Cambridge University Press, 2012.

Elmakias, Avraham, *The Naval Commanders of Early Islam: A Prosopographical Approach*, trans. Limor Yungman. Piscataway, NJ: Gorgias Press, 2018.

Fenton, Paul B., 'Jewish–Muslim Relations as Reflected in the Geniza Documents', in Mordechai A. Friedman (ed.), *Teʿuda XV: A Century of Geniza Research*, Tel Aviv: Tel Aviv University, 1999, pp 351–64 [Hebrew].

Fenton, Paul B., 'Jonah Ibn Ǧanāḥ's Medical Dictionary, the *Kitāb al-Talḫīṣ*: Lost and Found', *Aleph*, 16(1), 2016, pp. 107–43.

Fenton, Paul B., 'Maimonides, David ben Abraham', in Norman A. Stillman (ed.), *Encyclopedia of Jews in the Islamic World Online.* Leiden: Brill, 2013.

Finkel, Joshua, 'An Eleventh Century Source for the History of Jewish Scientists in Mohammedan Land (Ibn Ṣaʿid)', *Jewish Quarterly Review*, n.s., 18(1), 1927, pp. 45–54.

Finkel, Joshua, 'A Risāla of al-Jāḥiẓ', *Journal of the American Oriental Society*, 47, 1927, pp. 311–34.

Fischel, Walter J., 'Azarbaijan in Jewish History', *Proceedings of the American Academy for Jewish Research*, 22, 1953, pp. 1–21.

Fischel, Walter J., *The Origin of Banking in Mediaeval Islam: A Contribution to the Economic History of the Jews of Baghdad in the Tenth Century.* Hertford: Austin & Sons, 1933.

Fischel, Walter J., 'The Spice Trade in Mamluk Egypt: A Contribution to the

Economic History of Medieval Islam', *Journal of the Economic and Social History of the Orient*, 1(2), 1958, pp. 157–74.

Fleming, Robin, 'Writing Biography at the Edge of History', *American Historical Review*, 2009, 114(3), pp. 606–14.

Freimann, Hayyim A., 'The Genealogy of Moses Maimonides' Family', *Alumma*, 1, 1936, pp. 9–32 [Hebrew].

Frenkel, Miriam, 'Book Lists from the Geniza as a Source for the Culture and Social History of the Jews in Mediterranean Society', in Mordechai A. Friedman (ed.), *Teʿuda XV: A Century of Geniza Research*, Tel Aviv: Tel Aviv University, 1999, pp. 333–49 [Hebrew].

Frenkel, Miriam, *The Compassionate and Benevolent: The Leading Elite in the Jewish Community of Alexandria in the Middle Ages*. Jerusalem: Ben-Zvi Institute, 2006.

Frenkel, Miriam, 'The Leadership of the Community in Aleppo in the Eleventh and Twelfth Centuries', *Peamim: Studies in Oriental Jewry*, 66, 1996, pp. 20–42 [Hebrew].

Frenkel, Miriam, 'The Medieval Jewish Community of Aleppo', MA thesis, Hebrew University of Jerusalem, 1990.

Friedenwald, Harry, *The Jews and Medicine*. Baltimore: Johns Hopkins University Press, 1944.

Friedman, Mordechai A., 'A Bitter Protest about Elimination of Piyyutim from the Service – A Request to Appeal to the Sultan', *Peamim: Studies in Oriental Jewry*, 78, 1999, pp. 128–47 [Hebrew].

Friedman, Mordechai A., 'Did Maimonides Teach Medicine? Sources and Assumptions', in Carlos del Valle Rodríguez (ed.), *Maimónides y su época*. Madrid: Sociedad Estatal de Conmemoraciones Culturales, 2007, pp. 361–76.

Friedman, Mordechai A., 'The Family of Ibn al-Amshāṭī, the House of Maimonides' In-Laws', *Zion*, 69, 2004, pp. 271–97 [Hebrew].

Friedman, Mordechai A., 'Maimonides, Zūṭā and the Muqaddams: A Story of Three Bans', *Zion*, 70, 2005, pp. 472–527 [Hebrew].

Friedman, Mordechai A., 'Maimonides *Rayyis al-Yahūd* (Head of the Jews) in Egypt', in Uri Ehrlich, Howard Kreisl and Daniel Lasker (eds), *By the Well: Studies in Jewish Philosophy and Halakhic Thought Presented to Gerald J. Blidstein*. Beersheba: Gefen, 2008, pp. 413–35.

Gervers, Michael and Ramzi Jibran Bikhazi (eds), *Conversion and Continuity: Indigenous Christian Communities in Islamic Lands, Eighth to Eighteenth Centuries*. Toronto: Pontifical Institute of Mediaeval Studies, 1990.

al-Ghazūlī, ʿAlī b. ʿAbd Allāh al-Bahāʾī, *Maṭāliʿ al-Budūr fī Manāzil al-Surūr*. Cairo: Maktabat al-Thaqāfa al-Dīniyya, 2002.

Gil, Moshe, *In the Kingdom of Ishmael*. Jerusalem: Bialik Institute / Tel Aviv: Ministry of Defense, 1997 [Hebrew].

Gil, Moshe, 'The Jewish Merchants in the Light of Eleventh Century Geniza Documents', *Journal of the Economic and Social History of the Orient*, 46(3), 2003, pp. 273–319.

Gil, Moshe, *Jews in Islamic Countries in the Middle Ages*. Leiden: Brill, 2004.

Gil, Moshe, 'The Origin of the Karaites', in Meira Polliack (ed.), *Karaite Judaism: A Guide to its History and Literary Sources*. Leiden: Brill, 2003. pp. 73–118.

Gil, Moshe, *Palestine during the First Muslim Period (643–1099)*. Tel Aviv: Tel Aviv University / Ministry of Defense, 1983 [Hebrew]. English abridgement Cambridge: Cambridge University Press, 1992.

Gil, Moshe, 'The Rādhānite Merchants and the Land of Rādhān', *Journal of the Economic and Social History of the Orient*, 17(3), 1974, pp. 299–328.

Gil, Moshe, 'Review of Historical Research on the Geniza Documents', *World Union of Jewish Studies Newsletter*, 22, 1983, pp. 17–29.

Gil, Moshe, 'Shipping in the Light of the 11th Century Cairo Geniza Documents', in Tal Oren and Michael Winter (eds), *The Encounter of Crusaders and Muslims in Palestine: As Reflected in ʾArsūf, Sayyidunā ʿAlī and Other Coastal Sites*. Tel Aviv: ha-Kibbutz ha-Meuḥad, 2007, pp. 151–90 [Hebrew].

Gil, Moshe, *The Tustaris: Family and Sect*. Tel Aviv: Diaspora Research Institute, 1981.

Gil, Moshe and Ezra Fleischer, *Yehuda ha-Levi and His Circle*, Geniza Documents 55. Jerusalem: World Union of Jewish Studies, 2001.

Giladi, Avner, *Muslim Midwives: The Craft of Birthing in the Premodern Middle East*. New York: Cambridge University Press, 2015.

Gilliot, Claude, 'Prosopography in Islam: An Essay of Classification', *Medieval Prosopography*, 23, 2002, pp. 19–54.

Goitein, Shlomo D., 'The Biography of Rabbi Judah ha-Levi in the Light of the Cairo Geniza Documents', *Proceedings of the American Academy for Jewish Research*, 28, 1959, pp. 41–56.

Goitein, Shlomo D., 'Court Records from the Cairo Geniza in JNUL', *Kirjath Sepher*, 44(1), 1968, pp. 263–76.

Goitein, Shlomo D., 'The Exchange Rate of Gold and Silver Money in Fatimid and Ayyubid Times: A Preliminary Study of the Relevant Geniza Material', *Journal of the Economic and Social History of the Orient*, 8(1), 1965, pp. 1–46.

Goitein, Shlomo D., 'From the Mediterranean to India: Documents on the Trade to India, South Arabia, and East Africa from the Eleventh and Twelfth Centuries', *Speculum*, 29(2), 1954, pp. 181–97.

Goitein, Shlomo D., *Jewish Education in Muslim Countries.* Jerusalem: Ben-Zvi Institute, 1962.

Goitein, Shlomo D., 'Jewish Society and Institutions under Islam', in H. H. Ben-Sasson and Samuel Ettinger (eds), *Jewish Society through the Ages.* London: Vallentine, Mitchell, 1971, pp. 170–85.

Goitein, Shlomo D., *Jews and Arabs: Their Contacts through the Ages*, 3rd edn. New York: Schocken, 1974.

Goitein, Shlomo D., 'A Letter from Seleucia (Cilicia), Dated 31 July 1137', *Speculum*, 39(2), 1964, pp. 298–303.

Goitein, Shlomo D., 'A Letter of Historical Importance from Seleucia (Selefke), Cilicia, Dated 21 July 1137', *Tarbiz*, 27, 1958, pp. 521–35 [Hebrew].

Goitein, Shlomo D., *Letters of Medieval Jewish Traders.* Princeton, NJ: Princeton University Press, 1973.

Goitein, Shlomo D., 'A Maghrebi Living in Cairo Implores His Karaite Wife to Return to Him', *Jewish Quarterly Review*, n.s., 73(2), 1982, pp. 138–45.

Goitein, Shlomo D., 'Maimonides' Life in the Light of the Geniza Documents', *Peraqim*, 4, 1966, pp. 29–42.

Goitein, Shlomo D., 'The Medical Profession in the Light of the Cairo Geniza Documents', *Hebrew Union College Annual*, 34, 1963, pp. 177–94.

Goitein, Shlomo D., *A Mediterranean Society: The Jewish Communities of the Arab World as Portrayed in the Documents of the Cairo Geniza.* Berkeley: University of California Press, 1967–93.

Goitein, Shlomo D., '"Meeting in Jerusalem": Messianic Expectations in the Letters of the Cairo Geniza', *AJS Review*, 4, 1979, pp. 43–57.

Goitein, Shlomo D., 'Ministrants and Physicians as Booksellers', *Kirjath Sepher*, 44(1), 1968, pp. 125–8.

Goitein, Shlomo D., 'Minority Selfrule and Government Control in Islam', *Studia Islamica*, 31, 1970, pp. 101–16.

Goitein, Shlomo D., 'The Moses Maimonides–Ibn Sanāʾ al-Mulk Circle', in Moshe Sharon (ed.), *Studies in Islamic History and Civilization in Honour of Professor David Ayalon.* Jerusalem: Cana, 1986, pp. 399–405.

Goitein, Shlomo D., 'A New Autograph by Maimonides and a Letter to Him from his Sister Miriam', *Tarbiz*, 32(2), 1963, pp. 184–94.

Goitein, Shlomo D., 'The Oldest Documentary Evidence for the Title Alf Laila wa-Laila', *Journal of the American Oriental Society*, 78(4), 1958, pp. 301–2.

Goitein, Shlomo D., *Palestinian Jewry in Early Islamic and Crusader Times*. Jerusalem: Yad Yitshak Ben Zvi, 1980 [Hebrew].

Goitein, Shlomo D., 'The Qayrawan United Appeal for the Babylonian Yeshivoth and the Emergence of the Nagid Abraham Ibn 'Aṭā'', *Zion*, 27, 1962, pp. 156–64 [Hebrew].

Goitein, Shlomo D., 'A Report on Messianic Troubles in Baghdad in 1120–21', *Jewish Quarterly Review*, n.s., 43(1), 1952, pp. 57–76.

Goitein, Shlomo D. 'The Rise of the Near-Eastern Bourgeoisie in Early Islamic Times', *Journal of World History*, 3(3), 1956–7, pp. 583–604.

Goitein, Shlomo D., 'The Social Services of the Jewish Community as Reflected in the Cairo Geniza', *Jewish Social Studies*, 26(1), 1964, pp. 3–22.

Goitein, Shlomo D., 'Three Letters from Qayrawan Addressed to Joseph ben Jacob ben 'Awkal', *Tarbiz*, 34, 1965, pp. 166–7 [Hebrew].

Goitein, Shlomo D., 'The Title and Office of the Nagid a Re-Examination', *Jewish Quarterly Review*, n.s., 53(2), 1962, pp. 93–119.

Goitein, Shlomo D., *The Yemenites: History, Communal Organization, Spiritual Life – Selected Studies*, ed. Menahem Ben-Sasson. Jerusalem: Yad Yizhak Ben Zvi / Hebrew University of Jerusalem, 1983 [Hebrew].

Goitein, Shlomo D. and Mordechai A. Friedman, *India Book I: Joseph al-Lebdi, Prominent India Trader*. Jerusalem: Ben-Zvi Institute, 2009 [Hebrew].

Goitein, Shlomo D. and Mordechai A. Friedman, *India Book II: Maḍmūn Nafid of Yemen and the India Trade*. Jerusalem: Ben-Zvi Institute, 2010 [Hebrew].

Goitein, Shlomo D. and Mordechai A. Friedman, *India Book III: Abraham Ben Yijū – India Trader and Manufacturer*. Jerusalem: Ben-Zvi Institute, 2010 [Hebrew].

Goitein, Shlomo D. and Mordechai A. Friedman, *India Book IV/A: Halfon and Judah ha-Levi – the Lives of a Merchant Scholar and a Poet Laureate according to the Cairo Geniza Documents*. Jerusalem: Ben-Zvi Institute, 2013 [Hebrew].

Goitein, Shlomo D. and Mordechai A. Friedman, *India Book IV/B: Halfon the Travelling Merchant Scholar – Cairo Geniza Documents*. Jerusalem: Ben-Zvi Institute, 2013 [Hebrew].

Goitein, Shlomo D. and Mordechai A. Friedman, *India Traders of the Middle Ages: Documents from the Cairo Geniza*. Leiden: Brill, 2008.

Golb, Norman, 'The Topography of the Jews of Medieval Egypt', *Journal of Near Eastern Studies*, 24(3), 1965, pp. 251–70.

Golb, Norman, 'The Topography of the Jews of Medieval Egypt VI: Places of

Settlement of the Jews of Medieval Egypt', *Journal of Near Eastern Studies*, 33(1), 1974, pp. 116–49.

Golb, Norman, Neḥumah B. Wahb, Ma'mar ha-Sofer B. Isaac and Moses B. Solomon, 'Legal Documents from the Cairo Geniza', *Jewish Social Studies*, 20(1), 1958, pp. 17–46.

Goldberg, Jessica L., *Trade and Institutions in the Medieval Mediterranean: The Geniza Merchants and Their Business World.* Cambridge: Cambridge University Press, 2012.

Goldziher, Ignaz, 'Ibn Hūd, the Mohammedan Mystic, and the Jews of Damascus', *Jewish Quarterly Review*, 6(1), 1893, pp. 218–20.

Goskar, Tehmina, 'Material Worlds: The Shared Cultures of Southern Italy and Its Mediterranean Neighbours in the Tenth to Twelfth Centuries', *Al-Masāq*, 23(3), 2011, pp. 189–204.

Gottheil, Richard, 'Dhimmis and Moslems in Egypt', in Robert Harper, Francis Brown and George Foot Moore (eds), *Old Testament and Semitic Studies in Memory of William Rainey Harper*. Chicago: University of Chicago Press, 1908, vol. II, pp. 351–414.

Gottheil, Richard, 'A Distinguished Family of Fatimide Cadis (al-Nuʿmān) in the Tenth Century', *Journal of the American Oriental Society*, 27, 1906, pp. 217–96.

Gottheil, Richard, 'An Eleventh-Century Document Concerning a Cairo Synagogue,' *Jewish Quarterly Review*, 19(3), 1907, pp. 467–539.

Gottheil, Richard and William H Worrell, *Fragments from the Cairo Genizah in the Freer Collection*. London: Macmillan, 1927.

Gottschalk, Hans, *Die Mādarāiʾjjun: ein Beitrag zur Geschichte Ägyptens unter dem Islam*. Berlin and Leipzig: Walter de Gruyter, 1931.

Greenstone, Julius H., 'Two Memorial Lists from the Genizah', *Jewish Quarterly Review*, n.s., 1(1), 1910, pp. 43–59.

Grossman, Avraham, 'From Father to Son: The Inheritance of the Spiritual Leadership of the Jewish Communities in the Early Middle Ages', *Zion*, 50, 1985, pp. 189–220 [Hebrew].

Grossman, Avraham, 'The Relationship between the Social Structure and Spiritual Activity of Jewish Communities in the Geonic Period', *Zion*, 53, 1988, pp. 259–72 [Hebrew].

Guetta, Alessandro and Masha Itzhaki (eds), *Studies in Medieval Jewish Poetry: A Message upon the Garden*. Leiden: Brill, 2009.

Guthrie, Douglas, *Janus in the Doorway*. London: Pitman Medical, 1963.

Hacker, Joseph R., 'On the Character of the Cairo Mustaarib Community Leadership at the End of the Sixteenth Century', in Joseph R. Hacker and Yaron Harel (eds), *The Sceptre Shall Not Depart from Judah: Leadership, Rabbinate and Community in Jewish History*. Jerusalem: Bialik Institute, 2011. pp. 89–100 [Hebrew].

Ḥaddād, ʿAzrā (trans. & ed.), *Riḥlat Ibn Yūna al-Andalusī ilā Bilād al-Sharq al-Islāmī. Li-Binyāmīn b. Yūna al-Taṭīlī al-Nabārī*. Beirut: Dār Ibn Zaydūn, 1996.

Hamarneh, Sami, 'The Climax of Medieval Arabic Professional Pharmacy', *Bulletin of the History of Medicine*, 42(5), 1968, pp. 450–61.

Hamarneh, Sami, 'Development of Hospitals in Islam', *Journal of History of Medicine*, 17(3), 1962, pp. 366–84.

Hamarneh, Sami, 'Origin and Functions of the Ḥisba System in Islam and Its Impact on the Health Professions', *Sudhoffs Archiv für Geschichte der Medizin und der Naturwissenschaften*, 48, 1964, pp. 157–73.

Hamarneh, Sami, *The Physician, Therapist and Surgeon Ibn al-Quff (1233–1286): An Introductory Survey of His Time, Life and Work*. Cairo: Atlas Press, 1974.

Hamarneh, Sami, 'The Rise of Professional Pharmacy in Islam', *Medical History*, 6(1), 1962, pp. 59–6.

Hammer-Purgstall, Joseph Freiherr von, *Literaturgeschichte der Araber: von ihrem Beginne bis zu Ende des zwölften Jahrhunderts der Hidschret*. Vienna: Kaiserlich-königliche Hof- und Staatsdruckerei, 1850–6.

Harris, W. V., 'Popular Medicine in the Classical World', in W. V. Harris (ed.), *Popular Medicine in Graeco-Roman Antiquity: Explorations*. Leiden: Brill, 2016, pp. 1–64.

Hary, Benjamin and Marina Rustow, 'Karaites at the Rabbinical Court: A Legal Deed from Mahdiyya Dated 1073 (T-S 20.187)', *Ginzei Qedem*, 2, 2006, pp. *9–*36.

Hazan, Uri, 'Medical, Administrative and Financial Aspects of Hospitals in Medieval Islam 8th–15th Centuries'. PhD dissertation, Bar-Ilan University, 2004 [Hebrew].

Heynick, Frank, *Jews and Medicine: An Epic Saga*. Hoboken, NJ: Ktav, 2002.

Hirschberg, Julius, *The History of Ophthalmology, Vol. I: Antiquity*, trans. Frederic C. Blodi. Bonn: Wayenborgh, 1982.

Hirschberg, W. Z., *A History of the Jews in North Africa*. Leiden: E. J. Brill, 1974.

Hodgson, Marshall G. S., *The Venture of Islam: Conscience and History in a World Civilization, Vol. 1: The Classical Age of Islam*. Chicago: University of Chicago Press, 1974.

Hofer, Nathan, 'The Ideology of Decline and the Jews of Ayyubid and Mamluk Syria', in Stephan Conermann (ed.), *Muslim–Jewish Relations in the Middle*

Islamic Period: Jews in the Ayyubid and Mamluk Sultanates (1171–1517). Göttingen: V&R unipress, 2017, pp. 95–120.

Höglmeier, Manuela, *al-Ǧawbarī und seine Kašf al-asrār: ein Sittenbild des Gauners im arabischen-islamischen Mittelalter (7./13. Jahrhundert)*. Berlin: Klaus Schwarz, 2006.

Hoki, Yu, 'Dāniyāl ibn Shuʿyā's Ophthalmologic Question-and-Answer Textbook: A Study on Cairo Genizah Fragments of the Eleventh–Thirteenth Centuries', *Orient*, 53, 2018, pp. 69–93.

Hoki, Yu, 'Logic in Compound Drugs According to Medieval Arabic Medical Books and the Cairo Genizah', *Orient*, 52, 2017, pp. 59–78.

Humphreys, R. Stephen, *Islamic History: A Framework for Inquiry*, rev. edn. Princeton, NJ: Princeton University Press, 1991.

Ibn Abī Uṣaybiʿa, Aḥmad b. al-Qāsim, *ʿUyūn al-Anbāʾ fī ṭabaqāt al-aṭibbāʾ* ed. A. Müller. Cairo: al-Maṭbaʿa al-Wahhābiyya, 1882; Königsberg, 1884.

Ibn al-Furāt, Muḥammad b. ʿAbd al-Raḥīm, *Taʾrīkh Ibn al-Furāt [= Taʾrīkh al-Duwal wa-l-Mulūk]*, ed. Q. Zurayq. Beirut: al-Maṭbaʿa al-Amrīkānīyya, 1936–42.

Ibn al-Fuwaṭī, *Majmaʿ al-Ādāb fī Muʿjam al-Alqāb*, ed. Muḥammad al-Kāẓim. Tehran: Muʾasassa al-Ṭibāʿa, 1995–6.

Ibn Ḥajar al-ʿAsqalānī, Aḥmad b. ʿAlī, *Inbāʾ al-Ghumr bi-Abnāʾ al-ʿUmr*. Hayderabad: Dāʾirat al-Maʿārif al-ʿUthamaniyya, 1967; repr. Beirut: Dār al-Kutub al-ʿIlmiyya, 1986.

Ibn Ḥajar l-ʿAsqalānī, Aḥmad b. ʿAlī, *al-Durar al-Kāmina fī Aʿyān al-Miʾah al-Thāmina*, ed. Muḥammad Sayyid Jād al-Ḥaqq. Cairo: Dār al-Kutub al-Ḥadītha, 1966.

Ibn al-Hājj, *al-Madkhal ilā Tammiyat al-ʿAmāl bi-Taḥsin an-Niyya*. Cairo: al-Maṭbaʿa al-Miṣriyya bi-l-Azhar, 1929 [Arabic].

Ibn Ḥazm al-Andalusī, *Rasāʾil Ibn Ḥazm al-Andalusī*, ed. Iḥsān ʿAbbās. Beirut: al-Muʾassasa al-ʿArabiyya li-l-Dirāsat wa-l-Nashr, 1980–3.

Ibn Iyās, Muḥammad ibn Aḥmad, *Badāʾiʿ al-Zuhūr fī Waqāʾiʿ al-Dhuhūr*, ed. Mohammed Mustafa. Istanbul: Maṭbaʿat al-Maʿārif, 1936.

Ibn Juljul, Sulimān Bin Ḥasan, *Ṭabaqāt al-Aṭibbāʾ wa al-Ḥukmāʾ*. Beirut: Muʾasasat al-Risāla, 1985.

Ibn Jumayʿ, Hibbatallah b. Zayn, *Treatise to Ṣalāḥ ad-Dīn on the Revival of the Art of Medicine*, trans. & ed. Hartmut Fahndrich. Wiesbaden: Franz Steiner, 1983.

Ibn Kathīr, Ismāʿīl b. ʿUmar, *al-Bidāya wa-l-Nihāya*. Beirut: Dār al-Kutub al-ʿIlmiyya, 1993.

Ibn Khaldūn, *Tarʾīkh al-ʿAlāma Ibn Khaldūn: Kitāb al-ʿibar wa-Dīwān al-Mubtadaʾ*

wa-l-Khabar fī Ayyām al-ʿArab wa-l-ʿAjam wa-l-Barbar wa-man ʿĀṣarahum min Dhawī l-Sulṭān al-Akbar. Beirut: Dār l-Kitāb al-Lubnānī, 1958–9.

Ibn Murād, Ibrāhīm, *Buḥūth fī Taʾrīkh al-Ṭibb wa-l-Ṣaydaliyya ʿinda al-ʿArab*. Beirut: Dār al-Gharb al-Islāmī, 1991.

Ibn al-Qifṭī, Jamāl al-Dīn Abū al-Ḥasan ʿAlī ibn Yūsuf, *Taʾrīkh al-Ḥukamāʾ*, ed. Julius Lippert. Leipzig: Dieterich'sche Verlagsbuchhandlung, 1903.

Ibn Saʿīd, ʿAlī b. Mūsa, *al-Nujūm al-Zāhira fī Ḥulā Ḥaḍrat al-Qāhira*. Cairo: Maṭbaʿt Dār al-Kitāb, 1970.

Ibn Sahl, Sābūr, *The Small Dispensatory*, trans. Oliver Kahl. Leiden; Brill, 2003.

Ibn Taghrī Birdī, Abū al-Maḥāsin Yūsuf, *al-Manhal al-Ṣāfī wa-l-Mustawfā baʿda al-Wāfī*. Cairo: al-Hayʾa al-Miṣriyya al-ʿĀmma, 1984–2009.

ʿIsā Aḥmad Bek, *Muʿjam al-Atibbāʾ min Sanat 650 ilā Yawminā Hādhā: dhayl ʿUyūn al-Anbāʾ fī Ṭabaqāt al-Aṭibbāʾ li-Ibn-Abī- Uṣaybiʿa,* Cairo: Cairo University Press, 1942.

Isaacs, Haskell D., 'An Encounter with Maimonides', in Fred Rosner and Samuel S. Kottek (eds), *Moses Maimonides: Physician, Scientist, and Philosopher*. Northvale, NJ, and London: Jason Aronson, 1993, pp. 41–8, 240–2.

Isaacs, Haskell D,, *Medical and Para-medical Manuscripts in the Cambridge Genizah Collections*. Cambridge: Cambridge University Press, 1994.

Jacoby, David. 'Jewish Doctors and Surgeons in Crete under Venetian Rule', in Robert Bonfil, Menahem Ben-Sasson and Joseph R, Hacker (eds), *Culture and Society in Medieval Jewry: Studies Dedicated to the Memory of Haim Hillel Ben-Sasson*. Jerusalem: Historical Society of Israel, Zalman Shazar Center, 1989, pp. 431–44.

Jacquart, Danielle, *La Médecine médiévale dans le cadre parisien (XIVe–XVe siècle)*. Paris: Fayard, 1998.

Jacquart, Danielle, *Le Milieu médical en France du XIIe au XVe siècle*. Geneva: Droz, 1981.

Jacquart, Danielle, *Le Milieu médical en France du XIIe au XVe siècle: en annexe, 2e supplément au 'Dictionnaire' d'Ernest Wickersheimer*. Geneva: Droz; Paris, 1981.

Jadon, Samira, 'A Comparison of the Wealth, Prestige, and Medical Works of the Physicians of Salah al-Din in Egypt and Syria', *Bulletin of the History of Medicine*, 44(1), 1970, pp. 64–75.

Jadon, Samira, 'The Physicians of Syria during the Reign of Salāh Al-Din, 570–589 AH 1174–1193 AD', *Journal of the History of Medicine and Allied Sciences*, 25(3), 1970, pp. 323–40.

al-Jazarī, Shams al-Dīn Muḥammad, *Ḥawādith al-Zamān wa-Anbā'uhu wa-Wafayāt al-Akābir wa-l-A'yān min Abnā'ihi*. Beirut: al-Maktaba al-'Aṣriyya, 2006.

Jones, Peter Murray, 'Harley MS 2558: A Fifteenth-Century Medical Commonplace Book', in Margaret R. Schleissner (ed.), *Manuscript Sources of Medieval Medicine*. New York and London: Garland, 1995, pp. 35–54.

Kaḥāla, 'Umar Riḍā. *Mu'jam al-Mu'allifīn: Tarājim Muṣannifī al-Kutub al-'Arabiyya*. Beirut: Mu'assasa al-Risāla, 1993.

Kahl, Oliver, *The Dispensatory of Ibn al-Tilmīḏ*. Leiden: Brill, 2007.

Kahl, Oliver, 'Sābūr b. Sahl', in *The Encyclopedia of Islam*, new edn. Leiden: Brill, 1960–2007, vol. VIII, p. 694.

Kahl, Oliver, *Sābūr ibn Sahl's Dispensatory in the Recession of the 'Aḍudī Hospital*. Leiden: Brill, 2009.

Karmi, Ghanda, 'State Control of the Physicians in the Middle Ages: as Islamic Model', in Andrew W. Russell (ed.), *The Town and State Physician in Europe from the Middle Ages to the Enlightenment*. Wolfenbüttel, Germany: Herzog August Bibliothek, 1981. pp. 63–84.

Katsh, Abraham I., 'From the Moscow Manuscript of David ha-Nagid's Midrash on Genesis', *Jewish Quarterly Review*, n.s., 48(2), 1957, pp. 140–60.

Keats-Rohan, K. S. B. (ed.), *Prosopography Approaches and Applications: A Handbook*. Oxford: Unit for Prosopographical Research, 2007.

Kedar, Benjamin Z., 'The Frankish Period', in Alan D. Crown (ed.), *The Samaritans*, Tübingen: J. C. B. Mohr (Siebeck), 1989, pp. 82–94.

Kennedy, Hugh, *Muslim Spain and Portugal: A Political History of al-Andalus*. London and New York: Longman, 1996.

al-Khālidī, Khalid Yūnis, *al-Yahūd Taḥta Ḥukm al-Muslimīn fī al-Andalus 92-897, H, 711–1492*. Gaza: Dār al-Arqam lil-Tibā'ah wa-l-Nashr, 2000.

Khan, Geoffrey, *Arabic Legal and Administrative Documents in the Cambridge Genizah Collections*. Cambridge: Cambridge University Press, 1993.

al-Khazrajī, 'Alī b. al-Ḥasan, *al-'Uqūd al-Lu'lu'iyya fī Ta'rīkh al-Dawla al-Rusūliyya*. San'a: Markaz al-Dirāsāt al-Buḥūth al-Yamanī.

Klein-Franke, Felix and Zhu Ming, 'Rashīd al-Dīn as a Transmitter of Chinese Medicine to the West', *Le Muséon*, 109(3–4), 1996, pp. 395–404.

Kozodoy, Maud, 'The Jewish Physician in Medieval Iberia (1100–1500)', in Jonathan Ray (ed.), *The Jew in Medieval Iberia*. Boston, MA: Academic Studies Press, 2011, pp. 102–37.

Kraemer, Joel L., *Maimonides: The Life and World of One of Civilization's Greatest Minds*. New York: Doubleday, 2008.

Kraemer, Joel L., 'Six Unpublished Maimonides Letters from the Cairo Geniza', in Arthur Hyman (ed.), *Maimonidean Studies, Vol. II*. New York: Michael Scharf Publication Trust of Yeshiva University Press, 1991, pp. 61–94.

Krawulsky, Dorothea, *The Mongol Īlkhāns and their Vizier Rashīd al-Dīn*. Frankfurt: Peter Lang, 2011.

Lambourn, Elizabeth A., *Abraham's Luggage: A Social Life of Things in the Medieval Indian Ocean World*. Cambridge: Cambridge University Press, 2018.

Lane-Poole, Stanley, *A History of Egypt in the Middle Ages*, 4th edn. London: Frank Cass, [1925] 1968.

Langermann, Y. Tzvi, 'From My Notebooks: Masīḥ bin Ḥakam, a Jewish-Christian(?) Physician of the Early Ninth Century', *Aleph*, 4, 2004, pp. 283–97.

Langermann, Y. Tzvi, 'Three Singular Treatises from Yemeni Manuscripts', *Bulletin of the School of Oriental and African Studies*, 54(3), 1991, pp. 568–71.

Lasker, Daniel J., 'Ibn Simeon, Judah b. Joseph', in Norman A. Stillman (ed.), *Encyclopedia of Jews in the Islamic World Online*. Leiden: Brill, 2013.

Lasker, Daniel J., 'Israeli, Isaac ben Solomon', in Norman A. Stillman (ed.), *Encyclopedia of Jews in the Islamic World Online*. Leiden: Brill, 2013.

Lasker, Daniel J., 'Karaism and Jewish Studies', in *Shlomo Dov Goitein Memorial Lecture*. Tel Aviv: Tel Aviv University Press, 2000 [Hebrew].

Lasker, Daniel J,, 'Medieval Karaism and Science', in Gad Freudenthal (ed.), *Science in Medieval Jewish Cultures*. Cambridge: Cambridge University Press, 2011, pp. 427–37.

Le Strange, Guy, *Palestine under the Muslims: A Description of Syria and the Holy Land from* AD *650 to 1500, Translated from the Works of the Medieval Arab Geographers*. Beirut: Khayats, [1890] 1965.

Lecker, Michael, 'The Prosopography of Early Islamic Administration', *Jerusalem Studies in Arabic and Islam*, 34 (2008), pp. 1–5.

Leiser, Gary, 'Medical Education in Islamic Lands from the Seventh to the Fourteenth Century', *Journal of the History of Medicine and Allied Sciences*, 38, 1983, pp. 48–75.

el-Leithy, Tamer, 'Coptic Culture and Conversion in Medieval Cairo, 1293–1524 AD'. PhD dissertation, Princeton University, 2005.

Lev, Efraim, 'A Catalogue of the Medical and Para-Medical Manuscripts in the Mosseri Geniza Collection', *Journal of Jewish Studies*, 62(1), 2011, pp. 121–45.

Lev, Efraim, 'Drugs Held and Sold by Pharmacists of the Jewish Community of Medieval (11th–14th Centuries) Cairo According to Lists of *Materia Medica*

Found at the Taylor-Schechter Geniza Collection, Cambridge', *Journal of Ethnopharmacology*, 110(2), 2007, pp. 275–93.

Lev, Efraim, 'An Early Fragment of Ibn Jazlah's Tabulated Manual '*Taqwīm al-Abdān*' from the Cairo Genizah (T-S Ar.41.137)', *Journal of the Royal Asiatic Society*, 24(2), 2014, pp. 189–223.

Lev, Efraim, 'Mediators between Theoretical and Practical Medieval Knowledge: Medical Notebooks from the Cairo Genizah and their Significance', *Medical History*, 57(4), 2013, pp. 487–515.

Lev, Efraim, 'Medieval Egyptian Judaeo-Arabic Prescriptions (and the Edition of Three Medical Prescriptions)', *Journal of the Royal Asiatic Society*, 18(4), 2008, pp. 449–64.

Lev, Efraim, 'Work in Progress: The Research of Medical Knowledge in the Cairo Geniza – Past, Present and Future', in Stefan Reif, *The Written Word Remains: The Archive and the Achievement*. Cambridge: Taylor-Schechter Geniza Research Unit at Cambridge University Library, 2004, pp. 37–51.

Lev, Efraim and Zohar Amar, 'Ethnopharmacological Survey of Traditional Drugs Sold in Israel at the End of the 20th Century', *Journal of Ethnopharmacology*, 72(1–2), 2000, pp. 191–205.

Lev, Efraim and Zohar Amar, 'Ethnopharmacological Survey of Traditional Drugs Sold in the Kingdom of Jordan', *Journal of Ethnopharmacology*, 82, 2002, pp. 131–45.

Lev, Efraim and Zohar Amar, 'Practice versus Theory: Medieval *Materia Medica* According to the Cairo Geniza', *Medical History*, 51(4), 2007, pp. 507–26.

Lev, Efraim and Zohar Amar, *Practical Materia Medica of the Medieval Eastern Mediterranean According to the Cairo Geniza*. Leiden: Brill, 2008.

Lev, Efraim and Leigh Chipman, *Medical Prescriptions in the Cambridge Genizah Collections: Practical Medicine and Pharmacology in Medieval Egypt*. Leiden: Brill, 2012.

Lev, Efraim and Leigh Chipman, 'Texts/Documents/Translations: A Fragment of a Judaeo-Arabic Manuscript of Sābūr b. Sahl's *Al-Aqrābādhīn al-Ṣaghīr* Found in the Taylor-Schechter Cairo Genizah Collection', *Medieval Encounters*, 13, 2007, pp. 347–62.

Lev, Efraim, Leigh Chipman and Friedrich Niessen, 'Chicken and Chicory Are Good for You: A Unique Family Prescription from the Cairo Geniza (T-S NS 223.82–83)', *Jerusalem Studies in Arabic and Islam,* 35, 2008, pp. 335–52.

Lev, Efraim, Leigh Chipman and Friedrich Niessen, 'A Hospital Handbook for the Community: Evidence for the Extensive Use of Ibn Abī 'l-Bayān's *al-Dustūr al-bīmāristānī* by the Jewish Practitioners of Medieval Cairo', *Journal of Semitic Studies*, 53, 2008, pp. 103–18.

Lev, Efraim and Friedrich Niessen, 'Addenda to Isaacs's "Catalogue of the Medical and Para-medical Manuscripts in the Cambridge Genizah Collection" Together with the Edition of Two Medical Documents T-S 12.33 and T-S NS 297.56', *Hebrew Union College Annual*, 77, 2008, pp. 131–65.

Lev, Efraim and Renate Smithuis, 'A Preliminary Catalogue of the Medical and Para-Medical Manuscripts in the Rylands Geniza Collection, Together with the Partial Edition of Two Medical Fragments (A 589 and B 3239)', in Renate Smithuis and Philip S. Alexander (eds), *From Cairo to Manchester: Studies in the Rylands Genizah Fragments*. Oxford: Oxford University Press, 2013, pp. 157–97.

Lev, Yaacov, *Charity, Endowments, and Charitable Institutions in Medieval Islam*. Gainesville: University Press of Florida, 2005.

Lev, Yaacov, 'Persecutions and Conversion to Islam in Eleventh Century Egypt', *Asian and African Studies*, 22(1–3), 1988, pp. 73–91.

Lev, Yaacov, *Saladin in Egypt*. Leiden: Brill, 1999.

Levey, Martin, *Early Arabic Pharmacology: An Introduction Based on Ancient and Medieval Sources*. Leiden: Brill, 1973.

Levey, Martin, 'Ibn Māsawaih and his Treatise on Simple Aromatic Substances: Studies in the History of Arabic Pharmacology I', *Journal of the History of Medicine and Allied Science*, 16, 1961, pp. 394–410.

Levey, Martin, *Medical Ethics of Medieval Islam, with Special Reference to al-Ruhdwi's 'Practical Ethics of the Physician'*. Philadelphia: American Philosophical Society, 1967.

Levey, Martin, *The Medical Formulary or the ʾAqrābādhīn of al-Kindī*. Madison: University of Wisconsin Press, 1966.

Levey, Martin, 'The Pharmacology of Ibn Biklārish in the Introduction of His *Kitāb Al-Mustaʿīnī*', *Studies in Islam*, 6, 1969, pp. 98–104.

Levey, Martin and Noury al-Khaledy, *The Medical Formulary of al-Samarqandī*. Philadelphia: University of Pennsylvania Press, 1967.

Lévi-Provençal, Evariste, *Un Manuel hispanique de 'Ḥisba'*. Paris: Ernest Leroux, 1931.

Levtzion, Nehemia (ed.), *Conversion to Islam*. New York: Holmes & Meier, 1979.

Levtzion, Nehemia, 'Conversion to Islam in Syria and Palestine and the Survival of Christian Communities', in Michael Gervers and Ramzi Jibran Bikhazi (eds), *Conversion and Continuity: Indigenous Christian Communities in Islamic*

Lands Eighth to Eighteenth Centuries. Toronto: Pontifical Institute of Mediaeval Studies, 1990, pp. 289–311.

Levy-Rubin, Milka, 'New Evidence Relating to the Process of Islamization in Palestine in the Early Muslim Period: The Case of Samaria', *Journal of the Economic and Social History of the Orient*, 43(3), 2000, pp. 257–76.

Lewicka, Paulina B., 'Healer, Scholar, Conspirator: The Jewish Physician in the Arabic-Islamic Discourse of the Mamluk Period', in Stephan Conermann (ed.), *Muslim–Jewish Relations in the Middle Islamic Period: Jews in the Ayyubid and Mamluk Sultanates (1171–1517)*. Göttingen: V&R unipress, 2017, pp. 121–44.

Lewicka, Paulina B., *Medicine for Muslims? Islamic Theologians, Non-Muslim Physicians and the Medical Culture of the Mamluke Near East*, ASK Working Paper 3. Bonn: Annemarie Schimmel Kolleg, July 2012.

Lewicka, Paulina B., 'The Non-Muslim Physician in the Muslim Society: Remarks on the Religious Context of Medical Practice in Medieval Near East', in Agostino Cilardo (ed.), *Islam and Globalization: Historical and Contemporary Perspectives*. Leuven: Peeters, 2013, pp. 500–12.

Lewicka, Paulina B. and Gad Freudenthal, 'The Reception and Practice of Rationalist Medicine and Thoughts in Medieval Jewish Communities, East and West', in Josef Meri (ed.), *The Routledge Handbook of Muslim–Jewish Relations*. New York; Routledge, 2016, pp. 95–114.

Lewis, Bernard, *The Jews of Islam*. Princeton: Princeton University Press, 1984.

Lewis, Bernard, 'Palṭiel: A Note', *Bulletin of the School of Oriental and African Studies*, 30(1), 1967, pp. 177–81.

Little, Donald P., 'Coptic Conversion to Islam under the Baḥrī Mamlūks, 692–755/1293–1354', *Bulletin of the School of Oriental and African Studies*, 39(3), 1976, pp. 552–69.

Luṭf, ʿUmar Muṣṭafā, *Yahūd Miṣr al-Ayūbiyya: Dirāsa Taʾrīkhiyya Jadīda*. Riyadh: Kuliyyat al-Muʿallimīn, 2009.

Maimonides, Moses, *Treatise on Asthma*, ed. Suessman Muntner. Philadelphia: Lippincott, 1963.

Makdisi, George, *The Rise of Humanism in Classical Islam and the Christian West: With Special Reference to Scholasticism*. Edinburgh: Edinburgh University Press, 1990.

Mann, Jacob, *The Jews in Egypt and in Palestine under the Fatimid Caliphs*. New York: Ktav, 1970.

Mann, Jacob, *Texts and Studies in Jewish History and Literature*. Jerusalem: Ktav, 1972.

Mann, Jacob, *Texts and Studies in Jewish History and Literature, Vol. II: Karaitica.* Philadelphia: Hebrew Press of the Jewish Publication Society of America, 1935.

al-Maqqarī, Aḥmad b. Muḥammad, *Nafḥ al-Ṭīb fī Ghuṣn al-Andalus al-Raṭīb*, ed. Iḥsān ʿAbbās. Beirut: Dār Ṣādir, 1968.

al-Maqrīzī, Taqī al-Dīn Aḥmad b. ʿAlī, *Durar al-ʿUqūd al-Farīda fī Tarājim al-Aʿyān al-Mufīda.* Cairo: Dār al-Gharb al-Islāmī, 2002.

al-Maqrīzī, Taqī al-Dīn Aḥmad b. ʿAlī, *Ittiʿāẓ al-Ḥunafāʾ bi-Akhbār al-Aʾimma al-Faṭimiyyīn al-Khulafāʾ*, ed. Jamāl al-Dīn al-Shayyāl. Cairo: al-Majlis al-Aʿlā li-l-Shuʾūn al-Islāmiyya, 1967.

al-Maqrīzī, Taqī al-Dīn Aḥmad b. ʿAlī, *Kitāb al-Muqaffā al-Kabīr*, ed. Muḥammad al-Yaʿlāwī. Beirut, 1991.

al-Maqrīzī, Taqī al-Dīn Aḥmad b. ʿAlī, *Kitāb al-Sulūk li-Maʿrifa Duwal al-Mulūk*, ed. Muṣṭafā Ziyādah and Saʿīd ʿAbd al-Fattāḥ ʿĀshūr. Cairo: Lajnat al-Taʾlīf wa-l-Tarjama wa-l-Nashr, 1934–73.

al-Maqrīzī, Taqī al-Dīn Aḥmad b. ʿAlī, *al-Mawāʿiẓ wa-l-Iʿtibār bi-Dhikr al-Khiṭaṭ wa-l-Āthār fī Miṣr wa-l-Qāhira.* Cairo: Bulaq, 1854.

Margariti, Roxani Eleni, Aden and the Indian Ocean Trade: 150 Years in the Life of a Medieval Arabian Port. Chapel Hill: University of North Carolina Press, 2007.

Margariti, Roxani Eleni, 'Maritime Cityscapes: Lessons from Real and Imagined Topographies of Western Indian Ocean Ports', in: Roxani E. Margariti, Adam Sabra and Petra M. Sijpesteijn (eds), *Histories of the Middle East: Studies in Middle Eastern Society, Economy and Law in Honor of A. L. Udovitch.* Leiden: Brill, 2011, pp.101–26.

Margoliouth, G., 'Ibn Al-Hītī's Arabic Chronicle of Karaite Doctors', *Jewish Quarterly Review*, 9(3), 1897, pp. 429–43.

Marín, Manuela, 'Anthroponymy and Society: The Occupational *Laqab* of Andalusian *ʿulamāʾ*', in Jens Ludtke (ed.), *Romania Arabica: Festschrift für Reinhold Kontzi zum 70. Geburtstag.* Tübingen: Gunter Narr, 1996. pp. 271–9.

Marín, Manuela, 'Biography and Prosopography in Arab-Islamic Medieval Culture, Introductory Remarks', *Medieval Prosopography*, 23, 2002, pp. 1–17.

Martindale, J. R., 'The Prosopography of the Byzantine Empire', *Medieval Prosopography*, 17(1), 1996, pp. 169–91.

Martínez Delgado, José, 'Ibn Janāḥ', in Norman A. Stillman (ed.), *Encyclopedia of Jews in the Islamic World Online.* Leiden: Brill, 2013.

Martínez Delgado, José, 'Ibn Yashūsh, Isaac (Abū Ibrāhīm) Ibn Qasṭār', in Norman

A. Stillman (ed.), *Encyclopedia of Jews in the Islamic World Online*. Leiden: Brill, 2013.

Mazor, Amir, 'Asad al-Yahūdī', in Norman A. Stillman (ed.), *Encyclopedia of Jews in the Islamic World Online*. Leiden: Brill, 2013.

Mazor, Amir, 'Faraj Allāh ibn Ṣaghīr', in Norman A. Stillman (ed.), *Encyclopedia of Jews in the Islamic World Online*. Leiden: Brill, 2013.

Mazor, Amir, 'Ibn Ṣaghīr/Ibn Kūjik Family', in Norman A. Stillman (ed.), *Encyclopedia of Jews in the Islamic World Online*. Leiden: Brill, 2013.

Mazor, Amir, 'Jewish Court Physicians in the Mamluk Sultanate during the First Half of the 8th/14th Century', *Medieval Encounters*, 20(1), 2014, pp. 38–65.

Mazor, Amir, 'Maimonides' Apostasy According to Muslim and Jewish Sources', *Journal of Jewish Studies*, 70(2), 2019, pp. 318–31.

Mazor, Amir, 'Sadīd al-Dimyāṭī', in Norman A. Stillman (ed.), *Encyclopedia of Jews in the Islamic World Online*. Leiden: Brill, 2013.

Mazor, Amir and Efraim Lev, 'Dynasties of Jewish Physicians in the Fatimid and Ayyubid Periods', *Hebrew Union College Annual*, 89, 2019, pp. 225–65.

Mazor, Amir and Efraim Lev, 'The Phenomenon of Dynasties of Jewish Doctors in the Mamluk Period (1250–1517)', *European Journal of Jewish Studies*, 15, 2020, pp. 1–29.

Mazor, Amir and Efraim Lev, 'A Mosaic of Medieval Historical Sources – The Biography of the Egyptian Jewish physician Ibn Jumayʿ', *Revue des études juives* (forthcoming).

Meouak, Mohamed, 'Prosopography of the Political Elites and the "Sociography" of the Umayyad State of Cordoba', *Medieval Prosopography*, 23, 2002, pp. 167–84.

Meyerhof, Max, *Un Glossaire de matière médicale de Maimonide*. Cairo: Imprimerie de l'Institut Français d'Archéologie Orientale, 1940.

Meyerhof, Max, 'Jewish Physicians Contemporaries of Maimonides', *Koroth*, 7(5–6), 1977, pp. 392–400.

Meyerhof, Max, 'The Medical Work of Maimonides', in Salo W. Baron (ed.), *Essays on Maimonides*. New York: Columbia University Press, 1941, pp. 265–99.

Meyerhof, Max, 'Medieval Jewish Physicians in the Near East, from Arabic Sources', *Isis*, 28, 1938, pp. 432–60.

Meyerhof, Max, 'Notes sur quelques médecins juifs égyptiens qui se sont illustrés à l'époque arabe', *Isis*, 12(1), 1929, pp. 113–31.

Meyerhof, Max, 'Sultan Saladin's Physician on the Transmission of Greek Medicine to the Arabs', *Bulletin of the History of Medicine*, 18(2), 1945, pp. 169–78.

Meyerhof, Max, 'Von Alexandrien nach Bagdad: ein Beitrag zur Geschichte des Philosophischen und Medizinischen Unterrichts bei den Arabern', *Sitzungsberichte der Akademie der Wissenschaften*, 23, 1930, pp. 389–429.

Micheau, Françoise, 'Great Figures in Arabic Medicine, According to Ibn al-Qifṭī', in Sheila Campbell, Bert Hall and David Klausner (eds), *Health, Disease and Healing in Medieval Culture*. Basingstoke: Macmillan, 1992.

Micheau, Françoise, 'Hommes de sciences au prisme d'Ibn Qifti', *Cahiers de la Méditerranée*, 37, 1988, pp. 81–106.

Miller, Kathryn A., 'Doctors without Borders: Medicine in the Medieval Mediterranean World', in Joseph V. Montville (ed.), *History as Prelude: Muslims and Jews in the Medieval Mediterranean*. Lanham, MD: Lexington, 2011, pp. 109–30.

Miquel, Andre. 'Ibrāhīm b. Yaʿḳūb', in *The Encyclopedia of Islam*, new edn. Leiden: Brill, 1960–2007.

Mitchell, Piers D., *Medicine in the Crusades: Warfare, Wounds, and the Medieval Surgeon*. Cambridge: Cambridge University Press, 2004.

Molad-Vaza, Ora, 'Clothing in the Mediterranean Jewish Society as Reflected in the Documents of the Cairo Geniza, between the Middle of the 10th Century and the Middle of the 13th Century', PhD dissertation, Hebrew University of Jerusalem, 2010 [Hebrew].

Montgomery, James A., *The Samaritans, The Earliest Jewish Sect: Their History, Theology and Literature*. Eugene, OR: Wipf & Stock, [1907] 2006.

Moreen, Vera B., 'Rashīd al-Dīn Tabib', in Norman A. Stillman (ed.), *Encyclopedia of Jews in the Islamic World Online*. Leiden: Brill, 2013.

Morgan, David O., 'Rashīd al-Dīn Ṭabīb', in *The Encyclopedia of Islam*, new edn. Leiden: Brill, 1960–2007, vol. VII, pp. 443–4.

Morony, Michael G., 'The Age of Conversions: A Reassessment', in Michael Gervers and Ramzi Jibran Bikhazi (eds), *Conversion and Continuity: Indigenous Christian Communities in Islamic Lands, Eighth to Eighteenth Centuries*. Toronto: Pontifical Institute of Mediaeval Studies, 1990.

Mosseri, Jacques, *Catalogue of the Jacques Mosseri Collection*. Jerusalem: Jewish National and University Library, 1990.

Motzkin, Aryeh L., 'The Arabic Correspondence of Judge Elijah and His Family: A Chapter in the Social History of Thirteenth Century Egypt'. PhD dissertation, University of Pennsylvania, 1965.

Motzkin, Aryeh L., 'Elijah ben Zechariah, a Member of Abraham Maimuni's Court: A Geniza Portrait', *Revue des Études Juives*, 128, 1969, pp. 339–48.

Motzkin, Aryeh L., 'A Thirteenth-Century Jewish Physician in Jerusalem (A Geniza Portrait)', *Muslim World*, 60(4), 1970, pp. 344–9.

al-Muqaddasī, *ʾAḥsan al-Taqāsīm fī Maʿrifat al-ʾAqālīm*, ed. Michael J. de Goeje. Leiden: Brill, 1906.

Murray, Alan V., 'Prosopography', in Helen J. Nicholson (ed.), *Palgrave Advances in the Crusades*. New York: Palgrave Macmillan, 2005, pp. 109–29.

Nemoy, Leon, 'Samuel ben Moses al-Maghribi', *Harofe Haivri*, 25, 1952, pp. 150–3.

Netzer, Amnon, 'The Fate of the Jewish Community of Tabriz', in Moshe Sharon (ed.), *Studies in Islamic History and Civilization in Honour of Professor David Ayalon*. Jerusalem: Cana, 1986, pp. 411–19.

Netzer, Amnon, 'Rashīd al-Dīn and his Jewish Background', in Shaul Shaked and Amnon Netzer (eds), *Iranu-Judaica, Vol. III: Studies Relating to Jewish Contacts with Persian Culture throughout the Ages*, Jerusalem: Ben-Zvi Institute, 1994, pp. 118–26.

Neubauer, A., 'Egyptian Fragments: מגלות, Scrolls Analogous to That of Purim, with an Appendix on the First נגידים', *Jewish Quarterly Review*, 8(4), 1896, pp. 541–61.

Neubauer, Adolphe, 'Sur la lexicographie hébraïque', *Journal asiatique*, 19, 1862, pp. 244–67.

Neustadt, David, 'Contribution to the Economic History of the Jews in Egypt in the Middle Ages (Especially in the 12th–13th Centuries)', *Zion*, 2(3–4), 1937, pp. 216–55.

Nevins, Michael, *The Jewish Doctor: A Narrative History*. Northvale, NJ: Jason Aronson, 1984.

Nicolae, Daniel S., 'Jewish Physicians at the Court of Saladin'. MSt dissertation, University of Oxford, 2008.

Nicolae, Daniel S., 'A Medieval Court Physician at Work: Ibn Jumayʿ's Commentary on the Canon of Medicine'. PhD thesis, University of Oxford, 2012.

Northrup, Linda, *al-Bīmāristān al-Manṣūrī – Explorations: The Interface between Medicine, Politics and Culture in Early Mamluk Egypt*, ASK Working Paper 12. Bonn: Annemarie Schimmel Kolleg, September 2013.

al-Nuwayrī, Shihāb al-Dīn Aḥmad, *Nihāyat al-Arab fī Funūn al-Adab*. Cairo: al-Hayʾa al-Miṣriyya al-ʿAmma lil-Kitāb, 1992–8.

Olszowy-Schlanger, Judith, *Karaite Marriage Documents from the Cairo Geniza: Legal Tradition and Community Life in Mediaeval Egypt and Palestine*. Leiden: Brill, 1998.

Peacock, A. C. S., 'Introduction,' in A. C. S. Peacock (ed.), *Islamisation: Comparative Perspectives from History*. Edinburgh: Edinburgh University Press, 2017.

Perlman, Yaara, 'The Bodyguard of the Caliphs during the Umayyad and Abbasid Periods', *Al-Qantara*, 36(2), 2015, pp. 315–40.

Perlmann, Moshe, 'Notes on the Position of Jewish Physicians in Medieval Muslim Countries', *Israel Oriental Studies*, 2, 1972, pp. 315–19.

Perlmann, Moshe (trans. & ed.), 'Samau'al al-Maghribī, Ifḥām al-Yahūd: Silencing the Jews', *Proceedings of the American Academy for Jewish Research*, 32, 1964.

Petry, Carl F., *The Civilian Elite of Cairo in the Late Middle Ages*. Princeton, NJ: Princeton University Press, 1981.

Poliak, A. N. 'Nafīs b. David and Sa'd al-Dawla', *Zion*, 3(1), 1938, pp. 84–5 [Hebrew].

Polliack, Meira (ed.), *Karaite Judaism: A Guide to Its History and Literary Sources*. Leiden: Brill, 2003.

Polliack, Meira, 'Rethinking Karaism: Between Judaism and Islam', *AJS Review*, 30(1), 2006, pp. 67–93.

Pormann, Peter E., 'The Physician and the Other: Images of the Charlatan in Medieval Islam', *Bulletin of the History of Medicine*, 79(2), 2005, pp. 189–227.

Pormann, Peter E. and Emilie Savage-Smith, *Medieval Islamic Medicine*. Edinburgh: Edinburgh University Press, 2007.

Poznański, Samuel, 'Die jüdischen Artikel in Ibn al-Qifti's Gelehrtenlexikon', *Monatsschrift für Geschichte und Wissenschaft des Judentums*, 49(1), 1905, pp. 41–56.

Poznański, Samuel, 'Recent Karaite Publications', *Jewish Quarterly Review*, n.s., 2(3), 1912, pp. 445–51.

Prats, Arturo, 'Ibn 'Aknīn, Joseph b. Judah Jacob', in Norman A. Stillman (ed.), *Encyclopedia of Jews in the Islamic World Online*. Leiden: Brill, 2013.

Prats, Arturo, 'Moses ben Joseph ha-Levi', in Norman A. Stillman (ed.), *Encyclopedia of Jews in the Islamic World Online*. Leiden: Brill, 2013.

Prawer, Joshua, *The History of the Jews in the Latin Kingdom of Jerusalem*. Oxford: Clarendon Press, 1988.

Pummer, Reinhard, *The Samaritans*. Leiden: Brill, 1987.

Qāḍī, Wadād, 'Biographical Dictionaries: Inner Structure and Cultural Significance', in George N. Atiyeh (ed.), *The Book in the Islamic World: The Written Word and Communication in the Middle East*. Albany: State University of New York Press, 1995, pp. 93–122.

al-Qazwīnī, Zakriya ibn Muhammad, *'Ajā'ib al-Makhlūqāt wa-Gharā'ib al-Mawjūdāt*. Beirut, 1981.

Ragab, Ahmed, *The Medieval Islamic Hospital; Medicine, Religion, and Charity*. Cambridge, Cambridge University Press, 2015.

Ramaḍān, Hūwayda ʿAbd al-ʿAẓīm, *al-Yahūd fī Miṣr al-Islāmiyya ḥattā Nihāyat al-ʿAṣr al-Ayyūbī*. Cairo: al-Hayʿa al-Miṣriyya al-ʿĀmma lil-Kitāb, 2001.

al-Rāzī, Abū Baker Muḥammad b. Zakāriyyā, *Kītāb al-Tajārib: Maʿa Dirāsah fī Manhaj al-Baḥth al-ʿIlmī ʿinda al-Rāzī*, ed. Khālid Aḥmad Ḥarbī. Alexandria: Dār al-Wafāʾ li-Dunyā al-Ṭināʿah wa al-Nashr, 2006 [Arabic].

Rebenich, Stefan, 'Mommsen, Harnack, and the Prosopography of Late Antiquity', *Medieval Prosopography*, 17(1), 1996, pp. 149–67.

Reif, Stefan C., *A Jewish Archive from Old Cairo: The History of Cambridge University's Genizah Collection*. Richmond (London): Curzon, 2000.

Reif, Stefan C., *Published Material from the Cambridge Genizah Collections: A Bibliography, 1896–1980*. Cambridge: Cambridge University Press, 1988.

Reilly, Bernard F., *The Contest of Christian and Muslim Spain, 1031–1157*. Oxford: Blackwell, 1992.

Rejwan, Nissim, *The Jews of Iraq: 3000 Years of History and Culture*. London: Weidenfeld & Nicolson, 1985.

Reynolds, Dwight F. (ed.), *Interpreting the Self, Autobiography in the Arabic Literary Tradition*. Berkeley: University of California Press, 2001.

Richards, D. S., 'Arabic Documents from the Karaite Community in Cairo', *Journal of the Economic and Social History of the Orient*, 15, 1972, pp. 105–62.

Richards, D. S., 'A Doctor's Petition for a Salaried Post in Saladin's Hospital', *Social History of Medicine*, 5(2), 1992, pp. 297–306.

Richler, Binyamin, *Guide to Hebrew Manuscript Collections*. Jerusalem: Israel Academy of Sciences and Humanities, 1994.

Risse, Guenter B., *Mending Bodies, Saving Souls: A History of Hospitals*. New York: Oxford University Press, 1999.

Rosenthal, Franz, 'The Defense of Medicine in the Medieval Muslim World', *Bulletin of the History of Medicine* 43(6), 1969, pp. 519–32.

Rosenthal, Franz, 'The Physician in Medieval Muslim Society', *Bulletin of the History of Medicine*, 52(4), 1978, pp. 475–91.

Roth, Norman, 'Andalucia', in Norman Roth (ed.), *Medieval Jewish Civilization: An Encyclopedia*. New York: Routledge, 2003, p. 25–7.

Roth, Norman, 'Ibn ʿAknīn, Joseph b. Judah', in Norman Roth (ed.), *Medieval Jewish Civilization: An Encyclopedia*. New York: Routledge, 2003. pp. 344–8.

Roth, Norman, *Jews, Visigoths and Muslims in Medieval Spain: Cooperation and Conflict*. Leiden: E. J. Brill, 1994.

Roth, Norman, 'Māsarjawayh', in Norman Roth (ed.), *Medieval Jewish Civilization: An Encyclopedia.* New York: Routledge, 2003. pp. 432–3.

Roth, Norman, 'Medicine', in Norman Roth (ed.), *Medieval Jewish Civilization: An Encyclopedia.* New York: Routledge, 2003, pp. 433–42.

Roth, Norman, 'Sicily', in Norman Roth (ed.), *Medieval Jewish Civilization: An Encyclopedia.* New York: Routledge, 2003, pp. 606–11.

Russ-Fishbane, Elisha, *Judaism, Sufism, and the Pietists of Medieval Egypt. A Study of Abraham Maimonides and His Times.* Oxford: Oxford University Press, 2015.

Russell, Josiah C., 'The Population of Medieval Egypt', *Journal of the American Research Center in Egypt,* 5, 1966, pp. 69–82.

Rustow, Marina, 'At the Limits of Communal Autonomy: Jewish Bids for Intervention from the Mamluk State', *Mamlūk Studies Review,* 13(2), 2009, pp. 133–59.

Rustow, Marina, 'The Diplomatics of Leadership: Administrative Documents in Hebrew Script from the Geniza', in Arnold Franklin, Roxani Margariti, Marina Rustow and Uriel Simonsohn (eds), *Jews, Christians and Muslims in Medieval and Early Modern Times: A Festschrift in Honor of Mark R. Cohen.* Leiden: Brill, 2014, pp. 306–51.

Rustow, Marina, 'Formal and Informal Patronage among Jews in the Islamic East: Evidence from the Cairo Geniza', *Al-Qanṭara,* 29(2), 2008, pp. 341–82.

Rustow, Marina, *Heresy and the Politics of Community: The Jews of the Fatimid Caliphate.* Ithaca, NY: Cornell University Press, 2008.

Rustow, Marina, 'Judah ben Saʿadya', in Norman A. Stillman (ed.), *Encyclopedia of Jews in the Islamic World Online.* Leiden: Brill, 2013.

Rustow, Marina, 'Karaites Real and Imagined: Three Cases of Jewish Heresy', *Past and Present,* 197(1), 2007, pp. 35–74.

Rustow, Marina, 'Mevorakh ben Saʿadya', in Norman A. Stillman (ed.), *Encyclopedia of Jews in the Islamic World Online.* Leiden: Brill, 2013.

Rustow, Marina, 'Moses ben Mevorakh', in Norman A. Stillman (ed.), *Encyclopedia of Jews in the Islamic World Online.* Leiden: Brill, 2013.

Sabra, Adam, *Poverty and Charity in Medieval Islam: Mamluk Egypt, 1250–1517.* Cambridge: Cambridge University Press, 2000.

Saénz-Badillos, Angel, 'Ibn Muhājir, Abraham (Abū Isḥāq) ben Meʾir', in Norman A. Stillman (ed.), *Encyclopedia of Jews in the Islamic World Online.* Leiden: Brill, 2013.

al-Ṣafadī, Khalīl b. Aybak, *Aʿyān al-ʿAṣr wa-Aʿwān al-Naṣr,* ed. ʿAlī Abū Zayd et al. Beirut: Dār al-Fikr al-Muʿāṣir / Damascus: Dār al-Fikr, 1998.

al-Ṣafadī, Khalīl b. Aybak, *Kitāb al-Wāfī bi-l-Wafayāt*, ed. Aḥmad al-Arnāʾūṭ and Muṣṭafā Turkī. Beirut: Dār Iḥyāʾ al-Turāth al-ʿArabī, 2000.

al-Ṣafadī, Khalīl b. Aybak, *Kitāb al-Wāfī bi-l-Wafayāt*, various editors. Beirut: al-Maʿhad al-Almānī li-l-abḥāth al-Sharqiyya, 2008–10 [Arabic].

Safran, Janina M., 'Identity and Differentiation in Ninth-Century al-Andalus', *Speculum*, 76(3), 2001, pp. 573–98.

Sahner, Christian C., *Christian Martyrs under Islam: Religious Violence and the Making of the Muslim World.* Princeton, NJ: Princeton University Press, 2018.

Said, Hakim M. (ed.), *Al-Biruni's Book on Pharmacy and Materia Medica.* Karachi: Hamdard National Foundation, 1973.

al-Sakhāwī, Muḥammad b. ʿAbd al-Raḥmān, *al-Ḍawʾ al-Lāmiʿ li-Ahl al-Qarn al-Tāsiʿ*. Cairo: Maktabat al-Qudsī, 1935–6.

Salibi, Kamal S., 'The Banū Jamāʿa: A Dynasty of Shāfi'ite Jurists in the Mamluk Period', *Studia Islamica*, 9, 1958, pp. 97–109.

Salvatierra, Aurora O., 'Ibn Qamniʾel, Meʾir (Abū Ḥasan)', in Norman A. Stillman (ed.), *Encyclopedia of Jews in the Islamic World Online*. Leiden: Brill, 2013.

Sambari, Yosef ben Yitzhak, *Sefer Divrei Yosef*, ed. Shimon Shtober. Jerusalem: Ben-Zvi Institute, 1994 [Hebrew].

Sandford-Smith, John, *Eye Diseases in Hot Climates*, 2nd edn. Guildford: Wright, 1990.

Sarton, George, *Introduction to the History of Science*. Baltimore: Williams & Wilkins, 1931.

Savage-Smith, Emilie, 'Medicine', in Roshdi Rashed (ed.), *Encyclopedia of the History of Arabic Science.* London and New York: Routledge, 1996, vol. III, pp. 903–62.

Savage-Smith, Emilie, 'Ṭibb', in *The Encyclopedia of Islam*, new edn. Leiden: Brill, 1960–2007, vol. X, p. 455.

Sbath, Paul (ed.) 'Le Formulaire des hôpitaux d'Ibn abil Bayan, médecin du Bimaristan Annacery au Caire au XIIIe siècle', *Bullétin de l'Institut d'Egypte*, 15, 1932–3, pp. 9–78.

Schacht, Joseph, 'al-Subkī', in *The Encyclopedia of Islam*, new edn. Leiden: Brill, 1960–2007, vol. IX, p. 744.

Scheiber, Sándor, 'Unbekannte Gedichte von Aaron Ibn al-Ammani, dem Freunde Jehuda Hallevis', *Sefarad*, 27(2), 1967, pp. 269–81.

Scheindlin, Raymond P., 'The Jews in Muslim Spain', in Salma Khadra Jayyusi (ed.), *The Legacy of Muslim Spain*. Leiden: Brill, 1992.

Scheindlin, Raymond P., 'Judah (Abū 'l-Ḥasan) ben Samuel ha-Levi', in Norman

A. Stillman (ed.), *Encyclopedia of Jews in the Islamic World Online*. Leiden: Brill, 2013.

Schimmel, Annemarie, *Islamic Names*. Edinburgh: Edinburgh University Press, 1989.

Schirmann, Jefim, 'Studies of the Research Institute for Hebrew Poetry', *Jerusalem*, 6, 1945, pp. 265–88.

Schmidtke, Sabine and Jefim Schirmann, 'Samaw'al al-Maghribi', in Norman A. Stillman (ed.), *Encyclopedia of Jews in the Islamic World Online*. Leiden: Brill, 2013.

Schoenfeld, Andrew Jason, 'Immigration and Assimilation in the Jewish Community of Late Venetian Crete (15th–17th Centuries)', *Journal of Modern Greek Studies*, 25(1), 2007, pp. 1–15.

Schwarb, Gregor, 'Yūsuf al-Baṣīr', in Norman A. Stillman (ed.), *Encyclopedia of Jews in the Islamic World Online*. Leiden: Brill, 2013.

Segal, David Sinha, *The Book of Taḥkemonī: Jewish Tales from Medieval Spain*. London: Littman Library of Jewish Civilization, 2001.

Sela, Shulamit, 'The Head of the Rabbanite, Karaite and Samaritan Jews: On the History of a Title', *Bulletin of the School of Oriental and African Studies*, 57(2), 1994, pp. 255–67.

Sela, Shulamit, 'The Headship of the Jews in the Fatimid Empire in Karaite Hands: On the Karaite Leader David b. Isaac ha-Levi', in Ezra Fleischer, Mordechai A. Friedman and Joel A. Kramer (eds), *Mas'at Moshe: Studies in Jewish and Islamic Culture Presented to Moshe Gil*. Jerusalem: Bialik Institute, 1998, pp. 256–81 [Hebrew].

Serry, Yaron and Efraim Lev, 'A Judaeo-Arabic Fragment of Ibn-Biklārish's *Kitāb al-Musta'īnī*, Part of a Unique 12th-Century Tabular Medical Book Found in the Cairo Geniza (T-S Ar.44.218)', *Journal of the Royal Asiatic Society*, 20(4), 2010, pp. 407–40.

al-Shantarīnī, 'Alī b. Bassām, *al-Dhakhīra fī Maḥāsin Ahl al-Jazīra*, ed. Iḥsān 'Abbās. Beirut: Dār al-Thqāfa, 1978–9.

Shatzmiller, Joseph, *Jews, Medicine, and Medieval Society*. Berkeley: University of California Press, 1993.

al-Shayzarī, 'Abd al-Raḥmān ibn Nāṣir, *Nihāyat al-Rutba fī Ṭalab al-Ḥisba*. Cairo: Association of Authorship, Translations and Publications, 1946.

Shefer, Miri, 'Physicians in the Mamluk and Ottoman Courts', in David J. Wasserstein and Ami Aylon (eds), *Mamluks and Ottomans: Studies in Honour of Michael Winter*. Abingdon: Routledge, 2006, pp. 114–22.

Shilat, Isaacs (ed.), *Letters and Essays of Moses Maimonides*. Maaleh Adumim: Maaliyot, 1995 [Hebrew].

Shimmel, Annemarie, *Islamic Names*. Edinburgh: Edinburgh University Press, 1989.

Shivtiel, Avi and Friedrich Niessen, *Arabic and Judaeo-Arabic Manuscripts in the Cambridge Genizah Collections, New Series*. Cambridge: Cambridge University Press, 2006.

Shohetman, Eliav, 'New Sources from the Geniza on the Commercial Activities of the Ari in Egypt', *Peʿamim*, 16, 1983, pp. 56–64.

Silman, Yochanan, *Philosopher and Prophet: Judah Halevi, the Kuzari, and the Evolution of His Thought*. Albany: SUNY Press, 2012.

Simonsohn, Shlomo, *The Jews in Sicily. Vol. I: 383–1300*. Leiden: Brill, 1997.

Simonsohn, Uriel, 'Conversion, Exemption, and Manipulation: Social Benefits and Conversion to Islam in Late Antiquity and the Middle Ages', *Medieval Worlds*, 6, 2017, pp. 196–216.

Simonsohn, Uriel, 'Conversion to Islam: A Case Study for the Use of Legal Sources', *History Compass*, 11(8), 2013, pp. 647–62.

Sirat, Collette, *A History of Jewish Philosophy in the Middle Ages*. Cambridge: Cambridge University Press, 1985.

Sourdel, Dominique, 'Bukhtishūʿ', in *The Encyclopedia of Islam*, new edn. Leiden: Brill, 1960–2007, vol. I, p. 1298.

Steinschneider, Moritz, *Die Arabische Literatur der Juden: ein Beitrag zur Literaturgeschichte der Araber, Grossenteils aus Handschriftlichen Quellen*. Frankfurt: J. Kauffmann, 1902.

Steinschneider, Moritz, *Die Hebraeischen Übersetzungen der Mittelalters und die Juden als Dolmetscher*. Graz: Akademische Druck- und Verlagsanstalt, [1893] 1956.

Steinschneider, Moritz, 'An Introduction to the Arabic Literature of the Jews I (continued)', *Jewish Quarterly Review*, 9(4), 1897, pp. 604–30.

Steinschneider, Moritz, 'An Introduction to the Arabic Literature of the Jews I (continued)', *Jewish Quarterly Review*, 11(1), 1898, pp. 115–49.

Steinschneider, Moritz, 'An Introduction to the Arabic Literature of the Jews I (continued)', *Jewish Quarterly Review*, 11(2), 1899, pp. 305–43.

Steinschneider, Moritz, 'An Introduction to the Arabic Literature of the Jews I (continued)', *Jewish Quarterly Review*, 11(3), 1899, pp. 480–9.

Steinschneider, Moritz, 'An Introduction to the Arabic Literature of the Jews I (continued)', *Jewish Quarterly Review*, 11(4), 1899, pp. 585–625.

Steinschneider, Moritz, 'An Introduction to the Arabic Literature of the Jews II (continued)', *Jewish Quarterly Review*, 13(1), 1900, pp. 92–110.

Steinschneider, Moritz, 'An Introduction to the Arabic Literature of the Jews II (continued)', *Jewish Quarterly Review*, 13(2), 1901, pp. 296–320.

Steinschneider, Moritz, *Jewish Literature from the Eighth to the Eighteenth Century: With an Introduction on Talmud and Midrasch; a Historical Essay*. Hildesheim: G. Olms, 1967.

Stern, S. M., 'A Collection of Treatises by ʿAbd al-Laṭīf al-Baghdādī', *Islamic Studies*, 1(1), 1962, pp. 53–70.

Stern, S. M., *Corpus Codicum Hebraicorum Medii Aevi*. Copenhagen: E. Munksgaard, 1956, Part I, vol. III, pp. 12–21.

Stern, S. M., 'Maimonidis Commentarius', in Solomon D. Sassoon (ed.), *Mischnam*. Copenhagen: E. Munksgaard, 1961, pp. 27–8, plates XIV–XV.

Stillman, Norman A., 'The Eleventh Century Merchant House of Ibn ʿAwkal', *Journal of the Economic and Social History of the Orient*, 16(1), 1973, pp. 15–88.

Stillman, Norman A., 'Ibn ʿAṭāʾ, Abū Isḥāq Ibrāhīm (Abraham ben Nathan)', in Norman A. Stillman (ed.), *Encyclopedia of Jews in the Islamic World Online*. Leiden: Brill, 2013.

Stillman, Norman A., 'The Jew in the Medieval Islamic City', in Daniel Frank (ed.), *The Jews of Medieval Islam: Community, Society, and Identity*. Leiden: Brill, 1995. pp. 3–13.

Stillman, Norman A., 'The Jews in the Medieval Islamic City', in Ezra Fleischer, Mordechai A. Friedman and Joel A. Kramer (eds), *Masʾat Moshe: Studies in Jewish and Islamic Culture Presented to Moshe Gil*. Jerusalem: Bialik Institute, 1998, pp. 246–55 [Hebrew].

Stillman, Norman A., *The Jews of Arab Lands: A History and Source Book*. Philadelphia: Jewish Publication Society of America, 1979.

Stillman, Norman A., 'The Non-Muslim Communities: The Jewish Community', in Carl Petry (ed.). *The Cambridge History of Egypt, Vol. I: Islamic Egypt, 640–1517*. Cambridge: Cambridge University Press, 1998, pp. 189–210.

Stillman, Norman A. and Shlomo Pines, 'Abū al-Barakāt al-Baghdadī', in Norman A. Stillman (ed.), *Encyclopedia of Jews in the Islamic World Online*. Leiden: Brill, 2013.

Stone, Lawrence, 'Prosopography', *Daedalus*, 100(1), 1971, pp. 46–79.

Strauss, E., 'Documents for the Economic and Social History of the Jews in the Near East', *Zion*, 7, 1941–2, pp. 140–55 [Hebrew].

Stroumsa, Sarah, 'Between Acculturation and Conversion in Islamic Spain: The Case of the Banū Ḥasday', *Mediterranea*, 1, 2015, pp. 9–36.

Stroumsa, Sarah, *Maimonides in His World: Portrait of a Mediterranean Thinker*. Princeton, NJ: Princeton University Press, 2009.

Stroumsa, Sarah, 'On Jewish Intellectuals Who Converted in the Early Middle Ages', in Daniel Frank (ed.), *The Jews of Medieval Islam: Community, Society, and Identity*. Leiden: Brill, 1995, pp. 179–97.

Sublet, Jacqueline, 'La Prosopographie arabe', *Annales. Histoire, sciences sociales*, 25(5), 1970, pp. 1236–9.

Tabbaa, Yasser. 'The Functional Aspects of Medieval Islamic Hospitals', in Michael Bonner, Mine Ener and Amy Singer (eds), *Poverty and Charity in Middle Eastern Contexts*. Albany: State University of New York Press, 2003, pp. 95–119.

Talbot, Charles H. and Eugene A. Hammond, *The Medical Practitioners in Medieval England: A Biographical Register*. London: Wellcome Historical Medical Library, 1965.

Tannous, Jack, *The Making of the Medieval Middle East: Religion, Society, and Simple Believers*. Princeton, NJ: Princeton University Press, 2018.

Tenne, David, 'Ibn Janāḥ, Jonah', in Michael Berenbaum and Fred Skolnik (eds), *Encyclopedia Judaica*, 2nd edn. Farmington Hills, MI: Macmillan Reference USA, 2007, vol. IX, pp. 680–3.

Tobi, Yosef, 'Ben Solomon, Zechariah ha-Rofeh', in Norman A. Stillman (ed.), *Encyclopedia of Jews in the Islamic World Online*. Leiden: Brill, 2013.

Tobi, Yosef, *Between Hebrew and Arabic Poetry: Studies in Spanish Medieval Hebrew Poetry*. Leiden: Brill, 2010.

Tobi, Yosef, *The Jews of Yemen under the Shade of Islam since Advent to Nowadays*. Jerusalem: Misgav Yerushalaim, 2018 [Hebrew].

Udovitch, A. L., 'International Commerce and Society in Mid-Eleventh-Century Egypt and North Africa', in Haleh Esfandiyari and A. L. Udovitch (eds), *The Economic Dimensions of Middle Eastern History: Essays in Honor of Charles Issawi*. Princeton, NJ: Darwin Press, 1990, pp. 239–53.

Ullmann, Manfred, *Islamic Medicine*. Edinburgh: Edinburgh University Press, 1978.

al-ʿUmarī, Shihāb al-Dīn Aḥmad ibn Faḍl Allāh, *Masālik al-Abṣār fī Mamālik al-Amṣār*, ed. Kamāl Salmān al-Jabūrī. Beirut: Dār al-Kutub al-ʿIlmiyya, 2010.

Vorderstrasse, Tasha and Tanya Treptow (eds), *A Cosmopolitan City: Muslims, Christians, and Jews in Old Cairo*. Chicago: Oriental Institute of the University of Chicago, 2015.

Walker, Paul E., *Fatimid History and Ismaili Doctrine*. Aldershot: Ashgate, 2008.

Wasserstein, Abraham and David J. Wasserstein, *The Legend of the Septuagint: From Classical Antiquity to Today*. Cambridge: Cambridge University Press, 2006.

Wasserstein, David J., 'Conversion and the *Ahl al-Dhimma*' in Robert Irwin (ed.), *The New Cambridge History of Islam, Vol. IV: Islamic Cultures and Societies to the End of the Eighteenth Century*. Cambridge: Cambridge University Press, 2010. pp. 184–208.

Wasserstein, David J., 'Ibn Biklarish – Isra'ili', in Charles Burnett (ed.), *Ibn Baklarish's Book of Simples: Medical Remedies between Three Faiths in Twelfth-Century Spain*. London: Arcadian Library / Oxford: Oxford University Press, 2008, pp. 105–12.

Wasserstein, David J., 'Jewish Élites in al-Andalus', in Daniel Frank (ed.), *The Jews of Medieval Islam: Community, Society, and Identity*. Leiden: Brill, 1995. pp. 101–10.

Wasserstein, David J., *The Rise and Fall of the Party-Kings: Politics and Society in Islamic Spain, 1002–1086*. Princeton, NJ: Princeton University Press, 1985.

Wasserstein, David J., 'Samau'al ben Judah Ibn 'Abbās al-Maghribī', in Michael Berenbaum and Fred Skolnik (eds), *Encyclopedia Judaica*, 2nd ed. Farmington Hills, MI: Macmillan Reference USA, 2007, vol. XVII, pp. 741–2.

Wasserstein, David J., 'What's in a Name? 'Abdallāh b, Isḥāq b. al-Shanā'a al-Muslimānī l-Isrā'īlī and Conversion to Islam in Medieval Cordova', in Arnold E. Franklin, Roxani E. Margariti, Marina Rustow and Uriel Simonsohn (eds), *Jews, Christians and Muslims in Medieval and Early Modern Times: A Festschrift in Honor of Mark R. Cohen*. Leiden: Brill, 2014, pp. 139–54.

Wasserstrom, Steven M., *Between Muslim and Jew: The Problem of Symbiosis under Early Islam*. Princeton, NJ: Princeton University Press, 1995.

Wechsler, Michael G., 'Ibn Sughmar Family', in Norman A. Stillman (ed.), *Encyclopedia of Jews in the Islamic World Online*. Leiden: Brill, 2013.

Wedel, Gerhard, *Kitāb aṭ-Ṭabbāḫ des Samaritaners Abū l-Ḥasan aṣ-Ṣūrī*. Berlin: Freien Universität, 1987.

Wedel, Gerhard, 'Transfer of Knowledge and the Biographies of Samaritan Scholars: Careers of Samaritan Physicians under Muslim Patronage', *Samaritan Researches*, 5, 2000, pp. 3.75–3.83.

Weinberger, Leon J., 'Moses Dar'ī, Karaite Poet and Physician', *Jewish Quarterly Review*, n.s., 84(4), 1994, pp. 445–83.

Weisz, Yael, 'The Jewish Physicians – between al-Andalus and Christian Spain', *Jama'a*, 17, 2009, pp. 9–36.

Wickersheimer, Ernest, *Dictionnaire biographique des médecins en France au moyen age*. Paris: Droz, 1936.

Wiet, Gaston, *Cairo: City of Art and Commerce*. Norman: University of Oklahoma Press, 1964.

Wilson, Robertine B., 'The Bakhitishuʿ: Their Political and Social Role under the Abbasid Caliphs (AD 750–1100)', PhD dissertation, New York University, 1974.

Yaari, Avraham (ed.), *Massa Meshullam mi-Volterra be-Eretz-Israel bi-Shenath 141 (1481)*. Jerusalem: Mosad Bialik, 1948.

Yagur, Moshe, 'Between Egypt and Jerusalem: Geopolitics of the Jewish Community of Ashqelon in the Period of the Geniza'. MA thesis, Hebrew University of Jerusalem, 2011.

Yagur, Moshe, 'The Jews of Cyprus during the 16th Century', *Etmol*, 232, 2014, pp. 5–8.

Yahalom, Joseph and Joshua Blau, *The Wanderings of Judah Alharizi: Five Accounts of His Travels*. Jerusalem: Yad Izhak Ben-Zvi, 2002 [Hebrew].

Yarbrough, Luke, *The Sword of Ambition: Bureaucratic Rivalry in Medieval Egypt*. New York: New York University Press, 2019.

Yeroushalmi, David, *The Jews of Iran: Chapters in Their History and Cultural Heritage*. Costa Mesa, CA: Mazda, 2017.

Yeshaya, Joachim J. M. S., 'Darʿī, Moses ben Abraham', in Norman A. Stillman (ed.), *Encyclopedia of Jews in the Islamic World Online*. Leiden: Brill, 2013.

Yeshaya, Joachim J. M. S., *Medieval Hebrew Poetry in Muslim Egypt: The Secular Poetry of the Karaite Poet Moses ben Darʿī*. Leiden: Brill, 2011.

al-Yūnīnī, Quṭb al-Dīn Mūsā b. Muḥammad. *Early Mamluk Syrian Historiography: al-Yūnīnī's Dhayl Mirʾat al-Zamān*, trans. & ed. Guo Li. Leiden: Brill, 1998.

al-Zarhūnī, Nūr al-Dīn, *al-Ṭibb wa-l-Khidamāt al-Ṭibiyya fī al-Andalus khilāl al-Qarn al-Sādis al-Hijrī-al-Thānī-ʿAshar al-Mīlādī*. Alexandria: Muʾssasat Shabāb al-Jāmiʿa, 2006.

Zeldes, Nadia and Miriam Frenkel, 'The Sicilian Trade: Jewish Merchants in the Mediterranean in the Twelfth and Thirteenth Centuries', in Mina Rozen, Yehuda Nini and Solomon Simonsohn (eds), *Michael: On the History of the Jews in the Diaspora*. Tel Aviv: Diaspora Research Institute, 2009, vol. XIV, pp. 89–138 [Hebrew].

Zinger, Oded, 'Finding a Fragment in a Pile of Geniza: A Practical Guide to Collections, Editions, and Resources', *Jewish History*, 32(2–4), 2019, pp. 279–309.

Zinger, Oded, 'Women, Gender and Law: Marital Disputes According to Documents from the Cairo Geniza'. PhD dissertation, Princeton University, 2014.

Zonta, Mauro, 'Mineralogy, Botany and Zoology in Medieval Hebrew Encyclopaedias: "Descriptive" and "Theoretical" Approaches to Arabic Sources', *Arabic Science and Philosophy*, 6(2), 1996, pp. 263–315.

Zorgati, Ragnhild Johnsrud, *Pluralism in the Middle Ages: Hybrid Identities, Conversion, and Mixed Marriages in Medieval Iberia.* New York: Routledge, 2012.

List of Geniza Fragments

TS J1.43
TS K 3.6
TS K6 149
TS K6.177
TS K 15.6
TS K15.9
TS K 15.16
TS K15.49
TS K15.61
TS K15.66
TS K15.91
TS K15.92
TS K15.96
TS 8J1.2
TS 8J6.12
TS 8J6.15
TS 8J13.14
TS 8J15.20
TS 8J15.25
TS 8 J 16.22
TS 8J18.9
TS 8J19.30
TS 8K22.12
TS 10J6.6
TS 10J7.16
TS 10J7.6
TS 10J15.26
TS 10J17.19
TS 10J17.22
TS 10J17.27
TS 10J26.2
TS 13J3.27
TS 13J4.13
TS 13J6.25
TS 13J8.25
TS 13J14.25
TS 13J16.8
TS 13J20.27
TS 13J25.16
TS Ar. 4.7
TS Ar. 30.163
T-S Ar.30.286
T-S Ar. 34.94
T-S Ar. 38.131
TS Ar. 39.449
TS Ar. 41.81
TS Ar.44.218
T-S Ar. 44.51
TS Ar. 48.117
TS Ar. 51.144
TS Ar.53.55
TS Ar. 54.20
TS Ar. 54.21
TS Ar. 54.52
TS Ar. 54.91
TS 8.195
TS 12.487
TS 16.1
TS 16.176
TS 16.200
TS 16.261
TS 20.44
TS 20.47
TS 20.133
TS 24.76
TS Misc. 20.183
TS Misc.25.8
TS Misc. 26.2
TS NS 32.99
TS NS 69.52
TS NS 190.127
TS NS 224.17
TS NS 225.75
TS NS 226.30
TS NS 246.26.12
TS NS 304.4(a)
TS NS 313.17
TS NS 321.40
TS NS 321.77
TS NS 323.19
TS NS 324.47
TS NS 324.67
TS NS 324.7
TS NS 324.95
TS NS 338.39
TS NS J76
TS NS J 108a
TS NS J 151
TS NS J163
TS NS J260
TS NS J 315
TS NSJ422
TS AS 99.31
TS AS 145.9
TS AS 146.10
TS AS 146.24
TS AS 146.9
TS AS 147.23
TS AS 148.199
TS AS 149.17
TS AS 149.37
TS AS 150.30
TS AS 151.241
TS AS 151.5
TS AS 152.4
TS AS 153.31
TS AS 153.200
TS AS 155.229
TS AS 164.58
TS AS 202.396
CUL Or.1080 2.70
CUL Or. 1080 5.16
CUL Or. 1080 J2
CUL Or. 1080 J138
LG Misc 99
BL Or. 5535.3
BL Or. 10794.13
ENA 1290.1
ENA 2556
ENA 2558.4
ENA 2558.15
ENA 2558.20
ENA 2559.13
ENA 2591.6
ENA 2591.8
ENA 2592.14
ENA 2592.18
ENA 2592.22
ENA 2727.15e
ENA 2727.17a
ENA 2727.23b
ENA 2727.28

ENA 2727.30
ENA 2728.6
ENA 2730.2
ENA 2735.1
ENA 2738.1
ENA 2738.36
ENA 2748.2
ENA 2806.2
ENA 2967.3
ENA 3150.8
ENA 3846.6–7
ENA 4011.45
ENA 4020.54
ENA 4100.9(c)
ENA NS 18.17a
ENA NS 57.8
ENA NS 77.404
Bodl. MS heb. a. 2, fol. 14
Bodl. MS heb. a. 3, fol. 18
Bodl. MS. heb. b. 13, fol. 39
Bodl. MS heb. c. 13, fol. 6
Bodl. MS heb. c 28, fol. 47 (2876–47)
Bodl. MS heb. c. 50, fol. 17
Bodl MS heb. d. 65, fol. 8
Bodl. MS heb. d. 66, fol. 52
Bodl. MS heb. d. 66, fol. 57 (2878)
Bodl. MS heb. d. 68, fol. 101
Bodl. MS heb. e. 94, fol. 19
Bodl. MS heb. e. 94, fol. 21
Bodl. MS heb. e. 94, fol. 22
Bodl MS Heb. e. 101, fol. 13
Bodl. MS heb. e. 101, fol. 14
Bodl. MS heb. f. 22, fol. 25b–52b
Bodl. MS. heb. f. 56, fols. 13–19
Bodl. MS heb. f. 56, fol. 45
Bodl. MS heb. f. 56, fol. 50
Bodl. MS heb. f. 56, fol. 54
Bodl. MS heb. f. 56, fol. 55
Bodl. MS heb. f. 56, fol. 122
Bodl. MS heb. f. 56, fol. 126
Bodl. MS heb. f. 61, fol. 42
Bodl. MS heb. f. 61, fol. 50
Mosseri I.115.1
Mosseri V 392.3
Mosseri VIII.80.1
Mosseri II.195
Mosseri VII.9.5
Halper (CAJS) 354
Halper (CAJS) 464
Halper (Dropsie) 467
RNL Yevr. III B 669
RNL Yevr. Ar. II 1378
Wien, N: H 85 (PER H 85)

Index of People

Aaron b. Zedaqa b. Aaron ha-Rōfē al-ʿAmmānī, 40, 176, 177
Aaron ha-Levi ha-Rōfē ha-Sōfer ha-Mahir, 41, 371
Aaron ha-Levi Ibn al-Kirmānī, al-Kaḥḥāl *see* Abū al-Fakhr b. Abī al-Faḍl b. Abī Naṣr b. Abī al-Fakhr al-Yahūdī
Aaron ha-Rōfē al-ʿAmmānī, 41, 148, 176, 296, 364, 402
Aaron ha-Rōfē b. Samuel Ibn al-ʿAmmānī, 41, 119, 179
Aaron ha-Rōfē b. Yeshūʿā Ibn al-ʿAmmānī, 41, 179
Aaron ha-Rōfē b. Yeshūʿā ha-Rōfē Ibn al-ʿAmmānī, 41, 54, 128, 177, 178, 311, 318, 353, 354, 365, 389
Aaron ha-Rōfē al-Kāzrūnī, 41, 371, 405
Aaron Ibn al-ʿAmmānī *see also* Aaron ha-Rōfē b. Yeshūʿā ha-Rōfē Ibn al-ʿAmmānī
Abāqa, 181
ʿAbd Allāh (Taqī al-Dīn) b. Dāʾūd b. Abī al-Faḍl b. Abī al-Munajjab (*or* al-Mūnā) b. Abī al-Fityān (*or* al-Bayān) al-Dāʾūdi, 41, 151, 220–1, 275n1115, 299, 345, 348, 349, 370
ʿAbd al-ʿAzīz b. Maḥāsin al-Muwaffaq al-ʾIsrāʾīlī al-Mutaṭabbib (Uziel b. Obadia), 41, 206
ʿAbd al-ʿAzīz ha-Ḥazzān al-Ḥakīm, 41, 43, 113, 367
ʿAbd al-Bāqī al-ʿAṭṭār, 120
ʿAbd al-Dāʾim (al-Muwaffaq) b. ʿAbd al-ʿAzīz b. Maḥāsin ʾIsrāʾīlī al-Mutaṭabbib (Jekuthiel b. Uziel b. Obadia ha-Dayyān), 41, 207, 282, 283, 404
ʿAbd al-Ḥaqq, 120, 347, 399
ʿAbd al-Karīm b. ʿAbd al-Laṭīf, 42, 373, 400
ʿAbd al-Karīm b. Mūsā, 42, 373, 400
ʿAbd al-Laṭīf al-Baghdādī, 170, 232n77, 363
ʿAbd al-Laṭīf b. Ibrāhīm b. Shams al-Baghdādī, 42, 356, 396
ʿAbd al-Muʾmin, 52
ʿAbd al-Raḥīm b. ʿAlī al-Baysānī, 203
ʿAbd al-Raḥmān I 'the Immigrant', 374
ʿAbd al-Raḥmān III, 157–8, 296, 340, 357
ʿAbd al-Sayyid b. Isḥāq b. Yaḥyā al-Ḥakīm al-Faḍl Bahāʾ al-Dīn b. al-Muhadhdhab, al-Ṭabīb al-Kaḥḥāl, 43, 150, 208–9, 275n1115, 283, 294, 347, 348, 366, 370, 399
ʿAbd al-Sayyid the Dayyān, 81, 350
ʿAbd al-Wāḥid (Ibn al-Sīqānīyya) b. ʿAfīf b. ʿAbd Allāh al-Yahūdī al-Rabānī al-Mutaṭabbib ha-Kohen al-Ḥakīm, 41, 43, 113, 282
ʿAbdūn al-ʿAṭṭār, 120
Abraham al-ʿAṭṭār, 121
Abraham al-ʿAṭṭār b. Ṣadaqa al-Ḥanāwī, 121
Abraham b. al-F[...], 43
Abraham b. Daʿud, 57
Abraham b. David (b. Maimon), 94, 101, 392
Abraham b. Ezra, 46, 56, 171, 349–50
Abraham b. Hananiah ha-Rōfē, 43, 186, 187
Abraham b. Hillel ha-Ḥasid, 43, 311
Abraham b. Isaac ha-Kohen b. Furāt, 43, 165, 296, 327, 401
Abraham b. Maimon (Maimonides), 43, 59–60, 62, 74, 82, 83, 86, 91, 92, 93, 94, 96, 98, 101, 103, 107, 110, 118, 119, 148, 151, 162–4, 176, 179, 180, 183, 188, 205, 227, 281, 288, 294, 297, 300, 323, 326, 359, 362, 366, 367, 393, 428n484
Abraham b. Meʾir b. Muhājir *see* Abū Isḥāq (Abraham b. Meʾir b. Muhājir)
Abraham b. Meʾir Ibn Qamniʾel, 43, 45–6, 169
Abraham b. Moses ha-Rōfē, 43, 92, 111, 177, 178
Abraham b. Nathan *see* Abū Isḥāq Ibrāhīm b. ʿAṭā
Abraham b. Saʿadya, 43, 215
Abraham b. Saʿadya ha-Rōfē Darʿī, 43, 167, 385
Abraham b. Samuel Abulafia, 85
Abraham b. Sasson *see* Abū Isḥāq al-Maḥallī al-ʿAṭṭār
Abraham b. Yijū, 44, 315, 316, 385
Abraham ha-Kohen b. Isaac, 44
Abraham ha-Levi, 44, 372, 400
Abraham ha-Levi [Abū I]sḥāq al-Maḥallī al-ʿAṭṭār, 121
Abraham ha-Levi ha-Rōfē, 44, 371
Abraham ha-Rōfē, 44, 148, 167
Abraham ha-Rōfē b. ʿAlī, 44
Abraham ha-Rōfē b. Isaac al-Ghazūlī, 44
R. Abraham ha-Rōfē b. Jacob, 44, 216, 217
Abraham ha-Rōfē b. Simḥā, 192
Abraham ha-Rōfē b. Simḥā ha-Kohen, 44
Abraham ha-Sar ha-Rōfē, 45
Abraham Sakandarī, 44, 223, 224, 366
Abraham the Karaite, 45, 371
Abū Aḥmad Jaʿfar b. ʿAbīd, 153

Abū Aḥmar al-ʿAṭṭār, 121
Abū al-ʿAlā (Elazar b. Joseph), 121
Abū al-ʿAlā Levi, 58, 121, 124, 125
Abū al-ʿAlā Musallam al-ʿAṭṭār b. Sahl, 121
Abū ʿAlī ʿAlāʾ b. Zuhr, 45
Abū ʿAlī al-ʿAṭṭār, 121, 122, 127
Abū ʿAlī al-ʿAṭṭār (Rabbana Japheth), 121
Abū ʿAlī Ḥasan al-Mutaṭabbib al-Barqī, 45, 282
Abū ʿAlī al-Ṭabīb, 45
Abū al-ʿAmr b. al-Faraj, 160
Abū ʿAmr al-Ṭabīb, 45
Abū ʿAnān, 77, 386
Abū Asʿad al-Mutaṭabbib ha-Zāqēn, 45
Abū al-ʿAshāʾir Hibat-Allāh b. Zayn b. Ḥasan b. Ifrāʾīm b. Yaʿqūb b. Ismāʿīl Ibn Jumayʿ al-ʾIsrāʾīlī (Nethanel b. Samuel), 22, 23, 29, 45, 59, 75, 100, 150, 201, 202–4, 226, 288, 297, 303, 305, 309–10, 312, 322, 330, 332, 334, 336, 338, 352, 355, 359, 389–90, 448
Abū Ayyūb al-Yahūdī (al-ʾIsrāʾīlī) (Solomon b. al-Muʿallim), 45–6, 169, 297, 354, 379, 385
Abū al-Barakāt al-ʿAṭṭār, 121
Abū al-Barakāt b. Abū al-Kathīr, 72, 397
Abū al-Barakāt b. Joseph Lebdī, 63, 185
Abū al-Barakāt Hibat Allāh, 46, 171, 349
Abū al-Barakāt Hibat Allāh b. ʿAlī b. Malkā (or Malkān) al-Baladī b. al-Ṭabīb al-Faḍl (Nethanel Baruch b. Melekh), 22, 39, 46–8, 81, 297, 313, 328, 335, 336, 343, 344, 349, 352, 404
Abū al-Barakāt al-Quḍāʿī al-Muwaffaq, 48, 298
Abū al-Barakāt al-Ṭabīb b. al-Sharābī, 48, 142, 149, 191
Abū al-Barakāt Ibn Shaʿyā al-Muwaffaq, 48, 149, 195–6, 197, 371
Abū al-Bayān b. al-Mudawwar al-Sadīd, 48, 149, 200, 201, 283, 298, 337, 371
Abū al-Bayān Mūsā b. Abī al-Faḍl (Moses b. Mevōrākh b. Saʿadya), 48, 171, 172, 173, 297, 299–300, 362
Abū al-Bishr b. Aaron ha-Levi al-Kirmānī al-Ḥakīm, 48, 207, 282, 372
Abū al-Faḍāʾil (Jekuthiel b. Moses), 48, 174
Abū al-Faḍāʾil (Jekuthiel II b. Moses II ha- Rōfē), 48, 174–5, 317
Abū al-Faḍāʾil al-Ṭabīb, 49–50, 124
Abū al-Faḍl (Ḥasday b. Joseph b. Ḥasday), 88, 160, 296, 343, 344, 349, 354, 379
Abū Faḍl al-ʿAṭṭār, 122, 128
Abū al-Faḍl al-ʿAṭṭār b. Abū al-Ḥasan, 122
Abū al-Faḍl (Abū al-Faḍāʾil) b. al-Nāqid b. Obadia, al-Ṭabīb al-Muhadhdhab (Mevōrākh ha-Kohen), 49, 149, 184–5
Abū al-Faḍl b. al-Ṣarīḥ, 49, 398
Abū al-Faḍl Dāʾūd b. Sulaymān b. Abū al-Bayān al-ʾIsrāʾīlī al-Sadīd (David b. Solomon), 48, 201, 294, 298, 300, 305, 336, 353, 371, 454
Abū al-Faḍl al-Kallām, 287
Abū al-Faḍl Mubārak (Mevōrākh b. Saʿadya), 49, 75–6, 126, 127, 134, 136, 171–3, 289, 296, 300, 362, 367, 387, 390
Abū al-Faḍl al-Sharīṭī al-Ḥalabī ha-Rōfē (Benjamin al-Sharīṭī ha-Rōfē), 49, 397
Abū al-Faḍl al-Ṭabīb, 49, 128
Abū al-Faḍl al-Ṭabīb 2, 49, 76, 126, 127, 134, 136
Abū al-Fakhr (Yeshūʿā ha-Rōfē), 50
Abū al-Fakhr al-ʿAṭṭār, 122, 150, 205
Abū al-Fakhr al-ʿAṭṭār 2, 122, 125, 129, 130, 132, 201
Abū al-Fakhr al-ʿAṭṭār 3, 121, 122, 127
Abū al-Fakhr al-ʿAṭṭār b. al-Amshāṭī (Saʿadya b. Abraham), 50–1
Abū al-Fakhr b. Abī al-Faḍl b. Abī Naṣr b. Abī al-Fakhr al-Yahūdī (Aaron ha-Levi Ibn al-Kirmānī, al-Kaḥḥāl), 51, 207, 285, 372
Abū al-Fakhr Levi ʿAṭṭār, 58, 121, 124, 125
Abū al-Fakhr al-Ṭabīb, 51, 311
Abū al-Faraj al-ʿAṭṭār b. Abū al-Ḥasan al-ʿAṭṭār, 124, 205, 389
Abū al-Faraj b. Abū al-Barakāt, 51, 191–2
Abū al-Faraj b. Abū al-Faḍāʾil b. al-Nāqid, 51, 184–5, 285, 345, 348
Abū al-Faraj b. al-Kallām, 136, 204, 287, 332, 359
Abū al-Faraj b. Maʿmar al-Sharābī (Nethanel ha-Levi b. Amram), 66, 142–3, 288, 332
Abū al-Faraj b. al-Nashādirī, 58, 62, 87, 117, 319
Abū al-Faraj b. al-Raʾīs (Elijah b. Zechariah), 52, 176, 187–9, 206, 227, 297, 328, 366, 389, 390, 400
Abū al-Faraj Hārūn, 54
Abū al-Faraj al-Ṭabīb, 51
Abū al-Faraj al-Uṣṭūl, 51, 391
Abū al-Futūḥ al-ʿAṭṭār, 124
Abū al-Futūḥ al-Ṭabīb, 52, 234n137
Abū al-Ghālib, 66, 143, 288, 332
Abū al-Ḥajjāj (Granada), 109, 298
Abū al-Ḥajjāj Yūsuf b. Yaḥyā b. Isḥāq al-Sabatī al-Maghribī (Ibn Samʿūn) (Joseph b. Judah b. Simon), 22, 52–3, 74, 297, 331, 337, 345, 348, 382, 389, 397
Abū al-Ḥasan, 53, 191
Abū al-Ḥasan (Judah b. Samuel ha-Levi; Judah ha-Levi), 46, 53–4, 57, 80, 169, 171, 178, 314, 349, 353, 354, 378, 379, 381, 385, 387
Abū al-Ḥasan ʿAmmār ha-Rōfē, 54, 400
Abū al-Ḥasan ʿAṭṭār, 58, 87, 93, 124, 125
Abū al-Ḥasan al-ʿAṭṭār, 124
Abū al-Ḥasan al-ʿAṭṭār 2, 124
Abū al-Ḥasan al-ʿAṭṭār 3, 124, 150, 206, 298
Abū al-Ḥasan al-ʿAṭṭār 4, 124
Abū al-Ḥasan al-ʿAṭṭār b. Abū al-Fakhr, 124, 205
Abū al-Ḥasan b. Abū al-Sahl b. Abraham, 54
Abū al-Ḥasan b. Mūsā al-Fāṣid (the phlebotomist) al-ʿAṭṭār, 124, 125, 287
Abū al-Ḥasan b. al-Muwaffaq b. al-Najm b. al-Muhadhdhab Abī al-Ḥasan b. Samuel (al-Sheikh al-Muhadhdhab), 55, 283, 362
Abū al-Ḥasan b. Saʿīd al-Ṣārīfī Ibn al-Maṣmūdī, 55
Abū al-Ḥasan ha-Levi al-ʿAṭṭār (b. al-Dimyāṭī), 124, 391
Abū al-Ḥasan ha-Rōfē, 55
Abū al-Ḥasan Isḥāq b. Faraj b. Mārūth al-Ṣūrī, 76
Abū al-Ḥasan Saʿīd b. Hibat Allāh, 46, 335–7
Abū al-Ḥasan al-Ṭabīb, 55
Abū al-Ḥasan al-Ṭabīb 2, 55
Abū al-Ḥasan Yūsuf b. Josiah al-Tunisī (Joseph b. Isaiah), 56, 383
Abū Ibrāhīm b. Muwaril, 56, 168
Abū Ibrāhīm b. Qasṭār (Isaac b. Yashush), 56, 299, 378

Abū ʿImrān ʿAṭṭār, 58, 87, 93, 124, 125
Abū ʿImrān b. al-Lawī al-Ishbīlī (Moses b. Joseph ha-Levi), 57, 298
Abū ʿImrān Kohen ʿAṭṭār, 58, 121, 124, 125
Abū ʿImrān Levi ʿAṭṭār, 58, 121, 124, 125
Abū ʿImrān al-Ṭabīb)Ben Sumsuma(, 56
Abū Isḥāq, 43
Abū Isḥāq (Abraham b. Meʾir b. Muhājir), 57
Abū Isḥāq al-ʿAṭṭār, 117, 124, 125
Abū Isḥāq al-Ḥasid al-Ṭabīb, 58
Abū Isḥāq Ibrāhīm b. ʿAṭā (Abraham b. Nathan), 58, 296, 361, 362, 384
Abū Isḥāq Ibrāhīm al-Muṣannif *see* Ibrāhīm b. Faraj b. Mārūth al-Sāmirī al-Ṭabīb (al-Ḥakīm)
Abū Isḥāq al-Maḥallī al-ʿAṭṭār (Abraham b. Sasson), 125, 391
Abū al-ʿIzz al-ʿAṭṭār, 125
Abū al-ʿIzz b. Abū al-Maʿānī, 82, 318
Abū al-ʿIzz al-Kaḥḥāl, 58, 62, 87, 117, 121, 124, 125, 285
Abū al-ʿIzz al-Sharābī, 142
Abū al-ʿIzz Ṭabīb, 58, 87, 93, 124, 125
Abū al-ʿIzz al-Ṭabīb, 58, 61, 152
Abū Jaʿfar Joseph b. Aḥmad b. Ḥasday, 59, 160–1, 345, 348, 380
Abū al-Jūd Tobias, 59
Abū al-Khayr al-ʿAṭṭār, 68, 95, 125, 127
Abū al-Khayr al-Muhadhdhab b. al-Jalābnī, 59
Abū al-Khayr Salāma b. Mubārak b. Raḥmūn b. Mūsā al-Ṭabīb (Salāma b. Raḥmūn), 59, 148, 165, 175, 305, 335, 336
Abū al-Khayr al-Ṭabīb, 59
Abulafia family, 57
Abū al-Maʿālī (Abū al-ʿAlā) Tammām b. Hibat Allāh b. Tammām, 59, 75, 297, 337
Abū al-Maʿānī, 59–60, 74, 83, 86, 93, 96, 98, 108, 111, 118, 119, 205
Abū al-Maʿānī 2, 60, 74, 83, 86, 93, 96, 98, 108, 110, 118, 119, 205
Abū al-Maḥāsin b. al-Kāmukhī b. Abū al-Faḍāʾil, 60, 360
Abū al-Maḥāsin al-Sheikh al-Thiqa (Mishaʾel b. Josiah (Isaiah) ha-Levi ha-Rōfē ha-Sar) (b. Daniel, ha-Bāḥūr ha-Ṭōv), 60, 161–2
Abū al-Majd al-Ṭabīb, 122, 125, 129, 130, 132, 201
Abū al-Makārim al-Levi al-ʿAṭṭār b. Nāfiʿ, 126
Abū Manṣūr (Isaac), 60, 149, 185
Abū al-Manṣūr al-ʿAṭṭār, 126
Abū al-Manṣūr (Ablmanṣūr) al-ʿAṭṭār, 126
Abū Manṣūr b. Abī al-Futūḥ, 52, 60
Abū Manṣūr Muhadhdhab al-Dawla, 60, 99–100, 405
Abū Manṣūr al-Mutaṭabbib (Elazar b. Yeshūʿā ha-Levi), 60, 393, 220
Abū Manṣūr al-Mutaṭabbib (Shemarya b. ʿAlī ha-Rōfē), 61, 182
Abū Manṣūr Sulaymān b. Ḥaffāẓ (Solomon ha-Kohen), 61, 371
Abū Manṣūr al-Ṭabīb, 61
Abū Manṣūr al-Ṭabīb 2, 61
Abū Manṣūr, the Karaite, 61, 371
Abū al-Mufaḍḍal al-Muhadhdhab, 58, 61, 152
Abū al-Muḥāsan (Samuel b. Khalīfa), 61
Abū al-Munā al-ʿAṭṭār, 49, 76, 126, 127, 134, 136
Abū al-Munā al-ʿAṭṭār (Jacob b. David ha-Parnās), 126, 141
Abū al-Munā b. Abī Naṣr b. Ḥaffāẓ (al-Kohen al-ʿAṭṭār al-ʾIsrāʾīlī), 24, 61, 126, 140, 201, 353, 371
Abū al-Munā al-Sharābī, 49, 128
Abū al-Munā al-Ṭabīb, 61–2
Abū al-Munā al-Ṭabīb 2, 62
Abū al-Munajjā (Solomon b. Shaʿyā), 62, 197, 343, 344
Abū al-Munajjā al-ʿAṭṭār, 127
Abū al-Murajjā, 62
Abū al-Murajjā b. Daniel, 62
Abū al-Muẓaffar, 199
Abū Naṣr al-ʿAṭṭār, 127, 134
Abū Naṣr al-ʿAṭṭār 2, 49, 76, 126, 127, 134, 136
Abū Naṣr al-ʿAṭṭār 3, 127
Abū Naṣr al-ʿAṭṭār (Ibn Khalaf), 127
Abū Naṣr al-ʿAṭṭār b. Zubaybāt, 127
Abū Naṣr Hārūn b. Saʿadya, 62
Abū Naṣr al-Sadīd, 58, 62, 87, 117
Abū Naṣr Samawʾal b. Yaḥyā al-Maghribī (Samuel b. Judah b. ʿAbbās al-Maghribī), 46, 62, 170–1, 297, 343, 344, 349, 377, 382, 404, 405
Abū Naṣr al-Ṭabīb, 62
Abū Naṣr al-Ṭabīb 2, 62
Abū Naṣr al-Ṭabīb 3, 63
Abū Naṣr al-Ṭabīb b. al-Tinnīsī, 63, 185, 394
Abū al-Rabīʿ ʿAṭṭār, 91, 99, 108, 121, 122, 127, 134
Abū al-Riḍā al-ʿAṭṭār, 68, 95, 125, 127
Abū al-Riḍā ha-Levi, 314
Abū Riḍā al-Ṭabīb, 63, 65, 114
Abū al-Riḍā al-Ṭabīb (Joseph ha-Levi), 63, 289, 391–2
Abū Saʿd al-ʿAṭṭār, 128, 149, 192
Abū Saʿd al-ʿAṭṭār 2, 100, 122, 125, 128, 129, 130, 132, 201
Abū Saʿd al-Ḥarīrī, 128
Abū Saʿd al-Ṭabīb (al-Sadīd), 63
Abū Saʿd al-Ṭabīb 2, 64
Abū Sahl Dūnash b. Tamīm, 64, 305, 343, 344, 384
Abū Sahl Yedūthūn ha-Levi (Yedūthūn ha-Levi ha-Rōfē b. Levi ha-Levi), 64, 110
Abū Saʿīd, 128
Abū Saʿīd (al-Sheikh al-Muhadhdhab), 128
Abū Saʿīd al-ʿAṭṭār, 49, 122, 128
Abū Saʿīd b. al-ʿAṭṭār (Abū Saʿīd al-ʿAfṣī, Ben al-ʿAfṣī), 129, 135–6
Abū Saʿīd Khan, 181–2, 405
Abū Saʿīd of fusṭāṭ, 318
Abū al-Ṣalt Umayya b. ʿAbd al-ʿAzīz al-Andalusī, 175, 335
Abū Sulaymān Daʾūd Abī al-Munā, 228
Abū Sulaymān David, 57
Abū al-Surūr al-ʿAṭṭār (Peraḥya ha-Zaqēn ha-Talmid), 128
Abū al-Surūr b. Binyām ha-Levi, 128
Abū al-Surūr al-Sharābī, 49, 76, 126, 127, 134, 136, 142
Abū al-Surūr al-Ṭabīb (Sasson ha-Levi), 64
Abū al-Thanāʾ, 58, 62, 87, 117
Abū Yaʿqūb al-Baṣīr (Joesph b. Abraham) b. Nūḥ, 77
Abū Yaʿqūb al-Ḥakīm (Jekuthiel b. Moses ha-Rōfē), 64, 174, 282, 317

Abū Ya'qūb al-Ṭabīb *see* Isḥāq b. Mūsā b. El'āzār (Abū Ya'qūb al-Ṭabīb) (al-Mutaṭabbib)
Abū Yūsuf b. Ya'qūb, 74
Abū Zechariah b. Sa'ada, 65
Abū Zechariah Yaḥyā b. Sulaymān al-Dhamārī, 65
Abū Zikrī Kohen, 143
Abū Zikrī al-Sadīd b. Elijah b. Zecharia, 65, 176, 187–9, 227, 283, 297, 328
Abū Zikrī al-Ṭabīb (Judah b. Sa'adya), 65, 172–3, 296, 300, 362
Abū Zikrī al-Ṭabīb 2, 63, 65, 114
Abū Zikrī Yaḥyā (Sar Shālōm) (Zūṭā), 65, 182–4
al-'Āḍid li-Dīn Allāh, 50, 183
al-Afḍal (Fatimid), 197, 344
al-Afḍal (wazīr), 166, 309
al-Afḍal b. Badr al-Jamālī, 172
'Afīf (R. Joseph b. Ezra al-Miṣrī), 65, 402
'Afīf b. 'Abd al-Qāhir Sukra al-Yahūdī al-Ḥalabī al-Ṭabīb, 65, 193, 195, 298, 397
al-'Afīf b. Abī Sa'īd al-Sāwī, 65
'Afīf b. 'Imrān (Amram), 193
Aḥmad b. Ṭūlūn, 114
'Ala' al-Din 'Umar b. Muḥammad, 211
'Ala' al-Din Ibn Ṣaghir, 219
'Alī Abī al-Yamān al-Kindī, 198, 335, 336
'Alī b. Nathan, 65
Alī b. Sahl Rabban al-Ṭabarī, 89
'Alī b. Yūsuf b. Tāshufīn, 45, 73, 169, 297, 354, 379, 385
'Alī ha-Busmī, 128, 148, 166
'Alī ha-Rōfē, 65, 149, 182
'Alī Ibn Riḍwān, 24, 79, 161, 165, 173, 283, 309, 334–5, 336
Amato Lusitano, 68
Amīn al-Dawla Abū al-Ḥasan b. Ghazāl b. Abī Sa'īd al-Sāmirī (Wazīr al-Ṣāliḥ, and Sharaf al-Milla 'Glory of the Nation'), 66, 199–200, 298, 300, 337, 340, 345, 348, 349, 375, 396, 453
al-Āmir (Fatimid ruler), 172, 173
al-Amjad Bahrām Shāh, 198, 199, 298, 375
R. Amram b. Sa'īd b. Mūsā, 66, 143, 288, 332
Amram ha-Kohen ha-Rōfē b. Aaron, 66, 401
al-Amshāṭī family, 51
'Anan b. David, 167
Araḥ ha-Rōfē, 66
Arghūn Khān, 99–100, 341, 405
Aristotle, 30, 47, 90, 356
al-As'ad Abī al-Barakāt al-Ṭabīb, 66
As'ad al-Dīn (Ibn Ṣabra) al-Maḥallī al-Mutaṭabbib (Jacob b. Isaac), 66–7, 101, 116, 306, 309, 391, 398
Asad Ibn Jānī, 321
al-As'ad al-Mutaṭabbib, 67, 282
al-As'ad al-Ṭabīb, 67, 73
Asad al-Yahūdī (Usayda), 67, 285, 286, 298, 333, 364, 396, 397, 399, 402, 402
Asher Ben Jehiel, 90
al-Ashraf Khalīl b. Qalāwūn, 210, 382
al-Ashraf Mūsā b. al-'Ādil b. Ayyūb, 101, 298, 375, 396, 399
'Aṭiyya al-Qūṣī, 76
al-'Aṭṭār al-Ḥakīm (anonymous), 136, 283
'Awḍ, 67, 364, 366, 399
awlād al-Ra'īs (anonymous), 60, 74, 83, 86, 93, 96, 98, 108, 110, 118, 119, 205
'Awn Allāh b. Mūsā, 156
Ayāzkūj (Emir), 203–4
Azariah b. Ephraim, 68
al-'Azīz bi-Allah, 154

Badī' (Ṣadr al-Dīn) b. Nafīs b. Dā'ūd b. 'Anān al-Dā'ūdi al-Tabrīzī, 68, 218–19, 312
Bādīs, 58, 296, 361, 362, 384
Badr al-Jamālī, 173
Bahlawān, 170, 297
al-Bakrī, 77–8, 378
Baktamur al-Sāqī, 212
Banīn b. Da'ūd, 128, 254n689
Banū Jamā'a family, 146
Baqā' al-'Aṭṭār, 129
Barbosa the physician, 68, 401
Baruch (the physician from Damascus), 68, 398
Baybars al-Jāshnakīr, 7
Ben bū '[...]ā al-Ṭabīb, 68, 95, 125, 127
Ben ha-Sōfer ha-Dayyān (anonymous), 115, 311, 365
ben Maimon /Maimonidean family, 42, 43, 151, 161–4, 176, 183, 225, 227, 311, 370
Benjamin ha-Rōfē, 68, 119
Benjamin of Tudela, 49, 113, 170, 386, 389, 390, 391, 393, 394, 397, 398, 401
Benjamin al-Sharīṭī ha-Rōfē *see* Abū al-Faḍl al-Sharīṭī al-Ḥalabī ha-Rōfē
Benyām al-Rashīdī al-'Aṭṭār, 129, 136
Berākhōt b. Samuel, 68, 315
Berākhōt ha-Rōfē, 68
Berākhōt ha-Rōfē b. Sar Shālōm, 69, 108, 152
al-Bīyrūnī, 89
Bukhtīshū' family, 28, 228
Burhān al-Dīn Ibrāhīm, 69, 221

al-Dakhwār, Muhadhdhab al-Dīn 'Abd al-Raḥīm, 30, 191, 332, 338
Daniel al-Qūmisī, 430n524
Dāniyāl (Daniel) Ibn Sha'yā, 69, 196–7
Dā'ūd al-'Aṭṭār, 122, 125, 129, 130, 132, 201
Dā'ūd al-'Aṭṭār b. Abū al-Faḍl ha-Kohen, 129
David, 69
David al-Mukhammas, 69
David b. Abraham b. Moses b. Maimon, 55, 69, 151, 164, 327, 362, 402
David b. Daniel b. Azariah, 172, 390
David b. Jacob, 69, 92, 101, 151, 221
David b. Joshua Maimon (al-Maimūnī), 69, 164, 362, 396, 397
David b. Samuel Ibn Ṣaghīr, 69, 213, 215
R. David b. Shushan, 69, 400
David b. Solomon *see* Abū al-Faḍl Dā'ūd b. Sulaymān b. Abū al-Bayān al-'Isrā'īlī al-Sadīd
David ha-Rōfē, 69, 371
al-Dimashqī, 129
Dioscorides, 159, 178, 302, 311, 318
Dosa, the son of Saadia Gaon, 58, 160

Elazar)the king's physician(, 53, 69, 298, 397
R. Elazar, 70
Elazar b. Joseph see Abū al-'Alā (Elazar b. Joseph)
Elazar b. Judah b. Japheth he-Levi *see* Manṣūr b. Abī al-Futūḥ b. Abī al-Ḥasan

Elazar b. Tiqva ha-Levi ha-Sar ha-Nikhbād ha-Rōfē, 70, 205
Elazar b. Yeshūʿā ha-Levi *see* Abū Manṣūr al-Mutaṭabbib (Elazar b. Yeshūʿā ha-Levi)
Elazar ha-Levi ha-Zāqēn ha-Nikhbād ha-Rōfē, 70
Elazar ha-Rōfē, 70
Elazar Sakandarī, 70, 224, 366, 378, 453
Elazar the pharmacist, 129
Elias b. al-Mudawwar b. Ṣaddūd al-Yahūdī al-Ṭabīb al-Rundī, 70, 354, 379
Eliezer ha-Rōfē b. Obadia ha-Rōfē, 70, 217–18
Elijah b. Samuel, 78, 103, 168
Elijah b. Zechariah *see* Abū al-Faraj b. al-Raʾīs
Elijah ha-Kohen b. Solomon, 172
Elijah ha-Kohen ha-Rōfē, 70, 371
Elijah ha-R[ō]fē b. Samuel ha-Melammēd, 71, 318
Elisha ha-Rōfē, 71, 371
Ephraim al-ʿAṭṭār, 129, 389
Ephraim b. al-Ḥasan b. Isḥāq b. Ibrāhīm b. Yaʿqūb Abū Kathīr al-Zaffān (Ephraim b. al-Zaffān), 71, 148, 165–6, 173, 175, 296, 305, 309, 317, 334–5, 336
Ephraim b. Japheth, 71
Ephraim b. al-Zaffān *see* Ephraim b. al-Ḥasan b. Isḥāq b. Ibrāhīm b. Yaʿqūb Abū Kathīr al-Zaffān
Ephraim ha-Rōfē b. Isaac, 71
Ephraim ha-Rōfē b. Japheth b. Isaac, 71, 185
Euclid, 214

Faḍl b. Khalaf al-Raʾīs al-Sadīd, 71, 371
Falaṭīs the Indian, 90
Faraḥ b. Abū al-ʿAlā, 129–30, 134, 144
Faraj Allāh (Yeshūʿa) Ibn Ṣaghīr, 71, 212–13, 215, 299, 321, 331–2, 333, 335, 337, 350, 372
Farrukh Shāh, 198, 340
Fatḥ Allāh b. Muʿtaṣim b. Nafīs (Fatḥ al-Dīn), 71, 219–20, 301, 347, 453
Furāt b. Shaḥnāthā (Shaḥāthā) al-Yahūdī, 71, 333

Galen, 24, 46, 47, 90, 112, 161, 201, 203, 302, 310, 338, 352, 353, 380
al-Gaon al-Munā (anonymous), 60, 74, 83, 86, 93, 96, 98, 108, 110, 118, 119, 205
Gaykhātū, 181
Ghāzān Khān, 96, 181, 341, 405
al-Ghuzūlī, 47
Gregorios b. al-ʿIbrī, 399

al-Ḥāfiz (li-Dīn Allāh), 74–5, 186, 321–2, 362
Hai Gaon, 58, 361, 384
al-Ḥajjāj b. Yūsuf, 71
Ḥājī Khalīfa, 61, 93
al-Ḥakam II, 78, 157, 296, 340
al-Ḥākim bi-Amr Allāh, 72, 76, 104, 286, 296
al-Ḥakīm al-Iskandrī al-Murabbā al-Maghribī *see* Moses b. Abraham b. Saʿadya
al-Ḥakīm al-Ṣafī *see* Japheth b. David b. Samuel Ibn Ṣaghīr
Ḥalfon Abū Saʿīd b. Nethanel ha-Levi, 54
Ḥalfon b. Nethanel, 113, 381
Ḥalfon ha-Levi b. Manasseh, 61, 63, 116, 121, 125, 126, 127, 128, 130, 134
Ḥalfon ha-Levi b. Nethanel, 59, 71–2, 80, 381
Ḥalfon ha-Rōfē, 72
R. Hananel, 105
Hananiah b. Bezalel, 72, 397
Hananiah ha-Rōfē, 72, 186
al-Ḥaqīr al-Nāfiʿ al-Ṭabīb (al-Jirāḥī al-Miṣrī), 72, 286, 296
Hārūn (Aaron) b. Isaac of Cordova, 72–3, 296, 333, 336, 380
Hārūn b. Khulayf b. Hārūn, 130
Hārūn al-Rashīd, 89, 296
Ḥasan Abū Kanū?, 73, 297, 379
al-Ḥasan Hibat Allāh Mufaḍḍal al-Yahūdī, 73
al-Ḥasan Ṭabīb, 73
Ḥasday b. Joseph b. Ḥasday *see* Abū al-Faḍl (Ḥasday b. Joseph b. Ḥasday)
Ḥasday b. Shaprūṭ, 23, 73, 148, 157–60, 296, 300, 301, 340, 357, 361–3, 380, 454
Ḥayyīm b. Joseph Vital, 73, 327, 353, 400, 402
Ḥazqīl, 73
Hibat Allāh (Nethanel b. Moses ha-Levi), 73, 183, 184, 297, 306, 362
Hiba al-ʿAṭṭār, 130, 131
Hiba al-ʿAṭṭār 2, 122, 125, 129, 130, 132, 201
Hiba b. al-Kallām, 114, 287
Hippocrates, 24, 53, 90, 101, 161, 162, 203, 302, 309, 310, 322, 353, 380
Ḥunain b. Isḥāq, 115, 311
Ḥusayn al-ʿAṭṭār, 130

Ibn Abī al-Ḥawāfir, 228
Ibn Abī Uṣaybiʿa, 15, 25, 26, 46, 47, 48, 56, 66, 72, 75, 76, 88, 89, 116, 147, 155, 156, 158, 159, 160, 162, 163, 166, 170, 175, 184, 189, 190, 191, 193, 195, 197, 198, 199, 201, 203, 265n926, 268n988, 268n991, 270n1018, 281, 286, 288, 295, 303, 306, 309, 332, 333, 334, 337, 355, 404, 421n364, 424n414, 449
Ibn al-ʿAdīm, 195
Ibn Aḥmad b. al-Maghribī, 73, 211, 346
Ibn ʿAknīn (Joseph b. Judah b. Jacob), 53, 73–4, 337, 352, 378–9, 385–6
Ibn al-ʿAmmānī family, 176–80, 225, 227, 402
Ibn al-Athīr, 74
Ibn al-ʿAyn Zarbī, 334, 336
Ibn al-Bayṭār, 64, 89, 95, 286
Ibn Biklarish, 24
Ibn al-Dāʿī al-ʾIsrāʾīlī al-Irbilī al-Ḥakīm *see* Kamāl al-Dawla Abū ʿAlī b. Abī al-Faraj
Ibn Duqmāq, 197, 344
Ibn al-Fuwaṭī, 85, 180, 181, 283
Ibn al-Hājj, 119, 451
Ibn Ḥazm, 80, 381
Ibn al-Hītī, 69, 113, 213, 430n524
Ibn Hūd, 268n981
Ibn Iyās, 119, 120, 241n312
Ibn Jazla, 24
Ibn al-Julājilī, 60, 74, 83, 86, 93, 96, 98, 108, 110, 118, 119, 205
Ibn Juljul al-Andalusī, 89
Ibn Jumayʿ family, 202–4
Ibn Jumayʿ al-ʾIsrāʾīlī *see* Abū al-ʿAshāʾir Hibat-Allāh b. Zayn b. Ḥasan b. Ifrāʾīm b. Yaʿqūb b. Ismāʿīl Ibn Jumayʿ al-ʾIsrāʾīlī
Ibn Jumayʿ al-ʾIsrāʾīlī al-Ṭabīb *see* Mūsā b. Ifrāʾīm b. Dāʾūd b. Ifrāʾīm b. Yaʿqūb

Ibn Khaldūn, 77, 79, 109, 386
Ibn Khallikān, 48
Ibn al-Kirmānī family, 150, 207, 370
Ibn Kūjik, 74, 150, 151, 214, 215, 299, 371
Ibn Kūjik family, 196, 211, 213, 214–15, 275n1115, 370
Ibn al-Maghribī family, 210–11, 227, 275n1115, 294, 370
Ibn Māsawayh, 24
Ibn al-Mudawwar, 59, 75
Ibn Muṭrān, 190, 301, 323, 348
Ibn al-Nafīs, 212, 214, 273n1067, 331, 335, 337
Ibn al-Nāqid, 201, 305, 336
Ibn al-Nasṭās al-Naṣrānī, 104, 296
Ibn Qarqa (or Ibn Qirqah), 74–5, 186, 319, 321–2
Ibn al-Qifṭī, 15, 25, 26, 47, 49, 52, 53, 63, 142, 147, 154, 170, 280, 289, 331, 337, 382, 424n414
Ibn al-Quff, 24
Ibn al-Rūmī, 80
Ibn Rushd (Averroes), 310
Ibn Ṣaghīr Abī Faraj Allāh, 75, 212, 299, 335, 372
Ibn Ṣaghīr family, 150, 151, 196, 197, 210, 211–14, 227, 275n1115, 312, 344, 348, 370
Ibn Saʿīd al-Andalusī, 1043
Ibn Samʿūn *see* Abū al-Ḥajjāj Yūsuf b. Yaḥyā b. Isḥāq al-Sabatī al-Maghribī
Ibn Sanāʾ al-Mulk, 204, 332
Ibn Shaʿyā family, 149, 195–7, 214
Ibn Shortmeqash family, 57
Ibn Shūʿa (al-Muwaffaq), 59, 75, 297, 316, 355
Ibn Sīnā, 29, 30, 57, 61, 73, 89, 110, 203, 204, 207, 214, 338, 352, 380
Ibn Taghribirdī, 74
Ibn Taymiyya, 67, 96, 208, 333, 451
Ibn al-Tilmīdh, Amīn al-Dawla, 24, 47, 323
Ibn al-Ukhūwa, 338
Ibn Wāṣil, 214, 331
Ibn Zuhr (Avenzoar), Ibn Zuhr family, 228
Ibrāhīm, 75
Ibrāhīm al-ʿAṭṭār, 130, 132
Ibrāhīm b. Faraj Allāh b. ʿAbd al-Kāfī al-ʾIsrāʾīlī al-Yahūdī al-Dāʾūdi al-ʿAffānī (al-ʿAnānī), 76, 366, 372
Ibrāhīm b. Faraj b. Mārūth al-Sāmirī al-Ṭabīb (al-Ḥakīm) (Abū Isḥāq Ibrāhīm al-Muṣannif) (Shams al-Ḥukamāʾ), 76, 198, 282, 283, 297, 333–4, 335, 336, 375
Ibrāhīm b. Khalaf al-Sāmirī (the Samaritan), 76, 190–1, 199, 298, 335, 375, 398
Ibrāhīm b. Nūḥ al-Ṭabīb ha-Ḥākhām, 77, 371
Ibrāhīm b. Shūmalī, 77, 400
Ibrāhīm b. al-Tharthār, 77, 299, 339, 386
Ibrāhīm b. Yaʿqūb al-ʾIsrāʾīlī al-Ṭurṭūshī, 77–8, 378
Ibrāhīm b. Zarzar *see* Ibrāhīm b. al-Tharthār
Ibrāhīm ha-Rōfē, 49, 75–6, 126, 127, 134, 136
Ibrāhīm al-Mutaṭabbib b. Mukhtār (Ibn al-Yām), 75, 106, 282, 390
ʿImād al-Dawla Abū al-Khayr b. Muwaffaq al-Dawla Abū al-Faraj ʿAlī b. Abī al-Shujāʿ al-Hamadānī, 78, 181, 283
ʿImād al-Dīn al-Nābulsī, 213, 335, 337
ʿImrān b. Ṣadaqa al-ʾIsrāʾīlī al-Ḥakīm Awḥad al-Dīn al-ʾIsrāʾīlī (Moses b. Ṣedāqā), 78, 189, 190–1, 199, 282–3, 294, 298, 300, 332, 334, 335, 336, 398, 401
Iqbāl al-Dawla, 56, 296
ʿIsā b. Mūsā al-ʿAbbāsī, 71, 333
Isaac, 78, 372
Isaac Aldabi ha-Ḥasid, 90
Isaac b. Abraham b. Ezra, 46, 171, 349–50
Isaac b. Baruch ha-Rōfē, 78
R. Isaac b. Ḥalfōn, 164
Isaac b. ʿImrān, 79, 336, 384
Isaac b. Shoshan ha-Dayyān, 184
Isaac b. Solomon *see* Isḥāq b. Sulaymān al-ʾIsrāʾīlī
Isaac b. Yashush *see* Abū Ibrāhīm b. Qasṭār
Isaac ha-Kohen ha-Rōfē, 78, 166–7
Isaac ha-Kohen ha-Rōfē b. Furāt, 78, 148, 164–5, 301, 364, 401
Isaac ha-Rōfē, 78, 103, 168
Isaac ha-Rōfē 2, 78, 286, 401
Isaac ha-Sar ha-Adīr ha-Talmīd ha-Nikhbād ha-Rōfē ha-Ḥākhām, 79
Isaac Luria, 73, 327
R. Isaac Sholel, 65
Isḥāq b. Mūsā b. Elʿāzār (Abū Yaʿqūb al-Ṭabīb) (al-Mutaṭabbib), 65, 79, 154, 155, 156, 157, 296, 300, 362, 383–4
Isḥāq b. Sulaymān al-ʾIsrāʾīlī (Isaac b. Solomon), 23, 64, 79–80, 154, 296, 305, 313, 336, 351, 355, 384
Isḥāq al-Ruhāwī, 321
Ismāʿīl, 80
Ismāʿīl b. Abū al-Waqqār, 198, 335, 336
Ismāʿīl b. Faddād, 80
Ismāʿīl b. Mūsā b. Elʿāzār, 65, 80, 154, 156, 343, 344, 384
Ismaʿīl b. Yūnis, 80, 381
Israel b. Zechariah al-Ṭayfūrī, 80, 296
Israel ha-Dayyān al-Maghribī, 213
al-ʾIsrāʾīlī al-Ṣaydalānī, 130, 135, 137

Jacob, 80, 221
Jacob b. David ha-Parnās *see* Abū al-Munā al-ʿAṭṭār (Jacob b. David ha-Parnās)
Jacob b. Isaac *see* Asʿad al-Dīn (Ibn Ṣabra) al-Maḥallī al-Mutaṭabbib
Jacob b. Joseph, 80
Jacob b. Meʾir, 80, 379
Jacob ha-Rōfē, 72, 80, 381
Jacob ha-Rōfē 2, 80–1, 92, 103, 288, 400
Jacob ha-Rōfē b. Ayyūb, 81
Jacob ha-Rōfē b. Ḥalfon, 81
R. Jacob ha-Rōfē ha-Sar ha-Nikhbād ha-Zāqēn ha-[…] ha-Rōfē ha-[…], 81, 150, 216, 364
Jaʿfar al-Muqtadir, 77
al-Jāḥiẓ, 279
Jalāl al-Dīn b. al-Ḥazzān, 81, 181, 299, 367, 405
Jamāl al-Dīn ʿAbd Allāh b. ʿAbd al-Sayyid b. Isḥāq b. Yaḥyā, 81, 208, 209, 294
Jamāl al-Dīn Dāʾūd b. Abī al-Faraj b. Abī al-Ḥusayn b. ʿImrān al-Ṭabīb, 81, 346, 350, 399
Jamāl al-Dīn Ibrāhīm b. Shihāb al-Dīn Aḥmad (Sulaymān) al-Maghribī, 82, 210, 211, 212, 213, 294, 299, 301, 312, 341, 382
Japheth b. Araḥ ha-Rōfē, 66
Japheth b. David b. Samuel Ibn Ṣaghīr (al-Ḥakīm al-Ṣafī), 82, 213, 215, 282, 372

Japheth ([Abū] al-Maḥāsin) ha-Kohen b. Josiah, 82, 318
Japheth ha-Rōfē, 82, 389
Japheth ha-Rōfē b. Joseph ha-Parnās, 82
Japheth Levi ha-Rōfē b. Judah ha-Sōfer, 82
Jaqmaq, 42, 339
al-Jawbarī, Zayn al-Dīn, 139, 320–1
al-Jazarī, 81, 272n1062, 346
Jekuthiel b. Moses *see* Abū al-Faḍāʾil (Jekuthiel b. Moses)
Jekuthiel b. Moses ha-Rōfē *see* Abū Yaʿqūb al-Ḥakīm
Jekuthiel II b. Moses II ha- Rōfē *see* Abū al-Faḍāʾil (Jekuthiel II b. Moses II ha- Rōfē)
Jekuthiel b. Uziel b. Obadia ha-Dayyān *see* ʿAbd al-Dāʾim (al-Muwaffaq) b. ʿAbd al-ʿAzīz b. Maḥāsin ʾIsrāʾīlī al-Mutaṭabbib
Jekuthiel ha-Levi b. Petahya, 82, 205, 371, 398
R. Jonah Marinus *see* Marwān (Abūal-Walīd) Ibn Janāḥ al-Qurṭubī
R. Joseph, 70, 82
Joseph 2, 82
Joseph 3, 60, 74, 83, 86, 93, 96, 98, 108, 110, 118, 119
Joseph al-ʿAṭṭār, 130
Joesph b. Abraham *see* Abū Yaʿqūb al-Baṣīr (Joesph b. Abraham) b. Nūḥ
Joseph b. Abraham b. Waqār, 57
Joseph b. Abraham ha-Roʾeh *see* Yūsuf al-Baṣīr
R. Joseph b. Abraham Sakandarī (Iskandarī or Iskandarānī), 83, 151, 222, 223–4, 364, 366, 370, 378, 389
Joseph b. ʿAqnīn, 56, 168
Joseph b. al-Dayyān *see* Yūsuf ʿAbd al-Sayyid b. al-Muhadhdhab al-ʾIsrāʾīlī al-Mutaṭabib
Joseph b. Elazar al-ʿAṭṭār, 130, 134
R. Joseph b. Eliezer, 70, 82
R. Joseph b. Ezra al-Miṣrī *see* ʿAfīf (R. Joseph b. Ezra al-Miṣrī)
Joseph b. Isaac, 83, 400
Joseph b. Isaiah *see* Abū al-Ḥasan Yūsuf b. Josiah al-Tunisī
Joseph b. Jacob b. ʿAwkal, 58
Joseph b. Judah b. Jacob *see* Ibn ʿAknīn
Joseph b. Judah b. Simon *see* Abū al-Ḥajjāj Yūsuf b. Yaḥyā b. Isḥāq al-Sabatī al-Maghribī
R. Joseph b. Khalīfa *see* Joseph ha-Nagid b. Khalīfa
Joseph b. Meʾir b. Muhājir, 57
Joseph b. Migash, 54
Joseph b. Nissīn ha-Rōfē, 83
Joseph b. Simon (al-Maghribī), 53, 69
Joseph from Damascus, 83, 151, 221, 222, 399
Joseph al-Gazī, 83
R. Joseph ha-Dayyān, 80, 379
Joseph ha-Levi *see* Abū al-Riḍā al-Ṭabīb (Joseph ha-Levi)
Joseph ha-Nagid b. Khalīfa, 84, 299, 300, 362, 399
Joseph ha-Nāsī, 53
Joseph ha-Parnās ha-Rōfē, 84
Joseph ha-Rōfē, 84, 371
Joseph ha-Rōfē b. Isaac, 84
Joseph ha-Sar ha-Nikhbād ha-Rōfē, 84
Joseph (Abū ʿAmr) Ibn Qamniʾel, 84, 169
Joseph Ibn Ṣaddiq, 79, 355
R. Joseph Karo, 223
Joseph Sambari, 224
Joseph al-Ṭabīb, 83
Joshua Jacob al-ʿAṭṭār, 130, 136
Josiah Gaon, 129
Judah, 84
Judah b. Abūn /ʿAbbās *see* Yaḥyā b. ʿAbbās al-Maghribī
Judah b. Joseph b. Abī al-Thanā, 84–5, 334, 336, 403
Judah b. Moses *see* Yaḥyā Abū Zikrī al-Ṭabīb
Judah b. Mūsā b. Jacob, 85
Judah b. Saʿadya *see* Abū Zikrī al-Ṭabīb (Judah b. Saʿadya)
Judah b. Samuel ha-Levi *see* Abū al-Ḥasan (Judah b. Samuel ha-Levi)
Judah b. Tibbon, 54, 322, 329
Judah from Alexandria, 85, 286, 390
Judah from Damascus, 85, 222, 286, 399
Judah ha-Levi *see* Abū al-Ḥasan (Judah b. Samuel ha-Levi)
Judah ha-Melammēd b. Aaron ha-Rōfē Ibn al-ʿAmmānī, 62, 164, 176, 178, 179, 180, 227, 318, 367
Judah ha-Nāsī (son of Josiah ha-Nāsī), 84
Judah al-Ḥarīzī, 46, 49, 53, 68, 69, 72, 78, 80, 85, 90, 98, 191, 354, 379
Judah ha-Rōfē, 85, 397
Judah ha-Rōfē 2, 85
Judah ha-Rōfē b. Abraham Taurīzī, 85, 367, 373

Kamāl b. Mūsā, 86, 285, 288, 366, 400
Kamāl al-Dawla Abū ʿAlī b. Abī al-Faraj (Ibn al-Dāʿī al-ʾIsrāʾīlī al-Irbilī al-Ḥakīm), 85, 282, 298, 345, 348
al-Kaskarī, 320
Khāirbek al-Ashrafī, 120, 397
Khalaf al-Kaḥḥāl, 86, 285
Khan Hülegü, 85
Khiḍr, 86, 347
al-Kindī, 24
al-Kohen al-ʿAṭṭār al-ʾIsrāʾīlī *see* Abū al-Munā b. Abī Naṣr b. Ḥaffāẓ

al-Levi al-ʿAṭṭār ha-Zāqēn, 132

Maḥāsin (Obadia ha-Dayyān), 86, 150, 206, 207
Maḥāsin al-Ṭabīb, 86
al-Mahdī, 95
al-Mahdī ʿUbayd Allāh, 79, 384
Maḥfūẓ ha-Rōfē, 86, 397
Maḥfūẓ al-Ṭabīb, 86
Maimonides *see* Mūsā b. ʿAbd Allāh al-ʾIsrāʾīlī al-Qurṭubī
Makārim al-ʿAṭṭār, 122, 125, 129, 130, 132, 201
Makārim b. Isḥāq b. Makārim, 87, 285, 293, 294, 295, 324
Makārim Ibn al-Gadalī, 60, 74, 83, 86, 93, 96, 98, 108, 111, 118, 119, 205
Makārim al-Kaḥḥāl, 58, 62, 87, 117, 121, 124, 125, 285
Makārim Ṭabīb, 58, 87, 93, 124, 125
Makīn ʿAṭṭār, 132
Makīn (al-Sheikh) al-Ṭabīb, 87
al-Malik al-ʿĀdil, 59, 188, 190, 201, 260n806, 298
al-Malik al-Afḍal, 162, 261n823, 299

al-Malik al-ʿAzīz, 188
al-Malik al-Kāmil, 163, 188, 266n942, 297, 328
al-Malik al-Muʾayyad Abū al-Fidāʾ, 67, 364
al-Malik al-Muʿaẓẓam (ʿIsā), 188–9, 190, 328
al-Malik Naṣīr Naṣr Allāh, 81, 350
al-Malik al-Ṣāliḥ, 199, 200, 340, 349, 375, 396
al-Malik al-Ẓāhir al-Ghāzī, 52, 69, 298
al-Maʾmūn (Wazīr), 161
al-Manṣūr, 71, 333
Manṣūr al-ʿAṭṭār, 130, 132
Manṣūr b. Abī al-Futūḥ b. Abī al-Ḥasan (Elazar b. Judah b. Japheth he-Levi), 87
al-Manṣūr b. al-Qāʾim, 64, 384
al-Manṣūr bi-Ilāh, 154
al-Manṣūr Ismāʿīl, 80
al-Manṣūr Qalāwūn, 293, 362
al-Maqqarī, 70
Al-Maqrīzī, 55, 74, 76, 154–5, 156, 203, 220, 319
Marwān b. al-Ḥākam, 89
Marwān (Abū al-Walīd) Ibn Janāḥ al-Qurṭubī (R. Jonah Marinus), 56, 73, 87–9, 90, 94, 352, 356, 380, 454
Māsarjawayh, 89, 351
Masīḥ b. Ḥakam al-Dimashqī (ʿIsa), 89–90, 282, 296
Maṣlīaḥ, 90, 399
Maṣlīaḥ ha-Kohen ha-Gaon b. Solomon, 173, 186
al-Masʿūdī, 85, 114, 334
al-Mawlī al-Muhadhdhab (anonymuous), 60, 74, 83, 86, 93, 96, 98, 108, 110, 118, 119, 205
Meʾir b. Isaac Aldabi, 90–1, 400
Meʾir (Abū al-Ḥasan) Ibn Qamniʾel, 45, 56, 90, 148, 168–9, 297, 354, 385, 454
Menahem, 91, 393
Menahem b. Sarūq, 77, 157
Menahem ha-Kohen ha-Rōfē b. Zadok, 91, 109, 113
Menahem Ṭabīb, 91, 99, 108, 127, 134
Meshullam of Volterra, 82, 84, 104, 366, 399
Mevōrākh b. Saʿadya *see* Abū al-Faḍl Mubārak
Mevōrākh ha-Kohen *see* Abū al-Faḍl (Abū al-Faḍāʾil) b. al-Nāqid b. Obadia, al-Ṭabīb al-Muhadhdhab
Mevōrākh ha-Rōfē, 91, 371
Mishaʾel b. Josiah (Isaiah) ha-Levi ha-Rōfē ha-Sar *see* Abū al-Maḥāsin al-Sheikh al-Thiqa
R. Mishael ha-Rōfē, 91, 161
Möngke Khan, 85, 345
Moses b. Abraham b. Saʿadya, 78, 103, 215–16, 372, 389
Moses b. Abraham b. Saʿadya ha-Rōfē Darʿī, 78, 91, 92, 103, 148, 167–8, 191, 354, 371, 385, 389
Moses b. Elazar *see* Mūsā b. Elʿāzār al-ʾIsrāʾīlī
Moses b. Enoch, 160
Moses b. Ezra, 46, 53, 56, 57, 169, 354, 379, 433n558
Moses b. Jekuthiel ha-Rōfē *see* Mūsā b. Abī al-Faḍāʾil
Moses b. Joseph ha-Levi *see* Abū ʿImrān b. al-Lawī al-Ishbīlī
Moses b. Maimon *see* Mūsā b. ʿAbd Allāh al-ʾIsrāʾīlī al-Qurṭubī
Moses b. Mevōrākh b. Saʿadya *see* Abū al-Bayān Mūsā b. Abī al-Faḍl
Moses (Abū Saʿd) b. Nethanel ha-Levi, 91, 149, 182–3, 184, 281, 294, 297, 300, 359, 364
Moses b. Peraḥya b. Yijū, 91–2, 242n347, 366, 392
Moses b. Samuel, 75, 213
Moses b. Ṣedāqā *see* ʿImrān b. Ṣadaqa al-ʾIsrāʾīlī al-Ḥakīm Awḥad al-Dīn al-ʾIsrāʾīlī
Moses b. Yaḥyā ha-Bassāmi, 132, 133
Moses b. Yerushalayim ha-Kohen, 92, 101, 221
Moses ha-Levi, 78, 103, 168
Moses ha-Rōfē, 92
Moses ha-Rōfē 2, 92
Moses ha-Rōfē 3, 80, 92, 103, 288, 400
Moses ha-Rōfē b. Isaac ha-Rōfē, 78, 92, 103, 168
Moses Rōfē, 93
R. Moses Vidalish ha-Rōfē, 93, 400
al-Mu'ayyad Sheikh, 120, 220, 396
Mubārak b. Salāma b. Mubārak b. Raḥmūn b. Abū al-Khayr, 93, 175
Mubārak ha-Rōfē, 93
al-Mubashshir b. Fātik, 175, 335
Mufaḍḍal b. Mājīd b. Abī al-Bishr al-ʾIsrāʾīlī (al-Kātib), 93–4
Mufaḍḍal al-Mashmiʿa, 60, 74, 83, 86, 93, 96, 98, 108, 110, 118, 119, 205
Mufaḍḍ(al) Ṭabīb, 58, 87, 93, 124, 125
al-Muhadhdhab, 94, 101, 392
al-Muhadhdhab b. al-Naqqāsh (Muhadhdhab al-Dīn al-Naqqāsh), 30, 198, 335, 336
Muḥammad al-Lakhmī al-Shaqūrī, 77, 339
Muḥammad b. Malik-Shāh, 46
Muḥammad V al-Naṣrī, 77, 299, 339, 386
al-Muʿizz (Tunisia), 58, 296, 361, 362, 384
al-Muʿizz li-Dīn Allāh, 64, 154–5, 156, 157, 296, 351, 362, 384
Munā al-Ṭabīb, 94
Munajjā al-ʿAṭṭār b. Abū Saʿd al-ʿAṭṭār, 132, 192–3, 201
Munajjam (Menahem) b. al-Fawwāl, 88, 94, 352, 380
Munajjā al-Ṭabīb b. Hiba, 94
al-Muqaddasī, 279
al-Muqtadir b. Hūd, 154, 160
Mūsā ʿAṭṭār, 132
Mūsā al-ʿAṭṭār, 132
Mūsā b. ʿAbd Allāh al-ʾIsrāʾīlī al-Qurṭubī (Moses b. Maimon; Maimonides), 23, 30, 44, 45, 51, 52, 55, 59, 63, 70, 73–4, 75, 79, 94, 97, 109, 112, 129, 134, 140, 141, 151, 161, 162, 164, 169, 176, 184, 190, 198, 204, 225, 227, 242n347, 256n730, 260n795, 280, 281, 282, 289, 290, 294, 297, 299, 300, 304, 313, 314, 315, 317, 323, 326, 327, 330, 332, 334, 336, 339, 351, 352–3, 354, 355–6, 359, 362, 364, 366, 367, 378, 379, 384, 385–6, 409n96, 425n434, 428n484, 444n734, 454
Mūsā b. Abī al-Faḍāʾil (Moses b. Jekuthiel ha-Rōfē), 94, 148, 173, 174, 317, 364, 377
Mūsā b. Elʿāzār al-ʾIsrāʾīlī (Moses b. Elazar), 65, 94, 142, 148, 152, 153–5, 156, 157, 225, 227, 296, 300, 336, 340, 343, 351, 362, 364, 383–4
Mūsā b. Ifrāʾīm b. Dāʾūd b. Ifrāʾīm b. Yaʿqūb (Ibn Jumayʿ al-ʾIsrāʾīlī al-Ṭabīb), 95, 202, 204
Mūsā b. Isrāʾīl, 95
Mūsā b. Kūjik (Sharaf al-Dīn), 95, 214, 215
Mūsā b. Sayyār, 95
Mūsā (Abū al-Imrān) b. Yaʿqūb b. Isḥāq al-ʾIsrāʾīlī, 95, 154, 157, 296, 300, 384
Musallam al-ʿAṭṭār, 132

Musallam al-Ṭabīb, 95
al-Mustaʿīn biʾllāh Abū Jaʿfar Aḥmad b. Yūsuf al-Muʾtamin biʾllāh, 112
al-Mustaʿlī, 172, 173
al-Mustanjid biʾllāh, 46, 297, 404
al-Mustanṣir biʾllāh, 171, 172, 173
al-Muʿtamid, 57
al-Mutanabbī, 214
al-Mutawakkil, 80, 296
al-Muwaffaq Asʿad b. Iliyās b. al-Maṭrān, 190
Muwaffaq al-Dawla Abū al-Faraj ʿAlī b. Abī al-Shujāʿ al-Hamadānī, 95, 149, 180–1
al-Muwaffaq al-Kohen al-Ṭabīb, 68, 95, 125, 127, 283
Muwaffaq Mujāhid al-ʿĀmirī, 56, 296
al-Muwaffaq al-Qaṣīr al-Ṭabīb al-Yahūdī, 95, 283, 286, 333, 399
al-Muwaffaq Yaʿqūb al-Iksandrī, 102
al-Muẓaffar, 189

Nafīs b. Dāʾūd b. ʿAnān al-Tabrīzī, 95, 151, 218–19, 227, 275n1115, 299, 312, 347, 348, 349, 370, 372
al-Nafīs al-Sharābī, 58, 62, 87, 117, 142
Nagid Amram, 70, 82
Naḥman ha-Rōfē, 96, 397
Naḥum al-ʿAṭṭār, 118, 132
al-Naʿja al-Ṭabīb, 96
Najīb al-Dawla, 96, 182, 285, 299, 346
al-Najīb al-Kaḥḥāl (the ophthalmologist) al-Yahūdī, 96
Najīb Kohen Kamukhī, 60, 74, 83, 86, 93, 96, 98, 108, 110, 118, 119, 205
al-Najīb al-Ṭabīb b. al-Ḥāvēr b. Abū al-Mufaḍḍal, 96
Najm al-Dīn b. al-Munāfiḥ, 110
al-Naṣīr Dāʾūd, 190
Naṣīr al-Dīn al-Ṭūsī, 96, 207
al-Nāṣir Faraj, 220
al-Nāṣir Ḥasan, 219
al-Nāṣir Muḥammad b. Qalāwūn, 210, 211, 212, 213, 299, 321, 331, 341, 346, 382
Nathan b. Samuel, 54, 252n613, 289
Nathan of Damascus, 96, 222, 399
R. Nehorai, 96, 403
Nethanel b. Abraham, 97, 391
Nethanel b. Joseph ha-Sar ha-Nikhbād ha-Rōfē, 97
Nethanel b. Moses, 97
Nethanel b. Moses ha-Levi *see* Hibat Allāh (Nethanel b. Moses ha-Levi)
Nethanel b. Samuel *see* Abū al-ʿAshāʾir Hibat-Allāh b. Zayn b. Ḥasan b. Ifrāʾīm b. Yaʿqūb b. Ismāʿīl Ibn Jumayʿ al-ʾIsrāʾīlī
Nethanel Baruch b. Melekh *see* Abū al-Barakāt Hibat Allāh b. ʿAlī b. Malkā (or Malkān) al-Baladī b. al-Ṭabīb al-Faḍl
Nethanel ha-Levi b. Amram *see* Abū al-Faraj b. Maʿmar al-Sharābī
Nethanel ha-Rōfē, 97
R. Nethanel ha-Rōfē b. Abraham, 97, 216, 217
Nethanel ha-Rōfē b. Joseph b. al-Malī, 97
Nethanel ha-Rōfē ha-Sar Nikhbād ha-Yeshiva, 97
Nethanel ha-Rōfē Tifēret ha-Rōfēim, 97
Nethanel ha-Sar ha-Yaqar ha-Rōfē, 97

Nuʿmān b. Abī al-Riḍā b. Sālim b. Isḥāq, 97–8, 334, 337, 396
Nuʿmān family, 146
Nūr al-Dīn Zengī, 149, 193, 268n988, 291, 298

Obadia b. Ṣedāqā ha-Rōfē, 98
Obadia ha-Dayyān *see* Maḥāsin (Obadia ha-Dayyān)
Obadia ha-Rōfē, 98, 150, 217–18, 403
Obadia Kahana ha-Rōfē, 98
Obadia of Bartenura, 224
Ohev b. Muhājir, 57
Öljeitü Khān, 81, 181, 299, 405

Palṭiel b. Shephatiah (Shefaṭya), 155
Pantaleo de Aveiro, 68
Peraḥya ha-Zaqēn ha-Talmid *see* Abū al-Surūr al-ʿAṭṭār
Petahya ha-Levi ha-Rōfē, 98, 150, 205, 371, 398
Pinḥas, 98, 397
Plato, 90

al-Qāḍī al-Fāḍil, 162, 309, 339
Qaitbāy, 299, 363
al-Qalānisī, 89
Qalqashandī, 360
Qarāqūsh (Asad al-Dīn Saʿīd Qarāqūsh b. ʿAbd Allāh al-Asadī; Bahāʿ al-Dīn), 203
al-Qazwīnī, 77, 378
Qublāy, 219, 274n1093

Rabbana Japheth *see* Abū ʿAlī al-ʿAṭṭār (Rabbana Japheth)
Rabīb ha-Rōfē, 98, 386
al-Rabīb Kohen, 60, 74, 83, 86, 93, 96, 98, 108, 111, 118, 119, 205
Radbaz (R. David b. Zimra), 41, 43, 113
Raḍī b. Elijah b. Zecharia (the judge), 98, 188, 189
Raḍī al-Dīn al-Raḥbī, 190, 199, 335, 337
Rashīd, 98
al-Rashīd b. al-ʿAjamī ʿAṭṭār, 91, 99, 108, 127, 134
Rashīd al-Dīn al-Ṭabīb Faḍl Allāh b. al-Dawla, Abū al-Khayr b. ʿAlī Abū al-Hamadānī, 81, 96, 99, 180–2, 283, 294, 298, 301, 313, 341, 405, 453
Rashīd Ṭabīb, 91, 99, 108, 127, 134
al-Rāzī, Abū Bakr Muḥammad b. Zakariyya, 30, 31, 72, 89, 310, 338

Saʿadya, 100, 150, 215, 216, 370
Saʿadya 2, 100
Saʿadya b. Abraham *see* Abū al-Fakhr al-ʿAṭṭār b. al-Amshāṭī
Saʿadya b. Danān, 64, 384
Saʿadya b. Mevōrākh, 100, 148, 171–2, 173, 296, 297, 364
Saʿadya Gaon, 79, 355
Saʿadya ha-Rōfē Darʿī, 100, 167, 385
Ṣabra family, 66, 116, 391
Sābūr b. Sahl, 24
Saʿd (ʿIzz al-Dawla) b. Manṣūr b. Kammūna, 99, 346, 404
Saʿd al-Dawla b. Ṣafī b. Hibat Allāh b. Muhadhdhib al-Dawla al-Abharī, 60, 99–100, 294, 300, 341, 405
Ṣadaqa, 100, 372

Ṣadaqa al-ʿAṭṭār, 127, 134
Ṣadaqa b. ʿAbd al-Qāhir, 100
Ṣadaqa b. Abraham ha-Kohen, 92, 101, 221
Ṣadaqa (al-Faḍl) b. Munajjā b. Ṣadaqa al-Sāmirī al-Ṭabīb (Ibn al-Shāʿir), 67, 101, 298, 306, 309, 375, 396, 399
Ṣadaqa ha-Kohen b. Maṣlīaḥ, 130, 134
Ṣadaqa ha-Rōfē, 101
Ṣadaqa al-ʾIsrāʾīlī, 100, 149, 189, 190, 294, 298, 300
Ṣadaqa al-Shādhilī, 99
Ṣadaqa al-Ṭabīb, 100, 201
al-Sadīd, 94, 101
al-Sadīd al-Dimyāṭī al-Ṭabīb al-Yahūdī, 101, 212, 213, 213–14, 215, 283, 299, 331, 335, 337, 372, 391
al-Sadīd al-Ṭabīb, 100, 102, 149, 201
Ṣadr al-Dīn al-Zinjānī, 181, 405
al-Ṣafadī, Khalīl b. Aybak, 47, 41, 67, 211, 213, 214, 268n988, 331, 341
Sahlān b. Abraham, 134
Saʿīd al-Dawla Abū al-Fakhr, 102, 197
Saʿīd Ibn Hibat Allāh, 24
al-Sakanī family, 41
Saladin, 48, 52, 59, 69, 75, 76, 149, 162, 184, 188, 190, 193, 195, 198, 199, 200, 201, 202, 203, 204, 228, 268n988, n991, 295, 297, 298, 301, 303, 322, 330, 334, 348, 400, 401, 443n732
Ṣalāḥ al-Dīn Ibn Yūsuf al-Ḥamawī, 98, 334, 337
Salāma al-ʿAṭṭār, 49, 76, 126, 127, 134, 136
Salāma al-ʿAṭṭār (Solomon ha-Zāqēn), 134
Salāma b. Raḥmūn *see* Abū al-Khayr Salāma b. Mubārak b. Raḥmūn b. Mūsā al-Ṭabīb
al-Ṣāliḥ Ismāʿīl, 199
al-Samarkandī, 24
Samuel, 102
Samuel 2, 372, 373
Samuel b. Elazar ha- Rōfē, 102, 389, 393
Samuel b. ʿEli, 52
Samuel b. Elijah al-Sinnī, 78, 103, 168
R. Samuel b. Ḥakīm *see* R. Samuel ha-Levi ha-Zāqēn
Samuel b. Jacob b. Japheth b. Moses, 102, 103, 373
Samuel b. Japheth al-Rashīd, 102
Samuel b. Judah b. ʿAbbās al-Maghribī *see* Abū Naṣr Samawʾal b. Yaḥyā al-Maghribī
Samuel b. Khalīfa *see* Abū al-Muḥāsan (Samuel b. Khalīfa)
Samuel b. al-Mawlā al-Sheikh al-Muhadhdhab Abū al-Ḥasan al-Yahūdī al-Qarrāʾ al-Mutaṭabbib al-Shahīr bi-Alexandrī, 373
Samuel b. Moses b. Yeshūʿā b. Mordechai b. Amram b. Solomon b. Amram *see* Samuel b. Solomon al-Maghribī
Samuel b. Nagrila, 443n558
Samuel b. Saʿadya ha-Levi, 45, 50, 124, 134, 140, 193, 366
Samuel b. Saʿdūn, 102
Samuel b. Solomon al-Maghribī, 65, 102–3, 366, 372, 383
Samuel b. Tibbon, 322, 323, 367
Samuel ha-Kohen, 103, 372, 373
Samuel ha-Kohen ha-Rōfē, 78, 103, 168
Samuel ha-Levi b. Solomon, 103
R. Samuel ha-Levi ha-Zāqēn (R. Samuel b. Ḥakīm), 103, 283, 400
Samuel ha-Melammēd b. Joseph ha-Melammēd b. Yijū, 51
Samuel ha-Nagid b. Hananiah (Abū Manṣūr), 51, 54, 70, 72, 74–5, 103, 149, 182–3, 184, 186–7, 252n613, 287, 289, 298, 300, 322, 362, 364
Samuel ha-Rōfē, 80, 92, 103, 288, 400
Samuel ha-Rōfē 2, 104, 403
Samuel ha-Rōfē Ibn al-ʿAmmānī, 104, 178, 179, 389
Samuel Rakaḥ (Rakakh/Rabakh) (Solomon b. R. Joseph), 104, 299, 300, 363, 366
Samuel Sar ha-Sarīm, 104
Ṣanīʿat al-Malik Abū al-Ṭāhir Ismāʿīl, 104, 202, 204, 336
Ṣaqr (Shaqīr/Shuqayr) al-Ṭabīb, 104, 296
R. Sar Shālōm ha-Rōfē b. Abraham b. Jacob, 104, 216, 217
Sasson ha-Levi *see* Abū al-Surūr al-Ṭabīb
Sayf al-Dīn, 198
Sayyid al-Ahl al-ʿAṭṭār, 134
Sayyid al-Ahl b. Hiba, 129, 134–5, 144
Sayyid ʿAnān, 430n524
Seth b. Japheth, 105, 397
Shabbetay ha-Rōfē, 105, 392
Shabbetay ha-Rōfē 2, 105
Shahāda b. Abraham, 105, 285, 400
Shamlā al-ʿAṭṭār, 135, 396
Shams al-Dīn Aldajiz, 170
Shams al-Ḥukamāʾ *see* Ibrāhīm b. Faraj b. Mārūth al-Sāmirī al-Ṭabīb (al-Ḥakīm)
Sharaf al-Milla *see* Amīn al-Dawla Abū al-Ḥasan b. Ghazāl b. Abī Saʿīd al-Sāmirī
Sharaf al-Ṭūsī, 49
al-Sheikh Abū al-Faḍāʾil al-Ṭabīb, 50, 124
Sheikh Abū al-Qāsim, 166
al-Sheikh Joseph, 60, 74, 83, 86, 93, 96, 98, 105, 108, 110, 118, 119, 150, 205
al-Sheikh al-Muhadhdhab al-Ṭabīb (anonymous), 58, 62, 87, 117, 319
al-Sheikh al-Muwaffaq Shams al-Riʾāsa *see* Abū al-ʿAshāʾir Hibat-Allāh b. Zayn b. Ḥasan b. Ifrāʾīm b. Yaʿqūb b. Ismāʿīl Ibn Jumayʿ al-ʾIsrāʾīlī
al-Sheikh al-Ṣāliḥ Sharaf al-Dīn Maḥmūd, 95, 333
Shelah ha-Levi b. Yeshūʿā ha-Levi ha-Rōfē, 105
Shemarya b. ʿAlī ha-Rōfē *see* Abū Manṣūr al-Mutaṭabbib (Shemarya b. ʿAlī ha-Rōfē)
Shemtov b. Joseph b. Falaquera, 355
Shemtov Shaprūt b. Isaac of Tudela, 57
Shihāb al-Dīn Aḥmad (Sulaymān) al-Maghribī al-Ishbīlī, 105, 150, 210–11, 294, 299, 312, 346, 348, 382
Sitt al-Shām b. Ayyūb, 198, 375
Solomon b. Judah, 66, 165, 166, 401
Solomon b. Jacob, 106, 400
Solomon b. Jesse, 65, 107
Solomon b. R. Joseph *see* Samuel Rakaḥ
Solomon b. al-Muʿallim *see* Abū Ayyūb al-Yahūdī (al-ʾIsrāʾīlī)
Solomon b. Shaʿyā *see* Abū al-Munajjā (Solomon b. Shaʿyā)
Solomon ha-Kohen *see* Abū Manṣūr Sulaymān b. Ḥaffāẓ
Solomon ha-Levi, 106
Solomon ha-Levi ha-Rōfē b. Abraham ha-Levi, 106
Solomon ha-Nagid b. Joseph ha-Nagid, 84

Solomon ha-Rōfē, 106
Solomon ha-Rōfē 2, 106
Solomon ha-Rōfē b. ʿAlī, 106, 166
Solomon ha-Rōfē b. Rabīʿ, 106, 384–5
Solomon ha-Sar ha-Nikhbād ha-Talmīd ha-Rōfē b. Daniel ha-Sar ha-Nikhbād, 106
Solomon (Sulaymān) ha-Sar ha-Rōfē b. [...] ha-Rōfē, 75, 106
Solomon ha-Zāqēn *see* Salāma al-ʿAṭṭār (Solomon ha-Zāqēn)
Solomon Ibn Gabirol, 79, 355, 433n558
R. Solomon Luria, 106–7, 327, 400
Solomon Qāmīs, 107, 402
Subkī family, 146
Sufyān, 45
Sukra (ʿAbd al-Qāhir) al-Yahūdī al-Ḥalabī, 107, 149, 193–5, 275n1115, 298, 370, 397
Sulaymān al-ʿAṭṭār, 135
Sulaymān b. ʿAlī, 107, 400
Sulaymān b. Junayba, 276n1120, 312
Sulaymān b. Mūsā al-Yahūdī al-Mutaṭabbib, 107, 282
Sulaymān Ḥakīm, 107

al-Ṭabīb al-Maristān (Anonymous), 117, 125, 410n115
Tābit al-Ṭabīb, 107
Ṭāhir al-Ṭabīb, 107
al-Tamīmī al-Muqaddasī, 77, 154
al-Taqī Ibn al-Gadal, 60, 74, 83, 86, 93, 96, 98, 107–8, 111, 118, 119, 205
Tarifi family, 92, 168
Templar of Tyre, 104
Thābit b. Qurra, 85, 334, 336
al-Thiqa (al-Sheikh) al-Ṭabīb, b. al-Sheikh Dāʾūd, 91, 99, 108, 127, 134
Tiqva ha-Levi ha-Rōfē ha-Sar ha-Nikhbād, 108, 150, 205, 364
Tiqva ha-Rōfē b. Sar Shālōm, 69, 108, 152
Tobias ha-Rōfē b. Japheth, 108

ʿUmar b. ʿAbd al-ʿAzīz, 89
al-ʿUmarī, Ibn Faḍl Allāh, 47, 170, 193, 195, 211, 213, 214, 321, 331, 333, 350
ʿUthmān (son of Saladin), 48
Uziel b. Obadia *see* ʿAbd al-ʿAzīz b. Maḥāsin al-Muwaffaq al-ʾIsrāʾīlī al-Mutaṭabbib

Wazīr al-Ṣāliḥ *see* Amīn al-Dawla Abū al-Ḥasan b. Ghazāl b. Abī Saʿīd al-Sāmirī

al-Yahūdī al-ʿAṭṭār, 130, 135
Yaḥyā Abū Zikrī al-Ṭabīb (Judah b. Moses), 108, 384
Yaḥyā b. ʿAbbās al-Maghribī (Judah b. Abūn), 49, 108, 148, 169–70, 171, 382, 349, 378, 397, 404
Yaḥyā b. Isḥāq, 345, 348, 349
Yaḥyā b. Joseph b. Solomon, 108, 400
Yaḥyā b. al-Ṣāʾigh, 109, 298
Yaḥyā b. Sulaymān al-ʾIsrāʾīlī al-Ṭabīb al-Ḥakīm (Zechariah b. Solomon), 22, 109, 282, 406
Yaḥyā ha-Kohen ha-Rōfē b. Mevōrākh, 91, 109
Yaʿqūb b. Ghanāʾim (Abū Yūsuf) al-Sāmirī (Muwaffaq al-Dīn), 110, 375, 398
Yaʿqūb b. Isḥāq, 65, 110, 154, 156, 157, 384
Yaʿqūb Ibn Killis, 155
Yaʿqūb (Abū Yūsuf) ʿImrān al-Mutaṭabbib, 110, 282
Yazīd ha-Bassām, 135
al-Yazūrī (Qāḍī and Wazīr), 165
Yedūthūn, 110, 409n85
Yedūthūn ha-Levi ha-Rōfē b. Levi ha-Levi *see* Abū Sahl Yedūthūn ha-Levi
Yeshūʿā, 110
R. Yeshūʿā, 60, 74, 83, 86, 93, 96, 98, 108, 110–11, 118, 119, 205
Yeshūʿā b. Berākhōt ha-Rōfē, 68
R. Yeshūʿā b. Menahem, 111, 399
Yeshūʿā ha-Levi ha-Rōfē, 111
Yeshūʿā ha-Levi ha-Rōfē 2, 111
Yeshūʿā ha-Levi ha-Rōfē b. Elijah, 111
Yeshūʿā ha-Levi ha-Rōfē b. Hai ha-Levi, 111
Yeshūʿā ha-Rōfē *see* Abū al-Fakhr (Yeshūʿā ha-Rōfē)
Yeshūʿā ha-Rōfē b. Aaron al-ʿAmmānī, 43, 92, 111, 177, 178, 298
Yeshūʿā ha-Rōfē b. Aaron ha-Rōfē Ibn al-ʿAmmānī, 111, 179, 180
Yeshūʿā ha-Rōfē b. Judah, 111
al-Yūnīnī, 209
Yūsuf ʿAbd al-Sayyid b. al-Muhadhdhab al-ʾIsrāʾīlī al-Mutaṭabib (Joseph b. al-Dayyān), 111, 209, 294, 366
Yūsuf b. Abī Saʿīd b. Khalaf al-Sāmirī al-Muhadhdhab al-Ṭabīb (Wazīr al-Amjad), 76, 111, 198–9, 283, 298, 300, 334, 335, 336, 340, 375, 402
Yūsuf b. Abū al-Faraj b. Abū al-Barakāt al-Ṭabīb, 135, 191–2
Yūsuf b. Ibrāhīm, 112, 400
Yūsuf b. Isḥāq Ibn Biklārish, 24, 112, 352, 380–1, 454
Yūsuf b. al-Kazan, 113, 381
Yūsuf b. Nūḥ, 113, 372
Yūsuf b. Tāshufīn, 169, 297, 354, 385
Yūsuf b. Yaʿqūb b. Ghanāʾim, 375, 398
Yūsuf al-Baṣīr (Joseph b. Abraham ha-Roʾeh), 430n524
Yūsuf al-Kaḥḥāl, 113, 285

R. Zadok ha-Rōfē, 113, 397, 398
al-Zaffān family, 166
al-Ẓāhir (Egyptian Ayyubid), 199–200
al-Ẓāhir Barqūq, 119, 219–20, 347, 405
al-Ẓāhir Baybars, 273n1067
Al-Ẓahīr al-Bayhaqī, 47
Zakī al-Ḥakīm, 41, 43, 113
Zakkay Nāsī b. Yedīdyāhū Nāsī, 44
Zayn al-Dīn Khiḍr al-ʾIsrāʾīlī al-Zuwaylī, 113, 276n1120, 294, 312, 347
Zayn al-Ḥassāb, 200, 336
Zechariah b. Solomon *see* Yaḥyā b. Sulaymān al-ʾIsrāʾīlī al-Ṭabīb al-Ḥakīm
Zechariah (al-Raʾīs) the Alexandrian, 113, 149, 187, 227, 298, 317, 353, 364, 389, 402
Zūṭā *see* Abū Zikrī Yaḥyā (Sar Shālōm)

Index of Places

Abhar (Iran), 99, 294, 405
Abyār/Ibyār, 387
Acre/Akko, 55, 164, 402, 442n725
Aden, 143, 144, 311
Africa, 376
Aleppo, 49, 52–3, 65, 67, 69, 72, 85, 86, 96, 98, 105, 107, 113, 115, 120, 149, 164, 170, 193, 195, 231n58, 268n981, 277, 285, 286, 291, 297, 298, 345, 348, 358, 382, 394, 396–8, 402, 443n731, n733
Alexandria, 40, 41, 43, 45, 49, 52, 54, 59, 65, 70, 71, 72, 78, 82, 83, 85, 91, 92, 100, 102, 103, 104, 106, 110, 111, 112, 113, 114, 117, 118, 120, 124, 129, 135, 139, 143, 144, 148, 149, 150, 151, 167, 172, 176, 177, 178, 179, 180, 187, 188–9, 191, 192, 203, 204, 206, 215–16, 222, 223, 227, 277, 279, 282, 286, 289, 291, 296, 298, 305, 316, 317, 318, 345, 348, 354, 366, 367, 371, 372, 378, 379, 381, 383, 387, 389–90, 393, 402, 454
Algeria, 18, 105, 106, 385
Almeria, 80, 112, 113, 352, 377, 380, 381, 435–6n575
Amman, 41, 148, 176, 296, 401, 402, 442–3n726
Anatolia, 404
Ancona, 68, 401
Andalusia, 15, 23, 40, 43, 45, 48, 53, 56, 57, 59, 70, 72, 73, 77, 80, 83, 84, 87, 90, 94, 97, 109, 112, 113, 137, 139, 147, 148, 151, 152, 157, 158–60, 162, 168, 169, 170, 173, 222, 223, 228, 282, 317, 336, 340, 343, 345, 348, 354, 357, 363, 369, 374–82, 385, 389, 433n557, 433–4n558, 435n570
Archidona, 374
Ashkelon, 113, 187, 277, 389, 402, 443n728
Ashmūm (Egypt), 316
Asia Minor, 115, 313
Azerbaijan, 39, 81, 152, 170, 180, 282, 297, 299, 344, 348, 367, 377, 382, 403–5, 445n752, n753

Baalbek, 66, 101, 149, 198, 199, 298, 309, 340, 375, 396, 399, 402, 443n730
Babylonia, 18, 58, 105, 160, 363
Baeza, 377, 382
Baghdad, 15, 28, 46–8, 52, 62, 80, 95, 99, 108, 116, 148, 158, 170, 218, 291, 294, 297, 320, 336, 341, 343, 344, 345, 346, 348, 349, 361, 377, 382, 397, 399, 404, 444–5n742
al-Balad (Iraq), 46, 445n744
Banias, 81
Barcelona, 73–4, 352, 379, 385, 432n554
Baṣra, 13, 89
Bilād al-Shām, 282, 394–403; *see also* Syria, Lebanon, Jordan *and* Eretz-Israel
Bilbays (Egypt), 107, 279, 316, 390
al-Bīra/Birecik, 41, 86, 150, 206, 207, 227, 404, 445n748
Byzantium, 23, 114–15, 159, 327

Candia (Crete), 83, 85, 96, 151, 221, 222, 286, 399
Carmona, 377, 382
Castile, 53, 77, 339, 379
Catalonia, 432n548, n554
Ceuta (Morocco), 52, 382
China, 182
Chios, 115
Constantine (Algeria), 105
Constantinople, xi, 42, 105, 108, 115, 159, 357
Cordova, 72, 73, 87–8, 94, 148, 157–60, 162, 296, 333, 340, 352, 355, 356, 357, 361, 374, 377, 378, 380, 431n544, 432n556, 433n557, 434n561, 435n570, n571, 436n575
Crete, 23, 83, 85, 96, 151, 221, 222, 286, 399
Cyprus, 107, 402

Damascus, 15, 30, 43, 49, 66–7, 68, 69, 70, 73, 75, 76, 78, 81, 82, 83, 84, 85, 95, 96, 98, 100, 101, 110, 111, 113, 115, 120, 135, 146, 148, 149, 150, 151, 162, 164, 189, 190–1, 193, 194, 195, 198, 199, 205, 208–9, 221, 222, 228, 231n51, 267n959, 268n981, 272n1062, 273n1067, 277, 285, 286, 291, 294, 298, 306, 309, 316, 327, 333, 334, 335, 336, 340, 345, 346, 347, 349, 350, 353, 364, 366, 371, 374, 375, 394, 396, 397, 398–9, 401, 402, 410n106, 433n557, 443n731
Damietta/Dimyāṭ, 51, 316, 328, 390–1, 393
Dammūh, 75, 390
Dar'a, 167, 385

Dénia, 56, 259n789, 296, 378, 432n552
Dhamār (Yemen), 109, 406
Dhū Jibla, 44, 385
Diyarbakir (Turkey), 170, 344, 349

Egypt
Lower Egypt, 288, 391
Upper Egypt, 393
Egyptian periphery/rif/provincial Egypt, 63, 97, 116, 144, 282, 386–94, 454
Eretz-Israel, 40, 42, 43, 44, 52, 54, 58, 65, 66, 69, 73, 77, 78, 80, 83, 85, 86, 90, 92, 93, 103, 105, 106, 107, 108, 112, 139, 165, 187, 188, 190, 223, 327, 366, 369, 378, 379, 382, 392, 400, 401, 402
Europe, 28, 77, 79, 114, 147, 239n254, 295, 306, 328–30, 378, 382, 384, 400–1, 431n544

Famagusta, 107
Far East/'the East', 24, 281
Fez, 73–4, 77, 94, 108, 162, 170, 337, 345, 348, 355, 378, 379, 382, 385, 386, 404, 438n626
France, 322
Fusṭāṭ, 18–19, 43, 44, 45, 52, 54, 55, 59, 61, 62, 63, 71, 76, 83, 87, 105, 107, 108, 110, 115, 118, 120, 127, 142, 143, 144, 162, 165, 172, 174, 178, 185, 186, 191, 197, 202–3, 205, 265n916, 285, 288, 289, 291, 305, 306, 310, 317, 318, 321, 332, 345, 348, 362, 363, 368, 371, 378, 379, 381, 387, 390, 392, 393, 394, 401, 454

Gabès (Tunisia), 59, 323
Germany, 77, 378
Giza, 166, 335
Granada, 53, 64, 77, 109, 298, 299, 329, 339, 354, 377, 379, 384, 386, 433–4n558, 435n570

Hama, 67, 81, 120, 190, 285, 286, 299, 364, 396, 397, 399, 401, 402, 443n731
Hamadān, 48, 149, 180, 181, 294, 341, 352, 404, 405, 446n756
Ḥarrān, 90, 101, 298, 309, 375, 396, 399
Hebron, 111
Ḥijaz, 13, 291
Hilla (Iraq), 99, 346
Holy Land, 41, 374, 432n548; *see also* Eretz-Israel
Homs, 69, 78, 111, 190–1, 198, 209, 375, 399, 401

Iberia, 158, 159, 256n730, 349, 357, 374, 376, 377; *see also* Andalusia *and* Spain
India, 18, 24, 40, 44, 47, 52, 71, 128, 140, 143, 144, 174, 185, 281, 315, 316, 317, 320, 345, 348, 352, 385, 393
Indian Ocean, 143
Iran, 18, 24, 39, 40, 41, 46, 52, 60, 62, 68, 71, 78, 81, 95, 96, 99, 105, 120, 139, 144, 152, 170, 180, 181–2, 211, 228, 237n217, 282, 294, 315, 341, 344, 348, 349, 369, 371, 377, 397, 403–5, 445n752, n753, 446n756
Iraq, 18, 39, 40, 41, 46, 47, 52, 62, 64, 71, 80, 86, 89, 95, 99, 105, 108, 116, 139, 143, 152, 170, 172, 206, 207, 218, 230n42, 231n51, 261n823, 282, 291, 315, 320, 335, 345, 348, 349, 351, 354, 369, 376, 384, 397, 403–4, 443n733
Irbil (Iraq), 231n51
(modern Land of) Israel, 291, 394, 401, 402, 442n725, 443n728, n732; *see also* Eretz-Israel
Istanbul, 88; *see also* Constantinople
Italy, 13, 40, 73, 84, 94, 153, 155, 164, 327, 383, 400

Jaffa, 115, 327, 401, 402–3, 443n728, n732
Jerez, 377, 382
Jerusalem, 42, 44, 52, 54, 65, 66, 68, 69, 70, 73, 75, 77, 78, 80–1, 82, 83, 85, 86, 90, 92, 93, 103, 105, 106–7, 108, 112, 149, 165, 172, 187, 188–9, 223–4, 279, 285, 286, 288, 317, 324, 327, 353, 366, 372, 373, 378, 389, 392, 400–1, 402, 442n725, 443n728, n732, 444n738
Jordan, 176, 190, 291, 394, 399, 401, 442n726

Karak, 78, 190, 267n959, 399, 401
Kāzrūn (Iran), 41, 371, 405

Lebanon, 218, 394, 443n730, 444n736, n738
the Levant, 30, 144
Libya, 319, 323, 444n736
Lublin, 106, 327, 401
Lucena, 54, 87, 352, 356, 377, 380, 435n570

Maghrib, 40, 43, 44, 45, 52, 58, 59, 64, 77, 79, 80, 106, 108, 111, 112, 132, 139, 143, 150, 155, 156, 168, 169, 170, 210, 215, 216, 228, 277, 294, 348, 369, 381, 382–6, 389
al-Maḥalla (Egypt), 66–7, 97, 116–17, 121, 184, 391
al-Mahdiyya (Tunisia), 44, 58, 79, 80, 132, 133, 156, 316, 319, 383–5, 437n594
Malaga, 377, 382, 432n556
Mamṣūṣa (quarter in Cairo), 62, 87
Marāgha (Azerbaijan), 170, 297, 377, 405
Marrakesh, 45, 90, 148, 168–9, 297, 354, 379, 385, 438n624
Marseille, 70
Mazara, 91, 386
Mediterranean, 16, 18, 20, 21, 25, 28, 143, 174, 277, 278, 317, 328–9, 367, 374, 382, 383, 389, 390, 398, 400, 432n554, 435n575, 442n725, 444n738, 455
Mesopotamia, 42, 399; *see also* Babylon, Iraq *and* Turkey
Minyat Ghamr (Egypt), 91, 391–2
Minyat Ziftā (Egypt), 63, 91, 94, 101, 105, 114, 125, 314, 318, 366, 391–2, 441n684
Miṣyāf (Syria), 81
Mongolia, 85
Morocco, 18, 40, 52, 73, 77, 90, 94, 139, 162, 167, 169, 339, 354, 369, 382, 385, 386, 438n624, n626
Mosul, 46, 99, 231n58, 445n744
M'sila (Algeria), 106, 385
Muṭaylib, 392

Nablus, 374
Navarre, 159
Near-East, 20, 21, 31
Nile, 387, 390, 391, 393
Nile Delta, 316, 390, 391, 392
North Africa, 18, 143, 144, 210, 282, 345, 348, 354, 382–6, 403; *see also* Maghrib

Old Cairo *see* Fusṭāṭ
Oman, 143
Oria (Italy), 94, 153–5, 383

Palermo, 133, 313, 438n631
Palestine, 18, 165, 183, 363, 442n725; *see also* Eretz-Israel
Portugal, 107, 169, 402
Provence, 54

Qadis, 146
Qalyūb, 316, 321, 392–3
Qayrawān, 58, 64, 79, 94, 106, 108, 132, 133, 143, 153–4, 277, 296, 305, 313, 336, 340, 343, 344, 351, 355, 383–5, 437n594
Qūṣ (Egypt), 60, 102, 279, 389, 393

Ramle, 43, 66, 78, 148, 164, 165, 166, 296, 301, 401, 443n732
al-Raqqah, 84, 334, 336, 399, 403, 443–4n733
Rhodes, 115
Ronda (Spain), 70, 379, 432n556

Saged (Syria), 67
Safed, 65, 73, 75, 83, 107, 223–4, 285, 286, 353, 366, 378, 396, 397, 400, 402
Salman, 316
Salmūn, 393
Samarkand, 291
Saragossa, 45, 48, 59, 87–8, 90, 94, 97, 112, 148, 160, 168, 259n789, 296, 344, 345, 352, 354, 380, 385, 432n552, 435n571
Seleucia, 114–15, 313, 402
Seville, 45, 57, 90, 148, 168–9, 298, 352, 354, 377, 379, 385, 432n556, 434n561, 435n570
Sicily, 18, 40, 51, 91, 98, 132, 133, 143, 179, 277, 313, 383, 386, 389, 438n631
Spain, 18, 19, 45, 54, 56, 70, 72, 74, 94, 112, 113, 160, 162, 164, 167, 173, 175, 223, 239n254, 277, 296, 327, 333, 335, 355, 366, 377, 378, 379, 380, 381, 382, 385, 400, 433n557, n558, 435n570; *see also* Iberia
Christian Spain, 147
Muslim Spain, 147, 322, 377; *see also* Andalusia
Southern Spain, 18, 374–6; *see also* Andalusia
Spain, expulsion from, 19, 378
Syria, 15, 25, 31, 40, 41, 42, 43, 49, 52, 65, 66, 67, 68, 69, 70, 71, 72, 75, 78, 81, 82, 83, 84, 85, 86, 90, 95, 96, 97, 98, 100, 101, 104, 105, 107, 110, 111, 113, 114, 120, 135, 139, 152, 153, 161, 163, 164, 176, 189, 190, 193, 195, 198, 199, 205, 208, 209, 215, 217, 221, 222, 227, 228, 267n958, 279, 285, 286, 291, 315, 316, 319, 320, 329, 333, 334, 336, 337, 345, 348, 349, 356, 363, 364, 369, 371, 386, 394, 396, 397, 398, 401, 402, 403, 404, 443n731, n733, 449, 450

Tabriz, 60, 68, 71, 78, 81, 85, 96, 99, 149, 180, 181–2, 218, 219, 285, 294, 298, 299, 301, 341, 346, 347, 372, 373, 405, 445n752, n753
Ṭanān (Egypt), 91, 288, 393
Tiberias, 96, 164, 403, 444n734
the Tigris, 46, 445n744
Tinnīs (Egypt), 288, 393–4
Toledo, 53, 56, 80, 90, 354, 379, 400, 433n557, 435n571
Tortosa, 77, 378
Tripoli (Libya), 59, 102, 319, 323, 444n736
Tripoli (Syria), 70, 98, 150, 217–18, 227, 403, 444n736
Tunisia, 18, 44, 59, 91, 102, 106, 148, 152, 154, 296, 313, 316, 323, 343, 361, 362, 383, 437n594
Turkey, 68, 170, 399, 401, 445n748
Tyre, 104, 403

Venice, 222

(Christian) West, 64, 144, 182, 228, 329, 370; *see also* Europe
(Muslim) West, 18, 313, 351, 355, 454

Yemen, 18, 40, 71–2, 109, 119, 405–6

Zuwayla (neighbourhood in Cairo), 74, 203, 319

General Index

Abbasid rulers, dynasty and period, 13, 47, 57, 71, 80, 95, 143, 145, 296, 333, 339, 394, 398, 404, 442n725, 443n726, 442n742
(Rabbinic) Academy/college, 54, 58, 145, 160, 172, 183, 306, 363, 384, 444–5n742; *see also Yeshiva*
Aghlabī rulers, dynasty and period, 79, 296, 384
Almohad rulers, dynasty and period, 73–4, 376, 379, 385, 433n558, 434n561
Almoravid rulers and dynasty, 45, 56, 73, 148, 160, 168–9, 296, 297, 354, 376, 379, 385, 432n552, 433n558, 434n561, 435n570, 436n575, 438n624, n626
anatomy, 24, 90–1, 93, 203
Aragon, kingdom of, 435n571
Ayyubid rulers, dynasty and period, 18, 19, 25, 26, 27, 59, 67, 68, 87, 101, 147, 148, 149, 150, 161, 162, 183, 187, 188–9, 193, 195, 196, 197, 198, 199, 200, 201, 214, 225–6, 227, 228, 267n959, 280, 291, 295, 297, 298, 309, 312, 315, 319, 324, 326, 328, 339, 340, 343, 357, 360, 363, 364, 375, 394, 396, 398, 399, 443n726, 449, 454

Ben Ezra synagogue, 19
Berbers, 88, 432n556, 443n558
Bīmāristān see hospital
Byzantine Empire and period, 12, 115, 159, 290, 357, 396, 400, 443n726, n730

classical Geniza period, 19, 138, 166, 280, 307, 398
classical world or period, 30, 290
(Jewish) converts and conversion to Islam, 15, 18, 27, 41, 43, 46–7, 48, 51, 52, 59, 62, 65, 66, 68, 69, 71, 73, 74, 81, 82, 85, 86, 95, 96, 99, 105, 110, 111, 113, 120, 135, 149, 150, 151, 155, 157, 160, 161, 170–1, 180, 181, 184, 185, 193, 195, 197, 198, 199, 208–9, 210, 211, 213, 214, 215, 218–19, 220, 221, 226, 228, 275n1115, 276n1120, 281, 283, 285, 293, 294, 297, 299, 301, 312, 330, 333, 340, 341–50, 354, 366, 370, 372, 375, 377–8, 379, 381, 382, 385, 396, 397, 399, 404, 405, 448, 452, 454
court physicians, 18, 27, 28, 38, 42, 45, 46, 48, 52, 57, 58, 59, 64, 69, 71, 76, 77, 79, 80, 81, 84, 85, 95, 97, 101, 104, 109, 114, 120, 148, 149, 150, 151, 152–3, 154–5, 156, 157, 158, 161, 162, 163, 164, 165, 166, 169, 170, 171, 172–3, 176, 178, 180, 181, 186, 188, 189, 190, 193, 195, 197, 198, 199, 200, 201, 202, 210, 211, 212, 214, 215, 219, 225, 226, 227, 228, 257n746, 260n806, 264n883, 266n942, 275n1115, n1116, 278, 283, 289, 294, 295–302, 303, 305, 306, 309, 313, 315, 317, 323, 326, 327, 330, 334, 338, 339, 340, 341, 343, 346, 348, 351, 354, 357, 359, 363, 364, 367, 370, 377, 378, 379, 382, 383, 384, 385, 386, 387, 393, 396, 404, 405, 449–50, 451, 452, 453, 454, 455
Crusaders and Crusader Kingdom, 26, 31, 55, 162, 290, 394, 400, 401, 402, 432n548, 438n631, 442n725, 443n726, n728, n731, n732, 444n734, n736, n738, 445n748

dayyān, 39, 41, 67, 80, 81, 86, 91, 102, 104, 111, 115, 134, 140, 150, 176, 178, 184, 187, 206, 207, 208–9, 213, 223–4, 225, 227, 311, 350, 364, 365–6, 372, 379, 383, 399, 404, 442n720; *see also* judge
dhimmi, 27, 47, 75, 147, 190, 227, 277, 301, 315–16, 320, 329, 333, 337, 338, 339, 355, 449, 450, 451, 452
diagnosis, 24, 31, 72, 79, 144, 186–7, 191, 195, 201, 284, 289, 308, 332
diet, dietetics, 24, 31, 78, 79, 112, 290, 300, 351
dysentery, 165, 198, 284, 291

embryos, embryology, 24, 90
eye disease and treatment, 75, 95, 99, 115, 118, 129, 135, 144, 284–6, 306, 311, 314, 316, 322, 323, 324, 325, 355, 393

Fatimid rulers, dynasty and period, 18, 19, 26, 50, 64, 76, 79, 114, 115, 143, 146, 147, 148, 149, 153–5, 156, 157, 161, 162, 164, 165, 171, 172–3, 175, 183, 186, 195, 196, 197, 200, 203, 214, 225, 226, 227, 280, 296, 297, 298, 313, 326, 335, 340, 343, 344, 357, 360, 361, 362, 363, 364, 383–4, 391, 393, 394, 398, 403, 421n364, 428n482, 437n594, 443n726, 449
female practitioners, 29, 114, 281, 284, 306–8

fertilisation, 24
fever, 73, 79, 284, 291, 351, 380

Greeks, Greek science, etc., 25, 90, 178, 278, 281, 321, 443n730, 451

Head of the Diaspora (*Rosh Gola, Nagid ha-Gola*), 58, 218, 361, 384
Head of the Jews/Jewish community (*Ra'īs al-Yahūd, Ra'īs Ṭā'ifa al-Yahūd*), 42, 54, 74, 127, 148, 149, 155, 156, 157, 161, 162, 165, 172, 173, 178, 182, 183, 184, 186, 225, 226, 227, 265n916, 289, 296, 297, 298, 300, 321, 326, 356, 357, 359, 360–4, 367, 374, 378, 383, 384, 396, 401, 428n482, 450, 453; *see also Nagid*
Head of the Physicians, 42, 86, 107, 150, 151, 204, 210, 211, 212, 213, 218, 219, 226, 272n1062, 275n1116, 276n1120, 281, 285, 288, 294, 299, 312, 334, 341, 346, 347, 382, 400
Holy Roman Empire, 77, 159, 378
hospital, 18, 25–6, 28–9, 30, 31, 42, 47, 59, 87, 107, 117, 126, 140, 145, 147, 148, 149, 150, 165, 178, 180, 182, 200, 201, 203, 204, 208, 225, 228, 278, 279, 282, 284, 286, 287, 288, 289, 290–5, 297, 298 300, 302, 304, 305, 313, 324, 325, 332, 338, 339, 343, 353, 358, 390, 410n115, 452, 455
'Aḍudī hospital (Baghdad), 99, 294, 341
al-Bīmāristān al-Manṣūrī (Cairo), 273n1067, 292, 293
al-Bīmāristān al-Kabīr (Damascus), 190, 294, 298
the Cairo Hospital, 163
hospital of (New) Cairo, 295, 324
hospital of Saladin (Cairo), 204
Nāṣirī hospital, *al-Bīmāristān al-Nāṣirī* (Cairo), 201, 294, 295, 298, 353, 371
al-Nūrī hospital, *al-Bīmāristān al-Nūrī* (Damascus), 30, 191, 209, 294, 298, 347, 399, 401
the public hospital of Cairo, 211
Qalāwūn hospital (Cairo), 113, 294
Hūdid dynasty, 112, 380

internal medicine, 184, 284, 291, 357

(Jewish) judge, 16, 39, 43, 50, 76, 77, 98, 107, 124, 146, 148, 149, 151, 172, 176, 178, 179, 184, 188, 189, 205, 223, 227, 282, 289, 304, 305, 311, 316, 317, 318, 326, 327, 328, 353, 354, 359, 364, 365–6, 378, 390, 392, 400, 449, 366

Karaites, 39, 40, 41, 42, 43, 44, 45, 48, 51, 55, 61, 68, 69, 70, 71, 75, 76, 77, 78, 82, 84, 85, 89, 91, 92, 95, 98, 100, 101, 102, 103, 113, 126, 148, 149, 150, 151, 157, 167, 195, 197, 200, 201, 205, 207, 211, 212, 213, 214, 215, 218, 219, 220, 221, 275n1115, 282, 285, 298, 299, 301, 312, 331, 335, 348, 349, 350, 353, 354, 360, 366, 367, 368, 369–373, 374, 383, 385, 389, 391, 398, 400, 405, 430n524, 443n728
Kabbalah *see* mysticism
Khazars, 159

madrasa, 30, 209, 273n1067, 292, 303, 304, 309, 338, 381
Mamluk rulers, state and period, 18, 27–8, 30, 42, 65, 67, 86, 119, 120, 137, 146, 148, 149, 150, 151, 161, 193, 195, 196, 197, 200, 202, 204, 207, 208, 211, 212, 213, 214, 216, 217, 219, 220, 221, 222, 225, 226, 227, 228, 275n1115, 285, 286, 293, 299, 300, 312, 315, 319, 328, 328, 329–30, 333, 335, 337, 338, 340, 343, 345, 348, 357, 363, 364, 370, 374, 375, 393, 394, 398, 402, 442n725, 443n726, n732, 444n738, 450, 451–2, 454
Materia medica, 112, 138, 159, 292, 308, 380
Mongols/Mongol Īl-Khānate, 39, 85, 96, 99–100, 149, 182, 298, 299, 315, 341, 345, 348, 396, 399, 404, 445n753
Moors, 45, 57, 70, 72, 94, 160, 296, 298, 333, 380, 433n558
the *Muḥtasib*, 144, 303
Murabba'at al-'Aṭṭārīn, 137, 139; *see also Sūq al-'Aṭṭārīn*
mysticism, 36n86, 73, 79, 83, 85, 106, 109, 327, 353, 355, 402, 451, 453

Nagid, 42, 49, 51, 54, 55, 58, 65, 70, 72, 74, 75, 82, 84, 98, 103, 104, 126, 127, 134, 136, 155, 162, 164, 171–2, 173, 179, 180, 182, 183, 184, 186, 252n613, 287, 288, 289, 296, 297, 299, 311, 326, 327, 359, 360–4, 374, 384, 386, 387, 390, 393, 399, 402, 428n482, 450
Nāsī, 39, 44, 53, 57, 65, 84, 107, 159, 188, 357, 361, 363
Normans, 102

ophthalmology, ophthalmologist, 16, 24, 27, 48, 58, 67, 75, 86, 87, 96, 97, 99, 105, 113, 150, 152, 182, 184–5, 188, 196–7, 201, 207, 212, 226, 228, 283, 284–6, 288, 291, 292, 294, 299, 305, 307, 334, 345, 346, 366, 372, 442n720, 451
orthopaedics, 16, 284, 291
Ottoman Empire and period, 19, 21, 27, 30, 108, 285, 382, 394, 398, 400, 402

Pact of 'Umar, 315, 363
pathology, 24
phlebotomy/bloodletting/bleeding, 29, 109, 124, 125, 138, 287, 292, 306, 322, 359
pharmacology, 24, 112, 159, 178, 228, 283, 284, 303, 352, 380, 404
pharmacopoeia, 159, 284, 308
physiognomy, 80, 108, 381
physiology, 24, 90
prognosis, 24
psychology, 24, 74, 352, 385

Reconquista (of Spain), 376, 432n552, n554, 433n557, 434n558, n561, 435n570, n571
Roman Empire and period, 12, 259n778, 290, 374, 443n726, n730

Samaritans, 39, 40, 55, 66, 67, 76, 101, 110, 111, 149, 157, 198, 199, 282, 298, 306, 309, 334, 335, 340, 348, 349, 360, 368, 374, 394, 396, 398, 399, 402
Seljuks, 47, 230n42, 446n756
Sufi, Sufism, 26, 27, 53, 36n86, 208, 268n981, 330, 354, 451

Sūq al-ʿAṭṭārīn, 86, 108, 137, 288, 442n720
Sūq al-Qanādīl (Cairo), 203, 288
surgeon, surgery, 16, 24, 26, 27, 67, 72, 75, 85, 105, 222, 283, 284, 285, 286, 287, 291, 292, 329, 364, 390, 392, 399, 401

Taifa, 56, 57, 296, 376, 378, 431n544, 432n552, n556, 433n557, n558, 435n571, 436n575
Taylor-Schechter Geniza Research Unit at Cambridge University Library, 20, 308
therapy, 24, 197

Umayyad rulers, dynasty and period, 13, 89, 148, 157, 159, 228, 237n214, 239n254, 296, 340, 357, 374, 376, 378, 380, 394, 398, 401, 431n544, 433n557, n558, 437n594, 442n725, 443n726

Venetians, 13, 28, 85, 108, 115, 143, 286, 390, 403

wounds, treatment of, 16, 24, 63, 65, 72, 114, 115, 259n791, 286, 287, 329

Yeshiva, 52, 69, 97, 145, 146, 164, 165, 166, 172, 327, 361, 365, 444–5n742

Ẓāhirīs, 52

EU representative:
Easy Access System Europe
Mustamäe tee 50, 10621 Tallinn, Estonia
Gpsr.requests@easproject.com

www.ingramcontent.com/pod-product-compliance
Lightning Source LLC
Chambersburg PA
CBHW051552230426
43668CB00013B/1823
9781474483988